Health Insurance Today
A Practical Approach

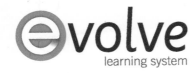
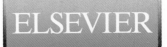

Fourth Edition

Health Insurance Today
A Practical Approach

Janet I. Beik, AA, BA, MEd
Southeastern Community College (retired)
Administrative Instructor
Medical Assistant Program
West Burlington, Iowa

ELSEVIER

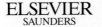

ELSEVIER
SAUNDERS

3251 Riverport Lane
St. Louis, Missouri 63043

HEALTH INSURANCE TODAY:
A PRACTICAL APPROACH, FOURTH EDITION   ISBN: 978-1-4557-0819-2

Notices

Knowledge and best practice in this field are constantly changing. As new research and experience broaden our understanding, changes in research methods, professional practices, or medical treatment may become necessary.

Practitioners and researchers must always rely on their own experience and knowledge in evaluating and using any information, methods, compounds, or experiments described herein. In using such information or methods they should be mindful of their own safety and the safety of others, including parties for whom they have a professional responsibility.

With respect to any drug or pharmaceutical products identified, readers are advised to check the most current information provided (i) on procedures featured or (ii) by the manufacturer of each product to be administered, to verify the recommended dose or formula, the method and duration of administration, and contraindications. It is the responsibility of practitioners, relying on their own experience and knowledge of their patients, to make diagnoses, to determine dosages and the best treatment for each individual patient, and to take all appropriate safety precautions.

To the fullest extent of the law, neither the Publisher nor the authors, contributors, or editors, assume any liability for any injury and/or damage to persons or property as a matter of products liability, negligence or otherwise, or from any use or operation of any methods, products, instructions, or ideas contained in the material herein.

Library of Congress Cataloging-in-Publication Data
Beik, Janet I.
    Health insurance today : a practical approach / Janet I. Beik. – 4th ed.
        p. ; cm.
    Includes bibliographical references and index.
    ISBN 978-1-4557-0819-2 (pbk.)
    I. Title.
    [DNLM: 1. Insurance, Health–United States. 2. Forms and Records Control–methods–United States. 3. Medical Records Systems, Computerized–United States. W 275 AA1]
    368.38'200973–dc23   2012014128

Executive Content Strategist: Susan Cole
Senior Content Development Specialist: Jennifer Bertucci
Content Manager: Linda Woodard
Publishing Services Managers: Julie Eddy and Hemamalini Rajendrababu
Project Managers: Kelly Milford and Srikumar Narayanan
Designer: Karen Pauls

Printed in China

Last digit is the print number: 9 8 7 6 5 4 3 2

To my husband, Lew, whose continued patience and encouragement have supported me through the writing and rewriting of this book.

To my former students, now successfully employed as medical assistants, billers, and coders, who have provided "vignettes" of their experiences that help "put a face" on actual occurrences in medical facilities.

To future students, both traditional and nontraditional, who may be inspired by this book and choose a rewarding career in healthcare.

To both veteran and novice instructors who dedicate their time and effort to inspire students to set far-reaching goals for exploring new possibilities in healthcare careers and promote lifelong learning.

Reviewers

S. Rehna Burge, CBCS
Medical Billing and Coding Instructor
Compass Career College
Hammond, Louisiana

Toni L. Clough, MBA
Business Instructor
Umpqua Community College
Roseburg, Oregon

Debra Downs, LPN, AAS, RMA (AMT)
Director/Instructor, Medical Assisting Program
Okefenokee Technical College
Waycross, Georgia

Robert Ekvall, PhD, CCS, CPC-H, CPC
College Instructor
UEI College
Chula Vista, California

Tracie Fuqua, BS, CMA (AAMA)
Program Director, Medical Assisting Program
Wallace State Community College
Hanceville, Alabama

Carol L. Jarrell, MLT, AHI
Lead Medical Assisting Instructor
Corinthian College
Merrillville, Indiana

Donna Maher, MS, RHIA, CMRS
Medical Coding Instructor
Renton Technical College
Renton, Washington

Nancy L. Maier, CMOA, MA
Medical Office Specialist Instructor
Kaplan College
Modesto, California

Ellen Pritchard, RN
Medical Program Coordinator
Douglas Education Center
Monessen, Pennsylvania

Theresa Rieger, CMA (AAMA), CPC
Manager
Mercy Health Northwest Family Clinic
Oklahoma City, Oklahoma

Karen Saba, CPC
Medical Careers Department
Spokane Community College
Spokane, Washington

Nerissa Tucker, MHA, CPC
Medical Coding and Billing Program
    Chair/Instructor
Allied Health Institute
North Lauderdale, Florida

Preface

As in the first three editions, this edition again follows my objective to present the complex issues of health insurance in such a manner that allows students to focus on what they need to know and how to function as a health insurance professional without excessive miscellaneous information that, although informative, can become burdensome to the reader.

Health Insurance Today: A Practical Approach, Fourth Edition, begins by introducing students to the history of insurance, providing some general facts regarding its origin, and describing the metamorphosis of health insurance into what we know it to be today.

While the textbook and workbook continue to address completing insurance claims using the universal paper claim form: the CMS-1500, more emphasis is given to submitting insurance claims electronically.

Organization of the chapters:
- Chapter Objectives
- Chapter Terms
- Opening Scenario
- Chapter Content
- Summary Check Points
- Closing Scenario
- Websites to Explore

SPECIAL CHAPTER FEATURES

"What Did You Learn?"

The chapters are broken into easy-to-learn sections, after which the students are asked, "What Did You Learn?" Several review questions are then presented, which reflect important "focus points" of that section.

Example:

> ### ⭐ What Did You Learn?
>
> 1. What is Medicaid?
> 2. When was the Medicaid program established?
> 3. Under what major act does the Medicaid program fall?

"Imagine This!"

The "Imagine this!" scenarios allow students to apply information to real-life situations, many of which have been taken from my actual experience in healthcare facilities. By applying what has been presented in each "Imagine This!" scenario, students can more easily relate the importance of the scenario and how it fits into real life, as well as determine the involved medical setting expectations.

Example:

> ### ⭐ Imagine This!
>
> Dr. Mueller is a nonPAR with Blue Cross and Blue Shield. The medical receptionist neglected to ask new patient Agnes Blank to assign benefits, so Blue Cross and Blue Shield sent the payment for Agnes' medical services directly to her. Agnes cashes the insurance check but fails to pay Dr. Mueller's bill. Statements mailed to Agnes are returned stamped "moved; no forwarding address."

"Stop and Think"

The "Stop and Think" exercises ask the student to read and study a particular paragraph, then apply critical thinking skills to resolve a problem or answer a question. Critical thinking is vital to individuals in the workplace, especially in a medical setting, where members of the healthcare team are often asked to think "on their feet" to resolve problems.

Example:

> ### 🕐 Stop and Think
>
> As a general rule, Dr. Vandenberg accepts Medicaid patients in her family practice. After seeing Harold Apple, a patient with an unpleasant personality, Dr. Vandenberg advises the medical receptionist not to schedule any further follow-up appointments for Mr. Apple. Is Dr. Vandenberg violating any Medicaid principles?

HIPAA Tips

A federal law, the Health Insurance Portability and Accountability Act (HIPAA), has presented challenges to both healthcare workers and patients. Although this textbook does not attempt to cover all the information included in HIPAA, it does give periodic applicable tips to help students better understand this important law.

Example:

> ### 📁 HIPAA Tip
>
> Medicaid HIPAA Compliant Concept Model (MHCCM) shows how HIPAA affects Medicaid and provides practical tools to help a state determine the best course of action for analyzing HIPAA's impact, determine implementation strategies, determine best practices, and validate what a state has accomplished.

APPENDIXES

There are three appendixes: A, B, and C. Appendix A is an example of a blank CMS-1500 (08/05) form. Appendix B presents nine examples of completed claim forms for a variety of payers along with step-by-step completion instructions. Appendix C presents the UB-04 institutional (hospital) claim form and completion instructions. .

STUDENT MATERIALS

Workbook

A comprehensive student workbook accompanies the textbook and is intended to supplement the material presented in the book. Each chapter follows a precise structure, beginning with a short introduction, workbook chapter objectives, a list of chapter terms, followed by a review test that allows the student to recall information presented in the book. Each workbook chapter ends with application and enrichment activities where students can apply what they have learned to today's healthcare environment. Most workbook chapters present at least one "Performance Objective." A performance (or learning) objective is a statement of what the students are expected to do when they have completed a specified course of instruction. It sets the conditions, behavior (action), and standard of task performance for the training setting. Performance objectives must be mastered to the predetermined criteria set by the instructor, institution, or organization. If the course is competency based, performance objectives may be repeated up to three times or until the student successfully meets the predetermined grading criteria.

One of the application exercises included in the student workbook involves creating a Health Insurance Professional's notebook. The purpose of this notebook is to allow the student to access information quickly and accurately when preparing insurance claims for some of the major third-party payers. If kept current, it will be an excellent resource later on the job.

EVOLVE Resources

The Evolve site (http://evolve.elsevier.com/Beik/today) is a free, interactive learning resource that works in coordination with the textbook. For students, it provides content-related resources that give them a chance to enhance their knowledge and practice their skills. The Evolve site gives students the chance to:

- Access the Evolve site on the Internet to research topics that are indicated by the Evolve icon in the chapters
- Use the Practice Management software Medisoft to practice completing duties as students would while working in a medical office

You will note that, throughout the textbook, the Evolve icon ⊝ appears, leading students to Internet links that provide for additional and/or updated information on the content presented. In those cases, the students should go to the Evolve site and find the Textbook references for that chapter. There they will find links to all referenced websites in the chapters.

The Evolve site also includes the following two distinct software offerings that support the teachings presented in this textbook.

Electronic Forms

Within the CMS-1500 Software, common health insurance forms, such as the CMS-1500 form and ledger card, are formatted in a very simple, straightforward way to electronically complete exercises in the Student Workbook. Using these basic forms, students can complete their exercises and turn in clean forms that are easier for the instructor to grade.

Guided Completion

A guided process to completing a CMS-1500 form, this software element corrects students as they complete a CMS-1500 form block-by-block. If any incorrect information is provided, the program corrects the student immediately. This software offers both direction and insight to students on how to complete a claim form correctly. This element accompanies select exercises and serves as an introduction to complete a CMS-1500 form.

INSTRUCTOR RESOURCES

TEACH Manual

This text is written in such a way so that it can be used in courses that range anywhere from 6 weeks in length to the more traditional 16-week semester. Sample course outlines and syllabi are included in the TEACH Manual on the Evolve site. If an instructor thinks that a particular chapter is not a good fit for his or her class, it can be eliminated from the course outline and substituted with other course material. Also, chapters do not have to be taught in the sequence they are presented.

The TEACH Manual contains an extensive amount of information and resources for both experienced and newer instructors. The Manual is a culmination of my education, work, and teaching experiences over the past 26 years. It answers such questions as "Where do I begin?," "How do I assess my students' work?," and "Are the students learning what they need to learn to successfully perform in the real world?" The Manual should be used to supplement the textbook and Student Workbook, which have been created for use in the following programs:

- Medical Assisting
- Health Information Management
- Medical Reimbursement Specialist
- Billing and Coding Specialist
- Medical Office Administration

Teaching is a complex task, and this Manual assists with instructional planning, delivery, and evaluation. A successful instructor must understand the various steps involved in effective teaching. To get the full benefit of this Manual, new and experienced instructors can adopt or adapt various teaching aids from the examples included in the various sections.

Test Bank

A comprehensive, customizable Test Bank can be found on the Evolve site; it includes true and false, multiple choice, matching, and short answer questions. Using ExamView, instructors can create customized tests or quizzes.

Powerpoint Presentations

PowerPoint slides are included with the TEACH instructor's material on the Evolve site. These slides are best used as visual summaries of chapter information to supplement oral presentations. Instructors are cautioned against using PowerPoint slides to completely replace lecture and interactive learning.

EVOLVE Resources

The Evolve site is a free, interactive learning resource that works in coordination with the textbook. In addition to those assets listed and described above, some of the outstanding instructor Evolve features include the ability to do the following:

- Post class syllabi, outlines, and lecture notes
- Set up virtual "office hours" and e-mail communication
- Share important dates and information through the online class calendar
- Encourage student participation through chat rooms and discussion boards

Evolve can play an integral part in how instructors teach, as well as how they interact with students, and it is my sincere hope that instructors take advantage of all the free, interactive Evolve resources that are available to them.

Janet I. Beik, AA, BA, MEd

A Word about HIPAA

HIPAA rings a bell for most people, but many do not know much about it other than they might have signed a form that contained this acronym when they visited their doctor. Those who are new to the world of health insurance, and intend on making a career in healthcare, need to know HIPAA's particulars.

HIPAA is an acronym for the Health Insurance Portability and Accountability Act of 1996 (August 21), Public Law 104–191, which amended the Internal Revenue Service Code of 1986. Also known as the Kennedy- Kassebaum Act, HIPAA includes a section, Title II, titled Administrative Simplification that requires the following:

1. Improved efficiency in healthcare delivery by standardizing electronic data interchange
2. Protection of confidentiality and security of health data through setting and enforcing standards

More specifically, HIPAA called on the Department of Health and Human Services (HHS) to publish new rules that ensure the following:

1. Standardization of electronic patient health, administrative, and financial data
2. Unique health identifiers for individuals, employers, health plans, and healthcare providers
3. Security standards protecting the confidentiality and integrity of "individually identifiable health information," past, present, or future

The bottom line is that HIPAA has resulted in extensive changes in most healthcare transaction and administrative information systems. Virtually all healthcare organizations are affected, including all healthcare providers, health plans, public health authorities, healthcare clearinghouses, and self-insured employers, as well as life insurers, information systems vendors, various service organizations, and colleges and universities.

To improve the efficiency and effectiveness of the healthcare system, HIPAA included "Administrative Simplification" provisions that required HHS to adopt national standards for electronic healthcare transactions. At the same time, Congress recognized that advances in electronic technology could erode the privacy of health information. Consequently, Congress incorporated provisions that mandated the adoption of federal privacy protections for individually identifiable or protected health information (PHI) into HIPAA.

When Congress enacted HIPAA in 1996, one of its main purposes was to protect private individual health information from being disclosed to anyone without the consent of the individual. Except under unusual circumstances, this consent needs to be in writing.

Title I of HIPAA protects health insurance coverage for workers and their families when they lose or change their jobs. According to Title II of HIPAA, the Administrative Simplification (AS) provisions require the establishment of national standards for electronic healthcare transactions and national identifiers for providers, health insurance plans, and employers. The AS provisions also address the security and privacy of health data. The purpose of all these standards is to improve the efficiency and effectiveness of the nation's healthcare system by encouraging the widespread use of electronic data interchange in healthcare.

Like everything else associated with healthcare, HIPAA introduces updates periodically. The following websites will help keep you current with HIPAA:

http://www.cms.gov/HIPAAGenInfo/01_Overview.asp

http://www.hdmcorp.com/federal-hipaa-law-update-2011/

About the Author

Janet Beik began her career in the healthcare field in 1964 when she was employed as a medical secretary and transcriptionist at the University of Iowa's Department of Medicine. After that, she worked as an administrative assistant in various medical facilities where she gained experience and expertise in all facets of "front office" work, including the preparation and submission of all types of insurance claims. In 1993 she began her teaching career as the administrative instructor in the Medical Assistant Program at Southeastern Community College in West Burlington, Iowa. During her tenure there, she acquired a master's degree in higher education from Iowa State University. Retiring in 2003, Ms. Beik began a career as a writer, first authoring several children's books, winning an achievement award for her story "Dolbee Creek—Elberta Trotsworth" from the National League of American Pen Women, Inc., Quad-Cities Branch. She was also a "master presenter" at the National Institute for Staff and Organizational Development (NISOD) at the University of Texas at Austin in May of 2000 for her master's thesis titled "Saving the Endangered Student."

Acknowledgments

I am pleased to present the fourth edition of my textbook, *Health Insurance Today: A Practical Approach*. I would like to thank the reviewers and the Elsevier staff, particularly Susan Cole, Jennifer Bertucci, Kelly Milford, Abby Hewitt, and Karen Pauls, who have provided valuable insight and guidance in preparing this fourth edition, which I greatly appreciate.

- Additionally, I would like to thank my daughter, Cynthia Bowen, a frequent collaborator and constant cheerleader, who assisted with the editing and updating of this fourth edition.
- A word of acknowledgment should also go out to my son, Jim, a computer engineer, who keeps my computers and printers running smoothly and resolves real and potential problems quickly and efficiently.

Janet I. Beik, AA, BA, MEd

Contents

UNIT I   BUILDING A FOUNDATION

Chapter 1   The Origins of Health Insurance

    What Is Insurance?, 1
    History, 3
    Metamorphosis of Medical Insurance, 4
    Key Health Insurance Issues, 7
        How Can People Obtain Health Insurance?, 7
        Access to Health Insurance, 7
        What Affects the Cost of Healthcare?, 9
        Cost Sharing, 10
    How Much is Enough?, 10
    Health Insurance Plans, 10

Chapter 2   Tools of the Trade: A Career as a Health (Medical) Insurance Professional

    Your Future as a Health Insurance Professional, 13
        Required Skills and Interests, 14
    Job Duties and Responsibilities, 17
    Career Prospects, 18
        Occupational Trends and Future Outlook, 18
        What to Expect as a Health Insurance Professional, 19
        Rewards, 20
    Is a Career in Healthcare Right for You?, 20
    Certification Possibilities, 20
    Career Focus for the Health Insurance Professional, 21
        Electronic Claims, 21
    CMS-1500 (08/05) Paper Form, 21

Chapter 3   The Legal and Ethical Side of Medical Insurance

    Medical Law and Liability, 26
        Employer Liability, 27
        Employee Liability, 27
    Insurance and Contract Law, 27
        Elements of a Legal Contract, 27
        Termination of Contracts, 28
    Medical Law and Ethics Applicable to Health Insurance, 28
    Important Legislation Affecting Health Insurance, 29
        Federal Privacy Act of 1974, 29
        Federal Omnibus Budget Reconciliation Act of 1980, 29
        Tax Equity and Fiscal Responsibility Act of 1982, 29
        Consolidated Omnibus Budget Reconciliation Act of 1986, 29
        Federal False Claim Amendments Act of 1986, 30
        Fraud and Abuse Act, 30
        Federal Omnibus Budget Reconciliation Act of 1987, 30
        The Patient Protection and Affordable Care Act, 30
    Medical Ethics and Medical Etiquette, 30

Medical Ethics, 30
Medical Etiquette, 31
Medical Record, 32
Purposes of a Medical Record, 32
Complete Medical Record, 32
Who Owns Medical Records?, 32
Retention of Medical Records, 32
Access to Medical Records, 33
Releasing Medical Record Information, 33
Documentation of Patient Medical Record, 33
Health Insurance Portability and Accountability Act and Compliance, 36
Impact of Health Insurance Portability and Accountability Act, 37
Enforcement of Confidentiality Regulations of Health Insurance Portability
   and Accountability Act, 38
Developing a Compliance Plan, 38
Confidentiality and Privacy, 39
Confidentiality, 39
Privacy, 39
Security, 39
Exceptions to Confidentiality, 40
Authorization to Release Information, 40
Exceptions for Signed Released of Information for Insurance Claims Submission, 40
Breach of Confidentiality, 41
Healthcare Fraud and Abuse, 41
Defining Fraud and Abuse, 41
Preventing Fraud and Abuse, 42

Chapter 4   Types and Sources of Health Insurance

Types of Health Insurance, 46
Indemnity (Fee-for-Service), 46
Managed Care, 47
Sources of Health Insurance, 47
Group Contract, 48
Individual Policies, 48
Medicare, 48
Medicaid, 48
TRICARE/CHAMPVA, 48
Standardized Benefits and Coverage Rule, 49
Disability Insurance, 49
Miscellaneous Healthcare Coverage Options, 50
Medical Savings Account, 50
Flexible Spending Account, 50
Health Reimbursement Arrangements, 51
Health Insurance Exchanges, 52
Accountable Care Organizations (ACOs), 52
Long-Term Care Insurance, 52
Dental Care, 53
Vision Care, 53
Consolidated Omnibus Budget Reconciliation Act, 53
Health Insurance "Watchdogs", 54
Other Terms Common to Third-Party Carriers, 54
Birthday Rule, 54
Coordination of Benefits, 55
Medical Necessity, 55
Usual, Reasonable, and Customary, 55
Participating Versus Nonparticipating Providers, 58
Miscellaneous Terms, 58

UNIT II   HEALTH INSURANCE BASICS

Chapter 5   Claim Submission Methods

Overview of the Health Insurance Claims Process, 62
  Two Basic Claims Submission Methods, 62
  Proposed Revisions to the CMS-1500 (08-05) Form, 63
Electronic Claims, 63
Health Insurance Portability and Accountability Act, 63
  Electronic Transactions and Code Set Requirements, 64
  Privacy Requirements, 64
  Security Requirements, 64
  National Identifier Requirements, 64
The New HIPAA 5010 Standards, 65
The Electronic Insurance Claims Process, 66
  Essential Information for Claims Processing, 66
  Verifying Insurance with New Technology, 73
Advantages of Electronic Claims, 75
Two Ways to Submit Electronic Claims, 75
  Claims Clearinghouses, 75
  Direct Claims, 76
  Clearinghouses Versus Direct, 76
The Universal Claim Form (CMS-1500), 77
  Format of the Form, 77
  Optical Character Recognition, 77
  Who Uses the Paper Form?, 78
  Proofreading, 79
  Claim Attachments, 79
  Tracking Claims, 80

Chapter 6   Traditional Fee-for-Service/Private Plans

Traditional Fee-for-Service/Indemnity Insurance, 85
How a Fee-for-Service Plan Works, 86
Health Care Reform and Preexisting Conditions, 87
  HIPAA and Credible Coverage, 88
Commercial or Private Health Insurance, 88
  Who Pays for Commercial Insurance?, 88
  High-Risk Pool, 88
  Coverage Mandate 2014, 89
  Health Insurance Exchange, 89
  What Is Self-Insurance?, 89
Blue Cross and Blue Shield, 90
  History of Blue Cross, 90
  History of Blue Shield, 90
  Blue Cross and Blue Shield Programs, 91
Participating Versus Nonparticipating Providers, 95
Submitting BCBS and Commercial Claims, 95
  Timely Filing, 95
  Filing Electronic Claims, 95
Commercial Claims Involving Secondary Coverage, 96
  Electronic Remittance Advice (ERA), 96

Chapter 7   Unraveling the Mysteries of Managed Care

What Is Managed Care?, 102
Common Types of Managed Care Organizations, 103
  Preferred Provider Organization, 104

Health Maintenance Organization, 105
Other Types of MCOs, 106
Advantages and Disadvantages of Managed Care, 106
Advantages, 106
Disadvantages, 106
Managed Care Certification and Regulation, 107
National Committee on Quality Assurance, 107
National Committee on Quality Assurance; Health Insurance Portability
and Accountability Act, 107
The Joint Commission, 107
URAC, 107
Utilization Review, 108
Complaint Management, 108
Preauthorization, Precertification, Predetermination, and Referrals, 108
Preauthorization, 109
Precertification, 109
Predetermination, 109
Referrals, 109
Health Insurance Portability and Accountability Act and Managed Care, 112
Impact of Managed Care, 115
Impact of Managed Care on the Physician-Patient Relationship, 115
Impact of Managed Care on Healthcare Providers, 115
Healthcare Reform's Impact on MCOs, 116
Future of Managed Care, 116

Chapter 8   Understanding Medicaid

What Is Medicaid?, 120
Evolution of Medicaid, 121
Temporary Assistance for Needy Families, 121
Supplemental Security Income, 121
Medicaid and Healthcare Reform, 123
Structure of Medicaid, 123
Federal Government's Role, 123
Mandated Services, 123
States' Options, 124
Community First Choice Option, 125
State Children's Health Insurance Program, 125
Fiscal Intermediaries/Medicaid Contractors, 126
Medicaid Integrity Contractors, 126
Other Medicaid Programs, 127
Maternal and Child Health Services, 127
Early and Periodic Screening, Diagnosis, and Treatment Program, 127
Program of All-Inclusive Care for the Elderly, 127
Medicaid Home and Community-Based Services Waivers, 127
Premiums and Cost Sharing, 128
Nonemergency Use of the Emergency Department, 129
Emergency Medical Treatment & Labor Act, 129
Payment for Medicaid Services, 129
Medically Necessary, 129
Prescription Drug Coverage, 129
Dual Eligibles, 129
Accepting Medicaid Patients, 130
Participating Providers, 130
Verifying Medicaid Eligibility, 130
Medicaid Identification Card, 131

Automated Voice Response System, 131
Electronic Data Interchange, 132
Point-of-Sale Device, 132
Computer Software Program, 132
Benefits of Eligibility Verification Systems, 132
Medicare/Medicaid Relationship, 132
Special Medicare/Medicaid Programs, 132
Medicare and Medicaid Differences Explained, 133
Medicaid Managed Care, 133
Medicaid Claims, 134
Completing the CMS-1500 Using Medicaid Guidelines, 134
Medicaid Secondary Claims, 134
Resubmission of Medicaid Claims, 134
Reciprocity, 134
Medicaid and Third-Party Liability, 135
Common Medicaid Billing Errors, 135
Medicaid Remittance Advice, 136
Special Billing Notes, 136
Time Limit for Filing Medicaid Claims, 136
Copayments, 136
Accepting Assignment, 138
Services Requiring Prior Approval, 138
Preauthorization, 138
Retention, Storage, and Disposal of Records, 138
Fraud and Abuse in the Medicaid System, 139
What Is Medicaid Fraud?, 139
Patient Abuse and Neglect, 139
Medicaid Quality Practices, 140

Chapter 9   Conquering Medicare's Challenges

Medicare Program, 144
Medicare Program Structure, 145
Enrollment, 150
Premiums and Cost-Sharing Requirements, 150
Medicare Part C (Medicare Advantage Plans), 151
Other Medicare Health Plans, 151
Medicare Part D (Medicare Prescription Drug Benefit Plan), 152
Changing Medicare Health or Prescription Drug Coverage, 152
Programs of All-Inclusive Care for the Elderly (PACE), 152
Medicare Combination Coverages, 153
Medicare/Medicaid Dual Eligibility, 153
Medicare Supplement Policies, 153
Medicare and Managed Care, 155
Medicare HMOs, 155
Advantages and Disadvantages of Medicare HMOs, 158
Why This Information Is Important to the Health Insurance Professional, 160
Preparing for the Medicare Patient, 160
Medicare's Lifetime Release of Information Form, 160
Determining Medical Necessity, 160
Advanced Beneficiary Notice, 161
Local Coverage Determination (LCD), 162
Health Insurance Claim Number and Identification Card, 162
Replacing the Medicare Card, 162
Medicare Billing, 164
Physician Fee Schedule, 164

Medicare Participating and Nonparticipating Providers, 165
Determining What Fee to Charge, 165
Filing Medicare Claims, 165
Electronic Claims, 165
Administrative Simplification Compliance Act (ASCA), 165
Transition to ASC X12 Version 5010, 167
Exceptions to Mandatory Electronic Claim Submission, 167
Small Providers and Full-Time Equivalent (FTE) Employee Assessments, 167
ASCA Enforcement of Paper Claim Submission, 167
Deadline for Filing Medicare Claims, 168
Using the CMS-1500 Form for Medicare Claims, 168
CMS-1500 Completion Guidelines, 168
Completing a Medigap Claim, 169
Medicare Secondary Payer, 169
Medigap Crossover Program, 171
Medicare/Medicaid Crossover Claims, 171
Medicare Summary Notice, 172
Information Contained on the MSN, 172
Medicare Remittance Advice, 172
Electronic Funds Transfer, 175
Medicare Audits and Appeals, 175
Audits, 175
Recovery Audit Contractor (RAC) Program, 176
Appeals (Fee-for-Service Claims), 176
Appeals Process (Medicare Managed Care Claims), 179
Quality Review Studies, 180
Quality Improvement Organizations, 181
Beneficiary Notices Initiative, 181
Beneficiary Complaint Response Program, 181
Hospital-Issued Notice of Noncoverage (HINN) and Notice of Discharge (NODMAR)
    and Medicare Appeal Rights Reviews, 181
The Center for Medicare and Medicaid Innovation (CMI), 182
Physician Review of Medical Records, 182
Physician Quality Reporting System (PQRS), 182
Medicare Billing Fraud, 182
Clinical Laboratory Improvement Amendments Program, 182

Chapter 10 Military Carriers

Military Health Programs, 187
TRICARE, 187
Military Health System, 188
TRICARE Management Activity (TMA), 188
TRICARE Regional Contractors, 188
Who is Eligible for TRICARE?, 188
Who Is Not Eligible for TRICARE?, 189
Losing TRICARE Eligibility, 189
TRICARE Program Options, 189
TRICARE Overseas Program (TOP), 189
TRICARE Young Adult (TYA) Program, 189
What TRICARE Pays, 190
TRICARE's Additional Programs, 190
TRICARE Dental Programs, 190
Supplemental TRICARE Programs, 193
TRICARE and Other Health Insurance (OHI), 193
TRICARE Standard Supplemental Insurance, 193

TRICARE For Life, 193
Verifying TRICARE Eligibility, 194
TRICARE-Authorized Providers, 194
TRICARE PARs and nonPARs, 196
Cost Sharing, 196
TRICARE Coding and Payment System, 196
TRICARE Claims Processing, 197
Who Submits Claims, 197
Submitting Paper Claims, 198
Deadline for Submitting Claims, 199
TRICARE Explanation of Benefits, 199
CHAMPVA, 199
Extending Eligibility, 202
Identifying CHAMPVA-Eligible Beneficiaries, 202
CHAMPVA Benefits, 203
CHAMPVA Cost Sharing, 203
Prescription Drug Benefit, 205
CHAMPVA In-house Treatment Initiative (CIT), 206
CHAMPVA-TRICARE Connection, 206
CHAMPVA-Medicare Connection, 206
CHAMPVA and HMO Coverage, 206
CHAMPVA Providers, 206
CHAMPVA For Life (CFL), 207
Filing CHAMPVA Claims, 207
CHAMPVA Preauthorization Requirements, 207
CHAMPVA Claims Filing Deadlines, 208
Instructions for Completing TRICARE/CHAMPVA Paper Claim Forms, 208
Claims Filing Summary, 209
CHAMPVA Explanation of Benefits, 209
Claims Appeals and Reconsiderations, 209
HIPAA and Military Insurers, 209

Chapter 11   Miscellaneous Carriers: Workers' Compensation and Disability Insurance

Workers' Compensation, 214
History, 214
Federal Legislation and Workers' Compensation, 215
Eligibility, 215
Workers' Compensation Claims Process, 217
Special Billing Notes, 222
Workers' Compensation and Managed Care, 224
Health Insurance Portability and Accountability Act and Workers' Compensation, 224
Workers' Compensation Fraud, 224
Online Workers' Compensation Service Center, 224
Private and Employer-Sponsored Disability Income Insurance, 224
Defining Disability, 225
Disability Claims Process, 225
Federal Disability Programs, 230
Americans with Disabilities Act, 231
Social Security Disability Insurance, 231
Supplemental Security Income, 232
State Disability Programs, 232
Centers for Disease Control and Prevention Disability and Health Team, 232
Ticket to Work Program, 233
Filing Supplemental Security Income and Social Security Disability Insurance Claims, 233

UNIT III   CRACKING THE CODES

Chapter 12 Diagnostic Coding

**Introduction to International Classification of Diseases
Coding System,** 239
Three Major Coding Structures, 239
History of International Classification of Diseases Coding, 240
Uses of Coded Data, 240
Two Diagnostic Coding Systems, 241
Comparing the Two Systems, 241
Guidelines, 241
ICD-9-CM Coding Manual, 242
Volume 2, Alphabetic List (Index), 242
Three Sections of Volume 2, 243
National Coverage Determinations and Local Coverage Determinations, 246
Process of Classifying Diseases, 246
Volume 1, Tabular List, 248
Supplementary Sections of Volume 1, 248
Locating a Code in the Tabular List (Volume 1), 249
Symbols and Conventions Used in Volume 1, 249
Typefaces, 250
Instructional Notes, 250
Essential Steps to Diagnostic Coding, 250
Special Coding Situations, 250
Coding Signs and Symptoms, 250
Etiology and Manifestation Coding, 251
Combination Codes, 252
Coding Late Effects, 252
Coding Neoplasms, 252
Coding Hypertension, 253
Overview of ICD-10 Coding System, 253
ICD-10-CM Code Structure, 253
Format of ICD-10-CM Manual, 253
Coding Steps for Alphabetic Index, 257
Tabular List, 258
Format and Structure of Codes, 258
Tabular List Conventions, 259
Manifestation Codes, 263
Morphology Codes, 263
Default Codes, 264
ICD-10-CM General Coding Guidelines and Chapter-Specific Guidelines, 264
Codes from A00.0 through T88.9, Z00-Z99.89, 264
Diagnostic Coding and Reporting Guidelines for Outpatient Services, 265
Selection of First-Listed Condition, 266
Outpatient Surgery, 266
Observation Stay, 266
Codes That Describe Symptoms and Signs, 266
Encounters for Circumstances Other than a Disease or Injury, 266
Level of Detail in Coding, 266
Code for Diagnosis, Condition, Problem, or Other Reason for Encounter/Visit, 266
Code All Documented Conditions That Coexist, 266
Health Insurance Portability and Accountability Act and Coding, 267
Code Sets Adopted as Health Insurance Portability and Accountability
Act Standards, 268
Implementation of ICD-10, 268
Importance of Learning Both Diagnostic Coding Systems, 268

Chapter 13 Procedural, Evaluation and Management, and HCPCS Coding

Overview of Current Procedural Terminology (CPT) Coding, 273
  Purpose of CPT, 274
  Development of CPT, 274
Three Levels of Procedural Coding, 274
CPT Manual Format, 275
  Introduction and Main Sections, 275
  Category II Codes, 275
  Category III Codes, 276
  Appendices A through N, 276
  CPT Index, 277
  Symbols Used in CPT, 277
  Modifiers, 278
  Unlisted Procedure or Service, 278
  Special Reports, 278
Conventions and Punctuation Used in CPT, 279
  Importance of the Semicolon, 279
  Section, Subsection, Subheading, and Category, 279
  Cross-Referencing with *See*, 279
Basic Steps of CPT Coding, 279
Evaluation and Management (E & M) Coding, 281
  Vocabulary Used in E & M Coding, 281
  Documentation Requirements, 283
  Three Factors to Consider, 283
  Key Components, 284
  Contributing Factors, 284
  Prolonged Services, 286
Subheadings of Main E & M Section, 286
  Office or Other Outpatient Services, 286
  Hospital Observation Services, 286
  Hospital Inpatient Services, 287
  Consultations, 287
  Emergency Department Services, 288
  Critical Care Services, 288
  Nursing Facility Services, 288
E & M Modifiers, 288
Importance of Documentation, 289
  E & M Documentation Guidelines: 1995 versus 1997, 289
  Deciding Which Guidelines to Use, 289
Overview of HCFA Common Procedure Coding System (HCPCS), 289
  HCPCS Level II Manual, 290
  Modifiers, 291
  Appendices, 291
National Correct Coding Initiative (NCCI), 291
Health Insurance Portability and Accountability Act (HIPAA) and HCPCS Coding, 292
  Crosswalk, 292
***Current Procedural Terminology, 5th Edition* (CPT-5)**, 292

UNIT IV   THE CLAIMS PROCESS

Chapter 14 The Patient

Patient Expectations, 296
  Professional Office Setting, 297
  Relevant Paperwork and Questions, 297
  Honoring Appointment Times, 297

Patient Load, 298
Getting Comfortable with the Healthcare Provider, 298
Privacy and Confidentiality, 298
Financial Issues, 298
Future Trends, 299
Aging Population, 299
Internet as a Healthcare Tool, 299
Patients as Consumers, 299
Health Insurance Portability and Accountability Act (HIPAA) Requirements, 299
Authorization to Release Information, 300
HIPAA and Covered Entities, 300
HIPAA Requirements for Covered Entities, 300
Patient's Right of Access and Correction, 301
Accessing Information through Patient Authorization, 301
Accessing Information through De-identification, 301
Billing Policies and Practices, 303
Assignment of Benefits, 303
Keeping Patients Informed, 304
Accounting Methods, 304
Electronic Medical Records, 306
Billing and Collection, 308
Billing Cycle, 308
Arranging Credit or Payment Plans, 308
Problem Patients, 310
Laws Affecting Credit and Collection, 311
Truth in Lending Act, 311
Fair Credit Billing Act, 311
Equal Credit Opportunity Act, 311
Fair Credit Reporting Act, 311
Fair Debt Collection Practices Act, 311
Collection Methods, 312
Collection by Telephone, 312
Collection by Letter, 313
Billing Services, 314
Collection Agencies, 314
Small Claims Litigation, 314
Who Can Use Small Claims, 315
How the Small Claims Process Works, 315

Chapter 15   The Claim

Introduction, 319
General Guidelines for Completing CMS-1500 Form, 319
Keys to Successful Claims, 319
First Key: Collect and Verify Patient Information, 320
Second Key: Obtain Necessary Preauthorization and Precertification, 321
Third Key: Documentation, 322
Fourth Key: Follow Payer Guidelines, 322
Fifth Key: Proofread Claim to Avoid Errors, 322
Sixth Key: Submit a Clean Claim, 322
Rejected Claims versus Denied Claims, 323
**Health Insurance Portability and Accountability Act (HIPAA) and National Standard
Employer Identifier Number,** 323
Claim Process, 323
Step One: Claim Is Received, 325
Step Two: Claims Adjudication, 325
Step Three: Tracking Claims, 325

Step Four: Receiving Payment, 328
Step Five: Interpreting Explanation of Benefits, 328
Step Six: Posting Payments, 330
Time Limits, 330
Processing Secondary Claims, 333
Real-Time Claims Adjudication, 334
Appeals, 334
Incorrect Payments, 334
Denied Claims, 334
Appealing a Medicare Claim, 335

UNIT V   ADVANCED APPLICATION

Chapter 16 The Role of Computers in Health Insurance

Introduction, 338
Impact of Computers on Health Insurance, 338
Role of Health Insurance Portability and Accountability Act (HIPAA) in Electronic Transmissions, 338
Electronic Data Interchange, 339
History of Electronic Data Interchange, 339
Benefits of Electronic Data Interchange, 339
Electronic Claims Process, 340
Methods Available for Filing Claims Electronically, 340
Enrollment, 340
Electronic Claims Clearinghouse, 340
Direct Data Entry Claims, 341
Clearinghouse versus Direct, 341
Advantages of Filing Claims Electronically, 342
Medicare and Electronic Claims Submission, 342
Additional Electronic Services Available, 343
Electronic Funds Transfer, 343
Electronic Remittance Advice, 344
Role of Computers in Transitioning to ICD-10 Diagnostic Coding System, 344
Electronic Medical Record, 344
Combination Records, 347
Digital Imaging Hybrid, 347
Potential Issues, 347
Future of Electronic Medical Records, 348
Privacy Concerns of Electronic Medical Records, 348
Federal Funding for Electronic Medical Record Trials and "Meaningful Use", 348

Chapter 17 Reimbursement Procedures: Getting Paid

Understanding Reimbursement Systems, 352
Types of Reimbursement, 353
Medicare and Reimbursement, 354
Medicare Prospective Payment System, 354
How the Medicare Prospective Payment System Works, 355
Other Systems for Determining Reimbursement, 356
Relative Value Scale, 356
Resource-Based Relative Value Scale, 356
Diagnosis-Related Groups, 357
Ambulatory Payment Classifications, 358
Resource Utilization Groups, 358

Transition of Medicare to Resource-Based Relative Value Scale, 359
  Setting Medicare Payment Policy, 359
  Medicare Inpatient Hospital Prospective Payment System, 359
  Medicare Long-Term Care Hospital Prospective Payment System, 359
Additional Prospective Payment Systems, 360
  Home Health Prospective Payment System, 360
  Inpatient Rehabilitation Facility Prospective Payment System, 360
  Significance of Reimbursement Systems to the Health Insurance Professional, 360
Peer Review Organizations and Prospective Payment Systems, 361
Understanding Computerized Patient Accounting Systems, 361
  Selecting the Right Billing System, 361
  Managing Transactions, 362
  Generating Reports, 364
Health Insurance Portability and Accountability Act and Practice Management
  software, 365

Chapter 18 Hospital Billing and the UB-04

Hospital Versus Physician Office Billing and Coding, 374
Modern Hospital and Health Systems, 374
  Emerging Issues, 374
Common Healthcare Facilities, 375
  Acute Care Facilities, 375
  Critical Access Hospitals, 375
  Ambulatory Surgery Centers, 376
  Other Types of Healthcare Facilities, 376
Legal and Regulatory Environment, 377
  Accreditation, 378
  Professional Standards, 379
  Governance, 379
  Confidentiality and Privacy, 379
  Fair Treatment of Patients, 380
Common Hospital Payers and Their Claims Guidelines, 381
  Medicare, 381
  Medicaid, 383
  TRICARE, 383
  CHAMPVA, 383
  Blue Cross and Blue Shield, 384
  Private Insurers, 384
National Uniform Billing Committee and the UB-04, 384
  UB-04 Data Specifications, 385
  837I: Electronic Version of the UB-04 Form, 385
Structure and Content of the Hospital Health Record, 387
  Standards in Hospital Electronic Medical Records, 388
  Standard Codes and Terminology, 388
Inpatient Hospital/Facility Coding, 388
  ICD-9-CM (Volume 3) Codes for Inpatient Hospital Procedures, 389
  Code Sets Used for Inpatient Hospital/Facility Claims in ICD-10-PCS, 389
  National Correct Coding Initiative, 392
  Recent Rule Changes Affecting Hospital Billing, 393
Outpatient Hospital Coding, 393
  Hospital Outpatient Prospective Payment System, 393
  Ambulatory Payment Classification Coding, 394
The Hospital Billing Process: Understanding the Basics, 394
  Informed Consent, 394
  Present on Admission (POA), 396
  Hospital Charges, 396

Electronic Claims Submission (ECS), 396
Health Information Management (HIM) Systems, 397
Payment Management, 397
HIPAA-Hospital Connection, 398
Billing Compliance, 398
Career Opportunities in Hospital Billing, 399
Training, Other Qualifications, and Advancement, 399
Job Outlook, 400

Appendix A Sample Blank CMS-1500 (08/05), 404

Appendix B CMS-1500 Claim Forms and Completion Instructions, 406

Appendix C UB-04 Claim Form and Completion Instructions, 425

Glossary, 430

CHAPTER **1**

The Origins of Health Insurance

Chapter Outline

I. What Is Insurance?
II. History
III. Metamorphosis of Medical Insurance
IV. Key Health Insurance Issues
    A. How Can People Obtain Health Insurance?
    B. Access to Health Insurance
        1. Identifying the Uninsured
        2. State Programs for the Uninsured

C. What Affects the Cost of Healthcare?
    1. Americans Are Living Longer Than Ever Before
    2. Advances in Medical Technology
    3. More Demand for Healthcare
    4. Media Intervention
D. Cost Sharing
V. How Much is Enough?
VI. Health Insurance Plans

CHAPTER OBJECTIVES

After completion of this chapter, the student should be able to:
1. Explain health (medical) insurance.
2. Discuss the early development of health insurance in the United States.
3. Outline the important changes in the evolution of health insurance.
4. List and explain today's key health insurance issues.
5. Explain how people can obtain health insurance, and what situations affect their access to it.
6. Examine issues affecting cost of healthcare.
7. Identify the basic types of health insurance plans.

CHAPTER TERMS

Accountable Care
   Organization
Consolidated Omnibus
   Budget Reconciliation
   Act (COBRA)
cost sharing
deductible
entity/entities

fee-for-service
group plans
health insurance
Health insurance
   exchange
Health Insurance Portability
   and Accountability Act
   (HIPAA)

Health Maintenance
   Organization (HMO) Act
indemnify
indemnity insurance
indigent
insurance
insured

insurer
managed healthcare
medical insurance
policy
preexisting conditions
premium
preventive medicine

WHAT IS INSURANCE?

To understand medical **insurance**, you have to know a little about insurance in general. First, let's look at a typical definition of insurance:

"The act or business, through legal means (normally a written contract), of protecting an individual's person or property against loss or harm arising out of specified circumstances in return for payment, which is called a **premium**."

The insuring party (called the **insurer**) agrees to **indemnify** (or reimburse) the **insured** for loss that occurs under the terms of the insurance contract.

Now that we know that insurance is basically financial protection against loss or harm, let's break it into smaller pieces. Insurance, as we know it, is a written agreement called a **policy**, between two parties (or **entities**), whereby one entity (the insurance company) promises to pay a

⟳ OPENING SCENARIO

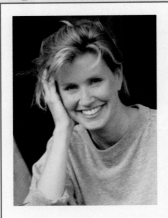

Joy Cassabaum, a single mother of two, has worked at a manufacturing plant in a Midwestern city for nearly 10 years. When the plant closed and moved its facilities out of the country, Joy found herself at the threshold of a new life and a new vocation. Joy decided she wanted a career change—something different from factory work, something more interesting and challenging. When Joy and her friend Barbara decided to attend a college career fair, Joy was intrigued by a presentation given by the healthcare instructors on medical insurance.

Joy was vaguely aware of what healthcare insurance was all about but never paid a lot of attention to it. Her former employer had provided excellent benefits, and when she or one of her children was ill or injured, they went to the doctor and basically forgot about it. If and when a bill came, she paid it, putting her trust in the doctor's staff. Now that she is unemployed, she has to not only make some smart career moves but also start thinking about things she had taken for granted before her layoff, and health insurance for her family had not even entered her mind until now.

Joy and Barbara signed up for the insurance billing specialist program at the local community college and eagerly began the first step on the path of their new careers. Let's follow them through their steps toward their goal of becoming health insurance specialists.

---

specific sum of money to a second entity (often an individual, or it could be another company) if certain specified undesirable events occur. Examples of undesirable events include a windstorm blowing a tree over on a house, a car being stolen, or—as in the case of medical insurance—an illness or injury. In return for this promise for financial protection against loss, the second entity (the insured) periodically pays a specific sum of money (premium) to the insurance company in exchange for this protection.

★ Imagine This!

John and Anna Smith buy a house for $150,000. That's a lot of money, and the Smiths have worked hard to save up for this purchase. Now, they look at the house and wonder, what if a strong wind blows the roof off? Or, worse yet, what if there is an electrical malfunction and the house catches fire? Along comes a neighbor who says, "Hey, I work for Colossus Insurance Company, and I'll write up an agreement saying that if you pay me $1000 a year, Colossus will foot the bills for any repair or replacement your house suffers in case of a storm, a fire, or most other bad stuff that can happen." The Smiths think, "This is great" and agree to the neighbor's offer. So, a contract (the insurance policy) is drawn up, John and Anna pay Colossus Insurance Company $1000 to satisfy their mortgage lender's requirement, their worries about their new house are relieved, and they sleep soundly each night. Homeowners' insurance protects people from having to pay large sums of money out of their own pockets to repair or replace their homes in the event of fire, storm, theft, or other hazards.

Now that you now have a better understanding of what insurance is in general, let's look at **medical insurance** (or **health insurance**, as it is frequently called). Medical insurance narrows down the "undesirable events" mentioned earlier to illnesses and injuries. The insurance company promises to pay part (or sometimes all, depending on the policy) of the financial expenses incurred as a result of medical procedures, services, and certain supplies performed or provided by healthcare professionals if and when an individual becomes sick or injured. Some insurance policies also pay medical expenses even if the individual is not sick or injured. Healthcare providers and companies that sell health insurance have determined that it is often less costly to keep an individual well or to catch an emerging illness in its early stages, when it is more treatable, than to pay more exorbitant expenses later on should that individual become seriously ill. This practice is referred to as **preventive medicine**.

The term *medical (health) insurance* should not cause students to become apprehensive when they hear it. A good analogy to put medical insurance into perspective might be to compare it with a picture puzzle. When the individual puzzle pieces are dumped onto a table, there is little meaning or continuity to the jumble of pieces lying haphazardly on the tabletop. Then slowly, as the pieces are assembled, a picture begins to take shape and the puzzle starts making sense. Similarly, medical insurance can be perplexing as individual concepts are presented, but when you "look at the whole picture," it becomes clearer and more understandable. As we begin to appreciate how the puzzle pieces fit together, we can understand the whole picture more easily when the puzzle is at last completed. Fig. 1-1 illustrates how the "medical insurance puzzle" is assembled.

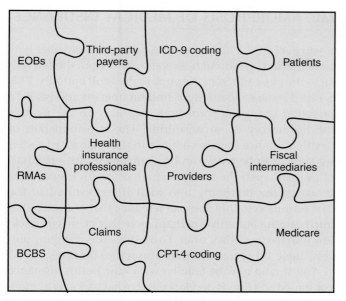

Fig. 1-1 The insurance "puzzle."

⭐ **Imagine This!**

It's ancient Babylon. Merchants are constantly being robbed or captured for ransom as their caravans cross the desert or as their ships sail off to trade with Egypt, India, and China. One wealthy businessman, who made loans to the traders—we'll call him Ali-baba Gosmere—conceived a clever plan. As the traders came to him to borrow money for their journeys, he told the merchants, "For two additional gold coins, I'll forgive your loan if you're robbed!" The traders thought, "Wow! How can we lose with this deal?" This clever lender, by collecting these "premiums" from many such traders, was able to absorb the losses of the few unfortunate ones who were robbed. And, as these stories go, everyone pretty much lived happily ever after. (According to documented history, this practice was later legalized in the Code of Hammurabi.)

🕐 **Stop and Think**

Read the paragraph again comparing health insurance with a picture puzzle. Can you think of other applicable analogies that would help make the various components of health insurance more understandable at this point?

💬 **What Did You Learn?**

1. Give a brief definition of insurance.
2. Medical insurance narrows down "undesirable events" to what two categories?
3. What is the term used when medical services and procedures are performed to keep a person well or prevent a catastrophic illness?

HISTORY

Insurance is not a recent phenomenon. The word *insurance* is derived from the Latin word *securitas,* which translates into the English word *security.*

From the beginning of time, people have looked for ways to ease some of the hardships of human existence. It has been common knowledge down through the ages that it has been difficult for any one individual to survive for long on his or her own. Prehistoric humans quickly learned that to survive, the resources of others must be pooled.

The beginnings of modern health insurance occurred in England in 1850, when a company offered coverage for medical expenses for bodily injuries that did not result in death. By the end of that same year in the United States, the Franklin Health Assurance Company of Massachusetts began offering medical expense coverage on a basis resembling health insurance as we know it now. By 1866, many other insurance companies began writing health insurance policies. These early policies were mostly for loss of income and provided health benefits for a few of the serious diseases that were common at that time—typhus, typhoid, scarlet fever, smallpox, diphtheria, and diabetes. People did not refer to these arrangements as insurance, but the concept was the same.

In the United States, the birth of health insurance came in 1929 when Justin Ford Kimball, an official at Baylor University in Dallas, Texas, introduced a plan to guarantee schoolteachers 21 days of hospital care for $6 a year. Other employee groups in Dallas soon joined the plan, and the idea caught on nationwide. This plan eventually evolved into what we now know as Blue Cross. The Blue Shield concept grew out of the lumber and mining camps of the Pacific Northwest at the turn of the 20th century. Employers, wanting to provide medical care for their workers, paid monthly fees to "medical service bureaus," which were composed of groups of physicians. The Blue Cross and Blue Shield plans traditionally established premiums by community rating—that is, everybody in the community paid the same premium.

To explore more interesting and detailed facts related to the history of insurance, refer to the list of websites at the end of this chapter.

HIPAA Tip

HIPAA amended the Employee Retirement Income Security Act (ERISA) to provide new rights and protections for participants and beneficiaries in group health plans. Understanding this amendment is important in decisions about future health coverage. HIPAA contains protections for health coverage offered in connection with employment (group health plans) and for individual insurance policies sold by insurance companies (individual policies).

What Did You Learn?

1. What is the Latin word for insurance, and what is its literal English translation?
2. State when and where the birth of health insurance occurred in the United States.
3. What did early insurance policies in the United States typically cover?

METAMORPHOSIS OF MEDICAL INSURANCE

If you ever took a biology course, you may remember how certain insects go through several stages—from the caterpillar to the pupa and from the pupa to the adult butterfly. This is called *metamorphosis*. By definition, metamorphosis is "a profound change in form from one stage to the next in the life history of an organism." The transformation of health insurance from what it was in the beginning to what we know it to be today can be compared to this metamorphosis, although the transformation of health insurance as it was in the beginning into what it has evolved in the 21st century certainly does not resemble that of a caterpillar into beautiful butterfly—perhaps more that of an ugly duckling into the proverbial swan. To illustrate this changing process, Table 1-1 presents a health insurance timeline.

You should now be familiar with how health insurance got started and how it developed into what we know as modern health insurance today. It is also important to know how it has changed throughout history and what caused these changes. As you might imagine, politics has played a big role in the development of health insurance in the United States. Support for government health insurance began when

TABLE 1-1	Health Insurance Timeline
1900s	American Medical Association (AMA) becomes a powerful national force. Membership increases from about 8000 physicians in 1900 to 70,000 in 1910—half of them in the U.S. This is the beginning of "organized medicine." Surgery is becoming more common. Physicians are no longer expected to provide free services to all hospital patients. United States lags behind European countries in finding value in insuring against costs of sickness. Railroads are the leading industry to develop extensive employee medical programs.
1910s	U.S. hospitals are now modern scientific institutions, valuing antiseptics and cleanliness, and using medications for the relief of pain. American Association for Labor Legislation (AALL) organizes first national conference on "social insurance." Progressive reformers gaining support for health insurance. Opposition from physicians and other interest groups and the entry of the United States into World War I in 1917 undermine reform front.
1920s	Reformers emphasize the cost of medical care instead of wages lost to sickness—the relatively higher cost of medical care is a new and dramatic development, especially for the middle class. Growing cultural influence of the medical profession—physicians' incomes are higher, and prestige is established. Rural health facilities are seen by many as inadequate. Penicillin is discovered, but it will be 20 years before it is widely used to combat infection and disease.
1930s	The Depression changes priorities, with greater emphasis on unemployment insurance and "old age" benefits. Social Security Act is passed, omitting health insurance. Against the advice of insurance professionals, Blue Cross begins offering private coverage for hospital care in dozens of states.
1940s	Penicillin comes into use. Prepaid group healthcare begins, seen as radical. To compete for workers, companies begin to offer health benefits, giving rise to the employer-based system in place today. Congress is asked to pass an "economic bill of rights," including the right to adequate medical care. President offers a single-system, national health program plan that would include all Americans.
1950s	Attention turns to Korea and away from health reform; United States has a system of private insurance for people who can afford it and welfare services for the poor. Federal responsibility for the sick is firmly established. Many more medications are available now to treat a range of diseases, including infections, glaucoma, and arthritis, and new vaccines become available that prevent dreaded childhood diseases, such as polio. The first successful organ transplantation is performed.
1960s	In the 1950s, the price of hospital care doubled. Now in the early 1960s, people outside the workplace, especially the elderly, have difficulty affording insurance. More than 700 insurance companies sell health insurance. Major insurance endorses high-cost medicine.

TABLE 1-1	Health Insurance Timeline—cont'd
	President signs Medicare and Medicaid into law. Number of physicians reporting themselves as full-time specialists grows from 55% in 1960 to 69%.
1970s	Prepaid group healthcare plans are renamed health maintenance organizations (HMOs), with legislation that provides federal endorsement, certification, and assistance. Healthcare costs escalate rapidly; U.S. medicine is now seen as in crisis. Growing complaints by insurance companies that the traditional fee-for-service method of payment to physicians is being exploited. Healthcare costs rise at double the rate of inflation. Expansion of managed care helps to moderate increases in healthcare costs.
1980s	Overall, there is a shift toward privatization and corporatization of healthcare. Under President Reagan, Medicare shifts to payment by diagnosis (DRG) instead of by treatment. Private plans quickly follow suit. Growing complaints by insurance companies that the traditional fee-for-service method of payment to physicians is being exploited. A specific fee or payment amount per patient (capitation) to physicians becomes more common.
1990s	Healthcare costs rise at double the rate of inflation. Expansion of managed care helps moderate increases in healthcare costs. By the end of the decade, 44 million Americans—16% of the nation—have no health insurance at all. Human Genome Project to identify all of the > 100,000 genes in human DNA gets under way. By June 1990, 139,765 people in the United States have HIV/AIDS, with a 60% mortality rate.
2000s	Healthcare costs continue to rise. Medicare is viewed by some as unsustainable under the present structure and must be "rescued." Changing demographics of the workplace lead many to believe the employer-based system of insurance cannot last. The Human Genome Project's identification of all of the > 100,000 genes in human DNA was completed in 2003, and all individual chromosome papers were completed in 2006; papers analyzing the genome continue to be published. Direct-to-consumer advertising for pharmaceuticals and medical devices is on the rise.

Theodore Roosevelt made national health insurance one of the major propositions of the Progressive Party during the 1912 presidential campaign, but the plan was eventually defeated. After 1920, opposition to government-sponsored plans was led by the American Medical Association (AMA) out of concern that government involvement in healthcare would lead to socialized medicine—a public tax-supported national healthcare system. During the middle of the 20th century, it became obvious that something needed to be done to provide medical care for the elderly. In 1965, during President Lyndon B. Johnson's administration, federal

legislation was enacted, resulting in *Medicare* for the elderly and *Medicaid* for the **indigent** (those having insufficient income or assets to be able to pay for adequate medical care). Since 1966, public and private health insurance has played a key role in financing healthcare costs in the United States. Medicare and Medicaid are examined more closely in later chapters.

Figs. 1-2 and 1-3 illustrate where U.S. health dollars come from and how they are spent.

The structure and system of care that is known today as *managed care* traces its history to a series of alternative

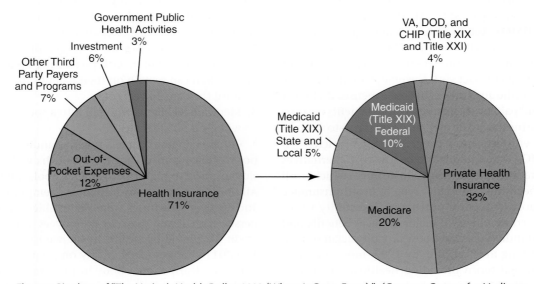

Fig. 1-2 Pie chart of "The Nation's Health Dollar: 2009 (Where It Came From)." (Courtesy Centers for Medicare and Medicaid Services, Office of the Actuary, National Health Statistics Group.)

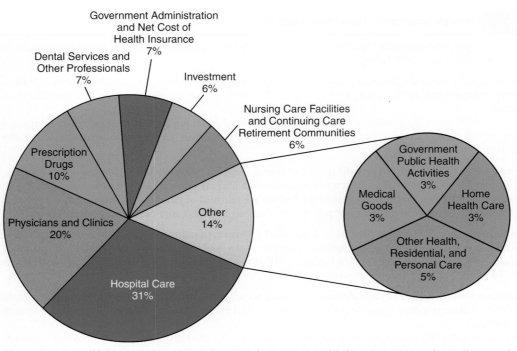

Fig.1-3 Pie chart of "The Nation's Health Dollar: 2009 (Where It Went)." (Courtesy Centers for Medicare and Medicaid Services, Office of the Actuary, National Health Statistics Group.)

healthcare arrangements that appeared in various communities across the United States in the 19th century. The goal of these arrangements was to help meet the healthcare needs of select groups of people, including rural residents and workers and families in the lumber, mining, and railroad industries. The enrollees paid a set fee to physicians, who delivered care under the terms of their agreement. In urban areas, such groups often were paid by charitable organizations to provide care to their members or charges. These prepaid group practices were a model for later entities that came to be known as *health maintenance organizations* (HMOs).

In 1973, Congress passed the **Health Maintenance Organization (HMO) Act**, which provided grants to employers who set up HMOs. An HMO is a plan that provides healthcare to its enrollees from specific physicians and hospitals that contract with the plan. Usually there are no **deductibles** (the amount of covered expenses that must be incurred and paid by the insured before benefits become payable by the insurer) to be met, no claim forms to be completed by the enrollee, and a geographically restricted service area. HMOs were intended to be low-cost alternatives to the more traditional **indemnity insurance**, which until recently has been the "standard" type of health insurance individuals most frequently purchased. Indemnity insurance provides comprehensive major medical benefits and allows insured individuals to choose any physician or hospital when seeking medical care. By 1997, more than 600 HMOs were in existence providing healthcare to nearly 70 million people in the United States. By 2010, the number of people enrolled in HMO and managed care plans had

decreased significantly as more alternative plan options became available. Currently, about 66 million people are covered by HMO health insurance policies. More detailed information on managed healthcare and HMOs is presented in Chapter 7.

In recent years the buzz word in healthcare is "reform." In 2010, two new healthcare laws were enacted, the Patient Protection and Affordable Care Act (Public Law No. 111-148) and the Health Care and Education Reconciliation Act (Public Law No. 111-152). These acts cover a number of issues and represent significant changes in America's healthcare industry. Although the legislation involves many pages, briefly, the following three major changes were made:

1. Insurance companies are no longer allowed to deny coverage to children with preexisting illnesses.
2. Children can remain on their parent's insurance policies until they are 26 years old.
3. Medicare recipients who fall into a specific coverage gap will get a $250 rebate.

Other changes include a rule that individuals who have not had health insurance for 6 months will receive a subsidy to enroll in high-risk insurance pools run by the states. All new insurance plans sold must exempt preventive care and specific screenings from deductibles, and small businesses with fewer than 25 employees will receive a tax credit for providing health insurance to their employees. The 2011 changes focus mostly on preparing for later updates. To learn more about healthcare reform, visit the Evolve site or enter the words "healthcare reform" in your search engine.

What Did You Learn?

1. How is the transformation of health insurance from what it was in the beginning to what it is today comparable with the metamorphosis of a caterpillar to a butterfly?
2. Why are some people and certain organizations in the United States opposed to the government getting involved in health insurance?
3. What two federal programs got their start in the 1960s during President Johnson's administration?
4. List the three major changes made to healthcare in 2010.

KEY HEALTH INSURANCE ISSUES

We know that health insurance is a constantly changing industry. Although key healthcare issues remain basically the same—confidentiality, patients' rights, and prescription drug coverage for the elderly—the focus remains on healthcare reform in the following areas:

- Expanding access for uninsured Americans
- Reducing costs while improving the healthcare system
- Regulation of managed care plans
- Revamping Medicare and Medicaid
- Restrictions on drug formularies (a list of prescription medications that a drug plan will pay for) and related pharmacy issues
- Expanding the use of electronic medical records (EMRs)
- Stabilizing emergency medical services

In the future, key issues might revolve around safeguarding individuals from the improper use of genetic information, creating precise definitions of "genetic tests" and "genetic information," genotherapy, and cloning. Meanwhile, this book focuses on healthcare issues that currently affect everyone.

How Can People Obtain Health Insurance?

Most people who have health insurance get it from one of two major sources: the government or private organizations. As mentioned earlier, the government provides health insurance programs to specific groups, such as the elderly and people who qualify because their income is below the federal poverty level. Many Americans get private health insurance through their employers. Still others purchase and pay for it themselves.

People pay for health insurance in a variety of ways. Many individuals who are employed full-time (or for a specific number of hours, e.g., 30 or 35, per week) are eligible for a **group plan** and have the cost of insurance premiums (or a certain portion of them) deducted from their paychecks. A group health insurance plan is one insurance policy that covers a group of people. Usually a business entity establishes a group health insurance plan to cover its employees; however, group plans are not limited to employers. Often clubs and organizations, chambers of commerce, special interest groups, trade associations, and church/religious groups organize healthcare for their members.

Until the early 1990s, employers, especially larger ones, commonly paid up to half of their employees' group health insurance premiums as an added benefit. In some cases, employers paid the entire cost of health insurance directly. As healthcare costs increased, however, along with medical insurance premiums, this practice became less common.

Individuals who do not have health insurance benefits through their employment or through government programs can purchase private health insurance policies directly from a commercial insurance company. In the case of the latter, premiums are usually much higher than those of employer-sponsored plans and individuals typically must complete a detailed healthcare questionnaire. Often (depending on the person's age and other factors), certain illnesses that were diagnosed or injuries that occurred before an effective date of the insurance policy are not covered. These are referred to as **preexisting conditions**.

Access to Health Insurance

A report generated and posted in September 2008 by the Henry J. Kaiser Foundation's Commission on Medicaid and the Uninsured stated that approximately 60% of people in this country younger than the age of 65 have health insurance as a work benefit. This number decreased to 44.6% in 2011. Millions of low-income Americans who do not have job-based coverage or cannot afford private insurance may qualify for coverage through public programs such as Medicare, Medicaid, and the State Children's Health Insurance Program (SCHIP). Gaps in this private/public system, however, still leave more than 40 million people younger than the age of 65 (nonelderly) uninsured. Those who fall into these "gaps" include low-wage workers who cannot afford private insurance, part-time employees who do not work enough hours to qualify for healthcare benefits, and employees hired by companies that cannot afford to (or do not) offer benefits often because of a low profit margin. Having no health insurance can seriously affect peoples' financial security, limiting their access to healthcare, which can ultimately affect their health.

Although millions of Americans lack health insurance because they cannot afford it, many others who can afford it cannot buy it because insurance companies consider them "high risk" owing to the fact that they may need expensive healthcare in the future. Private insurance companies assess the chances of whether applicants are likely to need expensive future medical care and group them into classes of risk. Individuals who are considered average or better than average risks (basically the young and healthy) usually can purchase insurance policies at a relatively affordable price. If the insurance company thinks an applicant presents too much risk, he or she is put into a high-risk pool; if the individual is allowed to enroll in the healthcare program, he or she is charged a much larger premium. Alternatively, the insurance company may refuse to insure a high-risk individual at all.

During the 1980s and 1990s, insurance companies, in an effort to keep costs down, began including a preexisting condition clause in their health insurance policies. This clause often denies access to anyone who already has a medical condition, or at least specifies that the insurer would not pay for medical expenses incurred as a result of that particular condition. As a general rule, preexisting condition clauses either are nonexistent or are limited to 1 to 2 years with employer-sponsored group plans.

⭐ Imagine This!

Fred Simmons had been a factory worker at Acme Auto Repair. After 20 years working on the line, Fred decided to open up his own body shop, repairing wrecked automobiles in his garage. Fred had previously been covered under Acme's group health insurance plan, but after he became self-employed, he applied for a private policy with Top-Notch Insurance. When the Top-Notch representative asked Fred to fill out an application form, one of the questions was, "Have you ever been treated for, or have had any symptoms of, heart disease?" Fred, honest man that he was, checked "yes," and for an explanatory note, stated, "I went to the emergency room in April of last year with chest pains." Top-Notch, afraid that Fred was in imminent danger of a heart attack, agreed to sell Fred an insurance policy but excluded payment for any treatment involving his heart, which they determined was a preexisting condition.

As a result of this preexisting condition clause, people found it difficult to change jobs if they, or any of their dependents, had a serious health condition. To get around this problem, Congress introduced the **Health Insurance Portability and Accountability Act (HIPAA)** of 1996, which (among other things) requires most employer-sponsored group health insurance plans to accept transfers from other group plans without imposing a preexisting condition clause. Additional information regarding HIPAA is presented in Chapter 3.

📁 HIPAA Tip

The four main provisions of HIPAA are that it:
1. Allows portability of health insurance coverage.
2. Protects workers and their families from preexisting conditions when they change or lose their jobs.
3. Establishes national standards for electronic healthcare transactions and national identifiers for providers, health plans, and employers.
4. Addresses the security and privacy of health data.
   Adopting these standards is intended to improve the efficiency and effectiveness of healthcare in the United States.

Another provision that serves to prevent people from losing their healthcare coverage is the **Consolidated Omnibus Budget Reconciliation Act (COBRA)**, a health benefit act that Congress passed in 1986. Under COBRA, when an employee quits his or her job or is laid off (or the hours are reduced) from a company with 20 or more workers, the law requires the employer to extend group health coverage to the employee and his or her dependents at group rates for 18 months and in some cases up to 36 months. Group health coverage for COBRA participants is usually more expensive than health coverage for active employees, because the employer usually pays a part of the premium for active employees, whereas COBRA participants generally pay the entire premium themselves. Coverage under COBRA is normally less expensive, however, than individual health coverage. *Note:* The American Recovery and Reinvestment Act (ARRA) provided a COBRA premium reduction for eligible individuals who were involuntarily terminated from employment through the end of May 2010. As a result, the COBRA premium reduction under ARRA is not available for employees who were involuntarily terminated after May 31, 2010. Individuals who qualified on or before May 31, 2010, however, may continue to pay reduced premiums for up to 15 months, as long as they are not eligible for another group health plan or Medicare. More information on COBRA is presented later in this text.

Identifying the Uninsured

In 2010, approximately 50 million people in the United States had no healthcare plan. The two top reasons for this, which are both related to cost, are:
- High premiums
- High costs of treatment

Uninsured workers are typically those who work in low-wage or blue-collar jobs, are employed by small firms, or work in service industries that do not offer healthcare coverage as a benefit. More than half of uninsured workers have no education beyond high school, which makes it difficult for them to get the higher-skilled jobs that normally do offer health insurance. Roughly two-thirds of uninsured families have incomes below 200% of the federal poverty level (FPL)—approximately $44,700 for a family of four in 2011.

The new healthcare legislation that took effect in 2010 affects the uninsured by:
- Providing immediate, temporary coverage for those individuals with preexisting conditions. (This coverage continues until 2014, when all the healthcare changes go into effect.)
- Extending Medicaid coverage (until 2014) to more categories of people, such as those who are low income and have no children.
- Allowing small businesses, the self-employed, and the uninsured (until 2014) to join together to buy less expensive policies.
- Assessing fines to those who do not purchase a healthcare plan and do not qualify under a hardship plan.

Additionally, the new healthcare law gives businesses incentives to cover more workers, such as the following:

- Businesses with fewer than 25 employees will get a tax credit up to 35% of the company's share of their total health care premium.
- Companies with 26 to 49 workers will not be affected.
- Businesses with 50 or more workers must offer coverage or pay $750 per worker. (That penalty applies for every employee if even one signs up for government-subsidized insurance.)

State Programs for the Uninsured

The new federal healthcare reform legislation expands coverage to people who do not currently qualify for state Medicaid programs. Effective 2014, all Americans with incomes up to 133% of federal poverty guidelines ($29,726 a year for a family of four in 2011) will be covered under this new, expanded program. Currently the states share the cost of the Medicaid program with the federal government; however, under the new law, the federal government will provide states with 100% financing for those individuals newly eligible for Medicaid for the first 3 years. This percentage decreases incrementally each year until 2020, at which time the federal government's share drops to 90%. For more information on Medicaid, see Chapter 8.

The Children's Health Insurance Program (CHIP) provides insurance for qualifying children who are ineligible for Medicaid but cannot afford private insurance. States receive a higher federal match to pay for CHIP coverage than for their Medicaid programs. All 50 states and the District of Columbia use Medicaid or CHIP to provide coverage beyond federal standards.

What Affects the Cost of Healthcare?

We all know that the costs of healthcare have increased a lot in recent years. In 1980, Americans spent nearly $250 billion on healthcare. By 1999, that figure had more than quadrupled to $1.2 trillion, and it was projected to reach $2.6 trillion (almost 16% of the gross domestic product) by 2010. Fig. 1-4 shows the growth in national health expenditures in the past 2 decades along with the projected expenditure for the present decade.

Many factors are to blame for this large increase in healthcare costs. Because of the complexity of the problem and the issues involved, it is easy to jump to conclusions that are not based on careful consideration of all the facts. Some blame the insurance companies for these rising costs, but one of the largest health insurance companies in the United States claims that, contrary to common opinion, administrative costs of processing claims and providing customer service for members amount to only a small portion of escalating premium dollars. The lion's share goes to pay for the medical care that members receive, and because the cost of this care keeps increasing, members' premiums keep increasing. Some reasons and explanations experts give to try to explain the increasing cost of healthcare are presented in the following paragraphs.

Americans Are Living Longer Than Ever Before

In 1900, the average life expectancy of Americans was about 50 years. In 2000, life expectancy was 76 years. You may have heard the phrase "the graying of America." During the 20th century, the number of people in the United States

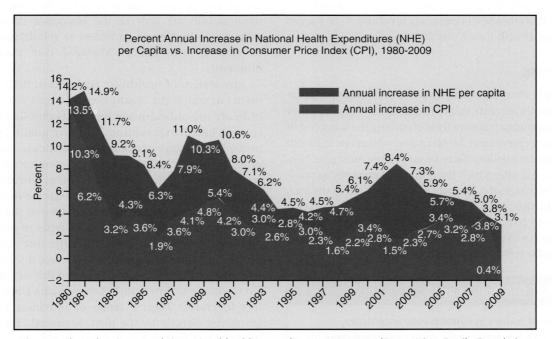

Fig. 1-4 Chart showing growth in national health expenditures, 1980-2009. (From Kaiser Family Foundation calculations using National Health Expenditure [NHE] data from the Centers for Medicare and Medicaid Services, Office of the Actuary, National Health Statistics Group; Kaiser Slides. http://facts.kff.org/chart.aspx?ch=212/.)

who were 65 years or older increased 11-fold. Because elderly people typically require more healthcare, when they join an insured group, the entire group's healthcare risks, along with the costs, rise accordingly.

Advances in Medical Technology

Until recent years when individuals had a serious disease, such as cancer or heart disease, there were no effective ways to treat it, and often they just died. Today, new technology (chemotherapy and organ and bone marrow transplants) and equipment (magnetic resonance imaging and robotics) provide treatments for medical conditions that were previously untreatable, but these new treatments are expensive.

More Demand for Healthcare

In years past, many people would treat their illnesses at home, reluctant to go to physicians, and many were actually afraid of hospitals. People tended to accept certain physical problems, such as sexual dysfunction, attention deficit disorder, and depression, as their "lot in life." Now, it seems that the trend is to see a physician for even minor medical problems. This increase in the general population's demand for healthcare has resulted in higher medical costs.

Media Intervention

The media is partly to blame. How many of us have watched a commercial on television in which someone has an ache or a pain? A charismatic voice announces that if you are suffering from this or that ailment, some new drug might be the answer, so, "Ask your doctor if *Cure-it-All* is right for you!" For more information on factors fueling rising healthcare costs, log on to the following website: http://www.americanhealthsolution. org/assets/Uploads/risinghealthcarecostsfactors2008.pdf/, for the Price Waterhouse Cooper study brochure ,"The Factors Fueling Rising Health Care Costs 2008."

Cost Sharing

Cost sharing (a situation in which insured individuals pay a portion of the healthcare costs, such as deductibles, coinsurance, or copayment amounts) is one method of curbing the rising cost of health insurance premiums. Most covered workers are in health plans that require a deductible to be met before most plan benefits are provided, after which the individual must pay a copayment or a percentage of coinsurance per encounter. In the past, a typical deductible was in the range of $250 to $500, and coinsurance 10% to 20%. Today, for affordable premiums, deductibles of $2500 or even $5000 are common. Coinsurance has remained in the 10% to 20% range, however.

❓ What Did You Learn?

1. List five of today's key health insurance issues.
2. Name four key factors that drive healthcare costs up.
3. How does "cost sharing" help keep healthcare costs down?

HOW MUCH IS ENOUGH?

We know why people need health insurance: to protect them from paying out large sums of money, sometimes to the point of bankruptcy, for quality medical care. In some parts of the United States, a 1-day stay in a hospital can cost up to $1000, and that is just for the room. If surgery is involved, this cost can easily zoom up to $10,000. Most Americans cannot afford to pay these kinds of medical bills out of their own pockets.

Although there is no way to know how much healthcare one individual will need in the future, insurance experts (called *actuaries*) use statistics to predict the healthcare costs of a large group. On the basis of these anticipated costs, an insurance company can establish premiums for the members of that group. The basic idea behind insurance is that each person who buys a policy with that particular insurance company technically agrees to pay a share of the group's total losses in exchange for a promise that the group will pay his or her healthcare costs if and when needed. By making this agreement, the group as a whole shoulders the burden of paying for expensive medical care for the few who may need it.

HEALTH INSURANCE PLANS

There are basically two categories of private insurance plans: indemnity plans, as discussed earlier, and managed care plans. The indemnity plan (also called **fee-for-service**) is the type of plan most Americans were covered under until the past 2 decades. Under this type of plan, patients can go to any healthcare provider or hospital they choose, medical bills are sent to the insurance carrier, and the patient (or healthcare provider) is reimbursed according to rules of the policy. Managed care plans function differently.

Any system of healthcare payment or delivery arrangements in which the health plan attempts to control or coordinate use of health services by its enrolled members to contain health expenditures, improve quality, or both falls under the category of **managed healthcare.** Arrangements often involve a defined delivery system of providers with some form of contractual arrangement with the plan. Under managed healthcare plans, patients see designated providers, and benefits are paid according to the structure of the managed care plan. With both types of plans, patients and the insurance company share the cost of services rendered. Lately, many people have become disillusioned with some managed healthcare plans, and this development has led to changes. Now, some of these plans allow their enrollees to choose from a range of providers who are not employed directly by the plan. Managed care is discussed in detail in Chapter 7.

As mentioned earlier, in addition to private healthcare plans, there are two government-funded plans: Medicare, which provides healthcare coverage for individuals age 65 and older and individuals with certain disabilities, and Medicaid, which provides healthcare coverage for qualifying low-income individuals. Both of these plans are discussed individually and in more detail in later chapters.

Additional types of healthcare plans are on the horizon. For example, recent healthcare reform proposes **health insurance exchanges**, a model intended to create a more organized and competitive market for health insurance by offering a choice of plans with common rules governing how each plan is offered and its cost and providing information to help consumers better understand the choices available to them. For more information on this topic, visit the Evolve site.

Another healthcare model that is currently being considered is the **Accountable Care Organization** (ACO). Authors of this coverage structure are formulating ACOs to provide a new, more efficient way to deliver care. Similar to an HMO, an ACO is a network of doctors and hospitals that shares responsibility for providing care to patients. Under the new healthcare law, ACOs would agree to manage all of the healthcare needs of a minimum of 5,000 Medicare beneficiaries for at least 3 years. Goals for an ACO are to determine how to successfully

- Keep patients within the ACO, and encourage them to stay healthy and take more responsibility for their own healthcare.
- Encourage patients to use healthcare providers that are part of the ACO network to keep the overall costs down within the organization.

🕐 Stop and Think

Compare the concept of today's health insurance "cost sharing" with the ancient sailors of Babylon.

💬 What Did You Learn?

1. Why do people need health insurance?
2. Name the two basic categories of health insurance.

SUMMARY CHECKPOINTS

▶ Medical insurance can be defined as financial protection from loss or harm as a result of medical care and treatment due to illness and injuries. When an individual purchases an insurance policy, the insuring company promises to pay a portion of the financial expenses incurred (as outlined in the policy) resulting from any medical procedures, services, and certain supplies performed or provided by healthcare professionals if and when the insured or his or her dependents become sick or injured. In return for this financial protection, the insured individual pays a monthly (or periodic) premium.

▶ The roots of modern health insurance began in England in 1850, when a company offered coverage for medical expenses for bodily injuries that did not result in death. Medical insurance in the United States began shortly after the turn of the 20th century as a result of a contract between schoolteachers and a hospital in Texas wherein the hospital agreed to provide certain services for a set number of days for a nominal fee.

▶ Medical insurance has gone through many stages to evolve into what we know it to be today. Politics has played a big role in this growth and change and is responsible for the advent of major government-sponsored plans—Medicare and Medicaid—and HMOs. Important changes include the following:
- Employer-sponsored group health plans
- Creation of Medicare and Medicaid
- Development of managed care
- HIPAA
- Healthcare reform

▶ People can get access to health insurance through two major sources: (1) government-sponsored programs and (2) private organizations.

▶ People on both ends of the health insurance spectrum—individuals who are poor or elderly and individuals who work and are eligible for benefits through an employer-sponsored group plan—tend to acquire access to medical insurance. Individuals in the middle—part-time workers and workers in low-wage jobs—are often left out.

▶ Healthcare costs and premiums have increased exponentially in recent years as a result of many factors, as follows:
- Americans are living longer than ever before
- Advances in medical technology, leading to more expensive equipment and methods of treatment
- More demand for healthcare
- Media intervention

▶ People buy health insurance to protect them from financial loss or ruin. Just one overnight stay in a hospital coupled with a surgical procedure can cost thousands of dollars.

▶ The two basic types of health insurance plans are indemnity (fee-for-service) and managed care.

CLOSING SCENARIO

After the orientation and the first several class sessions, Joy and Barbara believe they have made the right choice in enrolling in a health careers program in the community college. After completing the first chapter of the book, the women know that a health insurance professional career track is right for them. Joy is pleasantly surprised that the topic of insurance can be interesting, especially its history.

One of the most important things the women are experiencing is a growing "camaraderie" with other students in the class and the new friends they are making. During breaks and after class, the women share ideas, suggestions, and tips, and confide worries, concerns, and expectations with their peers.

WEBSITES TO EXPLORE

- For live links to related websites and additional URLs that provide more information on the topics discussed in this chapter, please visit the Evolve site at http://evolve. elsevier.com/Beik/today/
- If you are interested in learning more about the evolution of health insurance in the United States, log on to the PBS website and study the Healthcare Timeline table: http://www.pbs.org/healthcarecrisis/history.htm/
- For more information on HIPAA, log on to the following website: http://www.cms.hhs.gov/HIPAAGenInfo/
- It is important for the health insurance professional to know about COBRA. The following URL will direct your search to an informative website that includes the full text of COBRA: http://www.cobrainsurance.com/
- For a "primer" on "Key Information on Health Care Costs and Their Impact," log on to this website: http://www.kff.org/insurance/upload/7670_02.pdf/

- The Affordable Care Act became law in March of 2010. To learn more about this important legislation, log on to http://www.healthcare.gov/

Author's Note: Websites change frequently. If any of these URLs is unavailable, use applicable guide words in your Internet search to acquire additional information on the various subjects listed.

REFERENCES AND RESOURCES

http://www.gallup.com/poll/152621/fewer-americans-employer-based-health-insurance.aspx.

The Henry J. Kaiser Family Foundation: Key Facts: The Uninsured and the Difference Health Insurance Makes, 2008. http://www.kff.org/uninsured/upload/1420-10.pdf/.

United States Census Bureau: Facts for Features and Special Editions, April 19, 2002. http://www.census.gov/Press-Release/www/releases/archives/facts_for_features_special_editions/000807.html/.

United States Department of Health and Human Services: The 2009 HHS Policy Guidelines, *Fed Regist* 74(14), January 23, 2009. http://aspe.hhs.gov/POVERTY/09poverty.shtml/.

CHAPTER 2

Tools of the Trade: A Career as a Health (Medical) Insurance Professional

Chapter Outline

I. Your Future as a Health Insurance Professional
   A. Required Skills and Interests
      1. Education
      2. Preparation
II. Job Duties and Responsibilities
III. Career Prospects
   A. Occupational Trends and Future Outlook

B. What to Expect as a Health Insurance Professional
      1. Home-Based Careers
   C. Rewards
IV. Is a Career in Healthcare Right for You?
V. Certification Possibilities
VI. Career Focus of the Health Insurance Professional
   A. Electronic Claims
   B. CMS-1500 Paper Claim Form

CHAPTER OBJECTIVES

After completion of this chapter, the student should be able to:

1. List the entry-level skills necessary for success in the health insurance professional's career.
2. Discuss college courses typically included in a medical insurance billing and coding program.
3. Explain the importance of effective study skills and proper preparation to maximize learning.
4. Demonstrate the importance of time management by developing and using a time management chart.
5. Identify desirable personality traits and on-the-job skills health insurance professionals should possess to optimize career success.
6. Classify various job titles and their corresponding duties included under the general umbrella of "health insurance professional."
7. Explore career prospects and job opportunities for health insurance professionals.
8. Predict possible rewards of a career in medical-related fields.
9. Investigate certification possibilities related to the field of insurance billing and coding.
10. Compare the two methods of submitting insurance claims.

CHAPTER TERMS

application
autonomy
CMS-1500 claim form
certification
communication
comprehension
covered entity
diligence
electronic data interchange (EDI)

initiative
integrity
objectivity
paraphrase
prioritize
professional ethics
trading partners

YOUR FUTURE AS A HEALTH INSURANCE PROFESSIONAL

Before you begin any college or vocational program, you might want to ask yourself, "Where will this take me, and what career opportunities are available to a graduate of this type of program?" You should think about several things. Naturally, the first question in many individuals' minds is, "How much money can I make?" That question is logical, but other factors should be considered when choosing a career. One wise person said, "If you choose a job you love, you will never have to work a day the rest of your life."

OPENING SCENARIO

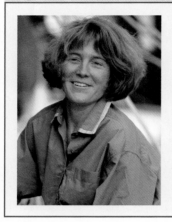

Joy and Barbara, two nontraditional students, are apprehensive about embarking on a new career path. The idea of becoming a health insurance professional sounded important and exciting, and they are willing and eager to learn. They share a common interest in the medical field, but neither one is interested in the clinical side of the profession.

When Joy attended the college career fair, she knew immediately that this was an ideal vocation for her. She considered herself an organized person who paid attention to detail. She was treasurer of the PTA at her children's school and took pride in her impeccable bookkeeping. Barbara, too, believed her organizational skills were one of her strong suits, but the idea of detailed, hand-kept records did not appeal to her. Working with computers is what spurred her interest. Was it possible that both women could find their niche as health insurance professionals? Their instructor assured them they could but that it would involve a lot of work and dedication.

Although there are many different career paths you can choose in the area of healthcare, this chapter refers to the domain of medical expertise of a "health insurance professional," sometimes referred to as a medical insurance specialist. The administrative health insurance professional plays a crucial role in healthcare and one that is increasingly in demand. Qualified health insurance professionals (also referred to as *medical billing and coding specialists*) are experts in generating, submitting, and tracking insurance claims for a variety of payers and ensure that insurance companies reimburse the healthcare provider (and/or patient) appropriately and in a timely manner for services rendered. Those trained as health insurance professionals are vital not only to healthcare providers but to health insurance companies as well. They also play an important role in patient advocacy. Although job opportunities in this career field are increasing because of the relatively complex nature of health insurance in general (particularly the coding process), the industry is placing great emphasis on training and experience. Certification is recommended and is available for various specialties in the allied health field. Certification tells prospective employers that the individual possesses the skills necessary in a particular area, which helps the office run efficiently and effectively and provides for each patient's specific needs. (See "Certification Possibilities" later.)

It should be noted here that although we refer to this career field as "health insurance professional," there is no nationally recognized title or acronym for this broad specialty.

Required Skills and Interests

Success as a health insurance professional requires a certain degree of competency or knowledge in general educational areas. To increase the potential for success, candidates entering this field should possess college entry–level skills in the following areas:

- Reading and **comprehension** (understanding what you have read)
- Basic business math
- English and grammar

- Oral and written **communication** (sending and receiving information through speech, writing, or signs that is mutually understood)
- Keyboarding and office skills
- Computer **application** skills (ability to use computer hardware and software, including Windows and Microsoft Word [or similar word processing software], and ability to use the Internet)

Education

Many community colleges and career training schools offer programs that provide graduates with the skills to become specialists in the health insurance field. Typically, students begin the program with core courses that are built on in the later stages of the program. They receive extensive hands-on training and practice in medical insurance billing and coding and in computerized patient account management. Box 2-1 lists courses included in a typical insurance billing professional program.

Program length for a health insurance professional is 2 to 4 years at community colleges and technical schools and 4 to 9 months at a career school. Most community colleges offer a 2-year associate degree in this discipline. A 4-year college typically awards a Bachelor of Science degree in health science, healthcare management, or whatever specific health fields are offered. Diplomas and certificates also can be obtained from correspondence or online courses and home study programs. A graduate of a health insurance professional or billing and coding program has opportunities for entry-level employment as a medical biller, medical coder, or other health insurance–related position in hospitals, nursing homes, physicians' offices, ambulatory care facilities, medical or surgical supply companies, or billing service companies.

Preparation

Another important key for success in any career, besides basic entry-level skills and applicable education, is proper preparation. You might have deduced from the scenario that Joy and Barbara have been out of school for several years. Both women think their study skills need sharpening. To succeed

Box 2-1

Courses in a Typical Insurance Billing Professional Program

Core Courses

Anatomy and Physiology
Medical Terminology
Keyboarding
Word Processing
Business English
Business Math
Medical Office Administrative Skills

Specialized Courses

Medical Transcription
Medical Records Management
Current Procedural Terminology (CPT) Coding
International Classification of Diseases, Clinical Modification, edition 10 (ICD-10-CM), Coding
Medical Insurance Billing
Computerized Office Management
Bookkeeping/Accounting

in any formal college or training program, you must have good study skills.

Schools today encourage "lifelong learning." This means that learning will not stop when you graduate from the college or career program you have chosen but that you will continue to learn for the rest of your career—or, ideally, the rest of your life. In healthcare, this is especially true because this discipline is constantly changing. Many students who have been out of school for several years find that their study skills may be a little rusty. Even if you have been out of school for only a short time, you still may need help to "get back in the groove" of studying. The following is a list of suggestions that may help you develop effective study skills to enhance your chances of success:

1. **Prioritize Your Life.** Develop a weekly time management schedule in which tasks and activities are **prioritized** (organized by importance). Make sure this schedule:
   - allows time for studying each specific subject,
   - spreads out study times throughout the week,
   - permits time for recreation and rest and family, and
   - grants periodic "rewards," such as watching TV or lunch out with friends.
   Make a list of the things you need to do (just as you make a list before you go grocery shopping). Do not create a schedule that is too detailed or rigid. As you progress, make adjustments as needed. Table 2-1 provides an example of a time management schedule.
2. **Learn How to Study.** Choose a quiet, suitable area where you
   - can concentrate,
   - will have minimal interruptions,
   - can be comfortable enough to focus on your work, and
   - are close to resources (e.g., computer, reference materials).
3. **Develop Positive Personality Traits.** Not everyone is suited to working in the field of medicine. Following

is a list of desirable personality traits and qualities of character that experts believe an individual should possess to be successful in this field:
- Self-discipline
- A positive attitude
- **Diligence** (sticking with a task until it is finished)
- **Integrity** (having honest ethical and moral principles)
- **Objectivity** (not influenced by personal feelings, biases, or prejudices)
- **Initiative** (readiness and ability to take action)
- Enthusiasm

🕐 Stop and Think

Reread the personality traits listed. Do you understand what each one means? Review the definition for each. Do you think you possess all of these personality traits? If there are any that you think you do not have or that you might need to improve on, list them along with ideas on how to develop these traits or make them better.

4. **Prepare for Class.** Getting the most out of the courses you take involves effort on your part. The time and effort you invest in your preparation before class and the time you spend in class greatly affect what you get out of your schooling:
   - Attend every class and be on time.
   - Become an active participator—ask questions and take notes.
   - Learn to recognize important points in the text and from lectures.
   - Outline, underline, highlight, or make notes in the text margins.
   - Work through questions/examples until you understand them.
   - Communicate with your instructor and other students.
   - Become a good listener.
   - Complete all homework and assigned readings on time.
   - Develop the ability to concentrate.
   - Enhance your reading comprehension. (After you read a section of the text, stop and ask yourself, "What are they trying to get across to me?")
   - **Paraphrase** (write down in your own words) important facts from lectures and readings.

🕐 Stop and Think

Think about each of the bulleted points. Why do you think each one is important to your success as a student and as a career professional? Develop a plan for effective studying. Compare your study plan with the plans of your peers and share ideas. Keep working on your study plan until you have developed one that works for you.

TABLE 2-1	Time Management Schedule						
TIME	**SUN**	**MON**	**TUES**	**WED**	**THURS**	**FRI**	**SAT**
6:00	Sleep	Shower/eat	Shower/eat	Shower/eat	Shower/eat	Shower/eat	Sleep
7:00	Personal	Personal	Personal	Personal	Personal	Personal	
8:00	Breakfast	Bus	Bus	Bus	Bus	Bus	Personal/breakfast
9:00	Family	Group discussion	Computer Lab	Group discussion	Computer Lab	Group discussion	Chores
10:00	Business Policy	Marketing Communications	Business Policy	Marketing Communications	Business Policy		
11:00	Self	Marketing Research	Library	Marketing Research	Library	Marketing Research	Self
12:00	Lunch	Lunch	Lunch	Lunch			
1:00	Lunch	Writing Lab	Lunch	Writing Lab	Lunch	Writing Lab	Chores
2:00	Group study	Group study/research	Group study/research	Shopping			
3:00	Expository Writing	Business and Professional Speaking	Expository Writing	Business and Professional Speaking	Expository Writing		
4:00	Chores	Bus	Sales Management	Bus	Sales Management	Bus	Recreation and rest
5:00	Dinner/recreation and rest	Bus	Dinner/recreation and rest	Bus	Dinner/recreation and rest		
6:00	Dinner	Chores	Dinner/recreation and rest	Chores	Dinner/recreation and rest	Write paper for Expository Writing	Family
7:00	Study	Study	Bus/shopping	Study	Chores	Recreation and rest	

In addition to the previously listed classroom skills, individuals experienced in working as health insurance professionals suggest that candidates for this field should be able to:

- Pay attention to detail.
- Follow directions.
- Work independently without supervision.
- Understand the need for and possess a strong sense of **professional ethics** (moral principles associated with a specific vocation).
- Understand the need for and possess strong people skills (ability to communicate effectively with all types of individuals at all levels).
- Demonstrate patience and an even temperament.
- Be empathetic without being sympathetic.
- Be organized but flexible.
- Be conscientious.
- Demonstrate a sense of responsibility.
- Possess manual dexterity.
- Understand and respect the importance of confidentiality.
- Demonstrate a willingness to learn.

In addition to these job skills, it is also important that a health insurance professional be proficient in using the computer and software programs, such as Word and Excel, for letter writing and creating reports.

What Did You Learn?

1. List five required classroom skills that help ensure success as a health insurance professional.
2. Why is "preparation" an important key to success?
3. List five "on-the-job" skills that experienced health insurance professionals should possess.

Imagine This!

Sandra Bence-Franklin works for New Beauty Products, Inc., a large cosmetics firm, where her responsibilities are limited to handling incoming calls on a complicated telephone system and greeting and directing customers. Although the pay and benefits are good, she has quickly become bored and disillusioned with her job. She desires more challenge and variety. Her cousin Lisa, a health insurance professional, has recently been hired at Oceanside Medical Center. Lisa talks constantly about the variety and challenges of her new job, remarking, "I'm doing something different every day. I'm learning so much, and it's so interesting! I really feel I'm making a difference when I help a patient understand the confusing issues of medical insurance."

At first, Sandra has paid little attention to Lisa's ramblings, but as time goes on and her job becomes more and more mundane, she begins to pay closer attention to what Lisa was saying. "Maybe," Sandra muses, "I should look into what a career as a health insurance professional has to offer me."

JOB DUTIES AND RESPONSIBILITIES

We mentioned earlier that there are different career options you can choose that are covered under the general umbrella term health insurance. The title we have chosen is "health insurance professional," which includes the knowledge and expertise associated with that of medical billing, generating insurance claims, and coding. Table 2-2 lists the various job titles under this specialty and their corresponding duties.

Another positive aspect of the health insurance professional's career is the variety of tasks and responsibilities it offers. These vary from office to office, depending on the number of employees, the degree of job specialization, and the type of practice; however, the variety of roles and job **autonomy** (working without direct supervision) make this profession attractive to many individuals. Typical duties of health insurance professionals might include, but are not limited to, the following:

- Scheduling appointments
- Bookkeeping and other administrative duties
- Explaining insurance benefits to patients
- Handling day-to-day medical billing procedures
- Adhering to each insurance carrier's guidelines
- Documenting all activities using correct techniques and medical terminology
- Keeping current on coding and compliance
- Completing insurance forms promptly and accurately
- Knowing and complying with laws and regulations
- Entering computer data
- Interpreting explanations of benefits (EOBs)
- Posting payments to patient accounts
- Corresponding with patients and insurance companies

TABLE 2-2	Roles Included Under the Umbrella of the Health Insurance Professional
SPECIALIZED FIELD	**ROLE/DUTIES**
Claims Assistant Professional (CAP)	Assists patients/consumers in obtaining full benefits from healthcare coverage under private or government health insurance and coordinates with healthcare providers to avoid duplication of payment and overpayment.
Medical Coder/Coding Specialist	Possesses expertise in assigning diagnostic and procedural codes using common coding manuals (ICD-9-CM and CPT).
Medical Claims Processor	Prepares and transmits claims by paper and electronically using the computer.
Reimbursement Specialist	Checks and verifies records, prepares insurance claims, posts ledger and general journal entries, balances accounts payable and accounts receivable records, and follows up on claims and delinquent reimbursements.
Billing Coordinator	Responsible for maintaining patient accounts and for collecting money. Also might create and file insurance claims and handle accounts receivable.
Patient Account Representative	Obtains patient insurance information, confirms appointments, verifies insurance eligibility, enters/updates insurance information into the records and computer.
Medical Claims Reviewer	Analyzes claims for "medical necessity" and valid policy coverage. Performs audits on charge entry for accuracy and HIPAA and Office of Inspector General compliance. Supports/maintains all forms of billing, payment posting, refunds, and credentialing and system issues.
Medical Claims Analyst	Assists with claim rule setup and maintenance, medical claim–related data mapping, claim analysis and other tasks related to supporting client's claims, and medical coding.
Electronic Claims Processor	Sets up and implements electronic claims processing (in standardized formats) via electronic modes and transmits claims to third-party payers.
Medical Collector	Handles inquiries regarding patient account balances and insurance submission dates. Proficient in collection laws and collection techniques used to settle delinquent accounts and maximize reimbursements.

What Did You Learn?

1. List at least eight of the various career options that are included under the general umbrella of a health insurance professional.
2. Why do you think autonomy might be attractive to some career-minded individuals?
3. List six typical duties of a health insurance professional.

CAREER PROSPECTS

Individuals who choose a career in a healthcare field, such as medical insurance, have an opportunity to work in a variety of professional locations, such as the following:

- Physicians' or dentists' offices
- Hospitals and urgent care facilities
- Pharmacies
- Nursing homes
- Home health agencies
- Mental health facilities
- Physical therapy and rehabilitation centers
- Insurance companies
- Health maintenance organizations (HMOs)
- Consulting firms
- Health data organizations

Successful completion of a health insurance program gives the student the training and skills to become a health insurance professional, which includes the various subspecialties. If an individual decides to become a medical coder, the education and knowledge of healthcare and disease processes he or she learned while taking educational courses or on the job gives the individual a good background if he or she chooses to become certified in this specialty. In the past, many coders were employed in hospitals; however, the growth of ambulatory care facilities and outpatient clinics has greatly increased the demand for employees with a solid background in coding and excellent computer skills.

HIPAA Tip

One goal of the administrative simplification provisions of HIPAA is to reduce the number of forms and methods of completing claims and other payment-related documents through the efficient use of computer-to-computer methods of exchanging standard healthcare information.

Stop and Think

The text stated that the numbers of ambulatory care facilities and outpatient clinics are increasing. What do you think has triggered this growth, and how does it affect health insurance professionals?

Occupational Trends and Future Outlook

Most healthcare providers in the United States today rely heavily on health insurance professionals and medical billing and coding specialists for better customer relations as well as assistance in maximum third-party reimbursement for their professional services. It is, therefore, important that those individuals wishing to enter this medical career specialty clearly understand the educational requirements, training, earning potential, and home business options. They should also be aware of any potential "downsides" of a career as a health insurance professional. Knowing what to expect and where the challenges lie will provide students with the right tools, which give them the best chance to succeed in their chosen career path.

Advancement opportunities in a health insurance career are virtually unlimited. Employment prospects exist in medical facilities ranging in size from a small staff of one or two healthcare providers to several hundred providers in a multispecialty group practice. An American Hospital Association survey showed that nearly 18% of billing and coding positions are unfilled because of a lack of qualified candidates.

As an alternative to working in a medical office as an employee, the health insurance professional has the option of working independently from a home-based office. Many electronic billing programs are available and can be set up through home office computers. Also, there is the possibility of becoming an independent insurance specialist or consultant, who contracts to do coding and claims submission for healthcare providers who do not have the ability or manpower to do it themselves. Another possibility would be to work as a consultant to help patients understand their insurance bills and what they should be paying.

The Health Insurance Portability and Accountability Act (HIPAA) of 1996 has created an opportunity for the healthcare industry to move from paper claims transactions to electronic transactions using one national standard format. This situation creates tremendous job opportunities for health insurance professionals to help noncompliant providers achieve HIPAA compliance. More information can be learned about HIPAA by logging onto and studying the websites listed at the end of this chapter.

HIPAA Tip

HIPAA, created to reduce healthcare costs and protect patient privacy (through the use of electronic data interchange), has established rigorous new standards and requirements for the maintenance and transmission of healthcare information. Healthcare providers, insurers, and clearinghouses need specialists with HIPAA training and HIPAA certification to ensure that medical facilities are in compliance with HIPAA's rules and regulations to help them avoid federal penalties.

What to Expect as a Health Insurance Professional

Following are nine steps explaining how to pursue a career as a health insurance professional and what to expect. These steps are provided for students to use as a guideline for success.

Step 1: Research Duties and Responsibilities. As mentioned previously, the student should be aware of the duties and responsibilities required to become a successful health insurance professional. When a patient receives healthcare services, each office visit and/or procedure performed must be assigned a specific code. Also, the patient's diagnosis (the reason he or she sought medical care) must be assigned a code. These codes, along with the corresponding charges, are submitted to the insurance company for payment decisions. After the insurer makes its decision, both the provider and patient receive notification of how the claim was adjudicated. An explanation of benefits (EOB) document is provided by the insurer that indicates the amount of the insurance payment and any remaining balance for which the patient is responsible. The health insurance professional is involved throughout this entire process.

Step 2: Enroll in a Formal Training Program. Education for health insurance professionals can vary, ranging from a diploma or certificate to an associate degree. Many community colleges and career schools offer a variety of allied health programs, both online classes and day, evening, and weekend classes, in an institutional environment. Associate of Applied Science degrees, which normally take 2 years to complete, can lead to higher salaries and expanded career opportunities.

Step 3: Become Certified. Numerous options are available for certification, depending on the employer's preferences and the individual's career goals. The American Medical Billing Association (AMBA) (www.ambanet.net) offers an examination to qualify as a Certified Medical Reimbursement Specialist (CMRS). An entry-level certification called Certified Coding Associate (CCA) is also available from the American Health Information Management Association (AHIMA) (www.ahima.org). The American Academy of Professional Coders (AAPC) also offers certifications for hospital, outpatient, and payer employees who use coding in their work. (See "Certification Possibilities" for further certification opportunities.)

Step 4: Obtain Employment. In addition to physicians' offices, insurance companies, hospitals, pharmacies, and government entities make use of health insurance professionals. An individual trained in this field but not yet certified may be able to acquire an entry-level position and pursue certification later. After acquiring a position within a medical facility, the person must work diligently to gain the experience needed to specialize in the field of health insurance professional. He or she should also be willing to learn and acquire new skills outside the job duties to enhance advancement opportunities.

Step 5: Learn and Perform Your Job Duties. It is important to study and learn the claims submission process from beginning to end. If a claim is rejected, determine the reason by reviewing the claim. The insurance usually offers a code that explains the specific reason for the rejection. Make any corrections or adjustments necessary, and resubmit all related charges. Making sure the claim is "clean" before submission will help you avoid losing valuable time. Always verify the correct spelling of the patient's (and the insured's) name, date of birth, sex, and Social Security number. Contact the patient if the information is not available in the file.

Step 6: Posting Payments. All payments received, either from the insurer or from the patient, should be posted promptly to the patient's account, and any contractual adjustments should be made as required by law. Sometimes insurance companies make errors when calculating payments; therefore it is important to check these amounts during the posting process to ensure accuracy. Follow the specific guidelines of the insurer for submitting original or corrected claims as well as for appealing rejected claims.

Step 7: Reporting Denied Charges to a Coding Specialist. The law requires that only certified coders make changes to a patient's medical codes once it is determined an error has occurred. If the health insurance professional is not a certified coder, all denied charges due to coding errors should be referred to the coding specialist in the appropriate department.

Step 8: Generate and Maintain a Log. It is recommended that health insurance professionals keep a detailed log of all conversations with either the patient or the insurance company. Such a log will provide detailed information to anyone who needs to examine the account for an accurate and up-to-date report of the status of the account. Many patient accounting software programs have features that allow this process.

Step 9: Benefit From Job Security and Flexibility. Advances in electronic billing have made it possible for some health insurance professionals and medical billing specialists to work from their homes. An experienced professional may be able to start a home business to provide insurance, billing, and coding services on a contractual basis. Home-based careers are discussed in more detail in the next section.

Home-Based Careers

With the advent of more sophisticated computer technology and the Internet, career opportunities in home-based medical billing and coding, as both part-time and full-time endeavors, are growing. Numerous online courses in this subspecialty are offered, as well as courses in career schools. Certification possibilities are available through the Medical Billing Network. Experts in this field suggest that if the idea of self-employment appeals to you, do some thorough research before you begin this venture.

The basics to get started are a personal computer (PC) (ideally no more than 2 years old) and access to the Internet via the most recent version of a Web browser (e.g., Internet Explorer, Netscape Navigator, or Firefox). Minimum requirements vary depending on personal preference and usage, but for basic e-mail, Internet access, word processing, and spreadsheet generation, at least a 1-GHZ processor (or better), a 2-GB minimum of memory (RAM), and an 80-GB hard drive are considered adequate. A DVD/CD-RW combo drive would enhance your system, if you can afford it. Keep in mind that these minimum requirements are upgraded every year or more often, and keeping your system as up to date as possible will enhance performance. After that, you need to find clients to support your home-based business. Consult with organizations for medical claims processors or medical billing businesses and with doctors in your community. Ask them about the medical billing field: How much of a need is there for this type of work? How much work does medical billing entail? What kind of training is required? Do they know anything about the promotion or promoter that you are interested in? Be aware of unsubstantiated dollar-earning possibilities, though. The Federal Trade Commission (FTC) has brought charges against promoters of medical billing opportunities for misrepresenting the earnings potential of their businesses and for failing to provide key preinvestment information required by law.

For additional information on home-based careers, explore the websites listed at the end of this chapter.

Rewards

Individuals working as health insurance professionals enjoy many benefits, such as job security, a good income, personal satisfaction, and challenges. One of the biggest rewards is the knowledge that they are helping people. As to earnings, at the turn of the 21st century, a graduate of a medical insurance professional program could expect to earn $20,000 to $30,000 a year on entry into the workforce, depending on his or her geographic area of the United States. This base wage typically increases rapidly as the individual gains experience and success in the field. Certified coders, at that same time, made on average between $24,000 and $60,000, depending on experience, credentials, location, and education. For income ranges in various allied health occupations, refer to the American Medical Association website listed in the websites at the end of this chapter.

❓ What Did You Learn?

1. How has HIPAA opened up opportunities for health insurance professionals?
2. What does the text suggest might be the biggest reward for health insurance professionals?

IS A CAREER IN HEALTHCARE RIGHT FOR YOU?

Health-related professions offer an exciting and satisfying career with exceptional challenges and opportunities for growth. With dozens of specialized health careers, an individual can use almost any talent he or she has. With such a variety of choices and specializations, there is a place in healthcare for anyone who chooses to follow this career path.

To see whether healthcare is a good career choice for you, take the following short quiz. When you are finished, add up the number of times you selected "yes." If you checked seven or more boxes "yes," a career in healthcare may be right for you!

YES	NO	
☐	☐	I am interested in health and sciences classes.
☐	☐	I am an active listener.
☐	☐	I enjoy helping people.
☐	☐	I might like helping people who are sick or injured.
☐	☐	I find working with equipment and technology appealing.
☐	☐	I am an even-tempered person.
☐	☐	I take satisfaction in working as a member of a team.
☐	☐	I find having responsibilities inviting.
☐	☐	I am an effective communicator.
☐	☐	I fare well under stress.
☐	☐	I perform competently in math.
☐	☐	I would prefer to have flexibility in my work schedule.
☐	☐	I enjoy meeting new people.
☐	☐	I am fascinated about the human body and how it works.
☐	☐	I delight in solving problems.
☐	☐	I take pleasure in carrying out instructions acceptably.
☐	☐	I am able to follow directions.
☐	☐	I aspire to work in a laboratory.

CERTIFICATION POSSIBILITIES

Graduates of a medical insurance professional program can be eligible for many different professional certifications that would enhance their careers. **Certification** is the culmination of a process of formal recognition of the competence possessed by an individual. In many vocational training institutions, certification is rewarded as recognition of the successful completion of a vocational training process, based on the time of training and practice and on the evaluated contents. Certification possibilities available to the health insurance professional include the following:

- Certified Medical Assistant
- Registered Medical Assistant
- Professional Association of Healthcare Coding Specialists
- American Academy of Professional Coders (AAPC)
- Certified Professional Coder (CPC)
- Certified Professional Coder for Hospitals (CPC-H)
- American Health Information Management Association (AHIMA)

- Certified Coding Specialist (CCS)
- Certified Coding Associate (CCA)
- Certified Coding Specialist for Physicians (CCS-P)

Additional national certifications for the health insurance professional are Nationally Certified Insurance Coding Specialist (NCICS) through the National Center for Competency Testing (NCCT), Certified Medical Reimbursement Specialist (CMRS) offered by the AMBA, and Certified Electronic Medical Biller (CEMB) available through instruction and testing from the Electronic Medical Billing Network of America, Inc.

AHIMA also offers certification in the other areas, such as:

- Health Information Management
- Registered Health Information Administrator (RHIA)
- Registered Health Information Technician (RHIT)
- Healthcare Privacy and Security
- Certified in Healthcare Privacy (CHP)
- Certified in Healthcare Privacy and Security (CHPS)
- Certified in Healthcare Security (CHS)

For additional possibilities of career-related certifications, explore the websites listed at the end of this chapter.

Individuals who are trained and certified as health insurance professionals, coders, and collection specialists have a basic goal: *to ensure that providers (and patients) get paid correctly the first time, every time, on time.* The ever-increasing complexity of diagnosis and treatment codes, coupled with the confusing and often seemingly contradictory guidelines for what various insurance carriers will accept as a claim, makes it almost impossible for healthcare providers to stay on top of the constantly changing healthcare scene and still maintain maximum cash flow.

The U.S. Department of Labor states that continued employment growth for health insurance professionals is spurred by the increased medical needs of an aging population and the number of healthcare practitioners. Federal regulations and confusing health insurance policies also have created a strong demand for professionals who can comprehend and perform successfully the demanding role of compliance and provider education.

Computers have dramatically transformed the medical insurance industry by enabling the health insurance professional to focus on accuracy and efficiency instead of the cumbersome task of manually processing each and every claim. This change has brought medical insurance billing into the limelight as one of the fastest growing disciplines in the workforce today. Health insurance professionals not only are in high demand but also have a secure future in the world of medicine.

CAREER FOCUS FOR THE HEALTH INSURANCE PROFESSIONAL

The focus of your career as a health insurance professional is the insurance claim. After completion of this course, you will be able to identify each health insurance payer, its individual rules, guidelines, and procedures, and the relevant information that must be collected in order to submit a claim.

Basically, there are two methods of claims submission, electronic and paper.

Electronic Claims

Since 2003, the Centers for Medicare and Medicaid Services (CMS)—the U.S. federal agency that administers Medicare, Medicaid, and the Children's Health Insurance Program—have required all physicians, providers, and suppliers who bill Medicare carriers, fiscal intermediaries (FIs), Medicare Administrative Contractors (MACs) for Parts A and B, and Durable Medical Equipment MACs (DME MACs) for services provided to Medicare beneficiaries to submit claims electronically (with a few exceptions) using HIPAA's standard ASC X12 version 4010A1 for HIPAA-covered transactions. (See Box 5-1, "Exceptions to Electronic Claim Submission Requirements," in Chapter 5.) In March 2009, the Secretary of the U.S. Department of Health and Human Services (HHS) adopted ASC X12 5010 (Version 5010) as the next standard for HIPAA-covered transactions. This change accommodates the new, expanded diagnostic coding system, International Classification of Diseases, 10th edition (ICD-10), which will be implemented in 2013. As of this writing, the date that all covered entities must be in full compliance with Version 5010 was June 30, 2012. The health information professional should check the CMS website periodically to see if this compliance date has extended further.

Level I compliance means that a **covered entity** (a healthcare provider, a health plan, or a healthcare claims clearing house) can clearly demonstrate the ability to successfully create and receive compliant transactions using the new 5010 version.

Level II compliance means that a covered entity has completed "end-to-end testing" with each of its **trading partners** (any business entity engaging in **electronic data interchange** [EDI]—the computer-to-computer exchange of structured information)—and is able to consistently transmit claims electronically using the new version of the standards.

Electronic claims submission using Version 5010 and the ICD-10 diagnostic coding system will be discussed in more detail later in the text. For an overview of Version 5010, visit the Evolve site. As mentioned above, the date for all covered entities to be in compliance with Version 5010 has been extended to June 30, 2012.

CMS-1500 (08/05) PAPER FORM

Even though CMS mandates that insurance claims be submitted electronically using the specific format as discussed in the previous section, there are exceptions to this rule. As a result, special attention is given in this book to completing the CMS-1500 paper form. After completing this course, you will be able to identify each health insurance payer; its individual rules, guidelines, and procedures; and the relevant information that must be included in each box of the **CMS-1500 claim form**, which is the standard insurance form used by all government and most commercial insurance payers (Fig. 2-1).

1500

HEALTH INSURANCE CLAIM FORM

APPROVED BY NATIONAL UNIFORM CLAIM COMMITTEE 08/05

PICA   PICA

1. MEDICARE MEDICAID TRICARE CHAMPUS CHAMPVA GROUP HEALTH PLAN FECA BLK LUNG OTHER	1a. INSURED'S I.D. NUMBER (For Program in Item 1)

(Medicare #)   (Medicaid #)   (Sponsor's SSN)   (Member ID#)   (SSN or ID)   (SSN)   (ID)

2. PATIENT'S NAME (Last Name, First Name, Middle Initial)

3. PATIENT'S BIRTH DATE   MM | DD | YY   SEX   M □   F □

4. INSURED'S NAME (Last Name, First Name, Middle Initial)

5. PATIENT'S ADDRESS (No., Street)

6. PATIENT RELATIONSHIP TO INSURED   Self □   Spouse □   Child □   Other □

7. INSURED'S ADDRESS (No., Street)

CITY   STATE

8. PATIENT STATUS   Single □   Married □   Other □

CITY   STATE

ZIP CODE   TELEPHONE (Include Area Code) (   )

Employed □   Full-Time Student □   Part-Time Student □

ZIP CODE   TELEPHONE (INCLUDE AREA CODE) (   )

9. OTHER INSURED'S NAME (Last Name, First Name, Middle Initial)

10. IS PATIENT'S CONDITION RELATED TO:

11. INSURED'S POLICY GROUP OR FECA NUMBER

a. OTHER INSURED'S POLICY OR GROUP NUMBER

a. EMPLOYMENT? (CURRENT OR PREVIOUS)   YES □   NO □

a. INSURED'S DATE OF BIRTH   MM | DD | YY   SEX   M □   F □

b. OTHER INSURED'S DATE OF BIRTH   MM | DD | YY   SEX   M □   F □

b. AUTO ACCIDENT?   PLACE (State)   YES □   NO □

b. EMPLOYER'S NAME OR SCHOOL NAME

c. EMPLOYER'S NAME OR SCHOOL NAME

c. OTHER ACCIDENT?   YES □   NO □

c. INSURANCE PLAN NAME OR PROGRAM NAME

d. INSURANCE PLAN NAME OR PROGRAM NAME

10d. RESERVED FOR LOCAL USE

d. IS THERE ANOTHER HEALTH BENEFIT PLAN?   YES □   NO □   *If yes,* return to and complete item 9 a-d.

READ BACK OF FORM BEFORE COMPLETING & SIGNING THIS FORM.
12. PATIENT'S OR AUTHORIZED PERSON'S SIGNATURE I authorize the release of any medical or other information necessary to process this claim. I also request payment of government benefits either to myself or to the party who accepts assignment below.

SIGNED _____ DATE _____

13. INSURED'S OR AUTHORIZED PERSON'S SIGNATURE I authorize payment of medical benefits to the undersigned physician or supplier for services described below.

SIGNED _____

14. DATE OF CURRENT: MM | DD | YY   ILLNESS (First symptom) OR INJURY (Accident) OR PREGNANCY(LMP)

15. IF PATIENT HAS HAD SAME OR SIMILAR ILLNESS. GIVE FIRST DATE   MM | DD | YY

16. DATES PATIENT UNABLE TO WORK IN CURRENT OCCUPATION   MM | DD | YY   FROM   TO   MM | DD | YY

17. NAME OF REFERRING PHYSICIAN OR OTHER SOURCE

17a.
17b. NPI

18. HOSPITALIZATION DATES RELATED TO CURRENT SERVICES   MM | DD | YY   FROM   TO   MM | DD | YY

19. RESERVED FOR LOCAL USE

20. OUTSIDE LAB?   YES □   NO □ $ CHARGES

21. DIAGNOSIS OR NATURE OF ILLNESS OR INJURY. (RELATE ITEMS 1,2,3 OR 4 TO ITEM 24E BY LINE)

1. |___.___   3. |___.___
2. |___.___   4. |___.___

22. MEDICAID RESUBMISSION CODE   ORIGINAL REF. NO.

23. PRIOR AUTHORIZATION NUMBER

24. A. DATE(S) OF SERVICE From MM DD YY To MM DD YY	B. PLACE OF SERVICE	C. EMG	D. PROCEDURES, SERVICES, OR SUPPLIES (Explain Unusual Circumstances) CPT/HCPCS	MODIFIER	E. DIAGNOSIS POINTER	F. $ CHARGES	G. DAYS OR UNITS	H. EPSDT Family Plan	I. ID. QUAL.	J. RENDERING PROVIDER ID. #
1										NPI
2										NPI
3										NPI
4										NPI
5										NPI
6										NPI

25. FEDERAL TAX I.D. NUMBER   SSN □ EIN □

26. PATIENT'S ACCOUNT NO.

27. ACCEPT ASSIGNMENT? (For govt. claims, see back)   YES □   NO □

28. TOTAL CHARGE $

29. AMOUNT PAID $

30. BALANCE DUE $

31. SIGNATURE OF PHYSICIAN OR SUPPLIER INCLUDING DEGREES OR CREDENTIALS (I certify that the statements on the reverse apply to this bill and are made a part thereof.)

SIGNED _____ DATE _____

32. SERVICE FACILITY LOCATION INFORMATION

a. NPI   b.

33. BILLING PROVIDER INFO & PH # (   )

a. NPI   b.

NUCC Instruction Manual available at: www.nucc.org

APPROVED OMB-0938-0999 FORM CMS-1500 (08/05)

CARRIER   PATIENT AND INSURED INFORMATION   PHYSICIAN OR SUPPLIER INFORMATION

Fig. 2-1 Copy of the CMS-1500 (08-05) Health Insurance Claim Form.

SUMMARY CHECKPOINTS

▶ College entry–level skills necessary for success as a health insurance professional include reading and comprehension, basic business math, English and grammar, oral and written communication, keyboarding and office skills, and computer application skills.

▶ Some college courses typically included in a medical insurance billing and coding program include, but are not limited to, the following:
- Medical Terminology
- Anatomy and Physiology
- Medical Law and Ethics
- Medical Records Management
- Current Procedural Terminology (CPT) Coding
- International Classification of Diseases, Clinical Modification, edition 10 (ICD-10-CM), Coding
- Medical Insurance Billing
- Computerized Office Management

▶ Effective study skills and proper preparation are important components for getting the most out of your education and optimizing your career potential. Success in these areas assists "lifelong learning."

▶ An effective plan that organizes and prioritizes study time along with other activities is important to the overall learning process.

▶ Time management schedules are excellent tools to help the student develop better study skills, but they should not be too detailed or rigid. Allow for adjustments, as needed, to accommodate not only time for studying but also for relaxation and rewards.

▶ Some of the personality traits and on-the-job skills health insurance professionals should possess to optimize career success include:
- self-discipline,
- a positive attitude,
- diligence,
- integrity,
- objectivity,
- initiative, and
- enthusiasm.

▶ Several different job titles, each with its corresponding duties, are included under the general umbrella of "health insurance professional." Job titles and duties vary from office to office, depending on the number of employees, the type of medical practice, and the degree of job specialization.

▶ Career prospects and job opportunities for health insurance professionals include, but are not limited to, physicians' or dentists' offices, hospitals, pharmacies, nursing homes, mental health facilities, rehabilitation centers, insurance companies, HMOs, consulting firms, and health data organizations.

▶ Health insurance professionals and similar healthcare careers offer job security, good income, personal satisfaction, challenges, and satisfying experiences as possible rewards, plus the most important reward of all—helping people.

▶ Professional certifications that enhance the careers of health insurance professionals include Certified Professional Coder (CPC) certification, the American Health Information Management Association (AHIMA) Certified Coding Specialist (CCS) and Certified Coding Associate (CCA) certifications, and National Center for Competency Testing (NCCT), Nationally Certified Insurance Coding Specialist (NCICS) certification.

▶ Two methods of submitting insurance claims are:
- Electronic submission using Version 5010 as required by CMS (with certain exceptions)
- CMS-1500 (08/05) universal paper form

🔄 CLOSING SCENARIO

Joy and Barbara now have a real feel not only for how to study and prepare for class but also for what to expect in their future careers as health insurance professionals. They were surprised to learn that there was such a demand for specialists trained in this field, and Joy finds the possibility of opening a home-based business particularly attractive because she still has young children at home. Barbara is optimistic that, after she has completed her schooling, job opportunities exist all over the United States. If her family is relocated because of her husband's job, she would be qualified to work in a variety of positions in many different kinds of health-related facilities in the country. Additionally, Joy and Barbara have decided to begin exploring certification possibilities.

WEBSITES TO EXPLORE

- For live links to related websites and additional URLs that provide more information on the topics discussed in this chapter, please visit the Evolve site at http://evolve.elsevier.com/Beik/today/
- For a listing of health-related careers and occupations, go to http://www.bls.gov/oco/
- AHIMA has a good website for health information technology careers. For more information, log on to http://www.ahima.org/careers/intro.asp/
- You also might want to explore this website created by coders for coders: http://www.codernet.com/
- For a professional outlook on medical coding and billing, go to http://www.skillsamherst.com/skills-career-education-center/medical-billing-and-coding-career-information/
- For additional possibilities of career-related certifications, explore these websites:
  www.aapc.com/
  www.phia.com/
  www.pmimd.com/
  http://www.ama-assn.org/ama/pub/category/6038.html/
- For a complete account of the HIPAA of 1996, log on to and peruse the following websites:
  http://www.cms.hhs.gov/hipaaGenInfo/
  http://www.hipaa.org/
- Additional websites to explore for certification possibilities:
  http://www.aama-ntl.org/
  http://www.amt1.com/
- Additional websites to explore for home-based careers:
  http://www.medicalbillingnetwork.com/
  http://www.capitalpublications.com/secure_html/free_medical_billing.html/

Author's Note: Websites change frequently. If any of these URLs is unavailable, use applicable guide words in your Internet search to acquire additional information on the various subjects listed.

REFERENCES AND RESOURCES

Degree Directory: *Medical Billing: How to Become a Medical Insurance Biller in 5 Steps*. Copyright 2003–2009. http://degreedirectory.org/articles/Medical_Billing_How_to_Become_a_Medical_Insurance_Biller_in_5_Steps.html/.
Mississippi Hospital Association Health Careers Center: *Health Care Career Guide*. Copyright 2003 MHA Careers Center. http://www.mshealthcareers.com/tools/careerguide.htm/.

CHAPTER 3

The Legal and Ethical Side of Medical Insurance

Chapter Outline

I. Medical Law and Liability
   A. Employer Liability
   B. Employee Liability
II. Insurance and Contract Law
   A. Elements of a Legal Contract
      1. Offer and Acceptance
      2. Consideration
      3. Legal Object
      4. Competent Parties
      5. Legal Form
   B. Termination of Contracts
III. Medical Law and Ethics Applicable to Health Insurance
IV. Important Legislation Affecting Health Insurance
   A. Federal Privacy Act of 1974
   B. Federal Omnibus Budget Reconciliation Act of 1980
   C. Tax Equity and Fiscal Responsibility Act of 1982
   D. Consolidated Omnibus Budget Reconciliation Act of 1986
   E. Federal False Claim Amendments Act of 1986
   F. Fraud and Abuse Act
   G. Federal Omnibus Budget Reconciliation Act of 1987
   H. The Patient Protection and Affordable Care Act
V. Medical Ethics and Medical Etiquette
   A. Medical Ethics
   B. Medical Etiquette
VI. Medical Record
   A. Purposes of a Medical Record
   B. Complete Medical Record
   C. Who Owns Medical Records?
   D. Retention of Medical Records
   E. Access to Medical Records
   F. Releasing Medical Record Information

VII. Documentation of Patient Medical Record
VIII. Health Insurance Portability and Accountability Act and Compliance
   A. Impact of Health Insurance Portability and Accountability Act
      1. Impact on the Health Insurance Professional
      2. Impact on Patients
      3. Impact on Providers
      4. Impact on Private Businesses
   B. Enforcement of Confidentiality Regulations of Health Insurance Portability and Accountability Act
   C. Developing a Compliance Plan
IX. Confidentiality and Privacy
   A. Confidentiality
   B. Privacy
   C. Security
   D. Exceptions to Confidentiality
   E. Authorization to Release Information
   F. Exceptions for Signed Released of Information for Insurance Claims Submission
      1. Medicaid-Eligible Patients and Workers' Compensation Cases
      2. Inpatient-Only Treatment
      3. Court Order
   G. Breach of Confidentiality
X. Healthcare Fraud and Abuse
   A. Defining Fraud and Abuse
      1. Who Commits Healthcare Insurance Fraud?
      2. How is Healthcare Fraud Committed?
      3. How Do Consumers Commit Healthcare Insurance Fraud?
   B. Preventing Fraud and Abuse

⟳ OPENING SCENARIO

Joy and Barbara are well entrenched into their course of study on becoming health insurance professionals. As they progress through the course, they are beginning to identify variations in their interests. Although their basic goals are similar, their individual interests are moving in different directions. Barbara determined early on that she prefers to work in a small facility; she intends to learn all aspects of managing an office. Joy has her heart set on a large, multiprovider office where she will more likely find opportunities to specialize in areas she finds interesting and exciting. One of these areas is the legal and ethical side of health insurance.

Before this course, Joy took a class in business law, which gave her a background in various legal processes. Their instructor relates the importance of a good, solid background in medical law and ethics to the class, and both women are convinced it is an important fundamental step in building a solid foundation of knowledge and understanding of health insurance. An in-depth study of how law and ethics affect the world of medical insurance intrigues Joy because a distant relative was involved in a medical lawsuit. For Barbara, law and ethics is a relatively foreign topic and she is curious to see how it relates to health insurance.

CHAPTER OBJECTIVES

After completion of this chapter, the student should be able to:

1. Discuss employer/employee liability.
2. List and explain the elements of a legal contract.
3. Name and briefly discuss important legislative acts affecting health insurance.
4. Compare and contrast medical ethics and medical etiquette, and explain their importance in the workplace.
5. State the basic purposes and components of a medical record.
6. Describe the issues of medical record ownership, retention, access, and release.
7. Discuss the requirements of appropriate medical record documentation.
8. List legal/ethical responsibilities of ancillary staff members.
9. Identify HIPAA's primary objectives.
10. Discuss HIPAA's impact on healthcare personnel and patients, providers, and businesses.
12. Demonstrate an understanding of privacy/ confidentiality laws.
13. List the exceptions to privacy/confidentiality laws.
14. Define and contrast fraud and abuse.
15. Analyze cause and effect of fraud and abuse in healthcare.
16. List ways to prevent fraud and abuse in the medical office.

CHAPTER TERMS

abandoning
abuse
acceptance
accountability
ancillary
binds

breach of confidentiality
competency
confidentiality
consideration
durable power of attorney
emancipated minor

ethics
etiquette
first party (party of the first part)
fraud
implied contract
implied promises
incidental disclosure
litigious
medical ethics
medical etiquette
medical (health) record

negligence
offer
portability
privacy
privacy statement
respondeat superior
second party (party of the second part)
subpoena *duces tecum*
third party

All there is to know about medical law and ethics would fill volumes of books. So as not to overwhelm you, this chapter attempts to zero in on what we think a health insurance professional should know to perform his or her job accurately and efficiently while maintaining confidentiality and sensitivity to patients' rights.

The practice of medicine is, after all, a business—not unlike an auto body shop. The auto body shop's goal is to fix cars; the medical facility's goal is to fix people. Although the medical facility may be more charitable, the bottom line of both (unless the medical facility qualifies as a nonprofit organization) is to produce revenue.

The primary goals of the health insurance professional are to complete and submit insurance claims and to conduct billing and collection procedures that enable him or her to generate as much money for the practice as legally and ethically possible that the medical record will support in the least amount of time. To do this, the health insurance professional must be knowledgeable in the area of medical law and liability.

MEDICAL LAW AND LIABILITY

Medical law and liability can vary widely from state to state; however, some rules and regulations affect medical facilities in the United States as a whole. The health insurance professional should become familiar with the medical laws and liability issues in his or her state and should follow them conscientiously. The following sections discuss various facets of medical law and liability.

Employer Liability

In our **litigious** (quick to bring lawsuits) society, people tend more and more to hold physicians to a higher standard than those in other professions, and the slightest breach of medical care can end up as a malpractice lawsuit. Often, these lawsuits are settled out of court—not because the healthcare provider was afraid he or she would be found negligent and wanted to avoid publicity, but because of cost.

⭐ Imagine This!

A well-known medical talk show host tells of a situation in which his TV crew was filming a critically ill patient in a California hospital. A woman in Texas saw the episode and, claiming that the patient was her mother who had recently died in a Texas hospital, sued. The film did not show the woman from the front, and the camera clearly showed items that accurately identified the hospital where the actual filming took place. The talk show host won the lawsuit, but it cost nearly $20,000 in court costs and legal fees to clear everything up.

Employee Liability

No matter what the employee's position is or how much education he or she has had, direct and indirect patient contact involves ethical and legal responsibility. Although we all know that professional healthcare providers have a responsibility for their own actions, what about the health insurance professional? Can he or she be a party to legal action in the event of error or omission? The answer is "yes"!

You may have heard the Latin term **respondeat superior** (*ree-spond-dee-at superior*). The English translation is "Let the master answer." *Respondeat superior* is a key principle in business law, which says that an employer is responsible for the actions of his or her employees in the "course of employment." For instance, if a truck driver for Express Delivery, Inc., hits a child in the street because of **negligence** (failure to exercise a reasonable degree of care), the company for which the driver works (Express Delivery) most likely would be liable for the injuries.

The **ancillary** members of the medical team (e.g., nurses, medical assistants, health insurance professionals, technicians) cannot avoid legal responsibility altogether. They also can be named as parties to a lawsuit. The healthcare provider usually bears the financial brunt of legal action, however, because he or she is what is referred to as the "deep pocket," or the person/corporation with the most money.

🕑 Stop and Think

Marcy Knox worked as a health insurance professional in a large medical center where there were many professional offices. One day, as she was delivering some paperwork to a psychiatrist's office on the same floor, she spotted a former teacher waiting in the reception area. At lunch, Marcy met Sherry, a former classmate. "You'll never guess who I saw in Dr. Pilova's office yesterday!" Marcy confided excitedly. Eager to share the news, Marcy didn't wait for her lunch partner to respond. "Our old instructor at Grassland Community College, Mrs. Bitterhaven!" Because Marcy was not employed by the psychiatrist's office, was she guilty of a breach of confidentiality in divulging this information to her friend?

❓ What Did You Learn?

1. What is the primary goal of the health insurance professional?
2. What does the Latin term *respondeat superior* mean?
3. List members of the healthcare team who would typically make up the "ancillary" staff.

INSURANCE AND CONTRACT LAW

Because a health insurance policy and the relationship between a healthcare provider and a patient are considered legal contracts, it is important that the health insurance professional become familiar with the basic concepts of contract law.

Elements of a Legal Contract

To understand insurance of any kind, you have to have a reasonable knowledge base of the legal framework surrounding it. In other words, you must learn some basic concepts about the law of contracts. The health insurance policy, being a legal contract, must contain certain elements to be legally binding. These elements are as follows:

1. Offer and acceptance
2. Consideration
3. Legal object
4. Competent parties
5. Legal form (written contracts only)

Let's take a closer look at each of these five contract elements and apply them to the health insurance contract. We will follow a fictitious character—Jerry Dawson, a self-employed computer consultant—through this process.

Offer and Acceptance

Jerry visits Ned Nelson of Acme Insurance Company and tells him that he wants to purchase a health insurance policy for his family. Jerry completes a lengthy application form detailing his family's medical history. Here, Jerry is making the **offer**—a proposition to create a contract with Ned's company. Ned sends the application to his home office; after verifying the information, someone at the home office might say, "This guy and his family are okay; we'll insure them." This is the **acceptance**; Acme Insurance has agreed to take on Jerry's proposition, or offer. The acceptance occurs when the insurance company **binds** (agrees to accept the individual[s] for benefits) coverage or when the policy is issued.

Consideration

Jerry receives his new insurance contract from Acme. The binding force in any contract that gives it legal status is the **consideration**—the *thing of value* that each party gives to the other. In a health insurance contract, the consideration of the insurance company lies in the promises that make up the contract (e.g., the promise to pay all or part of the insured individual's *covered medical expenses* as set forth in the contract). The promise to pay the premium is the consideration of the individual seeking health insurance coverage.

Legal Object

A contract must be *legal* before it can be enforced. If an individual contracts with another to commit murder for a specified amount of money, that contract would be unenforceable in court because its intent is not legal (murder is against the law). Are we confident that this insurance policy between Jerry, our computer expert, and Acme Insurance Company is legal? We can rest assured a contract is legal if it contains all the necessary elements and whatever is being contracted (the object) is not breaking any laws.

Competent Parties

The parties to the contractual agreement must be capable of entering into a contract in the eyes of the law. **Competency** typically enters into the picture in the case of minors (except for **emancipated minors**—individuals younger than 18 years who are independent and living away from home) and individuals who are mentally handicapped. The courts have ruled that if individuals in either of these categories enter into a contractual agreement, it is not enforceable because the individuals might not understand all of the legal ramifications involved.

Legal Form

Most states require that all types of insurance policies be filed with, and approved by, the state regulatory authorities before the policy may be sold in that state. This procedure determines whether the policy meets the legal requirements of the state and protects policyholders from unscrupulous insurance companies that might take advantage of them.

Termination of Contracts

A contract between an insurance company and the insured party can be terminated on mutual agreement or if either party defaults on the provisions in the policy. The insurance company can terminate the policy for nonpayment of premiums or fraudulent action. The insured individual usually can terminate the policy at his or her discretion.

The contract between a healthcare provider and a patient (referred to as an *implied contract,* discussed in the next section) can be terminated by either party; however, when the provider enters into this contractual relationship, he or she must render care as long as the patient needs it and follows the provider's instructions. The patient can terminate the contract simply by paying all incurred charges and not returning to the practice. The provider must have good reason to withdraw from a particular case and must follow specific guidelines in doing so. Some common reasons for a physician to stop providing care to a patient are

- the patient consistently fails to keep appointments;
- the patient's account becomes delinquent (typically 90 days) and makes no effort to arrange for payment; and
- the patient refuses to follow the physician's advice.

If it is determined that, for a specific reason, the physician desires to withdraw from a particular case, it is prudent that he or she

- notify the patient in writing of such a decision via certified mail with a return receipt to ensure the patient is aware of the decision;
- give the patient the names of other qualified healthcare providers, if the patient needs further treatment;
- explain the medical problems that need continued treatment; and
- state in writing the time (a specific date) of the termination.

It is important that these steps be followed to avoid a lawsuit for abandonment, because **abandoning** a patient—ceasing to provide care—is a breach of contract.

What Did You Learn?

1. Name and explain the necessary elements that make a contract legally binding.
2. "Competency" enters into the picture when what two categories of individuals are considered?
3. What governing bodies typically approve insurance contracts?

MEDICAL LAW AND ETHICS APPLICABLE TO HEALTH INSURANCE

Now that some of the fundamentals of contract law have been presented, we will take a brief look at basic medical law and liability as it applies to health insurance. First, it is important that the health insurance professional understand that the physician-patient relationship is a different kind of contract.

The contract (or policy) between our computer consultant and Acme Insurance was a written contract. The relationship between a healthcare provider and a patient is an **implied contract**—meaning that it is not in writing but it has all the components of a legal contract and is just as binding. You have the *offer* (the patient enters the provider's office in anticipation of receiving medical treatment) and *the acceptance* (the provider accepts by granting professional services). The *consideration* here lies in the provider's **implied promises** (promises that are neither spoken nor written but implicated by the individual's actions and performance) to render professional care to the patient to the best of his or her ability (this does not have to be in writing), and the patient's consideration is the promise to pay the provider for these services. This implied contract meets the *legal object* requirement because granting medical care and paying for it are within the limits of the law. The healthcare provider, of legal age and sound mind, and the patient (or the patient's parent or legal guardian, in the case of a minor or mentally handicapped individual) would constitute the competent parties—individuals with the necessary mental capacity or those old enough to enter into a contract. In an implied contract, however, there would be no *legal form* because it is not in writing.

> ### 🕐 Stop and Think
>
> Eleanor Stevens is a health insurance professional for Halcyon Medical Clinic. Clara Bartlett, a patient of the clinic, comes in for a physical examination. After the examination, Mrs. Bartlett approaches Eleanor and says, "Hon, my insurance company doesn't pay for doctor visits unless I'm sick or something. Dr. Forrest says I'm perfectly healthy, so I'll have to pay today's charge out of my own pocket. I'm a little short on money this month—the high cost of utilities and all—you understand, don't you? (Sigh.) I'm wondering if you could help me out just a little by fudging something on my claim so that my insurance will pay." How might Eleanor handle this situation?

You might have heard an insurance company referred to as a **third party**. In the implied contract between the physician and patient, the patient is referred to as the **party of the first part (first party)** in legal language and the healthcare provider is the **party of the second part (second party)**. Because insurance companies often are involved in this contract indirectly, they are considered the party of the third part (**third party**).

> ### 🕐 Stop and Think
>
> Ned Farnsworth takes a prescription to the local pharmacy. Ned lives in a small town where everyone knows everybody else, and he frequently plays golf with Archie, the pharmacist. After Archie fills Ned's prescription, Ned says, "Just put this on my bill, Arch. See you next Saturday on the links." Is this transaction a legally binding contract? If so, (1) what kind of a contract took place and (2) can you identify the four necessary components of this contract?

> ### 💬 What Did You Learn?
>
> 1. What is an *implied* contract?
> 2. True/False: An *implied* contract must be in writing to be enforceable.
> 3. Explain the function of a *third party* in a contract.

IMPORTANT LEGISLATION AFFECTING HEALTH INSURANCE

Several federal laws have evolved over the past few decades that regulate and act as "watchdogs" over the complicated and confusing world of health insurance.

Federal Privacy Act of 1974

The Federal Privacy Act of 1974 protects individuals by regulating when and how local, state, and federal governments and their agencies can request individuals to disclose their Social Security numbers (SSNs), and requiring that if that information is obtained, it be held as confidential by those agencies. Originally SSNs were to be used only for tax purposes; however, over the years, SSNs have been used for other things. With the growing problem of Social Security card fraud, individuals are encouraged to take steps to safeguard their SSNs. Many insurance companies formerly used SSNs for identification; however, in recent years, the trend is to use other numbering systems for identification.

Federal Omnibus Budget Reconciliation Act of 1980

The federal Omnibus Budget Reconciliation Act of 1980 (OBRA) states that Medicare is the secondary payer in the case of an automobile or liability insurance policy. If the automobile/liability insurer disallows payment because of a "Medicare primary clause" in the policy, however, Medicare becomes primary. In the event that the automobile/liability insurer makes payment after Medicare has paid, the provider (or the patient) must refund the Medicare payment.

Tax Equity and Fiscal Responsibility Act of 1982

The Tax Equity and Fiscal Responsibility Act (TEFRA) of 1982 made Medicare benefits secondary to benefits payable under employer group health plans for employees age 65 through 69 years and their spouses of the same age group.

Consolidated Omnibus Budget Reconciliation Act of 1986

The Consolidated Omnibus Budget Reconciliation Act (COBRA) of 1986 allows individuals to purchase temporary continuation of group health plan coverage if they are laid off, are fired for any reason (other than gross misconduct), or must quit because of an injury or illness. This coverage is temporary (18 months for the employee and 36 months for his or her spouse) and generally required by companies with 20 or more employees.

Federal False Claim Amendments Act of 1986

The Federal False Claim Amendments Act of 1986 expands the government's ability to control fraud and abuse in healthcare insurance. Its purpose is to amend the existing civil false claims statute to strengthen and clarify the government's ability to detect and prosecute civil fraud and to recover damages suffered by the government as a result of such fraud. The False Claims Amendments Act originally was enacted in 1863 because of reports of widespread corruption and fraud in the sale of supplies and provisions to the Union government during the Civil War.

Fraud and Abuse Act

The Fraud and Abuse Act addresses the prevention of healthcare fraud and abuse of patients eligible for Medicare and Medicaid benefits. It states that any person who knowingly and willfully breaks the law could be fined, imprisoned, or both. Penalties can result from the following:

- Using incorrect codes intentionally that result in greater payment than appropriate
- Submitting claims for a service or product that is not medically necessary
- Offering payment (or other compensation) to persuade an individual to order from a particular provider or supplier who receives Medicare or state health funds.
    Federal criminal penalties are established for individuals who
- knowingly or purposely defraud a healthcare program or
- knowingly embezzle, steal, or misapply a healthcare benefit program.

Federal Omnibus Budget Reconciliation Act of 1987

The federal Omnibus Budget Reconciliation Act of 1987 allows current or former employees or dependents younger than 65 years to become eligible for Medicare because of end-stage renal disease (ESRD). When the individual is diagnosed with ESRD and becomes eligible for Medicare, the employer-sponsored group plan is primary (pays first) for a period of up to 12 consecutive months, which begins when a regular course of dialysis is initiated or, in the case of a kidney transplant, the first month in which the individual becomes entitled to Medicare. If the individual's condition is due to a disability other than ESRD, group coverage is primary and Medicare is secondary. (This applies only if the company has at least 100 full-time employees.)

The Patient Protection and Affordable Care Act

The Patient Protection and Affordable Care Act (PPACA) is a *federal statute* that was signed into law in March 2010. This Act and the *Health Care and Education Reconciliation Act of 2010* (also signed into law in March 2010) make up the *health care reform* of 2010. The laws focus on reform of the private health insurance market, provide better coverage for those with preexisting conditions, improve prescription drug coverage in Medicare, and extend the life of the Medicare Trust fund by at least 12 years. The healthcare reform acts have also provided for a new patient's bill of rights. To learn more about this legislation and the new patient's bill of rights, visit the Evolve site.

> ### 🔎 What Did You Learn?
>
> 1. What legislation established that Medicare is the secondary payer in the case of an automobile/liability insurance policy?
> 2. For OBRA of 1987 to be applicable, how many employees must the employer have?
> 3. What is the name of the act that allows individuals the option of continuing their group coverage in case they are laid off or quit their jobs?
> 4. What did TEFRA of 1982 make Medicare benefits secondary to?

MEDICAL ETHICS AND MEDICAL ETIQUETTE

Most of us are familiar with the Oath of Hippocrates. It is a brief description of principles for physicians' conduct, which dates back to the 5th century BC. Statements in the Oath protect the rights of the patient and oblige the physician voluntarily to behave in a humane and selfless manner toward patients. Although there is no such written or recorded oath for health insurance professionals, certain codes of conduct are expected of all individuals who work in healthcare—referred to as *medical ethics* and *medical etiquette*.

Medical Ethics

The word ethics comes from the Greek word *ethos*, meaning "character." Broadly speaking, **ethics** are standards of human conduct—sometimes called "morals" (from the Latin word *mores*, meaning "customs")—of a particular group or culture. Although the terms ethics and morals often are used interchangeably, they are not exactly the same. *Morals* refer to actions, *ethics* to the reasoning behind such actions. Ethics are not the same as laws, and if a member of a particular group or culture breaches one of these principles or customs, he or she probably would not be arrested; however, the

I. A physician shall be dedicated to providing competent medical care, with compassion and respect for human dignity and rights.

II. A physician shall uphold the standards of professionalism, be honest in all professional interactions, and strive to report physicians deficient in character or competence, or engaging in fraud or deception, to appropriate entities.

III. A physician shall respect the law and also recognize a responsibility to seek changes in those requirements, which are contrary to the best interests of the patient.

IV. A physician shall respect the rights of patients, colleagues, and other health professionals, and shall safeguard patient confidences and privacy within the constraints of the law.

V. A physician shall continue to study, apply, and advance scientific knowledge, maintain a commitment to medical education, make relevant information available to patients, colleagues, and the public, obtain consultation, and use the talents of other health professionals when indicated.

VI. A physician shall, in the provision of appropriate patient care, except in emergencies, be free to choose whom to serve, with whom to associate, and the environment in which to provide medical care.

VII. A physician shall recognize a responsibility to participate in activities contributing to the improvement of the community and the betterment of public health.

VIII. A physician shall, while caring for a patient, regard responsibility to the patient as paramount.

IX. A physician shall support access to medical care for all people.

Fig. 3-1 Principles of medical ethics. (From the American Medical Association: Principles of Medical Ethics. Revised and adopted by the AMA House of Delegates, June 17, 2001. HSA:10-0390:9/10phy. www.ama-assn.org.)

group can levy a sanction (punishment) against this person, such as fines, suspension, or even expulsion from the group.

Ethics is a code of conduct of a particular group of people or culture. **Medical ethics** is the code of conduct for the healthcare profession. The American Medical Association (AMA) has long supported certain principles of medical ethics developed primarily for the benefit of patients. These are not laws but socially acceptable principles of conduct, which define the essentials of honorable behavior for healthcare providers. Fig. 3-1 provides a list of professional ethics from the AMA website.

The field of medical ethics is a current area of concern for practitioners and consumers. From the time an individual is conceived until death, there are ethical questions regarding healthcare at every juncture, such as:

- abortion,
- experimentation,
- prolongation of life,
- quality of life, and
- euthanasia.

It is often difficult to distinguish between absolute right and wrong in controversial medical issues. Although laws are universal rules to be observed by everyone, different cultures follow different moral and ethical codes. Who is to say whether or not these codes are right or wrong? It is sufficient to state here that it is important that all healthcare professionals follow the established standards of conduct issued by these professional organizations to guide their future course of action.

⭐ Imagine This!

Marian Grube worked in the spinal and brain injuries ward at Blessing Memorial Hospital. Often, she would relate the sad story of patients who lay there in a vegetative state, dying by inches, to close friends and family members. One such patient was a young man who had been severely injured as a result of a motorcycle accident. As a result of her experiences, Marian became an advocate for wearing helmets while riding motorcycles and bicycles. Once, during a public speaking engagement, she referred to this particular patient not by name, but by condition, using him as an example to drive her point home. The patient's family members complained, and Marian lost her job.

🕐 Stop and Think

In our scenario with Ned and Archie, identify the party of the first part and the party of the second part. Would there likely be a "third party" involved in this transaction; if so, who would it be?

Medical Etiquette

The word "etiquette" is derived from a mid-18th century French word for "ticket," likely from the custom of giving rules for behavior on a soldier's lodging ticket or on cards given out at the royal court. Although etiquette and ethics are closely related, there is a difference in their meaning. **Etiquette** consists of the rules and conventions governing correct or polite behavior in society in general or in a particular social or professional group or situation. In our society, etiquette dictates that we do not belch at the table. In the medical office, good etiquette is reflected in how the medical receptionist answers the telephone and greets patients. The health insurance professional can perform his or her duties well within the limits of medical ethics, but this does not mean that it is done so in a mannerly way. If the patient completes the information form incorrectly, causing a delay or rejection in the claim, the healthcare professional can resolve the situation in an ethical manner, but if he or she was rude or impatient with the patient in doing so, a breach of **medical etiquette** has occurred.

Ethics and etiquette are constantly evolving. What is acceptable behavior today might not have been okay 20, or even 10, years ago. In today's healthcare environment, patients are considered "customers," and they should be treated with respect and courtesy.

MEDICAL RECORD

The medical record (or health record) is an account of a patient's medical assessment, investigation, and course of treatment. It is a source of information and one component in the quality of patient care. The medical record is a chronological listing of medical-related facts regarding dates of an individual's injuries and illnesses; dates of treatment; and all notes, diagnostic test results, correspondence, and any other pertinent information regarding the medical care and treatment of the patient.

Purposes of a Medical Record

The medical record serves several important functions:
- It enables the healthcare provider to render medical care to the best of his or her ability.
- It provides statistical information for research.
- It offers legal protection for the healthcare team.
- It provides support for third-party reimbursement.

Complete Medical Record

The Joint Commission (not-for-profit organization that accredits healthcare programs in the U.S.) emphasizes four factors that improve the quality and usefulness of medical records, as follows:
- *Timeliness* (Entries, such as history and physical exam, must be made and updated as necessary within 24 hours of the encounter.)
- *Completeness* (documentation of patient problems and concerns, diagnostic tests performed and their results, diagnosis, treatment or recommended treatment, and prognosis)
- *Accuracy*
- *Confidentiality*

Typical components of a medical record include the following:
- Demographic information (patient information form, including insurance information)
- Current release of information form (signed and dated)
- Drug or other allergy flags
- Medical/health history
- Physical examination
- Chronological chart (progress) notes for all subsequent visits

- Medication sheet showing all prescriptions and over-the-counter drugs
- Results of diagnostic tests (x-rays, laboratory tests, electrocardiograms)
- Hospital records (if applicable)
- Correspondence

Who Owns Medical Records?

There is still some controversy regarding who actually owns the medical record. It has become an accepted opinion, however, that even though medical records contain a patient's personal and confidential information, medical records are the property of the physician providing the care or the corporate entity where the provider is employed. The information contained in the record is technically the patient's, however, because it cannot be divulged to anyone without the patient's written consent.

Retention of Medical Records

It is important that a medical facility have a policy regarding the retention of medical records. According to the AMA, physicians have an obligation to retain patient records that may reasonably be of value to a patient and that may offer guidelines to assist physicians in meeting their ethical and legal obligations to good patient care.

Statutes of limitation and other federal or state regulations may affect time requirements for retaining medical records. Other factors that affect record retention include
- expansion rate of records in the practice,
- space available for storage,
- volume of postactive uses, and
- costs of alternatives.

How long medical records are kept and how they are stored or disposed of vary from practice to practice and state to state. The records of any patient covered by Medicare (Title XVIII) should be kept for 5 years. Medicaid (Title XIX) and Maternal and Child Health (Title V) records should be kept for at least 6 years.

⭐ Imagine This!

Indiana law states that a provider must maintain health records for at least 7 years. A minor younger than 6 years of age has until the minor's eighth birthday to file a claim, however. It is advisable to retain the medical records of a minor younger than age 6 for longer than 7 years.

Some medical facilities go through medical records periodically and pull those that have had no activity for a certain number of years. Often these records are put into storage in another part of the office building. Sometimes the contents are microfilmed, and the actual physical records are destroyed. In all cases, medical records should be kept for at least as long as the length of time of the statute of limitations for medical malpractice claims. The statute of limitations is typically 3 or more years, depending on the state law. State medical associations and insurance carriers are the best resources for this information.

📁 HIPAA Tip

Every medical office should establish a policy for retention, storage, and disposal of old or inactive records. The health insurance professional should become familiar with the laws in his or her state that deal with retention of medical records and adhere to them. Check with the medical licensing board or medical society in your state for this information.

Access to Medical Records

As governed by The Joint Commission, access to medical records within an institution or practice is limited to situations involving the following:
1. Treatment
2. Quality assurance
3. Utilization review
4. Education
5. Research

Releasing Medical Record Information

Under no circumstances should any information from a patient's medical record (or from other sources) be divulged to any third party (including the patient's insurance carrier) without the *written* consent of the patient (parent or guardian in the case of a minor or mentally handicapped adult). Often, there is a place on the patient information form where the patient can sign to release information necessary to complete the insurance claim form so that his or her

insurance company can be billed; however, the HIPAA rules allow billing of third party insurers without patients' written authorization. This is referred to as "third party only" (TPO) billing. It is a good idea to advise the patient to specify the name of the insurer on the form. For information to be released to any other third party, a separate release of information should be used. Fig. 3-2 shows a typical information release form that can be used for a range of reasons.

🕐 Stop and Think

Ellen Porter walks out of an examination room and overhears a physician talking to a patient about treatment as they exit from the adjacent room. Is this a violation of the privacy law?

🕐 Stop and Think

A patient, waiting at the pharmacy pick-up counter, overhears a pharmacist talking to another patient about her prescription. Is this a violation of HIPAA privacy standards?

🕐 Stop and Think

Dr. Wallace, a long-time family practitioner, decided to retire and sell his practice to another, younger physician. Among the assets were all the medical records of Dr. Wallace's former patients accumulated over the years, which he sold to the new physician for $5 each. Was this sale legal without the patients' consent?

💬 What Did You Learn?

1. List four purposes of a medical record.
2. According to The Joint Commission, what are the four factors that improve the quality and usefulness of medical records?
3. What items should be included in a medical record?
4. Who owns medical records?
5. Why is a retention policy important?

DOCUMENTATION OF PATIENT MEDICAL RECORD

A **medical (health) record** is a clinical, scientific, administrative, and legal document of facts containing statements relating to a patient. It incorporates scientific data and

MEDICAL RECORD	Authorization for the Release of Medical Information

INSTRUCTIONS: Complete this form in its entirety and forward the original to the address below:

NATIONAL INSTITUTES OF HEALTH
MEDICAL RECORD DEPARTMENT
ATTN: MEDICOLEGAL SECTION
10 CENTER DRIVE, ROOM 1N208   TELEPHONE: (301) 496-3331
MSC1192   FACSIMILE: (301) 480-9982
BETHESDA, MD 20892-1192

IDENTIFYING INFORMATION:

Patient Name	Daytime Telephone	Date of Birth

REQUEST INFORMATION: Information is to be released to the following individual or party:

Name	Telephone
Address	

The purpose or need for disclosure (charges will be determined based on purpose of disclosure):

_____

Date Range of Information to be Released: from _____ to _____

Please check specific information to be released:

☐ Discharge Summary   ☐ Radiology Reports   ☐ EKG Reports
☐ History & Physical   ☐ Radiology Films   ☐ Echocardiogram Reports
☐ Operative Reports   ☐ Tissue Exam Reports   ☐ Heart Diagnostic Reports
☐ Outpatient Progress Notes ☐ Tissue Slides   ☐ Nuclear Medicine Reports
☐ Length of Stay Verification ☐ Lab Results   ☐ Nuclear Medicine Scans

☐ Other (Please Specify): _____

_____

AUTHORIZATION: Permission is hereby granted to the Warren Grant Magnuson Clinical Center to release medical information to the individual/organization as identified above.
(Note: submission of this form authorizes the release of the information specified within one year from date of signature.)

Patient/Authorized Signature	Print Name	Date

If other than patient, specify relationship: _____

Patient Identification	Authorization for the Release of Medical Information NIH-527 (02-01) P.A. 09-25-0099 File in Section 4: Correspondence

Fig. 3-2 National Institutes of Health (NIH) release of information authorization form.

sprained left ankle FA 12/27/12

12/23/2012   Rachel is seen again in the office today for follow up of her ~~sprained right ankle~~. She is able to put some weight on it, and swelling has subsided. Gradually increase activity. Continue ibuprofen for pain as needed. Recheck in two weeks. (s) Frances Akers, MD

Fig. 3-3 Example of a properly corrected chart entry.

scientific events in chronological order regarding the case history, clinical examination, investigative procedures, diagnosis, treatment, and the response to the treatment. Health records are extremely valuable, not only to healthcare providers and the scientific community, but also to patients and third-party carriers. Properly documented health records expand knowledge and improve the standard of medical care.

Health records are kept for two basic purposes:

1. They document the interaction between the healthcare provider and the patient so that a permanent record of what was said and done exists.
2. They show the ongoing process of patient care.

A health record must be accurate in every detail. It should be identifiable, it should be detailed, and it should be stored in a safe place. A health record is considered privileged communication, and any information in it should not be disclosed without written consent of the patient except if required by law. Records are the property of the healthcare provider and should be preserved for as long as the state's statutes require, typically at least 5 years (10 years in legal cases).

It is important that all members of the healthcare team know the correct methods for maintaining health records. Timely, accurate, and complete documentation is crucial to patient care. Thorough and accurate documentation

- facilitates claims review and payment,
- assists in utilization review and quality-of-care evaluations,
- provides clinical data for research and education, and
- serves as a legal document to be used as verification that care was provided.

Every medical facility should have a policy in place to ensure that health record entries are accurately documented and signed in a timely manner. If additional information needs to be added to the record, it should be in the form of an appropriate addendum that has been prepared in accordance with this policy. Fig. 3-3 shows the correct method of correcting an erroneous health record entry.

The physician does not always perform all patient record documentation. Some medical practices assign the task of documenting the chief complaint (CC) and history of present illness (HPI) to ancillary staff members. In such cases, it is important that the staff member understands the process of evaluation and management coding. Adequate and complete documentation helps establish medical necessity for the visit and the level of service, which justify the fee charged.

In addition to charting the CC and HPI, documentation that the ancillary medical staff might be responsible for includes the following:

- Patient contact, such as office visits and telephone calls
- Routine vital signs: blood pressure, pulse, respirations, weight, and height
- Applicable patient education—verbal instructions and written materials
- Communication or follow-up (either by phone or in writing) to patients who have failed to keep appointments, referrals, or scheduled tests
- Prescription refills authorized by the healthcare provider (some states require the physician's initials in the chart for every prescription refill)

The medical staff also should verify that all laboratory and diagnostic test results are read and signed by the healthcare provider and filed in the patient's chart in a timely manner. (The Office of the Inspector General [OIG] interprets "timely" as 24 hours.)

Appropriate documentation serves as the basis for the defense of malpractice claims and lawsuits (Fig. 3-4). Many insurance carriers now conduct record reviews in an effort to ensure proper documentation of services billed. Lack of proper documentation could result in reduced or denied claim payments. A common saying among healthcare professionals is "If it isn't documented, it didn't happen."

1. All medical record entries should be complete, accurate, and legible and contain the date of when the entry was made.
2. Only authorized individuals will make entries into medical records.
3. Entries should be made using a black ink (not felt tip) pen.
4. The author of every medical record entry shall be identified in the entry, and all clinical entries shall be individually authenticated by the responsible practitioner. Other entries will be authenticated as specified by medical staff bylaws or as required by state or federal law or regulation.
5. All authorized individuals who make entries into medical records will make every effort to create such entries in accordance with this policy, applicable medical staff bylaw provisions, and all applicable state and federal laws, regulations, and guidelines. Any questions concerning creation of medical record entries should be directed to appropriate personnel for clarification.
6. All final diagnoses and complications should be recorded without the use of symbols or abbreviations.
7. Only the abbreviations, signs, and symbols approved by the medical staff shall be used in medical records.

Fig. 3-4 Principles of documentation.

HEALTH INSURANCE PORTABILITY AND ACCOUNTABILITY ACT AND COMPLIANCE

The Health Insurance Portability and Accountability Act (HIPAA) was signed into law in 1996 by the Clinton Administration and congressional healthcare reform leaders. This act has four primary objectives:

1. To ensure health insurance portability
2. To reduce healthcare fraud and abuse
3. To enforce standards for health information
4. To guarantee security and privacy of health information for patients

Let's break this first objective down so that we can understand it better. The word **portability** means people with preexisting medical conditions cannot be denied health insurance coverage when moving from one employer-sponsored group healthcare plan to another. This law also helps individuals who need to switch health insurance companies in the event of job termination, job relocation, or quitting a job. Basically, HIPAA states that no one should be denied healthcare coverage. Accountability refers to the responsibility the healthcare profession has to others, specifically to patients, so that a feeling of confidence exists between patient and provider. **Accountability** applies more to patient rights, the billing process, and other aspects of the medical office.

Fig. 3-5 shows a flow chart illustrating who must comply with HIPAA standards. The series of easy "yes" and "no" questions is designed to be a simple test to help providers determine whether or not they must comply with the privacy, security, transactions, and other related standards of HIPAA.

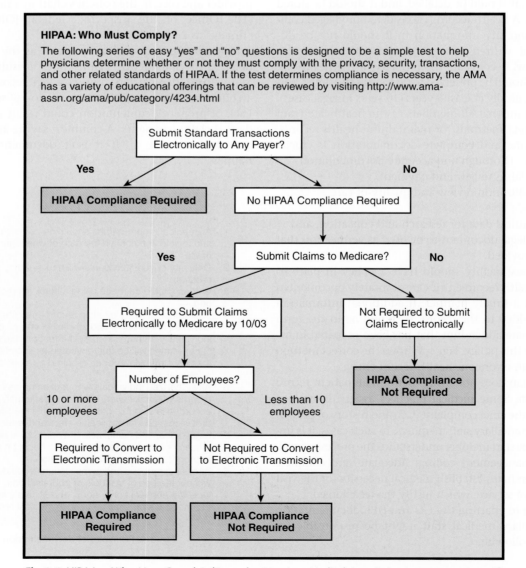

HIPAA: Who Must Comply?

The following series of easy "yes" and "no" questions is designed to be a simple test to help physicians determine whether or not they must comply with the privacy, security, transactions, and other related standards of HIPAA. If the test determines compliance is necessary, the AMA has a variety of educational offerings that can be reviewed by visiting http://www.ama-assn.org/ama/pub/category/4234.html

Fig. 3-5 HIPAA – Who Must Comply? (From the American Medical Association, www.ama-assn.org/.)

Impact of Health Insurance Portability and Accountability Act

HIPAA's regulations affect more than just the healthcare provider and his or her patients. The impact is felt across the board in professional, business, and private worlds. The following paragraphs discuss some of the more pertinent areas.

Impact on the Health Insurance Professional

Health insurance professionals who work in an office with more than 10 employees are likely to submit insurance claims to major government payers (Medicare and Medicaid) using a standardized electronic format, simplifying and creating efficiency via HIPAA's "Electronic Health Transactions Standards." These standards affect health insurance claims processing, health plan eligibility, payments, and other related transactions. The idea behind these standards is to make processing these records more efficient, more accurate, and less costly. In the past, most health, financial, and insurance records in medical offices were paper documents. Because more and more records are becoming computerized, concern has been raised regarding patient privacy and how it will be maintained in electronic media. It is crucial that a serious effort be made to engage providers and consumers in keeping personal health information private. As a result, health insurance professionals have become involved in setting up privacy standards. Patients now have the ability to view their medical records and to be informed about who else has viewed them and why. For this reason, the "Standards for Privacy"—a set of specific rules to ensure confidentiality—should be considered.

Because HIPAA imposes specific responsibilities on everyone who works in the healthcare field, major changes were required for medical institutions to become HIPAA compliant. Changes were needed on all levels—management of information, patient records, patient care, security, and coding. The health insurance professional must be aware of what these requirements are and why they are necessary. Examples include, but are not limited to, the following:

- Arranging patient charts in the receptacle outside the examination room door in such a way that patient names are not visible
- Locking the physician's office door when confidential laboratory reports and other documents are placed on his or her desk for review
- Closing the window separating the reception area from the waiting room when not in use
- Positioning computer screens so that someone standing at the reception desk cannot view them
- Changing computer security passwords routinely
- Avoiding transfer of confidential information via fax or electronic methods to unsecured locations, such as schools, hotel lobbies, and businesses

Fig. 3-6 illustrates "How to HIPAA," a list of the top 10 tips offered by the AMA website.

1. Understand the deadlines and move to compliance.
2. Know your compliance requirements.
3. Prioritize your compliance activities.
4. Ask the right questions.
5. Choose and use consultants wisely.
6. Learn from trusted sources.
7. Separate fact from fiction.
8. Visit website resources often for the latest updates.
9. Talk to your patients.
10. Look to the AMA for updates.

Fig. 3-6 How to HIPAA – Top 10 Tips. (From the American Medical Association, www.ama-assn.org/go/hipaa/.)

📁 HIPAA Tip

Healthcare providers are not required to monitor actively the means by which a business associate carries out the safeguards of the contract.

Impact on Patients

When patients see their healthcare providers, they are given a **privacy statement** at each location they visit. Patients are asked to read it, ask necessary questions for clarification, and sign the statement. Beyond that, there is little obvious evidence of any change from the patient's standpoint. Patients typically view the statement from both ends of the spectrum. On one end, a patient considers it as just one more piece of paper to sign, glances at it, and likely throws it away. On the other end, a patient reads it word for word, questions areas he or she is not clear on, and files it carefully away for future reference.

The statement includes not only information about who the physician or pharmacy shares health information with and why but also what rights patients have to access their own health information. The only real change brought about by HIPAA is in presentation. Patients were able to do all those things before HIPAA came into effect, but it was not brought to their attention in this manner and in printed form. Many patients view the principles behind HIPAA as good, in some cases, but think the implementation of those principles goes too far. For one thing, the statement tends to be wordy and can be difficult for some people to understand, especially the elderly.

Another way HIPAA has changed patient routines in many offices is that when patients sign in at the reception desk, they may no longer see a clipboard with the names of people who have signed in before them (commonly referred to as the "community sign-in sheet"). There are no privacy precautions in the reception room, however, if two patients happen to know each other. In most offices, medical personnel still continue to call the patient by name. That kind of exposure is called **incidental disclosure**, which is specifically allowed under HIPAA.

Stop and Think

You receive a phone call from Abner L. Smith, a local attorney. He is representing Patricia Lane, a patient of your practice, who was recently involved in a rear-end auto collision. Mr. Smith wants to know the results of Ms. Lane's recent MRI of her neck because it is important to the case. He tells you that Ms. Lane is sitting in his office and says it's okay for you to give him this information. What should you do?

In the long run, HIPAA regulations benefit patients by ensuring that their medical information is not accessible by anyone who is not entitled to view it. They also benefit patients by ensuring confidentiality.

Stop and Think

Sally Sergeant is seen in the physician's office for confirmation of a suspected pregnancy. After Sally left, her husband phones and inquires as to the results of the examination. Can any member of the medical staff give Sally's husband these results?

Impact on Providers

Providers are required to have business associate agreements with every company they exchange patient information with, including insurance companies, attorneys, financial institutions, and other providers. The idea behind these agreements is to reassure providers that the people they do business with are also complying with HIPAA regulations.

Providers no doubt feel HIPAA's impact mostly in their checkbook. Before the implementation of the HIPAA laws, it was estimated that the cost to bring medical facilities into compliance would be more than $66 billion. Further estimates indicate it is costing each physician practice $10,000 to $250,000, depending on the size of the practice, and the costs to hospitals are substantially greater.

HIPAA Tip

Employers should determine what type of computer security, such as a device that blocks unauthorized access, needs to be put into place for risk management purposes to ensure that health information is not used in the employment process.

Impact on Private Businesses

Businesses have the same obligation to protect medical records as government, medical, and human resource officials. Businesses need to ensure there is uniformity in application of HIPAA requirements. Employees typically receive a letter notifying them of any changes stemming from HIPAA. One of the most significant changes is that health records must now be kept separate from routine personnel records. Some companies were already doing that. Although the average worker might not have felt the effects of the HIPAA privacy requirements on the job, he or she no doubt felt them indirectly in the wallets.

HIPAA Tip

Health insurance professionals need to know how to apply for new provider identification numbers for physicians and other healthcare providers. Health insurance professionals also might be in charge of security measures for computers, which include virus protection, password maintenance, and ensuring that confidential information stays secure.

What Did You Learn?

1. Name the four primary objectives of HIPAA.
2. How does HIPAA affect claims submission and processing?
3. Define *incidental disclosure*.
4. How does HIPAA benefit patients?

Enforcement of Confidentiality Regulations of Health Insurance Portability and Accountability Act

One of the primary purposes of HIPAA is continuity of health insurance coverage if an individual changes jobs, but it also provides for standards for health information transactions and confidentiality and security of patient data. This confidentiality portion has had a considerable impact on the day-to-day workflow among medical institutions. HIPAA is complaint driven, however. If no one complains, there probably would not be an investigation. If a deliberate violation of the regulations were found, action would be taken. The Office of Civil Rights enforces the HIPAA regulations, and there are civil penalties of $100 per violation up to $25,000 per year. Criminal penalties are also possible, including $50,000 or a year in prison or both for wrongful disclosure or $250,000 or 10 years in prison or both for the intent to sell information. For more information about HIPAA, go to the website listed at the end of this chapter or type "HIPAA" into your search engine.

Developing a Compliance Plan

A written compliance plan can help protect a medical practice and can be the best defense against trouble. Compliance programs are a significant tool in reducing the potential for healthcare fraud and abuse; however, they must be adapted and implemented appropriately to be effective. The OIG recommends that the medical facility review its existing standards and procedures to determine whether it is in compliance with HIPAA laws and regulations using the following seven steps:

Step 1: Conduct internal auditing and monitoring.

Step 2: Establish standards and procedures.

Step 3: Designate a compliance officer/contact person.

Step 4: Conduct appropriate training and education.

Step 5: Respond to detected offenses and develop corrective action initiatives.

Step 6: Develop open lines of communication.

Step 7: Enforce disciplinary standards through well-publicized guidelines.

> ### ? What Did You Learn?
>
> 1. What is the best defense against committing violations against HIPAA guidelines?
> 2. What entity recommends that all medical facilities review standards and procedures to determine whether they are in compliance?
> 3. State the steps that are specifically important in developing and maintaining a compliance program.

CONFIDENTIALITY AND PRIVACY

The words "confidentiality" and "privacy" are sometimes used interchangeably, but there is a distinction between the two. **Privacy** "denotes a zone of inaccessibility" of mind or body, the right to be left alone and to maintain individual autonomy, solitude, intimacy, and control over information about oneself. **Confidentiality** "concerns the communication of private and personal information from one person to another." The key ingredients of confidentiality are trust and loyalty. Professionals rely on the promise of confidentiality to inspire trust in their clients and patients. In the case of healthcare providers, lawyers, and clergy, communications are legally designated "privileged." The following paragraphs examine these two terms separately as they affect healthcare.

Confidentiality

Confidentiality is the foundation for trust in the patient-provider relationship. Physicians have always had an ethical duty to keep their patients' confidences. Even before HIPAA came into being, the AMA's *Code of Medical Ethics* stated that the information disclosed to a physician during the course of the patient-physician relationship or discovered in connection with the treatment of a patient is strictly confidential. The basic reason for this is so that the patient feels comfortable to disclose, fully and frankly, any and all information to the provider. This full disclosure enables the physician to diagnose conditions more effectively and to treat the patient appropriately.

All healthcare organizations and providers must guarantee confidentiality and privacy of the healthcare information they collect, maintain, use, or transmit. Confidentiality means that only certain individuals will have the right to access the information and that it is secure from others. Confidentiality is at risk when the potential for improper access to information exists.

This obligation of confidentiality extends to health insurance professionals. Each member of the healthcare team has a responsibility to uphold confidentiality for patients. In a busy medical office setting or clinic, maintaining confidentiality might be difficult. Voices carry from the reception work area to waiting patients in chairs and through thin walls of examination rooms. Elevator or cafeteria discussions of Mrs. Brown's cancer or Mr. Lewis's heart attack are common, and this careless practice is prohibited. The person next to you could be a patient's friend, or relative, or someone else who is not entitled to this privileged information. Permission must be received from the patient before *any* disclosure.

Any information the health insurance professional learns while caring for a patient or performing administrative duties, such as completing insurance claims, must remain strictly confidential unless the professional is authorized in writing by the patient or ordered by law to reveal it. Section 164.506 of the HIPAA privacy regulations permits release of information for treatment, payment, or healthcare operation purposes *without a specific patient authorization*. However, most healthcare facilities believe it is good practice to have the patient's written authorization to release information necessary to process an insurance claim or to complete a treatment report for precertification, and there may be circumstances when authorization is required.

Privacy

As mentioned previously, privacy is different from confidentiality. It refers to an individual's right to keep some information to himself or herself and to have it used only with his or her approval. The American public's privacy concerns are of more recent origin, dating back to events in the 1960s and early 1970s that led to the Privacy Act of 1974.

Under HIPAA, physicians must use and disclose only the minimum amount of patient information needed for the purpose in question. Patients can request a copy of their medical records and can request amendments to incorrect records. Additionally, patients must receive notification of their privacy rights.

Security

HIPAA also requires administrative procedures for guarding data confidentiality, integrity, and availability with formal procedures for implementation. Physical safeguards are required and include the following:

- Maintaining a system for keeping and storing critical data safe, such as locked, fireproof file cabinets

- Reporting and responding to any attempts to "hack" into the system
- Assessing the security risks of the system
- Developing a contingency plan for data backup and disaster recovery
- Training in security awareness
- Ensuring that the data are secure by monitoring access and protecting the use of passwords or other methods used to ensure security

Exceptions to Confidentiality

Certain situations and classes of patients do not come under the umbrella of confidentiality. Additionally, certain medical information by law must be reported to state and local governments, where it is maintained in databases for research and public safety. Exceptions to confidentiality include, but are not limited to, the following:

- Treatment of minors
- Human immunodeficiency virus (HIV)–positive patients and health care workers
- Abuse of a child (or, in most states, an adult)
- Injuries caused by firearms or other weapons
- Communicable diseases
- Billing third-party-only (TPO) insurance

> ### ⭐ Imagine This!
>
> A California psychologist requested that University of California campus police arrest a patient of his who he believed was going to kill a woman. The patient was arrested but subsequently released after assuring the police that he would stay away from the woman. The woman was never notified of the impending danger, and the patient killed her 2 months later (*Tarasoff vs. Regents of the University of California*).

Some states allow disclosure of the following types of mental health information without patient consent to
- other treatment providers,
- healthcare services payers or other sources of financial assistance to the patient,
- third parties that the mental health professional feels might be endangered by the patient,
- researchers,
- agencies charged with oversight of the healthcare system or the system's practitioners,
- families under certain circumstances,
- law enforcement officials under certain circumstances, and
- public health officials.

Authorization to Release Information

We discussed earlier in this chapter the importance of obtaining a signed release of information before any information is divulged to any third party, including the patient's insurance carrier. Most states agree on the typical elements of a valid general release of information, which are as follows:

- Patient's name and identifying information
- Address of the healthcare professional or institution directed to release the information
- Description of the information to be released
- Identity of the party to be furnished the information
- Language authorizing release of information
- Signature of patient or authorized individual
- Time period for which the release remains valid

Failure to obtain an appropriate release for disclosing medical records information to a third party can result in serious consequences. Twenty-one states punish disclosure of confidential information by revoking a physician's medical license or taking other serious disciplinary action.

Exceptions for Signed Released of Information for Insurance Claims Submission

In a few situations, a signed release of information is not always required, as discussed in the following paragraphs.

Medicaid-Eligible Patients and Workers' Compensation Cases

When completing an insurance claim form for a Medicaid recipient or a patient being treated as a result of an on-the-job illness or injury (workers' compensation), a written release of information is not usually required. The reason is that the contract in these cases is actually between the healthcare provider and the government agency sponsoring that specific program, and the patient is the third party. In both cases, however, the patient cannot be billed for medical procedures or services, unless it is determined that he or she is ineligible for benefits for those particular dates of service. More information is given on Medicaid and workers' compensation in later chapters.

Inpatient-Only Treatment

Another group of patients for which the normally required signed release of information for filing insurance claims is waived comprises those who are seen in the hospital but do not come to the office for follow-up care. It is considered that the release of information signed by the patient for hospital services also covers the physician's services, and the health insurance professional can simply insert the phrase "Signature on file" in block 12 of the CMS-1500 claim form. An example would be when the healthcare provider sees a patient only for consultation purposes.

Court Order

If a patient's record is subpoenaed by a court of law as evidence in a lawsuit, it may be released to the court without the patient's approval. A **subpoena duces tecum** is a legal document that requires an individual to appear in court with a piece of evidence that can be used or inspected by the court. The judge determines whether the evidence is relevant to the controversy or issues that must be resolved between the parties of the lawsuit.

Breach of Confidentiality

When confidential information is disclosed to a third party without patient consent or court order, a **breach of confidentiality** has occurred. The disclosure violation can be oral or written, made by telephone, faxed, or transmitted electronically. As mentioned earlier, the release of private health information in a patient's medical record to third parties is allowed only if the patient has consented, in writing, to such disclosure. This rule includes the following categories of individuals:

- Attorneys
- Clergy
- Insurance companies
- Relatives (except when a relative has a **durable power of attorney**, meaning he or she has been named as an agent to handle the individual's affairs if the patient becomes incapacitated)
- Employers (except in the case of workers' compensation cases)
- All other third parties

State law governs who can give permission to release medical record information. Usually, the authority to release medical information is granted to

- the patient, if he or she is a competent adult or emancipated minor;
- a legal guardian or parent, if the patient is a minor child or is incompetent;
- an individual to whom the patient has granted power of attorney possessing legal authority to act for the patient in legal and business matters to make such decisions; or
- the administrator or executor of the patient's estate if the patient is deceased.

🕐 Stop and Think

Dr. Smithers, another provider in the same clinic, is seeing Ms. Sergeant (see previous Stop and Think box) for severe acne and needs information to prescribe certain medication. Can this information be provided to Dr. Smithers without Ms. Sergeant's signing a release of information?

❓ What Did You Learn?

1. What is the term for the foundation for trust in the patient-provider relationship?
2. Define *confidentiality*.
3. Whose responsibility is it to uphold patient confidentiality?
4. List the exceptions to confidentiality.
5. Before divulging confidential patient information to any third party, what must the health insurance professional do?

HEALTHCARE FRAUD AND ABUSE

Stories about the growing incidence of healthcare fraud and abuse can be found in newspapers and on television. Fraud and abuse in healthcare are widespread and costly to the U.S. healthcare system. Federal investigations have identified fraud and abuse in all areas of healthcare, including physicians' offices and clinics, hospitals, clinical laboratories, durable medical equipment suppliers, hospices, and home health agencies. Medicare and Medicaid scams cost taxpayers more than $60 billion a year. More recent legislation has enhanced enforcement capabilities, and even more government enforcement activity is expected in the future. Because physicians and members of their healthcare teams are not immune to such government actions, they (and others involved in providing patient care) need to know how to comply with the federal laws to guard against potential liability in fraud enforcement actions.

Defining Fraud and Abuse

Fraud can be defined any number of ways. The National Healthcare Anti-Fraud Association (NHCAA) defines fraud as an intentional deception or misrepresentation that the individual or entity makes, knowing that the misrepresentation could result in some unauthorized benefit to the individual, or the entity, or to another party.

Examples of health insurance fraud include billing for services that were not rendered and falsifying a patient's diagnosis to justify tests, surgery, or other procedures that are not medically necessary.

Abuse, although similar to fraud, is considered less serious when applied to healthcare. Abuse can be defined as improper or harmful procedures or methods of doing business that are contradictory to accepted business practices. Often, it is impossible to establish that the abusive acts were done with intent to deceive the insurance carrier.

Examples of health insurance abuse include charging for services that were not medically necessary, do not conform to recognized standards, or are unfairly priced. Another example of abuse is performing a laboratory test on large numbers of patients when only a few patients should have had the test.

Although no exact dollar amount can be determined, some authorities contend that health insurance fraud and abuse constitute a $100 billion/year problem. The U.S. General Accounting Office (GAO) estimates that $1 out of every $7 spent on Medicare is lost to fraud and abuse and that, in 1 year, Medicare typically loses nearly $12 billion to fraudulent or unnecessary claims. Private insurers estimate the dollar amount lost to health insurance fraud and abuse to be 3% to 5% of total healthcare dollars spent. When the annual U.S. healthcare expenditure totals $1 trillion, the amount lost to fraud and abuse translates to an estimated annual loss of $30 to $50 billion.

Who Commits Healthcare Insurance Fraud?

Just about anyone can commit health insurance fraud—physicians, hospitals, medical suppliers, pharmacies, nursing homes—the list goes on and on. Dishonest healthcare providers are not the only ones who commit fraud. Patients and insured individuals also commit health insurance fraud and abuse. Most healthcare providers, however, are caring, honest, and ethical professionals.

How is Healthcare Fraud Committed?

The most popular schemes for committing healthcare fraud include the following:
- Billing for services, procedures, and supplies that were not provided to the patient
  Example: Billing for a diagnostic test that was not performed
- Upcoding—billing for a more expensive service or procedure than what was provided
  Example: Charging for a comprehensive office visit when a shorter, routine visit occurred
- Unbundling of charges or code fragmentation—billing services separately that are usually included in a single service fee
  Example: Making separate charges for each component of a total abdominal hysterectomy; this operation typically has one code, which includes preoperative and postoperative procedures and a lesser fee than coding each component separately
- Misrepresenting services—misrepresenting or falsifying the diagnosis to obtain insurance payment on something that is not covered
  Example: Using a diagnosis of benign cataracts for a routine eye examination with refraction because many insurance policies do not cover this procedure

How Do Consumers Commit Healthcare Insurance Fraud?

The patient can agree or encourage the provider to inflate or misrepresent the services provided. An example is a patient who is seeing a psychiatrist who charges $150 for 1 hour of therapy. The patient, whose policy only covers 50% of psychotherapy charges, suggests that the therapy session be coded for 1½ or 2 hours so that the insurer pays more of the charges. Other methods consumers use to commit fraud are creating fake receipts and claims and modifying an actual receipt to gain more claim dollars.

Preventing Fraud and Abuse

As a health insurance professional, you can do your part to prevent fraud and abuse in the medical office. The following are some general principles to follow:
- Create a file for every major third-party payer your office deals with, and keep current providers' manuals, claims completion guidelines, and publications up to date to aid you in generating timely and accurate claims.
- Develop a list of "hot" phone numbers of these carriers to use when questions arise.
- Use the most current coding manuals, and code to the greatest specificity.
- Take advantage of every opportunity to improve your coding skills by attending seminars, continuing education, or both.
- Discuss questions or potential problems regarding diagnoses, procedures and services, and fees charged with the physician or other healthcare provider.
- Notify your superior immediately if you suspect fraud or abuse.

SUMMARY CHECKPOINTS

▶ The health insurance professional should have a basic knowledge of medical law and ethics to aid in accurate claims completion and submission and conduct himself or herself appropriately in and out of the medical facility.

▶ The elements necessary to constitute a legal contract are
  - offer and acceptance,
  - consideration,
  - legal object,
  - competent parties, and
  - legal form (written contracts only).

▶ The relationship between patient and healthcare provider is an implied contract, meaning it is not in writing, but it is just as legally binding in the eyes of the law.

▶ The federal laws that regulate health insurance include the following:

- Federal Privacy Act of 1974
- OBRA (1980)
- TEFRA (1982)
- COBRA (1986)
- Federal False Claim Amendments Act of 1986
- Fraud and Abuse Act
- OBRA (1987)
- The Patient Protection and Affordable Care Act
- New Patient's Bill of Rights

▶ Displaying proper medical ethics and etiquette in the workplace is important for the protection and well-being of the patients and the entire healthcare team. In today's complicated healthcare world, experts recommend that patients be regarded as "customers" who are vital to the practice and should be treated with courtesy and respect. When proper medical ethics and etiquette are shown in the workplace, the practice is more likely to avoid potential legal problems.

▶ Accurate, complete, and concise documentation in medical records is essential to the delivery of quality medical care and serves the following important purposes:
- It provides information about the patient's condition, the treatment, the patient's response to this treatment, and the patient's progress.
- It serves as a legal document, which can protect and defend the provider in the event of legal action.
- It provides information necessary for third-party reimbursement.
- It can be used in clinical research under certain circumstances.

▶ The four primary objects of HIPAA are to
- ensure health insurance portability,
- reduce healthcare fraud and abuse,
- enforce standards for health information, and
- guarantee security and privacy of health information for patients.

▶ HIPAA affects various categories of people involved with healthcare, including
- health insurance professionals,
- patients,
- healthcare providers, and
- private business entities.

▶ Confidentiality is the foundation for trust in the patient-provider relationship. Every healthcare organization and provider must guarantee confidentiality and privacy of the healthcare information they collect, maintain, use, and transmit. This obligation of confidentiality extends to every member of the healthcare team.

▶ Exceptions to confidentiality include
- minors (under specific circumstances),
- HIV-positive patients and HIV-positive healthcare workers,
- abuse of a child or adult,
- injuries inflicted by firearms or other weapons,
- communicable diseases, and
- TPO insurance.

▶ Fraud and abuse in healthcare are widespread in the U.S. healthcare system. Not only healthcare providers but also consumers commit fraud and abuse; however, most providers and consumers are honest and ethical. Fraud and abuse result in millions of wasted healthcare dollars. Health insurance professionals can do their part to prevent fraud and abuse in the medical office in numerous ways, such as
- creating and maintaining a file for each major third-party payer's guidelines,
- developing a list of "hot" phone numbers to use when questions arise,
- using the most current coding manuals and coding to the greatest specificity,
- keeping coding skills by attending seminars, continuing education, or both,
- discussing questions or potential problems with healthcare providers, and
- reporting suspected fraud or abuse.

CLOSING SCENARIO

The intricacies of contract law as it applies to health insurance have been an interesting and informative topic for Joy and Barbara. The fact that the relationship between a patient and the healthcare provider is an actual contract and falls under the rules of contract law puts this important relationship in a whole new light. The class Joy previously took in business law had given her a basic background in the legal process, and with the additional information acquired from this chapter, Joy believes she now has an excellent foundation from which

she can apply appropriate directives and rules of conduct to the world of health insurance.

Ethics and etiquette, too, have taken on a new meaning for the women. As these terms are applied to becoming a health insurance professional, Joy and Barbara have a better understanding of all the things they should strive for in their careers and professional lives. As Barbara put it, "Ethics and etiquette illustrate not only the manner in which we do our jobs, but our character while we are on the job."

WEBSITES TO EXPLORE

- For live links to the following websites, please visit the Evolve site at http://evolve.elsevier.com/Beik/today/.
- For extensive and up-to-date information on HIPAA, log on to the following websites:
  http://www.hhs.gov/ocr/privacy/
  http://www.cms.hhs.gov/hipaaGenInfo/
  http://www.hhs.gov/ocr/hipaa/
- The activities of the GAO are designed to ensure the executive branch's accountability to Congress under the Constitution and the government's accountability to the American people. You will find many interesting facts and information on medical insurance and healthcare on their website at
  http://www.gao.gov/.
- For more information on the Federal Privacy Act of 1974, research the following websites:
  http://www.usda.gov/
  http://www.ftc.gov/foia/privacy_act.htm/
- To learn more about healthcare fraud and abuse, log on to the following websites:

http://www.ama-assn.org/
http://oig.hhs.gov/publications/hcfac.asp/

- To learn more about exceptions to HIPAA confidentiality laws, go to the following website:
  http://privacy.health.ufl.edu/faq/hipaa_disclosures.shtml/.
- To access AHIMA's article on Defining the Legal Health Record, go to
  http://library.ahima.org/xpedio/groups/public/documents/ahima/bok1_048604.hcsp?dDocName=bok1_048604/.

Author's Note: Websites change frequently. If any of these URLs is unavailable, use applicable guide words in your Internet search to acquire additional information on the various subjects listed.

REFERENCES AND RESOURCES

Fallon LF Jr: Patient Confidentiality. Encyclopedia of Surgery. Copyright 2009 Advameg, Inc. http://www.surgeryencyclopedia.com/Pa-St/Patient-Confidentiality.html/.

Calloway SD: *Record Retention Periods*, HIPAAdvisory. http://www.hipaadvisory.com/regs/recordretention.htm/.

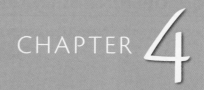

Types and Sources of Health Insurance

Chapter Outline

I. Types of Health Insurance
   A. Indemnity (Fee-for-Service)
   B. Managed Care
II. Sources of Health Insurance
   A. Group Contract
      1. Advantages
      2. Disadvantages
   B. Individual Policies
      1. Advantages
      2. Disadvantages
   C. Medicare
   D. Medicaid
   E. TRICARE/CHAMPVA
   F. Standardized Benefits and Coverage Rule
   G. Disability Insurance
      1. Private
      2. Social Security Disability Insurance
      3. Workers' Compensation

III. Miscellaneous Healthcare Coverage Options
   A. Medical Savings Account
   B. Flexible Spending Account
   C. Health Reimbursement Arrangements
   D. Health Insurance Exchanges
   E. Accountable Care Organizations
   F. Long-Term Care Insurance
   G. Dental Care
   H. Vision Care
IV. Consolidated Omnibus Budget Reconciliation Act
V. Health Insurance "Watchdogs"
VI. Other Terms Common to Third-Party Carriers
   A. Birthday Rule
   B. Coordination of Benefits
   C. Medical Necessity
   D. Usual, Reasonable, and Customary
   E. Participating Versus Nonparticipating Providers
   F. Miscellaneous Terms

CHAPTER OBJECTIVES

After completion of this chapter, the student should be able to:

1. Describe the two basic types of health insurance plans and how each functions.
2. Compare a group insurance contract with an individual policy.
3. List the major sources of health insurance and briefly explain each.
4. Assess the benefits of the various optional healthcare plans.
5. Discuss the purpose and function of the Consolidated Omnibus Budget Reconciliation Act (COBRA).
6. Evaluate the importance of the health insurance "watchdogs."
7. Define terms common to third-party carriers.

CHAPTER TERMS

Accountable Care Organization (ACO)
balance billing
birthday rule
cafeteria plan
CHAMPVA
CMS-1500 form
coinsurance
comprehensive plan
Consolidated Omnibus Budget Reconciliation Act (COBRA)
coordination of benefits (COB)

deductible
disability insurance
enrollees
exclusions
flexible spending account (FSA)
group contract
health insurance exchanges
indemnity (fee-for-service)
insured
maintenance of benefits (MOB)
managed care
Medicaid

⟳ OPENING SCENARIO

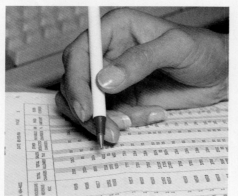

Barbara has volunteered to work two evenings a week for the free clinic in her rural community. On the basis of Barbara's interest in health insurance and her computer experience from her former job, the physician in charge has agreed to let her assist in the billing and insurance department. Barbara realizes there is still a lot she has to learn about insurance, but the knowledge she has acquired from these few early weeks in class has given her a good foundation on which to begin her volunteer work. She informs the physician that she prefers to watch and learn for a few weeks before actually performing any billing and insurance tasks, and as she gains more confidence, she will begin completing and submitting claims.

At first, the work is challenging, but Barbara becomes more comfortable each day that she works at the clinic. The new terms she's learned take on a much clearer meaning as she applies them to actual situations. Barbara enjoys helping new patients fill out the patient information form and is able to guide them and answer questions relating to primary and secondary insurance coverage. She is especially diligent about each patient having an up-to-date release of information in his or her record and confidently explains the rationale of this important document to patients who inquire. It surprises her that so many patients are willing to put their signature on a document without really knowing the reason why.

Being able to relate her real experiences in the clinic to what she is learning in the classroom allows Barbara to understand better the complexities of health insurance and "puts a face" on many of the issues and topics she is learning. Patient education is quickly becoming her area of special interest because it is obvious that many patients do not know their rights.

---

medically necessary
medical savings account (MSA)
Medicare
Medicare Supplement plans
Medigap
nonparticipating provider (nonPAR)
out-of-pocket maximum
participating provider (PAR)

policyholder
preexisting conditions
premium
Social Security Disability Insurance (SSDI)
TRICARE
usual, customary, and reasonable (UCR)
workers' compensation

TYPES OF HEALTH INSURANCE

Most people in the United States know how important it is to have health insurance in today's world of spiraling medical costs. You may have heard a lot of confusing terms when people speak of health insurance, such as "major medical," "comprehensive," and "managed care." Acronyms such as HMOs, PPOs, and POS make things even more confusing.

In Chapter 1, we learned how insurance got its start. Chapter 2 discussed the education and preparation necessary for becoming a health insurance professional and what job duties and responsibilities are common in this field. Chapter 2 also explained various career opportunities and certification possibilities. Chapter 3 provided a solid background on medical law and ethics. This chapter is the last step in building the foundation in medical insurance. Here, we look at the different types of health insurance and the various ways an individual (and his or her family) may be entitled to or eligible for health insurance benefits. We also explore the different types of health insurance and their sources and things that are common to all carriers. By the end of this chapter, we hope that you will begin to make sense of a lot of this medical insurance jargon.

The two basic types of health insurance plans today typically are described as **indemnity** (also called **fee-for-service**) and **managed care**. These two types of plans differ in their basic approach to paying healthcare benefits in three primary ways:

• Choice of providers
• Out-of-pocket costs for covered services
• How bills are paid

Indemnity (Fee-for-Service)

Indemnity (fee-for-service) is the traditional kind of healthcare policy in which patients can choose any healthcare provider or hospital they want (including specialists) and change physicians at any time. With indemnity plans, the **insured** (or **policyholder**) typically pays a monthly fee called a **premium**. Premiums are based on the policy type and coverage, and the better the coverage, the higher the premium. The patient also pays a certain amount of money up front each year toward his or her medical expenses, known as the **deductible**, before the insurance company begins paying benefits. Historically, this deductible amount was $100 to $500 per year; however, as health insurance costs continue to increase, deductibles of $1000 to $5000 per year are commonly seen. Typically, the higher the deductible, the lower the premiums. In policies that cover whole families, it is common that at least two people in the family must meet this yearly deductible before benefits begin; however, this differs from policy to policy and from one insurance company to another. Additionally, not all medical expenses count toward the deductible, but only those covered in the policy.

After the yearly deductible is met, the patient shares the bill with the insurance company in an arrangement called **coinsurance**. The policy may have an 80/20 coinsurance clause, which means that after the deductible is met, the patient must pay 20% of covered medical expenses and the insurance company pays 80%. This payment is based on what is referred to as **usual, customary, and reasonable (UCR)** rates. UCR rates are the part of a provider's charge that the insurance carrier allows as covered expenses. The UCR value of the provider's service is based on historical data developed from the following criteria:

- How much the provider charges his or her patients for the same or a similar service
- The variance in the charges by most providers for the same service in the same geographic area
- Whether the procedure requires more time, skill, or experience than it usually requires
- The value of the procedure in comparison with that of other services

Resource-based relative value scale (RBRVS) is a formula which assigns a value to every medical procedure to calculate Medicare's fee schedule allowance. RBRVS is utilized by many health plans in negotiating fee schedules with in-network physicians. RBRVS is discussed in detail in Chapter 17.

Fee-for-service policies generally have an **out-of-pocket maximum**. This means that when medical expenses reach a certain amount, the UCR fee for covered benefits is paid in full by the insurer. Additionally, there might be lifetime limits as to how much an insurance company pays under the policy (e.g., $1 million).

For the medical bills to be paid, the patient or the healthcare provider must fill out forms and send them to the insurance carrier. The form that is most commonly used is referred to as the **CMS-1500 form**, a universal form created by the government for Medicare claims and since adopted by most third-party carriers. The CMS-1500 may be submitted in paper form or electronically. To view both the back and front of the CMS-1500, see Appendix A.

Two kinds of fee-for-service coverage exist: basic and major medical. Basic coverage pays toward the costs of room and care while the patient is hospitalized. It also may cover some hospital services and supplies, such as x-rays and prescribed medicine. Basic coverage also pays toward the cost of surgery, whether it is performed in or out of the hospital, and for some physician visits. Major medical coverage takes over where basic coverage leaves off. It covers the cost of long and high-cost illnesses or injuries. Some policies combine basic and major medical coverage into one plan referred to as a **comprehensive plan**. Sometimes the insurance policy does not cover certain medical conditions. These are known as **exclusions** (illnesses or injuries not covered by the policy) and may be due to a **preexisting condition**, which is a physical or mental condition of an insured person that existed before the issuance of a health insurance policy or that existed before issuance and for which treatment was received. Preexisting conditions are excluded from coverage under some policies, or a specified length of time must elapse before the condition is covered.

★ Imagine This!

Larry Burton, a self-employed carpenter, injured his back in a skiing accident, requiring surgery and extensive treatment and therapy. Larry's medical expenses were covered through an individual policy with HealthNet Insurance Company. Several years later, because of HealthNet's rising premiums, Larry decided to apply for coverage under American Carpenter's Indemnity (ACI), which had lower premiums. ACI required Larry to complete an application form, which included an extensive questionnaire regarding his medical history. Eventually, ACI granted Larry coverage but excluded payment for treatment of future medical services or procedures involving his back and spine.

Managed Care

The term "managed care" is often heard on the news to describe certain medical plans, and many people do not know what it means. **Managed care** is medical care that is provided by a corporation established under state and federal laws. This corporation makes medical decisions for its **enrollees** (people who are covered under the managed care plan). A managed care provider tells patients which physicians they can see, monitors the medications and treatments prescribed, and ensures enrollees that their costs will remain as low as possible. For these services, enrollees pay a set insurance premium each year and a small copayment with each visit. To perform these services satisfactorily, the corporation typically hires a medical staff (physicians, nurses, and other healthcare providers). These "employees" are under contract and, to some degree, take their orders from corporate management. Many types of managed care organizations are available. For more detailed information on managed care, see Chapter 7.

? What Did You Learn?

1. Name the two basic types of health insurance plans today.
2. List the three primary ways these two types of insurance are different.

SOURCES OF HEALTH INSURANCE

Individuals can obtain healthcare coverage in today's insurance markets in several ways. Many individuals are eligible for coverage through their employers. Self-employed individuals and individuals who are ineligible for coverage through their employer should contact a professional health insurance agent and apply for a private policy. Additionally, government programs, such as Medicare and Medicaid, are available for qualifying individuals.

Group Contract

A **group contract** is a contract of insurance made with a company, a corporation, or other groups of common interest wherein all employees or individuals (and their eligible dependents) are insured under a single policy. The group policy is issued to the company or corporation, and everyone receives the same benefits. Often, when one thinks of a group healthcare plan, the first thing that comes to mind is coverage that is acquired through an individual's employment.

Group healthcare plans through an employer or other group have many advantages and some disadvantages.

Advantages

- Group policies are usually less expensive than individual policies.
- Everyone is usually eligible for coverage regardless of health status.
- Coverage is typically comprehensive.
- Premiums can be deducted from paychecks (if it is the policy of the employer).
- Coverage generally cannot be terminated because of frequent claims.
- Protection under the Health Insurance Portability and Accountability Act (HIPAA) allows an individual to move from one job to another without the fear of exclusions owing to preexisting conditions.

Disadvantages

- Individuals have little or no choice in the type of coverage provided under the group contract.
- Individuals must accept whatever coverage the group policy provides; modifications are not optional.
- Individuals often lose comprehensive coverage when they no longer belong to the "group," even though they may have "conversion" privileges (see the section on COBRA).
- Premiums for conversion policies tend to be much higher.

Some professions, such as the American Association of Professional Engineers, and individuals sharing a common occupation (e.g., farmers or labor union members) offer group health insurance plans for their members.

Individual Policies

If a person is self-employed or if the company with whom he or she is employed does not offer a group policy, the individual may need to buy individual health insurance. Individual health insurance policies can be purchased from most commercial insurers and companies such as Blue Cross and Blue Shield. As with group policies, there are advantages and disadvantages of having an individual health insurance policy.

Advantages

- The individual can select the type of policy that best fits the individual's (and his or her dependents') situation.
- The policy can be "individualized" to the individual's (or family's) needs.
- The individual controls the insurance contract.
- The individual usually does not lose coverage if he or she changes occupations.

Disadvantages

- Requirements are usually more restrictive.
- Premiums are typically higher and often depend on the individual's age and health risk.
- There are lower limits for certain coverages (e.g., mental health, substance abuse).
- Preexisting conditions are often excluded, or there is a waiting period before coverage begins.
- Exclusions are more common.
- The insurer can terminate some individual healthcare policies under certain circumstances.

Medicare

Medicare is a federal health insurance program that provides benefits to individuals 65 years or older and individuals younger than 65 years with certain disabilities. In many parts of the United States, Medicare-eligible patients now have a choice between managed care and indemnity plans. For individuals who enroll in the traditional Medicare plan, private insurance options help cover some of the gaps in Medicare coverage. These supplemental policies are called **Medigap** or **Medicare Supplement plans**. These policies must cover certain expenses, such as deductibles and the daily coinsurance amount for hospitalization. Some Medicare managed care policies may offer additional benefits, such as coverage for preventive medical care, prescription drugs, or at-home recovery, that original Medicare does not cover. For more details on Medicare, Medigap, and Medicare Supplement plans, see Chapter 9.

Medicaid

Medicaid covers some low-income individuals (particularly children and pregnant women) and certain disabled individuals. Medicaid is a joint federal-state health program that is administered by the individual states. Medicaid coverage differs from state to state. See Chapter 8 for more extensive information on Medicaid.

TRICARE/CHAMPVA

TRICARE is the U.S. military's comprehensive healthcare program for active-duty personnel and eligible family members, retirees, and family members younger than 65 years and survivors of all uniformed services (i.e., Army, Air Force,

Marines, Navy). The TRICARE program is managed by the military in partnership with civilian hospitals and clinics. It is designed to expand access to care, ensure high-quality care, and promote medical readiness. All military hospitals and clinics are part of the TRICARE program.

The Civilian Health and Medical Program of the Department of Veterans Affairs (**CHAMPVA**) is a health benefits program in which the Department of Veterans Affairs (VA) shares the cost of certain healthcare services and supplies with eligible beneficiaries. CHAMPVA is managed by the VA's Health Administration Center in Denver, Colorado, where applications are processed, eligibility is determined, benefits are authorized, and medical claims are processed. Military insurance programs are discussed in detail in Chapter 10.

Standardized Benefits and Coverage Rule

In August 2011, the Department of Health and Human Services (HHS) announced a new rule that will help consumers choose new and/or understand their existing health insurance policies. Starting in March 2012, all insurance vendors will be required to provide consumers with a standard four-page "summary of benefits and coverage," along with a universal glossary of common health insurance terms (e.g. "deductible," "copay," etc.). The summary will spell out what the policy does and does not cover, the cost of the monthly premium, what the deductible is, and how much an individual should expect to pay in out-of-pocket costs. The Rule is part of the Affordable Care Act, disclosed by the Centers for Medicare and Medicaid Services (CMS).

Under this Rule, if an insurance company wants to make major changes to a policy, policyholders would have to be notified of the changes 60 days in advance. Prior to the Rule, insurers offered policy information in a lengthy, often difficult-to-understand, document called a "certificate of coverage," generally provided after the policy was purchased. This summary also will contain real-life examples explaining what proportion of healthcare expenses a policy will cover, such as having a baby, treating breast cancer, and managing diabetes. Those who are shopping for or enrolled in a healthcare plan can request a copy of the Summary of Benefits and Coverage and must receive it within 7 days. The uniform glossary will be made available upon request, as well as in a link provided in the coverage label by the plan or insurance company. Refer to the Evolve site for links to the uniform glossary.

Disability Insurance

Disability insurance is a form of insurance that pays the policyholder a specific sum of money in place of his or her usual income if the policyholder cannot work because of illness or accident. It is not health insurance coverage, per se. Usually, policies begin paying after a waiting period stipulated in the policy and pay a certain percentage of the policyholder's usual income. Sometimes disability insurance is provided by employers, but it also is available as individual private coverage. Several types of disability insurance are available.

Private

An individual can purchase a private disability insurance policy or can be covered by a disability policy offered by his or her employer. Disability insurance does not cover illnesses or injuries related to one's employment. It is designed to replace 45% to 60% of an individual's gross income on a tax-free basis should an illness unrelated to the job prevent him or her from earning an income. Disability insurance policies vary from one insurance company to another, and each can be different. Disability insurance can provide short-term or long-term benefits, depending on the stipulations of the policy. Private disability insurance can be costly; however, some employers offer it to their employees at more reasonable rates. There is often a waiting period (e.g., 30 days) before benefits begin.

Social Security Disability Insurance

Social Security Disability Insurance (SSDI) is an insurance program for individuals who become unable to work. It is administered by the Social Security Administration (SSA) and is funded by Federal Insurance Contributions Act (FICA) tax withheld from workers' pay and by matching employer contributions. SSDI pays qualifying disabled workers cash and healthcare benefits. Workers who have worked and paid FICA tax for at least 5 of the 10 years before the date they become disabled typically are covered by SSDI. In other words, applicants must have worked 20 out of the 40 calendar quarters immediately preceding the onset date of disability to be covered. Younger workers can qualify with fewer years of work. A person can apply for SSDI benefits at any SSA office. A free booklet entitled *Social Security Disability Benefits* (SSA Publication No. 05-10029) is available at any Social Security office or through the SSA toll-free phone number: 800-772-1213. Individuals can apply via the Internet, at www.ssa.gov, but the procedure is relatively new, and there are still some "bugs" in the system.

The supplemental security income (SSI) disability program has marked similarities to SSDI. Both programs are run by the SSA, both offer disability benefits, and both use the same legal definition of "disability." The programs differ significantly, however, in their financial qualifications and benefits.

Workers' Compensation

Workers' compensation insurance pays workers who are injured or disabled on the job or have job-related illnesses. Laws governing workers' compensation are designed to ensure that employees who are injured or disabled on the job are provided with fixed monetary awards, eliminating the need for litigation. These laws also provide benefits for dependents of workers who die as a result of work-related accidents or illnesses. Some laws also protect employers and fellow workers by limiting the amount an injured employee can recover from an employer and by eliminating the liability of coworkers in most accidents. State workers' compensation statutes establish this framework for most employment and differ from state to state. Federal statutes are limited to federal employees or workers employed in some significant aspect of interstate commerce.

The Federal Employment Compensation Act provides workers' compensation for nonmilitary federal employees. Many of its provisions are typical of most workers' compensation laws. Awards are limited to "disability or death" sustained while in the performance of the employee's duties but not caused willfully by the employee or by intoxication. The act covers medical expenses resulting from the disability and may require the employee to undergo job retraining. In other words, if the employee is unable to return to his or her original position because of a particular disability, the employee is trained to perform in a different position, ideally at an equal level of pay. A disabled employee receives two-thirds of his or her normal monthly salary during the disability period and may receive more for permanent physical injuries or if he or she has dependents. The act provides compensation for survivors of employees who are killed. The Office of Workers' Compensation Programs administers the act.

The Federal Employment Liability Act, although not a workers' compensation statute, provides that railroads engaged in interstate commerce are liable for injuries to their employees if they have been negligent. Disability insurance and workers' compensation are discussed in Chapter 11.

MISCELLANEOUS HEALTHCARE COVERAGE OPTIONS

Medical Savings Account

A **medical savings account (MSA)**, sometimes referred to as a Health Savings Account (HSA), is a special tax shelter set up for the purpose of paying medical bills. Known as the Archer MSA, it is similar to an IRA (individual retirement account, which allows an individual to make tax-deferred contributions to a personal retirement fund) and works in conjunction with a special low-cost, high-deductible health insurance policy to provide comprehensive healthcare coverage at the lowest possible net cost for individuals who qualify. MSAs currently are limited to self-employed individuals and employees of small businesses comprising fewer than 50 employees where a small group MSA health plan is in place.

Here's how an MSA works. Instead of buying high-priced health insurance with low copays and a low deductible, the individual or business purchases a low-cost policy with a high deductible for the big bills and saves the difference in the MSA to cover smaller bills. Money deposited into the MSA account is 100% tax deductible (as with a traditional IRA) and can be easily accessed by check or debit card to pay most medical bills tax free (even expenses not covered by insurance, such as for dental and vision care). The funds that are not used for medical bills stay in the MSA account and keep growing on a tax-favored basis to cover future medical bills or to supplement retirement. An MSA plan offers (1) lower premiums, (2) lower taxes, (3) freedom of choice, and (4) more cash at retirement.

Funds can be withdrawn for other purposes but if that is done, the individual will face both increased income taxes and a 20% penalty. (Currently, the penalty does not apply to people over age 65.)

> ### 📁 HIPAA Tip
>
> Medical savings accounts under HIPAA provide federal tax deductions for contributions to multiyear savings accounts established for medical purposes.

Flexible Spending Account

The **flexible spending account (FSA)** is an IRS Section 125 **cafeteria plan**. A plan falls into the cafeteria category when the cost of the plan (premium) is deducted from the employee's wages before withholding taxes are deducted. This allows employees the option of pretax payroll deduction for some insurance premiums, unreimbursed medical expenses, and child/dependent care expenses. Cafeteria plans are among the fastest-growing employee benefits. Employers save when employees elect for pretax payroll deduction because lower adjusted gross income also reduces matching FICA and federal unemployment tax. Employees benefit because expenses for such items as health insurance premiums and unreimbursed medical, vision, dental, and child/dependent care expenses paid before the tax deduction result in immediate tax savings. When employees switch expenses to "before tax," they save on Social Security tax, federal income tax, and state and local tax (in most states). There are obvious advantages associated with FSAs. Consequently, the government has placed certain restrictions on plans of this type in exchange for the favorable tax treatment.

During the year, FSA participants may change the amount of their contribution designation only if there is a change in the health premium or the employee's family status, which includes

- marriage,
- divorce,
- change of employment by spouse,
- birth or adoption of a child,
- death of a spouse or a child, and
- change in employment status (i.e., from full-time to part-time)

The previous "use it or lose it" rule, whereby the individual had to forfeit any funds left over at the end of the year, has been removed. There is a new "use it or lose it" rule. At the beginning of each plan year, individuals designate a certain portion of their before-tax salary to the FSA for dependent care and medical expenses. Any funds left over in either category at the end of the year are forfeited. As of May 18, 2005, the IRS allows employers to give FSA participants up to an additional 2½ months to spend money left over in their FSAs at year's end on qualified health and dependent care expenses. Starting in 2011, over-the-counter (OTC) medicines will no longer be eligible for reimbursement unless their use is expressly directed by the healthcare provider. In 2013, a federally mandated $2500 cap on FSA contributions will take effect.

For more information on MSAs/HSAs and FSAs, visit the Evolve site.

Health Reimbursement Arrangements

Health reimbursement arrangements (HRAs), also known as "health reimbursement accounts" or "personal care accounts," are a type of health insurance plan that reimburses employees for certain qualifying medical expenses. The U.S.

Department of the Treasury set up guidelines on HRAs in June 2002. HRAs consist of funds set aside by employers to reimburse employees for "qualified" medical expenses, just as an insurance plan reimburses covered individuals for the cost of services incurred. Employers can deduct the cost of an insurance plan, including an HRA, as a business expense under Internal Revenue Code section 162.

HRAs are open to employees of companies of any size, unlike medical savings accounts (MSAs), which are available only to small business employees. An HRA provides "first-dollar" medical coverage until funds are used up. For example, if an employee has a $250 qualifying medical expense, the full amount will be covered by the HRA if this amount is available in the account. Under an HRA, the employer provides the funds, not the employee. All unused funds are rolled over at the end of the year. Former employees, including retirees, can have continued access to unused reimbursement amounts. HRAs remain with the originating employer and do not follow an employee to new employment. Table 4-1 compares key features of MSAs, FSAs, and HRAs.

TABLE 4-1	Comparison of Key Features of Health Spending Accounts		
	FLEXIBLE SPENDING ACCOUNT (FSA)	**MEDICAL SAVINGS ACCOUNT (MSA)**	**HEALTH REIMBURSEMENT ARRANGEMENT (HRA)**
Initial legislation or regulation	Revenue Act of 1978	Health Insurance Portability and Accountability Act of 1996	U.S. Department of the Treasury Revenue Ruling 2002-41
Date effective	January 1, 1979	January 1, 1997	June 26, 2002
IRS code reference	Internal Revenue Code section 125	Internal Revenue Code section 106(b)	Internal Revenue Code section 105-106
Eligibility	All employees except self-employed	Self-employed or employee of a small business (50 or fewer employees) (Must be covered by high-deductible health plan)	All employees
Qualified medical expenses	Unreimbursed medical care expenses as defined by Internal Revenue Code section 213, excluding premiums for health insurance coverage and long-term care expenses	Unreimbursed medical care expenses as defined by Internal Revenue Code section 213 Health insurance premiums under a continuation of coverage arrangement (such as COBRA) Health insurance premiums when the patient is receiving unemployment compensation Qualified long-term care insurance premiums	Unreimbursed medical care expenses as defined by Internal Revenue Code section 213
Nonqualified medical expenses	Expenses not defined by Internal Revenue Code section 213 Health insurance premiums under a continuation of coverage arrangement (such as COBRA) Health insurance premiums when the patient is receiving unemployment compensation Qualified long-term care insurance premiums	Expenses not under Internal Revenue Code section 213 Employer may set additional restrictions	Expenses not under Internal Revenue Code section 213

Continued

TABLE 4-1	Comparison of Key Features of Health Spending Accounts—cont'd		
	FLEXIBLE SPENDING ACCOUNT (FSA)	**MEDICAL SAVINGS ACCOUNT (MSA)**	**HEALTH REIMBURSEMENT ARRANGEMENT (HRA)**
Patient must be covered by a health insurance plan?	No	Yes	No
Contributor	Employee, employer, or both	Employee or employer, but not both	Employer
Contribution limits	No statutory limit; limits may be set by employer	Single coverage—65% of deductible Family coverage—75% of deductible	No statutory limit; limits may be set by employer
Funds carried over to next year?	No	Yes	Yes
Portability	Account cannot be maintained if the employee is no longer working for the employer	Continued access to unused account balance if the employee is no longer working for the employer Withdrawals for nonmedical purposes are subject to income tax and a 15% penalty tax Once the account holder reaches age 65 (the Medicare eligibility age), becomes disabled, or dies, withdrawals for nonmedical purposes are subject to income tax only, with no penalty	At employer discretion

From U.S. Department of Labor Statistics: Health Spending Accounts. Washington, DC. http://www.bls.gov/opub/cwc/cm20031022ar01p1.htm/.

HIPAA Tip

HIPAA mandates that when an employee's healthcare coverage is terminated, the employer automatically sends the employee, on the coverage's cancellation, a Certificate of Credible Coverage.

Health Insurance Exchanges

As discussed in Chapter 1, additional types of healthcare plans are on the horizon, such as the **health insurance exchange**. The intention of this model is to create a more organized and competitive market for health insurance by offering a choice of plans with common rules governing how each plan is offered, its cost, and providing information to help consumers better understand the choices available to them. For more information on this topic, visit the Evolve site.

Accountable Care Organizations (ACOs)

Another healthcare model that is currently being considered is the **Accountable Care Organization (ACO)**. Authors are designing this coverage model to provide a

new, more efficient way to deliver care. Similar to a Health Maintenance Organization (HMO), an ACO is a network of doctors and hospitals that shares responsibility for providing care to patients. Under the new healthcare law, the ACO would agree to manage all of the healthcare needs of a minimum of 5000 Medicare beneficiaries for at least 3 years. Goals for an ACO are to determine how to successfully

- Keep patients within the ACO, encouraging them to stay healthy and take more responsibility for their own healthcare
- Encourage patients to use healthcare providers that are part of the ACO network to keep the overall costs down within the organization

Long-Term Care Insurance

When we are healthy, it is easy to take activities of daily living (ADLs), such as bathing, dressing, and feeding ourselves, for granted. When an individual is stricken with a degenerative condition, however, such as a stroke or Alzheimer's disease, performing these ADLs becomes impossible without the assistance of another person. This type of care is referred to as *long-term care;* it is ongoing and quickly becomes expensive. Long-term care is not medical care but, rather, custodial care. Custodial care involves providing an individual with assistance or supervision or both with ADLs that he or she no longer can perform. Long-term care can be provided in many settings, including nursing homes, one's own home, assisted living facilities, and adult day care.

Today, long-term care insurance typically covers a broad range of services, including nursing home care, assisted living facilities, certain types of home healthcare, and adult day care. Similar to any insurance product, long-term care insurance allows the insured to pay an affordable premium to protect himself or herself in case of an unaffordable catastrophic event.

Dental Care

A health insurance plan may or may not cover dental care. Even if it does, it might not cover all procedures, such as orthodontics (teeth straightening) and cosmetic dentistry. Because dental care can be expensive, a separate dental insurance policy can be purchased. Health insurance plans typically cover dental restoration work needed because of disease or accident.

Vision Care

As with dental care, a health insurance plan may or may not cover vision care. General eye care, such as refractions (vision tests), are typically provided by an optometrist, a professional who is trained and licensed to examine eyes, checks for eye diseases and problems, and prescribes corrective lenses. More serious vision problems are normally handled by an ophthalmologist—a medical doctor specializing in eye diseases.

📁 HIPAA Tip

The Health Insurance Reform Act, incorporated within HIPAA, includes consumer protections for purchasers of long-term care insurance and clarifications that make treatment of private long-term care insurance identical to that of health insurance coverage.

CONSOLIDATED OMNIBUS BUDGET RECONCILIATION ACT

Congress passed the **Consolidated Omnibus Budget Reconciliation Act (COBRA)** health benefit provisions in 1986. The law amends the Employee Retirement Income Security Act, the Internal Revenue Code, and the Public Health Service Act to provide continuation of group health coverage that otherwise would be terminated when an individual leaves his or her place of employment. The law generally covers group health plans maintained by employers with 20 or more employees in the prior year. It applies to plans in the private sector and plans sponsored by state and local governments. The law does not apply, however, to plans sponsored by the U.S. government and certain church-related organizations. Under COBRA, a group health plan is ordinarily defined as a plan that provides medical benefits for the employer's own employees and their dependents through insurance or otherwise (e.g., a trust, health maintenance organization, self-funded pay-as-you-go basis, reimbursement, or combination of these).

COBRA contains provisions that give certain former employees and retirees, as well as their spouses and dependent children, the right to temporary continuation of health coverage at group rates. Currently, most people working for qualifying employers can continue their coverage for 18 months under the COBRA program when they lose their jobs. COBRA premiums can be expensive, however, because the ex-employee must pay the share of premiums once covered by the employer as well as his or her own share from the previous group health plan.

Events that can cause workers and their family members to lose group health coverage and that may result in the right to COBRA coverage include the following:

- Voluntary or involuntary termination of the covered employee's employment for reasons other than gross misconduct
- Reduced hours of work for the covered employee
- Covered employee becoming entitled to Medicare
- Divorce or legal separation of a covered employee
- Death of a covered employee
- Loss of status as a dependent child under plan rules

COBRA coverage generally starts on the date of the qualifying event, and benefits can last for the maximum coverage period, which varies according to the type of triggering event:

- 18-month maximum coverage period
- Reduction of hours (includes leave without pay and layoff)
- 36-month maximum coverage period (for specific qualifiers)
- Death of employee/retiree
- Divorce or legal separation
- Child's no longer meeting eligibility rules

Employee/retiree entitlement to Medicare does not apply because entitlement to Medicare does not result in loss of coverage.

⭐ Imagine This!

Mary is an employee covered under Southeast Medical Clinic's group health plan. When her employment terminates, she elects COBRA. Her maximum coverage period is 18 months. On the last day of the tenth month of her COBRA coverage, Mary gives birth. Her child is a qualified beneficiary. The child's maximum coverage period is the remaining 8 months of Mary's maximum coverage period.

Medical benefits provided under the terms of the plan and available to COBRA beneficiaries may include, but are not necessarily limited to, the following:

- Inpatient and outpatient hospital care
- Physician care
- Surgery and other major medical benefits
- Prescription drugs
- Any other medical benefits, such as dental and vision care

📁 HIPAA Tip

HIPAA does not set premium rates, but it does prohibit plans and issuers from charging an individual more than similarly situated individuals in the same plan because of health status. Plans may offer premium discounts or rebates for participation in wellness programs.

HEALTH INSURANCE "WATCHDOGS"

The following organizations are instrumental in recognizing and assessing healthcare plans and certifying the quality of the care they provide, functioning as "watchdogs":

- The Joint Commission—Evaluates and accredits nearly 20,000 health care organizations and programs, including almost 12,000 hospitals and home care organizations, and more than 7,000 other health care organizations that provide long term care, behavioral healthcare, laboratory and ambulatory care services. The Joint Commission also accredits health plans, integrated delivery networks, and other managed care entities.
- National Committee for Quality Assurance/NCQA— Accredits HMOs and other managed care organizations.
- American Accreditation HealthCare Commission/ (formerly Utilization Review Accreditation Commission/ URAC)—Accredits preferred provider organizations (PPOs) and other managed care networks.
- Accreditation Association for Ambulatory Health Care— Accredits outpatient healthcare settings such as ambulatory surgery centers, radiation oncology centers, and student health centers.
- Community Health Accreditation Program—Accredits community, home health, and hospice programs; public health departments; and nursing centers.
- Consumer Coalition for Quality Health Care—A national, nonprofit organization of consumer groups advocating for consumer protections and quality assurance programs and policies.

Several of these organizations are discussed in later chapters.

💬 What Did You Learn?

1. Who qualifies for a medical savings account?
2. Explain how a medical savings account operates.
3. What are the benefits of a flexible spending account?
4. What happens to leftover funds in a flexible spending account at the end of the year?
5. What type of healthcare typically falls in the category of long-term care?
6. To whom does the COBRA law generally apply?
7. List the various events that qualify an employee for COBRA coverage.
8. What medical benefits are included under COBRA?

OTHER TERMS COMMON TO THIRD-PARTY CARRIERS

Many terms are used commonly in the medical provider, hospital, and healthcare industries. A few of the more commonly used terms are discussed here. In the Websites to Explore at the end of this chapter, several URLs for accessing a comprehensive list of health insurance terms and their definitions are given.

Birthday Rule

The **birthday rule** is an informal procedure used in the health insurance industry to help determine which health plan is considered "primary" when individuals (usually children) are listed as dependents on more than one health plan. This scenario occurs frequently among divorced parents. Sometimes, parents include their children on each other's insurance plan to maximize coverage and, if they are divorced, to ensure that the children will be covered when visiting the other parent. The insurance plans need to coordinate benefits so that the claim is paid properly. To prevent overpayment, one parent's plan is designated as the primary plan and the other as a secondary plan. The birthday rule determines which plan is primary. It states that *the health plan of the parent whose birthday comes first in the calendar year will be considered the primary plan.*

Exceptions to the birthday rule are as follows:

- Parents who share the same birthday
- Active employees
- Different plan types

When parents have the same birthday, the parent who has had his or her plan longer pays first. When parents are divorced or separated, the plan of the parent who has legal custody is considered primary. If the custodial parent remarries, the new spouse's plan would be considered secondary. The plan of the parent without custody would pay any additional expenses not covered. If one spouse is currently employed and has insurance and the other spouse has coverage through a former employer (COBRA), the plan of the currently employed spouse would be primary. Group plans are considered primary over individual plans.

These are generally accepted rules, not laws. It is important to keep in mind that these practices are common among insurance companies, but they are not governed by law. Practices may vary from one insurer to another. It is important that people read their policies carefully to make sure they understand how their insurance company handles dual coverage. Additionally, a prudent health insurance professional should discuss this situation with the patient's parent or guardian as it arises.

🕐 Stop and Think

Helen and Paul Jackson are recently divorced. Hunter, their 7-year-old son, comes to the office with a broken wrist. Helen informs the health insurance professional that she is the custodial parent but the court has named Paul as the party responsible for all medical bills. After the divorce, Helen had quit her job to become a stay-at-home mom, and she and Hunter are still covered on a COBRA policy through Packers United; Paul is covered by a Blue Cross/Blue Shield PPO group plan. Helen's birth date is listed on the patient information form as May 24, 1964. Hunter's father's birth date is September 5, 1959. To which third-party insurer should the insurance claim be sent first?

Coordination of Benefits

Coordination of benefits (COB) came into being several years ago when it was common for a husband and wife to each have the same or similar group health insurance benefits but on different policies. This was commonly referred to as "overinsurance." Possible sources of overinsurance include the following:
- The husband and the wife are employed and eligible for group health coverage, and each lists the other as a dependent.
- A person is employed in two jobs, both of which provide group health insurance coverage.
- A salaried or professional person who has group health insurance coverage with an employer also has an association group health plan.

The historical concept of COB has been to limit the total benefits an insured individual can receive from both group plans to not more than 100% of the allowable expenses. This prevents the policyholders from making a profit on health insurance claims.

Under COB, the primary plan pays benefits up to its limit, then the secondary plan pays the difference between the primary insurer's benefits and the total incurred allowable expenses (historically 100% of the allowed expenses) up to the secondary insurer's limit. Each state may have different COB regulations based on the National Association of Insurance Commissioners and variations in the language used to assist consistent claim administration. When this situation arises, the health insurance professional must rely on the patient (or his or her parent or guardian if a minor) to state which policy is primary. It is not the health insurance professional's responsibility to make this determination.

Maintenance of benefits (MOB) is a relatively new term. MOB allows patients to receive benefits from all health insurance plans they are covered under, while maintaining responsibility for coinsurance and/or copay amounts on these coverages. The total combined payment from all sources cannot be more than the total charge for all services. With MOB processing, secondary payers allow benefits only up to their own maximum allowable for the specific service(s). If the primary carrier's payment is equal to or more than what the secondary carrier's payment would have been as primary, no additional benefits will be remitted. With this arrangement, patients may have out-of-pocket expenses, something not usually seen with COB processing.

Medical Necessity

Most third-party payers do not pay for medical services, procedures, or supplies unless
- they are proper and needed for the diagnosis or treatment of a patient's medical condition;
- they are provided for the diagnosis, direct care, and treatment of a medical condition;
- they meet the standards of good medical practice in the local area; and
- they are not mainly for the convenience of the patient or the healthcare provider.

When medical services, procedures, or supplies meet these criteria, they are said to be **medically necessary** or meet the standards of "medical necessity." For treatment of Medicare patients, it is sometimes necessary to complete a certificate of medical necessity (Fig. 4-1).

Usual, Reasonable, and Customary

We learned earlier in this chapter that usual, reasonable, and customary (UCR) is a calculation of what certain third-party payers believe is the appropriate fee for healthcare providers to charge for a specific service or procedure in a certain geographic area. The fee is based on a consensus of what most local hospitals, physicians, or laboratories typically charge for a similar procedure or service in the geographic area in which the provider practices. The state and federal governments do not regulate UCR charges, but Medicare publishes its own fee schedules using RBRVS.

Healthcare providers' actual charge may be different from the UCR (allowable) charge of the third-party payer. When an insurance carrier has a UCR charge that is below the actual provider's charge, the patient may be responsible for paying this difference. This is called **balance billing**.

U.S. DEPARTMENT OF HEALTH & HUMAN SERVICES
CENTERS FOR MEDICARE & MEDICAID SERVICES

FORM APPROVED
OMB NO. 0938-0679

CERTIFICATE OF MEDICAL NECESSITY

DMERC 01.02A

HOSPITAL BEDS

SECTION A   Certification Type/Date: INITIAL ___/___/___   REVISED ___/___/___

PATIENT NAME, ADDRESS, TELEPHONE and HIC NUMBER

(___ ___ ___)___ ___ ___-___ ___ ___ ___ HICN _____

SUPPLIER NAME, ADDRESS, TELEPHONE and NSC NUMBER

(___ ___ ___)___ ___ ___-___ ___ ___ ___ NSC # _____

PLACE OF SERVICE _____
NAME and ADDRESS of FACILITY if applicable (See reverse)

HCPCS CODE

_____
_____
_____
_____

PT DOB ___/___/___; Sex ____ (M/F); HT. ____ (in.); WT. ____ (lbs.)

PHYSICIAN NAME, ADDRESS (Printed or Typed)

PHYSICIAN'S UPIN: _____

PHYSICIAN'S TELEPHONE #: (___ ___ ___) ___ ___ ___-___ ___ ___ ___

SECTION B   Information in this Section May Not Be Completed by the Supplier of the Items/Supplies.

EST. LENGTH OF NEED (# OF MONTHS): _____ 1-99 (99=LIFETIME) | DIAGNOSIS CODES (ICD-9): _____ _____ _____ _____

ANSWERS	ANSWER QUESTIONS 1, AND 3-7 FOR HOSPITAL BEDS
	(Circle **Y** for Yes, **N** for No, or **D** for Does Not Apply)
	QUESTION 2 RESERVED FOR OTHER OR FUTURE USE.
Y N D	1. Does the patient require positioning of the body in ways not feasible with an ordinary bed due to a medical condition which is expected to last at least one month?
Y N D	3. Does the patient require, for the alleviation of pain, positioning of the body in ways not feasible with an ordinary bed?
Y N D	4. Does the patient require the head of the bed to be elevated <u>more than 30 degrees</u> most of the time due to congestive heart failure, chronic pulmonary disease, or aspiration?
Y N D	5. Does the patient require traction which can only be attached to a hospital bed?
Y N D	6. Does the patient require a bed height different than a fixed height hospital bed to permit transfers to chair, wheelchair, or standing position?
Y N D	7. Does the patient require frequent changes in body position and/or have an immediate need for a change in body position?

NAME OF PERSON ANSWERING SECTION B QUESTIONS, IF OTHER THAN PHYSICIAN (Please Print):
NAME: _____ TITLE: _____ EMPLOYER: _____

SECTION C   Narrative Description Of Equipment And Cost

(1) <u>Narrative</u> description of all items, accessories and options ordered; **(2)** Supplier's charge; and **(3)** Medicare Fee Schedule Allowance for <u>each</u> item, accessory, and option. *(See Instructions On Back)*

SECTION D   Physician Attestation and Signature/Date

I certify that I am the physician identified in Section A of this form. I have received Sections A, B and C of the Certificate of Medical Necessity (including charges for items ordered). Any statement on my letterhead attached hereto, has been reviewed and signed by me. I certify that the medical necessity information in Section B is true, accurate and complete, to the best of my knowledge, and I understand that any falsification, omission, or concealment of material fact in that section may subject me to civil or criminal liability.

PHYSICIAN'S SIGNATURE _____ DATE ____/____/____ (SIGNATURE AND DATE STAMPS ARE NOT ACCEPTABLE)

CMS-841 (04/96)

Fig. 4-1 Certificate of medical necessity. **A,** Front;

Continued

SECTION A: **(May be completed by the supplier)**

CERTIFICATION
TYPE/DATE: If this is an initial certification for this patient, indicate this by placing date (MM/DD/YY) needed initially in the space marked "INITIAL." If this is a revised certification (to be completed when the physician changes the order, based on the patient's changing clinical needs), indicate the initial date needed in the space marked "INITIAL," and also indicate the recertification date in the space marked "REVISED." If this is a recertification, indicate the initial date needed in the space marked "INITIAL," and also indicate the recertification date in the space marked "RECERTIFI-CATION." Whether submitting a REVISED or a RECERTIFIED CMN, be sure to always furnish the INITIAL date as well as the REVISED or RECERTIFICATION date.

PATIENT
INFORMATION: Indicate the patient's name, permanent legal address, telephone number and his/her health insurance claim number (HICN) as it appears on his/her Medicare card and on the claim form.

SUPPLIER
INFORMATION: Indicate the name of your company (supplier name), address and telephone number along with the Medicare Supplier Number assigned to you by the National Supplier Clearinghouse (NSC).

PLACE OF SERVICE: Indicate the place in which the item is being used; i.e., patient's home is 12, skilled nursing facility (SNF) is 31, End Stage Renal Disease (ESRD) facility is 65, etc. Refer to the DMERC supplier manual for a complete list.

FACILITY NAME: If the place of service is a facility, indicate the name and complete address of the facility.

HCPCS CODES: List all HCPCS procedure codes for items ordered that require a CMN. Procedure codes that do not require certification should not be listed on the CMN.

PATIENT DOB, HEIGHT,
WEIGHT AND SEX: Indicate patient's date of birth (MM/DD/YY) and sex (male or female); height in inches and weight in pounds, if requested.

PHYSICIAN NAME,
ADDRESS: Indicate the physician's name and complete mailing address.

UPIN: Accurately indicate the ordering physician's Unique Physician Identification Number (UPIN).

PHYSICIAN'S
TELEPHONE NO: Indicate the telephone number where the physician can be contacted (preferable where records would be accessible pertaining to this patient) if more information is needed.

SECTION B: **(May not be completed by the supplier. While this section may be completed by a non-physician clinician, or a physician employee, it must be reviewed, and the CMN signed (in Section D) by the ordering physician.)**

EST. LENGTH OF NEED: Indicate the estimated length of need (the length of time the physician expects the patient to require use of the ordered item) by filling in the appropriate number of months. If the physician expects that the patient will require the item for the duration of his/her life, then enter 99.

DIAGNOSIS CODES: In the first space, list the ICD9 code that represents the primary reason for ordering this item. List any additional ICD9 codes that would further describe the medical need for the item (up to 3 codes).

QUESTION SECTION: This section is used to gather clinical information to determine medical necessity. Answer each question which applies to the items ordered, circling "Y" for yes, "N" for no, "D" for does not apply, a number if this is offered as an answer option, or fill in the blank if other information is requested.

NAME OF PERSON
ANSWERING SECTION B
QUESTIONS: If a clinical professional other than the ordering physician (e.g., home health nurse, physical therapist, dietician), or a physician employee answers the questions of Section B, he/she must print his/her name, give his/her professional title and the name of his/her employer where indicated. If the physician is answering the questions, this space may be left blank.

SECTION C: **(To be completed by the supplier)**

NARRATIVE
DESCRIPTION OF
EQUIPMENT & COST: Supplier gives **(1)** a narrative description of the item(s) ordered, as well as all options, accessories, supplies and drugs; **(2)** the supplier's charge for each item, option, accessory, supply and drug; and **(3)** the Medicare fee schedule allowance for each item/option/accessory/supply/drug, if applicable.

SECTION D: **(To be completed by the physician)**

PHYSICIAN
ATTESTATION: The physician's signature certifies **(1)** the CMN which he/she is reviewing includes Sections A, B, C and D; **(2)** the answers in Section B are correct; and **(3)** the self-identifying information in Section A is correct.

PHYSICIAN SIGNATURE   After completion and/or review by the physician of Sections A, B and C, the physician must sign and date the CMN in Section D, verifying the Attestation appearing in this Section. The physician's signature also certifies the items ordered are medically necessary for this patient. Signature and date stamps are not acceptable.

Fig 4-1—cont'd   **B,** back. (Courtesy U.S. Department of Health & Human Services, Centers for Medicare & Medicaid Services.)

Participating Versus Nonparticipating Providers

A **participating provider (PAR)** is one who contracts with the third-party payer and agrees to abide by certain rules and regulations of that carrier. In doing so, the provider usually must accept the insurance carrier's allowable fee as payment in full (after patient deductibles and coinsurance are met) and may not bill the patient for the balance. Some insurance companies offer certain incentives to providers if they agree to become PARs, such as processing claims more quickly and furnishing claims with preidentifying information. Another advantage of becoming a PAR is that payment from the insurer is paid directly to the provider rather than to the patient.

A **nonparticipating provider (nonPAR)** has no contractual agreement with the insurance carrier; the provider does not have to accept an insurance company's reimbursement as payment in full. Patients can be billed for the difference between the insurance carrier's allowed fee and the provider's actual fee. (Medicare limits how much a nonPAR can charge, however.) One disadvantage of being nonPAR is that, typically, insurance payments are sent to the patient, rather than to the provider.

Miscellaneous Terms

Copayment—A way of sharing medical costs often associated with managed care. Here, the patient pays a flat fee every time he or she receives a medical service (for example, $15 for every visit to the doctor). The healthcare plan typically pays the rest of covered expenses.

Covered Expenses—Covered healthcare services are those medical procedures the health plan (insurer) agrees to pay, which are listed in the health insurance policy.

Non-cancellable Policy—A policy that guarantees the patient/insured can receive health insurance coverage as long as the premiums are paid on time—also called a guaranteed renewable policy.

Primary Care Physician (PCP)—A family physician, internist, obstetrician-gynecologist, or pediatrician who is usually the patient's first contact for healthcare. A PCP monitors the patient's health, diagnoses and treats routine health problems, and refers the patient to a specialist if another level of healthcare is needed. *Note:* Many health plans pay for a specialist only if the patient is referred by his or her PCP.

Provider—Any person (doctor, nurse, dentist) or institution (hospital or clinic) that provides medical care.

Third-Party Payer—Any payer for healthcare services other than the patient. This can be an insurance company, a managed care organization (HMO or PPO), or the federal government.

What Did You Learn?

1. When a child is listed on both parents' health plans, which one pays first?
2. List some exceptions to the birthday rule.
3. What are some possible sources of overinsurance?
4. Name the four stipulations that determine medical necessity.

SUMMARY CHECKPOINTS

▶ The two basic types of health insurance plans are indemnity (fee-for-service) and managed care. Under the indemnity type of plan, the patient may visit any healthcare provider, such as a physician or hospital. The patient or the medical provider sends the bill to the insurance company, which typically pays a certain percentage of the fee after the patient meets the policy's annual deductible. A fee-for-service plan might pay 80% of a medical bill. The patient would pay the remaining 20% of the bill—an amount often called coinsurance. Managed care organizations finance medical care in a way that provides incentives for patients to maintain good health. Most managed care plans designate which healthcare providers and facilities patients can receive treatment from. Managed care plans also attempt to make patients and physicians aware of the costs associated with their healthcare decisions. Advocates of managed care claim that by emphasizing health maintenance and illness prevention, managed care organizations reduce the number of expensive medical treatments in the long run.

▶ **Group health insurance** involves one insurance policy covering a group of people. Usually a company establishes a group health insurance plan to cover its employees; however, health insurance plans are not limited to employers. Many different specialized groups can obtain a group health insurance plan for their members, such as clubs/organizations, special interest groups, trade associations, and church/religious groups. An individual health insurance policy covers one person, or a family, on one plan.

▶ The advantages of group health insurance are as follows:
• Group policies are usually less expensive than individual policies.
• Everyone usually is eligible for coverage regardless of health status.
• Coverage is typically comprehensive.
• Premiums can be deducted from paychecks (if it is the policy of the employer).
• Coverage generally cannot be terminated because of frequent claims.

- Protection under HIPAA allows an individual to move from one job to another without the fear of exclusions because of preexisting conditions.

▶ The disadvantages of group health insurance are that:
- Individuals have little or no choice in the type of coverage provided under the group contract.
- Individuals must accept whatever coverage the group policy provides; modifications are not optional.
- Individuals often lose comprehensive coverage when they no longer belong to the "group," even though they may have "conversion" privileges (e.g.; COBRA).
- Premiums for conversion policies tend to be much higher.

▶ The major sources of health insurance are as follows:
- *Medicare*—A federal health insurance program for individuals 65 years old and older and individuals younger than 65 with certain disabilities.
- *Medicaid*—A joint federal-state health insurance program that is run by the individual states. Medicaid covers some low-income individuals and certain categories of disabled individuals.
- *TRICARE/CHAMPVA*—TRICARE is the U.S. military's comprehensive healthcare program. TRICARE covers active duty personnel and their eligible family members and retirees and their qualifying family members. CHAMPVA is a healthcare benefits program for the spouse or widow (or widower) and children of certain qualifying categories of veterans.
- *Disability insurance*—Insurance that is designed to replace a portion of an individual's gross income in the case of an accident or illness that is unrelated to his or her employment.
- *Social Security Disability Insurance (SSDI)*—An insurance program administered by the SSA and funded by a combination of FICA taxes withheld from employees' pay and matching contributions of the employer. SSDI pays healthcare benefits to qualifying disabled workers.
- *Workers' compensation*—A type of insurance that pays workers who are injured or disabled on the job or suffer from job-related illnesses.

▶ Miscellaneous healthcare coverage options include:
- *Medical savings account*—A health insurance option for certain qualifying self-employed individuals and small businesses consisting of two components: a low-cost, high-deductible insurance policy and a tax-advantaged savings account. Individuals pay for their own healthcare up to the annual deductible by withdrawing funds from the savings account or paying medical bills out of pocket. The insurance policy then pays for most or all costs of covered services after the deductible is met.
- *Flexible spending account*—Offers tax advantages to the employer and the employee. Provides reimbursement for medical expenses that are not typically covered by a high-deductible, major medical policy, e.g., insurance premiums, dental, vision, and child care.
- *Health insurance exchange*—Proposes a choice of plans with common rules governing how the plan is offered, its cost, and providing information to help consumers better understand the choices available to them.
- *Accountable care organizations*—A network of doctors and hospitals similar to an HMO that shares responsibility for providing care to patients. ACOs would agree to manage all of the healthcare needs of a minimum of 5000 Medicare beneficiaries for at least 3 years. Goals for an ACO are to determine how to successfully
  - keep patients within the ACO, encouraging them to stay healthy and take more responsibility for their own healthcare and
  - encourage patients to use healthcare providers that are part of the ACO network to keep the overall costs down within the organization.

▶ Health insurance "watchdogs" include the following:
- The Joint Commission evaluates and accredits health care organizations and programs, including hospitals, home care organizations, and other healthcare organizations that provide long-term care, behavioral care, and laboratory and ambulatory care services.
- National Committee for Quality Assurance (NCQA) accredits HMOs and other managed care organizations.
- American Accreditation HealthCare Commission/ URAC accredits PPOs and other managed care networks.
- Accreditation Association for Ambulatory Health Care accredits outpatient health care settings, such as ambulatory surgery centers, radiation oncology centers, and student health centers.
- Community Health Accreditation Program accredits community, home health, and hospice programs; public health departments; and nursing centers.
- Consumer Coalition for Quality Health Care is a national, nonprofit organization of consumer groups advocating for consumer protections and quality assurance programs and policies.

▶ COBRA gives workers and their dependents who lose their health insurance benefits the right to continue group coverage temporarily under the same group health plan sponsored by their employer in certain instances when coverage under the plan would otherwise end. The law generally covers group health plans maintained by employers with 20 or more employees in the prior year.

CLOSING SCENARIO

Barbara and Joy have learned much about the fundamentals of medical insurance. The first four chapters have given them a good foundation of knowledge regarding health insurance in general. The legal and ethical side of health insurance has been particularly informative, and the women are aware of the importance of having a sound footing in this area. On their own, they have researched the HIPAA rules and regulations extensively. Joy is considering enrolling in a business law course in the evenings to enhance her understanding of law as it pertains to healthcare.

The two women have become involved in the Student Health Careers Club and developed an "activity board" to encourage other students to take part in a health fair being sponsored by the free clinic where Barbara volunteers. The main theme they have chosen is, "Educating Patients about Their Rights." They intend to apply what they have learned in class and through their research to a short presentation to clinic visitors.

WEBSITES TO EXPLORE

- For live links to the following websites, please visit the Evolve site at
  http://evolve.elsevier.com/Beik/today/
- For a comprehensive list of health insurance terms and their definitions, log on to the following websites:
  http://www.cms.hhs.gov/apps/glossary/
  http://www.bcbs.com/glossary/glossary.html/
  http://www.valleyhealth.biz/glossary.html/
- For more information on healthcare in general, explore these websites
  http://www.cms.hhs.gov/
  http://www.ahima.org/
  http://www.hipaa.org/

- Browse this CMS website to learn more about HIPAA:
  http://www.cms.hhs.gov/hipaa/

Author's Note: Websites change frequently. If any of these URLs is unavailable, use applicable guide words in your Internet search to acquire additional information on the various subjects listed.

REFERENCES AND RESOURCES

The White House of President Barack Obama: *The American Recovery and Reinvestment Act of 2009,* Washington, DC, February 13, 2009. http://www.whitehouse.gov/administration/eop/ostp/library/compliance/recoveryact/.

United States Department of Labor: *Notice of Changes Under HIPAA to COBRA Continuation Coverage Under Group Health Plans,* Washington, DC. www.dol.gov/ebsa/publications/cobra.html/.

CHAPTER 5

Claim Submission Methods

Chapter Outline

I. Overview of the Health Insurance Claims Process
  A. Two Basic Claims Submission Methods
  B. Proposed Revisions to the CMS-1500 (08-05) Form
II. Electronic Claims
III. Health Insurance Portability and Accountability Act (HIPAA)
  A. Electronic Transactions and Code Set Requirements
  B. Privacy Requirements
  C. Security Requirements
  D. National Identifier Requirements
IV. The New HIPAA 5010 Standards
V. The Electronic Insurance Claims Process
  A. Essential Information for Claims Processing
    1. Patient Information Form
      a. New Patient Information
      b. Insurance Section
      c. Additional Insurance
      d. Insurance Authorization and Assignment

    2. Patient Insurance Identification Card
    3. Patient Health Record
    4. Encounter Form
    5. Patient Ledger Card
  B. Verifying Insurance with New Technology
VI. Advantages of Electronic Claims
VII. Two Ways to Submit Electronic Claims
  A. Claims Clearinghouses
  B. Direct Claims
  C. Clearinghouses Versus Direct
VIII. The Universal Claim Form (CMS-1500)
  A. Format of the Form
  B. Optical Character Recognition
    1. Using OCR Format Rules
  C. Who Uses the Paper Form?
  D. Proofreading
  E. Claim Attachments
  F. Tracking Claims

CHAPTER OBJECTIVES

After completion of this chapter, the student should be able to:

1. Explain how HIPAA's technology standards influence electronic claims
2. Explain how technology influenced electronic claims
3. Discuss the impact of HIPAA on claims submission
4. Determine the rationale for the new HIPAA 5010 Standards
5. Outline the electronic billing process and list the information necessary for the process
6. Identify the advantages of electronic claims submission
7. Compare and contrast the use of a clearinghouse versus direct claims submission
8. Explain the origin and evolution of the CMS-1500 form

CHAPTER TERMS

ASCII (American Standard Code for Information Interchange)
assign(s) benefits
beneficiary
claim attachments
claims clearinghouse
clean claims
CMS-1500 form
demographic information
dial-up(s)
direct claim submission
electronic protected health information (e-PHI)

employer identification number (EIN)
encounter form
guarantor
HIPAA-covered entity
insurance billing cycle
medical necessity
mono-spaced fonts
national provider identifier (NPI)
OCR scannable
optical character recognition (OCR)

OPENING SCENARIO

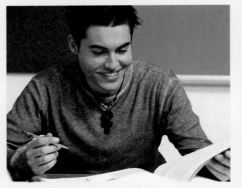

Emilio Sanchez and Latisha Howard are enrolled in a health insurance course at a career school in their area. Emilio graduated from high school just last year and knew immediately what career path he wanted to pursue—health insurance administration. Latisha has worked in the healthcare field for 5 years as a nursing assistant, but she injured her back lifting a patient and had to give up her job at a long-term care facility. Because her experience lies in healthcare, she decided to stay in this discipline but pursue a different avenue that did not involve physical exertion.

In the class in which they are enrolled, the facilitator allows students to progress at their own speed, and Emilio and Latisha found that they not only work well together but also work at about the same pace. Both students feel comfortable that they know the material covered in Unit I well enough to move on to Unit II and continue with their learning experience in health insurance.

After reading over the outline for Chapter 5, Emilio and Latisha discuss how electronic innovations have affected the lives of Americans. They agree they are not surprised that advances in technology have also impacted healthcare and how insurance claims are submitted. They are convinced there are advantages to using practice management software to streamline the day-to-day functions of a medical office. There is so much to learn about claim submission methods, and they are anxious to begin this chapter. The student version of the Medisoft program allows them to follow the steps of how data is entered into the various screens, eventually generating an electronic claim that can be transmitted quickly, accurately, and efficiently for payment.

patient ledger card
practice management software
protected health information
(PHI)

release of information
small (entity) provider
third-party payer
waiver

OVERVIEW OF THE HEALTH INSURANCE CLAIMS PROCESS

The health insurance claims process is an interaction between the healthcare provider and an insurance company (**third-party payer**). Sometimes referred to as the **insurance billing cycle**, this interaction can take anywhere from several days to several months to complete, depending on the number of exchanges in communication required. The cycle begins when a patient visits a healthcare provider, where a medical record is created or an existing one is updated. This record contains **demographic information** including, but not limited to, the patient's name, address, Social Security number, date of birth, sex, telephone number(s), and insurance identification number(s). Also included in the record are examination details, medication prescribed, diagnoses, and suggested treatment. If the patient is a minor, information of the **guarantor** (a parent or an adult related to, or legally responsible for the patient) is recorded. The medical record can be paper, electronic, or a combination of both. It is a legal document and the information it contains is protected by privacy laws.

Once the patient visit is over, the health insurance professional (or medical biller) transmits information from the record to the insurance company in the form of a claim. Historically, claims were submitted using a paper form—the

CMS-1500 form—named for its originator, the Centers for Medicare and Medicaid Services (CMS) (see later). After federal legislation was passed in 1996 (Health Insurance Privacy and Portability Act [HIPAA]), CMS directed providers who submitted claims to Medicare to do so electronically, with few exceptions. However, some providers, for example, dentists and small, rural practices, may still be using the paper form.

After the insurance company receives the claim, it is reviewed, evaluated for validity—patient eligibility, provider credentials, and **medical necessity**—and processed. (To meet the medical necessity criteria, services or supplies must be appropriate and necessary for the symptoms, diagnosis, and/or treatment of the medical condition and they meet the standards of good medical practice.) Approved claims are reimbursed according to pre-negotiated rates between the provider and the insurance contract. Failed claims are rejected, and notice is sent to both the provider and the patient. An explanation of benefits (EOB) or a remittance advice (RA) is generated for both approved and rejected claims. EOBs and RAs are discussed in a later chapter.

Two Basic Claims Submission Methods

In this chapter, we will talk about the two basic methods of submitting health insurance claims, electronic and paper. Submission of claims has gone through a metamorphosis just as health insurance itself has. Prior to the electronic age, providers submitted claims on paper through the mail. Every insurance carrier had its own specialized type of paperwork for submitting claims. Imagine the frustration a health insurance professional must have felt trying to figure out how to complete all these different forms properly. Then, in the mid-1970s, the Health Care Financing Administration (HCFA, pronounced "hick-fa") created a new form for Medicare claims, called the *HCFA-1500*. The form was approved by the American Medical Association Council on Medical Services and was subsequently adopted by all government healthcare programs. Although the HCFA-1500 originally was developed for submitting Medicare claims, it eventually was accepted by most commercial/private insurance carriers to assist the standardization of the claims process. Because HCFA is now called the CMS, the form is called the CMS-1500; however, it is basically the same document as the original. The CMS-1500 has gone through several updates, the most recent being CMS-1500 (08-05).

Because many medical offices currently submit claims electronically, we will discuss the electronic claims submission process first; because some providers still use the paper claim form, submission of claims using the CMS-1500 is also discussed. The information needed for claims processing, however, is the same whether it is a paper or electronic claim.

Proposed Revisions to the CMS-1500 (08-05) Form

The National Uniform Claims Committee (NUCC) is proposing certain data reporting revisions in the Version 005010 837 professional electronic claim transaction. As of this writing, immediate changes are not anticipated to the paper CMS-1500 form; however, after considering several options for revising the form, the NUCC decided to proceed with making "minor changes" to the existing form. Also, a revised NUCC *1500 Health Insurance Claim Form Reference Instruction Manual* is available as of July 2011. For a list of the proposed changes and to view a mock-up of the "cleaned" form, log on to the NUCC website at http://www.nucc.org/. The health insurance professionals should keep up to date with these potential changes to the 1500 form by periodically logging on to the NUCC website.

? What Did You Learn?

1. The health insurance claims process is an interaction between _____ and _____.
2. After the patient visit, information from the record is transmitted to the insurance company in the form of a _____.
3. Provide an accurate definition for "medical necessity."
4. Name the two basic claim submission methods.

ELECTRONIC CLAIMS

With the development and growth of computer technology, specifically medical **practice management software** (a type of software that deals with the day-to-day operations of a medical practice), the way claims are generated and processed has changed. Practice management software allows users to enter patient demographic information, schedule appointments, maintain lists of insurance payers, perform billing tasks, and generate reports. Also known as health information systems, this category of software has made it possible to manage large numbers of insurance claims with various payers accurately and efficiently. Currently, many companies offer such software programs. Computer technology has also made claims submission faster and more accurate at a cost savings to the practice using it.

Although new technologies improved some facets in the administration of healthcare, others made it more complex. Just as in dealing with the many types of paper insurance claim forms and specific standards for completing each, payers once more developed individualized methods for providers to submit claims electronically. The result was added administrative costs for providers and the necessity for their staffs to learn various, often complicated, computer programs.

HEALTH INSURANCE PORTABILITY AND ACCOUNTABILITY ACT

A very significant change that impacted medical billing was the legislation passed by Congress in 1996—the Health Insurance Portability and Accountability Act (HIPAA). HIPAA initiated changes to promote uniformity in healthcare claim submission by adopting standards for electronic health information transactions. This adoption eliminated most of the unique forms used by individual health insurance carriers and the different requirements for processing claims. By October 2003, every **HIPAA-covered entity** (healthcare plans, healthcare providers, and healthcare clearinghouses) was asked to begin using these standard formats for processing claims and payments as well as for the maintenance and transmission of electronic healthcare information and data. Prior to HIPAA, there were over 400 different ways to submit a claim. With HIPAA there are only two—submitting them electronically using the new standard transaction formats or (if the provider meets certain criteria) using the universal CMS-1500 paper form (discussed later in this chapter). This standardization of submitting claims and simplifying the processes involved makes getting paid quicker, easier, and less costly. The HIPAA mandates also help providers take advantage of new technologies, ultimately improving their overall business practices.

As a result of HIPAA, CMS directed all healthcare providers to submit Medicare claims electronically in a HIPAA-compliant format beginning in October 2003. Recognizing that this ruling could generate some challenging situations, the Administrative Simplification Compliance Act (ASCA) of 2001 identified limited exceptions to this requirement, which include:

- Roster billing of Medicare-covered vaccinations
- Dental claims
- Claims in which there are two or more primary plans and Medicare is secondary
- Service interruptions beyond the control of the provider

Also qualifying for exemption are **small entities, or small providers**—those with 25 or fewer full-time employees (FTEs)—and physicians, practitioners, and suppliers with 10 or fewer FTEs. This small entity exemption applies only to billing Medicare electronically, not to implementing HIPAA transactions and code sets.

The intent of HIPAA's Administrative Simplification law was to provide consumers with greater access to healthcare insurance, to protect the privacy of healthcare data, and to promote more standardization and efficiency in the healthcare industry. Although HIPAA covers a number of important healthcare issues, this chapter focuses on the Administrative Simplification portion of the law—specifically HIPAA's Electronic Transactions and Code Sets requirements. There are four parts to HIPAA's Administrative Simplification:

- Electronic transactions and code sets standards requirements
- Privacy requirements
- Security requirements
- National identifier requirements

Following is a brief summary of each of these four parts. For more detailed information on HIPAA's Administrative Simplification Act, visit the Evolve site.

📁 HIPAA Tip

An organization that routinely handles protected health information in any capacity is, in all probability, considered a covered entity.

⭐ Imagine This!

The Rolling Prairie Health Clinic holds a senior health fair every fall. Many Medicare beneficiaries come to the clinic for their annual flu and/or pneumonia shots. Amelia, Rolling Prairie's health insurance professional, uses roster billing as a quick and convenient way to bill Medicare for these vaccinations. Nina, the clinic manager, reminds Amelia that when submitting a roster bill, the provider must have given the same type of vaccination to five or more people on the same date of service and that each type of vaccination must be billed on a separate roster bill. Amelia cannot combine pneumococcal pneumonia vaccines (PPVs) and flu vaccines on the same roster bill.

Electronic Transactions and Code Set Requirements

HIPAA requires every provider who conducts business electronically to use the same healthcare transactions, code sets, and identifiers. HIPAA has identified 10 standard transactions for Electronic Data Interchange (EDI) for the transmission of healthcare data. Claims and encounter information, payment and remittance advice, and claims status and inquiry are some of these standard transactions that affect medical billing and claim submission. The *Current Procedural Terminology, 4th Edition* (CPT-4) and *International Classification of Diseases, 10th Revision* (ICD-10) codes (see Chapters 12 and 13) are examples of code sets for procedure and diagnosis coding, respectively. Other code sets adopted under the Administrative Simplification provisions of HIPAA include those used for claims involving medical supplies, dental services, and drugs.

Privacy Requirements

The *Standards for Privacy of Individually Identifiable Health Information* (Privacy Rule) establishes a set of national standards for the protection of certain health information. The U.S. Department of Health and Human Services (HHS) issued the Privacy Rule to implement one of the HIPAA main requirements. These standards address the use and disclosure of an individual's health information—referred to as **protected health information (PHI)**—as well as standards for an individual's privacy rights to understand and control how his or her health information is used. Within HHS, the Office for Civil Rights (OCR) is responsible for implementing and enforcing the Privacy Rule in regard to voluntary compliance procedures and civil penalties.

A major goal of the Privacy Rule is to ensure that individuals' health information is properly protected while allowing the flow of health information needed to provide and promote high-quality healthcare and to protect the public's health and well-being. The objective is to strike a balance between the uses of information and protecting a patient's privacy.

Security Requirements

The *Security Standards for the Protection of Electronic Protected Health Information* (Security Rule) established a national set of security standards for protecting certain health information that is held or transferred in electronic form. This rule addresses the technical and non-technical safeguards that covered entities must put in place to secure individuals' **electronic protected health information (e-PHI)**. As with the Privacy Rule, the OCR is responsible for enforcing the Security Rules.

A major goal of the Security Rule is to protect the privacy of individuals' health information while allowing covered entities to adopt new technologies to improve the quality and efficiency of patient care.

National Identifier Requirements

HIPAA requires the adoption of a standard unique identifier for every healthcare provider, health plan, and employer that identifies the entity on standard transactions. The Final Rule, issued in January 2004, adopted the **national provider identifier (NPI)** as this standard. The NPI is a 10-digit *intelligence free* number, meaning the number does not carry any information about the provider, such as the state in which he or she practices or the type of specialization. The NPI replaced healthcare identifiers used prior to the onset of this rule, which included Medicare legacy IDs (unique identifiers specific to Medicare), unique provider identification numbers (UPINs), provider identification numbers (PINs), and National Supplier Clearinghouse (NSC) identifiers. NPIs remain with the provider and do not change even if he or she changes locations or specialties.

The NPI should not be confused with the **employer identification number (EIN)**, which is a unique, 9-digit number issued to businesses for use by the Internal Revenue Service (IRS) in the administration of tax laws. Both the NPI and the EIN are used in claims submission.

What Did You Learn?

1. What type of software was instrumental in the expansion of electronic claims?
2. Name the important legislation Congress passed in 1996 that significantly impacted medical billing and claims submission.
3. List who is included in the designation "covered entity."
4. What are the 4 exceptions to ASCA's electronic claims submission requirement?
5. Name the 4 parts to HIPAA's Administration Simplification.
6. *True or False:* The NPI and the EIN are basically the same and can be used interchangeably on claims.

THE NEW HIPAA 5010 STANDARDS

Up until January 2012, HIPAA required the use of Standard X12 transactions to report and inquire about healthcare services. Providers who submitted claims electronically used the 4010/4010A1 version of HIPAA transactions, which are nearly a decade old. A new transaction standard–Version 5010–will be implemented in 2012, and the old Version 4010A1 will no longer be valid. Currently, the date for all entities to be in full compliance with Version 5010 is June 30, 2012; however, it is important that the health insurance professional check the CMS site periodically to see if the compliance date has changed. This new version addresses many of the deficiencies in the former version and accommodates the reporting of NPIs and the new ICD-10 codes (see Chapter 12). The following entities are affected by the switch to Version 5010:

- Hospitals
- Physicians
- Dentists
- Third-party payers
- Vendors
- Billing services
- Laboratories
- Clearinghouses

The following transactions are included in the 5010 Final Rule:

- Healthcare claims for professional, institutional and dental services
- Eligibility for a health plan (inquiry and response)
- Referral certification and authorization
- Healthcare claim status (inquiry and response)
- Enrollment and disenrollment in a health plan
- Healthcare payment and remittance advice
- Healthcare premium payments
- Coordination of benefits
- Healthcare services—request for review and response

Providers who submit claims electronically must use Version 5010 unless they qualify for Exceptions to Electronic Claim Submission Requirements (Box 5-1). Non-compliant transactions received after the compliance deadline, will be rejected as directed by CMS.

Although HIPAA does not require healthcare providers to use electronic transactions, ASCA does impose such a requirement for those who bill Medicare. ASCA requires that all claims submitted to the Medicare program be submitted in electronic form, with limited exceptions. The implication

Box 5-1

Exceptions to HIPAA's Electronic Claim Submission Requirement

- A small provider billing a Medicare fiscal intermediary that has fewer than 25 full-time equivalent (FTE) employees, and a physician, practitioner, or supplier with fewer than 10 FTEs that bills a Medicare carrier
- A dentist
- A participant in a Medicare demonstration project in which paper claim filing is required to report data essential for the demonstration
- A provider that conducts mass immunizations, such as flu injections, and may be permitted to submit paper roster bills

- A provider that submits claims when more than one other payer is responsible for payment prior to Medicare payment
- A provider that furnishes services only outside the United States
- A provider experiencing a disruption in electricity and communication connections that are beyond its control
- A provider that can establish existence of an "unusual circumstance" that precludes electronic submission of claims

of this requirement is that because the claims are submitted electronically, they are also required to comply with HIPAA. Physicians who qualify for exemption under the small provider exemption may continue sending paper claims. A small provider or supplier is defined *as a provider of services with fewer than 25 full-time equivalent employees or a physician, practitioner, facility, or supplier (other than a provider of services) with fewer than 10 full-time equivalent employees* (see Box 5-1).

For more detailed information about 5010, visit the Evolve site to find the link to a CMS article in *MLN Matters*, entitled "An Introductory Overview of the HIPAA 5010."

📁 HIPAA Tip

Small providers who can use paper forms (i.e., CMS-1500 and UB-04) for submitting claims can continue to do so, because the most recent versions of these paper claim forms accommodate the relevant data reported in Version 5010.

💬 What Did You Learn?

1. After January 2010, providers who submit claims electronically must use Standard Version _____.
2. List the entities that are affected by the switch to the new HIPAA Standards Version.
3. The new Standards Version supports the reporting of _____ and the new _____ codes.
4. *True or False:* ASCA requires that all claims submitted to the Medicare program be submitted in electronic form, with no exceptions.
5. Physicians who qualify for exclusion under the _____ exemption may continue sending paper claims.

THE ELECTRONIC INSURANCE CLAIMS PROCESS

Regardless of how claims are submitted, the insurance claims process begins when the patient arrives at the medical facility, at which time he or she is given various forms to read and fill out. The front office staff then enters the information into the medical facility's computer using the practice management software that meets electronic filing requirements as established by the HIPAA claim standards. It is from this information that the claim is generated through the internal functioning of the software.

Essential Information for Claims Processing

The following sections discuss the various forms and documents from which necessary data for generating claims are gathered along with illustrations showing sample data entry screens.

Patient Information Form

A *patient information form,* sometimes referred to as a *patient registration form,* is a document (typically one page) that patients are asked to complete for the following reasons:

1. to gather all necessary demographic information to aid the healthcare professional in providing appropriate treatment,
2. to have a record of current insurance information for claim preparation and submission,
3. to keep health records up to date, and
4. to give the physician/provider authorization to release medical information and to accept assignment for insurance benefits.

When the form is completed, it becomes an integral part of the patient's health record. This information form is considered a legal document, and the information should be updated at least once a year. It is a good idea to ask returning patients whether there have been any changes since they were last in the office. Fig. 5-1 shows a typical patient information form.

New Patient Information

Look at this section in the example patient information form in Fig. 5-1. Note that it asks for general demographic information, such as name, address, Social Security number, and employment. Financial status and self-pay amounts might also need to be identified and communicated completely, clearly, and accurately. The front office staff is also responsible for obtaining treatment consents, release of information consents, necessary authorizations, and assignments. Fig. 5-2 illustrates how demographic information appears on the patient entry screen in a typical type of practice management software.

Medical facilities normally request that patients provide their Social Security numbers. In this age of identity theft, patients may appear reluctant to do so. It is the responsibility of the health insurance professional, or whoever is gathering personal data, to assure the patient that all information will remain strictly confidential.

Insurance Section

The second section contains questions regarding the patient's insurance. Having the patient fill out the blanks in this section is important, but it is also necessary to request and make photocopies of the front and the back of the patient's insurance ID card. The ID card often lists additional information that patients might not routinely include on the form, such as telephone numbers for preauthorization or precertification. Also, it is common for patients to transpose or omit identifying alphabetical characters or numbers or both. It is also recommended to make a copy of the patient's driver's license, or other picture identification, for verification to make certain that the person is not using someone else's insurance card.

ACCOUNT # _____

PATIENT # _____

NEW PATIENT INFORMATION *DATE* _____

PATIENT'S NAME (PLEASE PRINT)	S.S. #	MARITAL STATUS					SEX		BIRTH DATE	AGE
		S	M	W	D	SEP	M	F		

STREET ADDRESS PERMANENT TEMPORARY	CITY AND STATE		ZIP CODE	HOME PHONE#
PATIENT'S EMPLOYER	OCCUPATION (INDICATE IF STUDENT)	HOW LONG EMPLOYED	BUS. PHONE # EXT. #	
EMPLOYER'S STREET ADDRESS	CITY AND STATE		ZIP CODE	
DRUG ALLERGIES, IF ANY	PHARMACY		PHARMACY PHONE #	
SPOUSE OR PARENT'S NAME	S.S. #		BIRTH DATE	
SPOUSE OR PARENT'S EMPLOYER	OCCUPATION (INDICATED IF STUDENT)	HOW LONG EMPLOYED	BUS. PHONE #	
EMPLOYER'S STREET ADDRESS	CITY AND STATE		ZIP CODE	
*SPOUSE'S STREET ADDRESS, IF DIVORCED OR SEPARATED	CITY AND STATE	ZIP CODE	HOME PHONE #	

PLEASE READ: ALL CHARGES ARE DUE AT THE TIME OF SERVICES. IF HOSPITALIZATION IS INDICATED, THE PATIENT IS RESPONSIBLE FOR FURNISHING INSURANCE CLAIM FORMS TO THE OFFICE PRIOR TO HOSPITALIZATION.

REFERRED BY	STREET ADDRESS, CITY, STATE	ZIP CODE	PHONE #
BLUE SHIELD (GIVE NAME OF POLICYHOLDER) ☐	☐ ALLIANCE ☐ OTHER ☐ ALLIANCE SELECT	BIRTH DATE	POLICY #
OTHER (WRITE IN NAME OF INSURANCE COMPANY) ☐	NAME OF POLICYHOLDER	BIRTH DATE	POLICY #
OTHER (WRITE IN NAME OF INSURANCE COMPANY) ☐	NAME OF POLICYHOLDER	BIRTH DATE	POLICY #

MEDICARE # ☐	RAILROAD RETIREMENT # ☐	MEDICAID # ☐

INDUSTRIAL ☐	WERE YOU INJURED ON THE JOB? ☐ YES ☐ NO	DATE OF INJURY	INDUSTRIAL CLAIM #
ACCIDENT ☐	WAS AN AUTOMOBILE INVOLVED? ☐ YES ☐ NO	DATE OF ACCIDENT	NAME OF ATTORNEY

WERE X-RAYS TAKEN OF THIS INJURY OR PROBLEM? ☐ YES ☐ NO	IF YES, WHERE WERE X-RAYS TAKEN? (HOSPITAL, ETC.)	DATE X-RAYS TAKEN

HAS ANY MEMBER OF YOUR IMMEDIATE FAMILY BEEN TREATED BY OUR PHYSICIAN(S) BEFORE? INCLUDE NAME OF PHYSICIAN AND FAMILY MEMBER.

NEAREST RELATIVE OR FRIEND NOT RESIDING WITH YOU	STREET ADDRESS, CITY, STATE	ZIP CODE	PHONE #

ALL PROFESSIONAL SERVICES RENDERED ARE CHARGED TO THE PATIENT. NECESSARY FORMS WILL BE COMPLETED TO HELP EXPEDITE INSURANCE CARRIER PAYMENTS. HOWEVER, THE PATIENT IS RESPONSIBLE FOR ALL FEES, REGARDLESS OF INSURANCE COVERAGE. IT IS ALSO CUSTOMARY TO PAY FOR SERVICES WHEN RENDERED UNLESS OTHER ARRANGEMENTS HAVE BEEN MADE IN ADVANCE WITH OUR OFFICE BOOKKEEPER.

INSURANCE AUTHORIZATION AND ASSIGNMENT

Name of Policy Holder_____   HIC Number _____

I request that payment of authorized Medicare/Other Insurance company benefits be made either to me or on my behalf to _____
for any services furnished me by that party who accepts assignment/physician. Regulations pertaining to Medicare assignment of benefits apply.
I authorize any holder of medical or other information about me to release to the Social Security Administration and Health Care Financing Administration or its intermediaries or carriers any information needed for this or a related Medicare claim/other Insurance Company claim. I permit a copy of this authorization to be used in place of the original, and request payment of medical insurance benefits either to myself or to the party who accepts assignment. I understand it is mandatory to notify the health care provider of any other party who may be responsible for paying for my treatment. (Section 1128B of the Social Security Act and 31 U.S.C. 3801-3812 provides penalties for withholding this information.)

Signature_____   Date_____

Accounts past 60 days will accrue an interest charge.   NEW PATIENT INFORMATION

Fig. 5-1 A typical patient information form.

Additional Insurance

In some cases, patients may be covered under more than one insurance policy. For example, a Medicare patient might have supplemental coverage through another payer. Most patient information forms have a separate section where additional insurance is listed. Information from a secondary insurance policy should be noted in this section, including the name of the policy, the policyholder's name, and the policy numbers. It is important for the health insurance professional to confirm that the "additional insurance" is

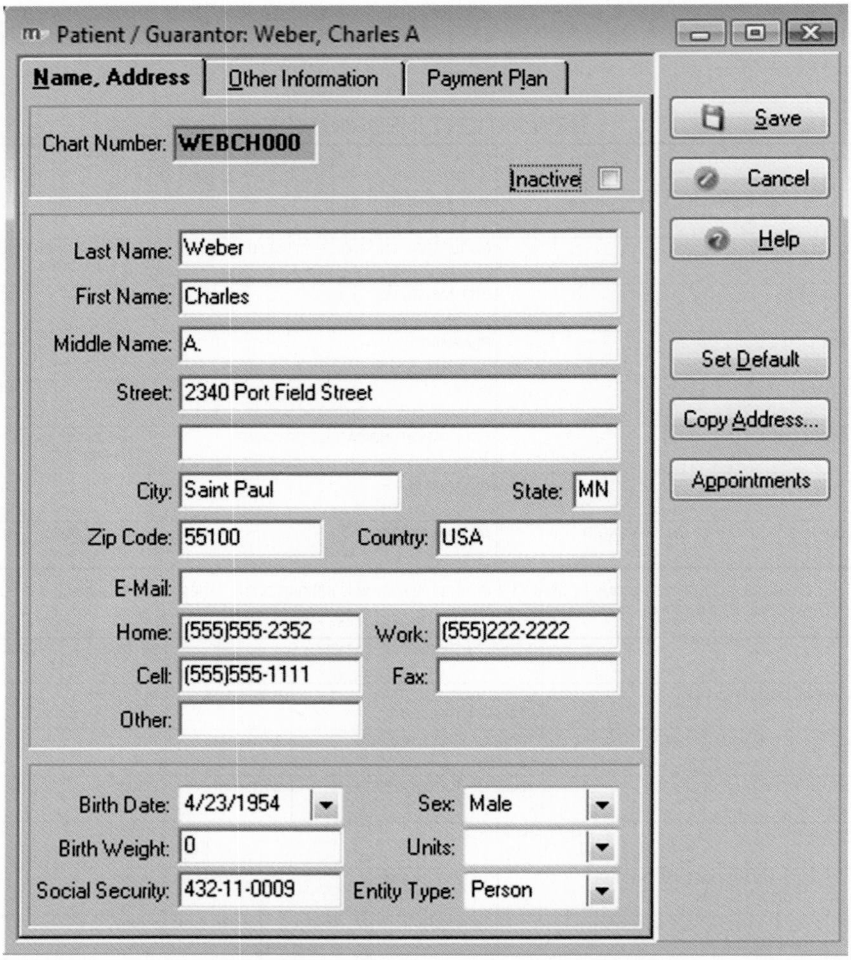

Fig. 5-2 Patient entry screen using practice management software. (Screenshot used by permission of MCKESSON Corporation. All Rights Reserved. ©MCKESSON Corporation 2012.)

secondary. Some patients, particularly elderly ones, can become confused over the technicalities of dual insurance coverage. If the patient is uncertain which of the policies is primary and which is secondary, the health insurance professional may have to do some detective work, such as telephoning one or both of the insuring agencies, to find out. Fig. 5-3 shows the screen where insurance information is entered.

Insurance Authorization and Assignment

The section on insurance authorization and assignment should be completed and signed by the patient or responsible party, in the case of a minor or mentally disabled individual. This section gives the healthcare professional the authorization to release the information necessary to complete the insurance claim form. It also **"assigns benefits"**—that is, it authorizes the insurance company to send the payment directly to the healthcare professional. This authorization should be updated at least once a year, unless it is a "lifetime" **release of information** worded specifically for Medicare claims.

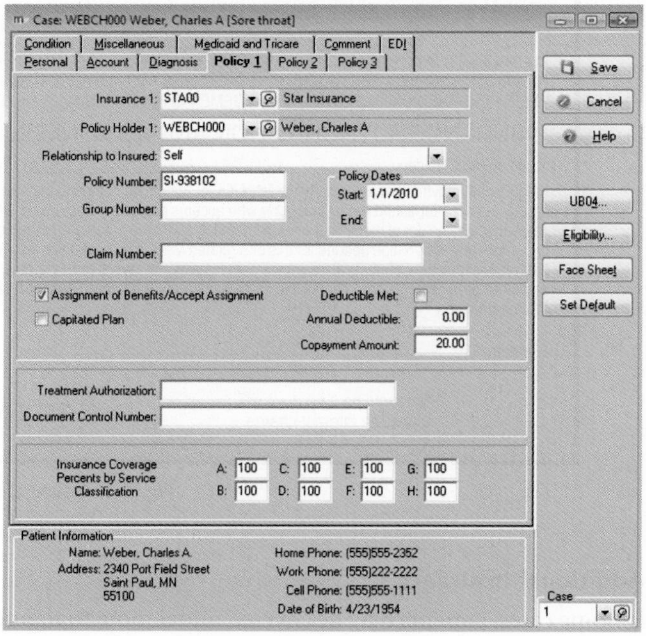

Fig. 5-3 Insurance information using practice management software. (Screenshot used by permission of MCKESSON Corporation. All Rights Reserved. ©MCKESSON Corporation 2012.)

Patient Insurance Identification Card

Every insurance company has a unique identification card that it issues to its subscribers. With Medicare, every individual (referred to as a **beneficiary**) has his or her own individual card. Other insurers, such as Blue Cross and Blue Shield, may issue a card that covers not only the subscriber but also his or her spouse and any dependents included on the policy; this arrangement is referred to as a *family plan*. As mentioned previously, at the same time the patient completes the information form, the health insurance professional should ask to see his or her insurance ID card and make a photocopy of it to keep in the health record. It is important to always make sure to copy both front and back of the ID card if there is information on the back. On subsequent visits, the health insurance professional should ask the patient whether there is any change in coverage. If so, he or she should ask for and make a copy of the new card. The rationale for this procedure is to have complete and correct insurance information on file for the purpose of accurate claims submission. It is also helpful for obtaining telephone numbers to contact for preauthorization/precertification from the carrier if certain procedures or inpatient hospitalization is required. Fig. 5-4 shows the front and back of a typical insurance ID card.

Patient Health Record

After the patient information form is completed, the health insurance professional should examine it to ensure that all necessary information has been entered and that the entries are legible. The form is customarily either placed in the patient's paper health record near the front or scanned into an electronic medical record (EMR) after the information is typed into the data fields of the EMR, so that the health insurance professional has easy access to it when it is time to complete and submit a claim. Details of the patient medical record are discussed in Chapter 3. To review, a medical record is an account of a patient's medical assessment, investigation, and course of treatment. It is a source of information and a vital component in quality patient care. A complete medical record should

- outline the reason for the patient's visit to the healthcare professional,
- document the healthcare professional's findings,
- include a detailed discussion of the recommended treatment,
- provide information to any referring physician or other healthcare provider,
- serve as a teaching or research tool (or both), and
- provide a means for assessing the quality of care by the practitioner or other healthcare provider.

The clinical chart note illustrated in Fig. 5-5 is a typical example taken from a patient's health record.

★ Imagine This!

Tammy Butler visited Dr. Harold Norton, her family care provider, on February 10 for her yearly wellness examination plus routine diagnostics. Dr. Norton's health insurance professional submitted the claim the day after the visit. A month later, Tammy received an EOB from her health insurer indicating that the services were not covered under her policy. Assuming that her policy did not cover wellness examinations, Tammy forgot about it. During Christmas vacation of that same year, Tammy again visited Dr. Norton for a case of sinusitis. The claim was denied again by her insurer. Puzzled that a second claim had been denied, Tammy contacted Dr. Norton's office and, after some extensive research, learned that they had filed her claims under an old ID number from a previous employer. The problem was that it was now January of a new year—past the deadline for filing claims for the previous year. The health insurance professional at Dr. Norton's office informed Tammy that she was responsible for the charges.

Iowa Med Co.

	HOSPITAL CO-PAY	EMERGENCY ROOM CO-PAY
GROUP NUMBER 17098-020-00004	$ .00	$ 50.00

MEMBER
LINDA L. FUHR

MEMBER NUMBER
H-550-XX-5072-02

PRIMARY CARE PHYSICIAN
GEOFF LOMAN

OFFICE VISIT
CO-PAY
$10.00

ABC INSURANCE COMPANY
P.O. BOX 12340
FRESNO   CA   93765

**IMPORTANT
INFORMATION
ON REVERSE**

FOR BENEFITS, ELIGIBILITY AND
CLAIMS CALL MEMBER SERVICES: 1-800-XXX-XXXX
FOR PRECERTIFICATION AND
REFERRALS CALL: 1-800-XXX-XXXX

PAYER NUMBER   60054 0106

RX COPAY $10.00   RX GROUP NUMBER 0067-0000   PHARMACY PLAN

For mental health services, call 1-800-424-4047

Member: Co-pays and higher benefits apply to services rendered by your primary care physician (PCP) or through your PSP's referral. Call your PCP in advance for an appointment. If a life threatening emergency exists, seek immediate attention. If admitted, call Member Services within 48 hours. When not referred by your PCP, you are responsible for any precertification required by your plan. For you or your physician to obtain precertification, call Member Services. Failure to obtain precertification may result in reduced benefits.
Providers: Call Member Services to verify eligibility; this card does not guarantee coverage. In case of an emergency, notify Member Services the next business day.
This plan is administered by ABC Insurance Company.

Smith & Co. Health Plans

Fig. 5-4 Insurance ID card.

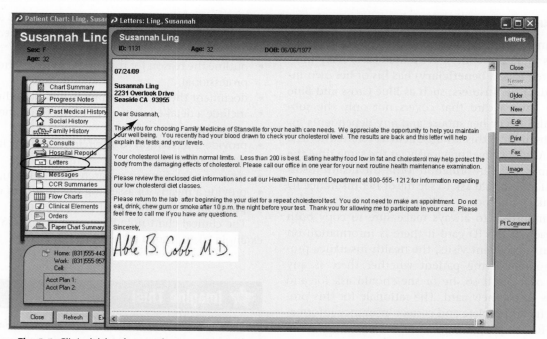

Fig. 5-5 Clinical (chart) notes from a patient's health record. (Screenshot used by permission of MCKESSON Corporation. All Rights Reserved. ©MCKESSON Corporation 2012.)

Stop and Think

In the previous scenario described in Imagine This!, do you agree with Dr. Norton's health insurance professional that Tammy is responsible for the charges on the two visits in question? What should the health insurance professional have done to prevent this?

Note: For offices that have switched from paper records to electronic medical records (EMRs), this process may be different. EMRs are discussed in detail in Chapter 16.

Encounter Form

We have discussed three of the items necessary for generating an insurance claim. Now we look at a document used by most medical practices that is often referred to as the **encounter form**. This multipurpose billing form is known by many names (e.g., superbill, routing form, patient service slip). The encounter form can be customized to medical specialties and preprinted with common diagnoses and procedures for that particular specialty. Encounter forms can be either paper or electronic. Fig. 5-6 shows an example of a paper encounter form; Fig. 5-7 illustrates an electronic version of this form.

Typically, the encounter form is clipped to the front of the patient's paper medical record before the patient is seen in the clinical area. (If the medical facility utilizes EMRs, this information would be available on the selected screen.) Note the variety of information included on the form shown in both figures:

- demographic,
- accounting,
- professional services rendered,
- procedure (CPT) codes
- professional fees, and
- return appointment information.

It is important that the sections dealing with professional services and diagnostic and procedure codes be updated annually so that revised codes are changed, new codes are added, and old codes are deleted.

The following is a typical routine in many medical offices. Each morning, the medical records clerk (or whichever member of the healthcare team is in charge of this task) prepares the health records for the patients who are to be seen that day. An encounter form is attached to the front of each record, and any areas on the form regarding the date of service, patient demographics, and accounting information are filled out. (If computerized patient accounting software is used, this information is printed automatically on the form.) Each encounter form has a number (usually at the top) that serves as an identifier for that particular patient visit.

As each patient is seen in the clinical area, the healthcare provider indicates on the form what services or procedures were performed along with the corresponding fees. The provider signs the encounter form and indicates whether and when the patient needs to return or have any follow-up tests. It is important that the encounter form is checked for accuracy, after which the front office staff totals the day's charges, enters any payment received, and calculates the balance due. The patient receives a copy of the completed encounter form, and a copy is retained in the medical office for accounting purposes and future reference in case any question comes up regarding that particular visit. Many offices file these forms by number within files that are separated into months and days. Medical offices are subject to

Tri-State Medical Group
400 North 4th Street • Anytown, Iowa 50622
Phone: 319-555-5734 • Fax: 319-555-5758
Fed. Tax I.D. # 42-1435XXX

008112

ACCOUNT NO.		DOB		DATE OF SERVICE	
PATIENT NAME			PROVIDER		
INSURANCE ID #-PRIMARY			SECONDARY		

DESCRIPTION	CODE		FEE	DESCRIPTION	CODE	FEE	DESCRIPTION	CODE	FEE
OFFICE VISIT	NEW	ESTAB.		DT, Pediatric	90702		Removal Skin Tags up to 15 Lesions	*11200	
Minimum	99201	99211		MMR	90707		Exc. Malignant Lesion, Trunk, Arm or Leg		
Brief	99202	99212		Oral Polio	90712		Exc. Malignant Lesion, Face, Ear, Eyelid, Nose		
Limited	99203	99213		IVP Polio	90713		Exc. Malignant Lesion, Scalp, Hand, Neck, Feet		
Extended	99204	99214		Varicella	90716		Lacer, Repair 2.5cm or Less/Location:	*12001	
Comprehensive	99205	99215		Td, Adult	90718		Scalp, Nk, Axille, Ext. Genitalia, Trk, Hands/Feet		
Prenatal Care		59400		DTP & HIB	90720		Lacer, Repair 2.5cm or Less/Location:	*12011	
Global		99024		Influenza	90659		Face, Ears, Eyelids, Nose, Lips & Mucous Mem.		
PREVENTIVE	NEW	ESTAB.		Hepatitis B, Newborn to 11 Years	90744		Burn w/Dressing, w/o Anesth. Small	16020	
Infant	99381	99391		Hepatitis B, 11-19 Years	90747		Wart Removal	*17110	
Age 1-4	99382	99392		Hepatitis B, 20 Years & Above	90746		Removal FB Conjunct. Ext. Eye	*65205	
Age 5-11	99383	99393		Pneumococcal	90732		Removal FB Ext. Auditory Canal	69200	
Age 12-17	99384	99394		Hemophilus Infl. B	90645		Ear Lavage	69210	
Age 18-39	99385	99395		Therapeutic:	90782		Tympanometry	92567	
Age 40-64	99386	99396		Allergy Inject Single	95115		EKG Tracing Only w/o Interp. & Rept	93005	
Age 65 & Over	99387	99397		Allergy Inject Multiple	95117		Nebulizer Therapy (x)	94640	
OFFICE CONSULTATION				B-12	J3420		Pulse Oximetry	94760	
Limited		99241		Injection / Aspiration	20600		Cryosurgery		
Intermediate		99242		Small joint-Finger, Toes, Ganglion			Debridement	11041	
Extended		99243		Injection / Aspiration	20605		Excise Ingrown Toenail	11730	
Comprehensive		99244		Intermediate jt-Wrist, Elbow, Ankle			Colposcopy w/Biopsy	57454	
Complex		99245		Injection / Aspiration	20610		Leep	57460	
LABORATORY PROCEDURES				Major jt. - Shoulder, Hip, Knee			Endometrial Bx	58100	
Venipuncture		36415		Inject Tendon/Ligament	20550		Cryotherapy	57511	
Routine Urinalysis w/o Microscopy		81002		Aristacort	J3302		Peak Flow Measurement	94160-52	
Hemoccult		82270		Depo Provera	J1055		Intradermal Tests CMI # Doses =	95025	
Glucose Blood Reagent Strip		82948		Rocephin	J0696		Intradermal Tests/Allergens	95024	
Wet Mount		87210		OFFICE PROCEDURE / MINOR SURGERY			Intravenous Access	36000	
PAP Smear		88155		I & D Abscess	10060		Immunotherapy/Single Injection	95120	
Urine Pregnancy		81025		Removal FB Subcutaneous	*10120		Immunotherapy/Double Injection	95125	
Other:		99000		I & D Hematoma	10140		Regular Spirometry	94010	
X-RAY				Puncture Aspiration Abscess	10160		Spirometry Read by Physician	94010-26	
X-ray Cervical Spine		75052		Exc. Ben. Lesion #:			Spirometry w/pre & Post Bronchodilator	94060	
X-ray Thoracic Spine		72070		Location:			Spirometry/Bronchodilator read by Doctor	94060-26	
X-ray Lumbar Spine (2)		72100		Exc. Ben. Lesion #:			Skin Prick Test: # of Tests =	95004	
X-ray Lumbar Spine (Comp)		72110		Location:			Vial Preparation	95165	

X-ray Pelvis (1 view)	72170	**HOSPITAL ORDERS**	
X-ray Sacrum & Coccyx	72220		
X-ray Clavicle (Complete)	73000	☐ OB Non-Stress Test	☐ Cystogram	☐ Physical Therapy
X-ray Shoulder (2) or	73030	☐ OB Ultrasound-Diagnostic	☐ MRI	
X-ray Humerus (2 views)	73060	☐ OB Ultrasound-Routine	☐ CT Scan _____	
X-ray Elbow (AP & LATE)	73070	☐ Biophysical Profile	☐ Chest X-ray	☐ Diet Consultation
X-ray Forearm (AP & LA)	73090	☐ Mammogram-Diagnostic	☐ X-ray _____	
X-ray Wrist (AP & LATE)	73100	☐ Mammogram-Routine	☐ Bone Densitometry	
X-ray Wrist (3 Views)	73110		☐ EKG	☐ Laboratory
X-ray Hand (2 Views)	73120	☐ Ultrasound _____	☐ Holter Monitor	
X-ray Hand (3 Views)	73130	☐ Gallbladder Ultrasound	☐ Echocardiogram	
X-ray Finger (2 Views)	73140	☐ Pelvic Ultrasound	☐ Treadmill _____	
X-ray Hip (2 Views)	73510	☐ Doppler Studies _____	☐ Thallium Stress Test	
X-ray Hips (Bilateral)	73520		☐ Doppler Studies_____	
X-ray Scoliosis (2 AP & LA)	72069	☐ IVP	☐ PFT-Partial	
X-ray Femur (AP & LATE)	73550	☐ Upper GI	☐ PFT-Complete	
X-ray Knee (AP & LATE)	73560	☐ Lower GI	☐ Cardiac Rehab	
X-ray Knee (3 Views)	73564	☐ Barium Enema		

X-ray Tibia & Fibula	73590
X-ray Ankle (3 Views)	73610
X-ray Foot (AP & LATER)	73620
X-ray Foot (AP. LA.,)	73630
X-ray Calcaneus (2 Views)	73650
X-ray Toes	73660
X-ray Pelvis & Hip Inf	73540
Elbow, Minimum of 3 Views	73080
IMMUNIZATIONS & INJECTIONS	
PPD Intradermal TB Tine	86580
DTaP	90700

☐ Barium Swallow

AUTHORIZATION TO PAY BENEFITS AND RELEASE INFORMATION TO TRI-STATE MEDICAL GROUP: I hereby authorize payment directly to the undersigned Physician of all Surgical and / or Medical Benefits, if any, otherwise payable to me for his / her services as described above. I have read and understand the Financial Policy and that I am financially responsible for charges not covered by this insurance. I also authorize the undersigned Physician to release any information acquired in the course of my examination or treatment.

Signed: _____

Date: _____

Provider's Signature   Date

PREVIOUS BALANCE	
CHARGES TODAY	
TOTAL	
AMOUNT PAID	
BALANCE DUE	

DX or Other Information	Samples:
	Your next appointment is:

BILLING COPY

Fig. 5-6 Sample paper encounter form.

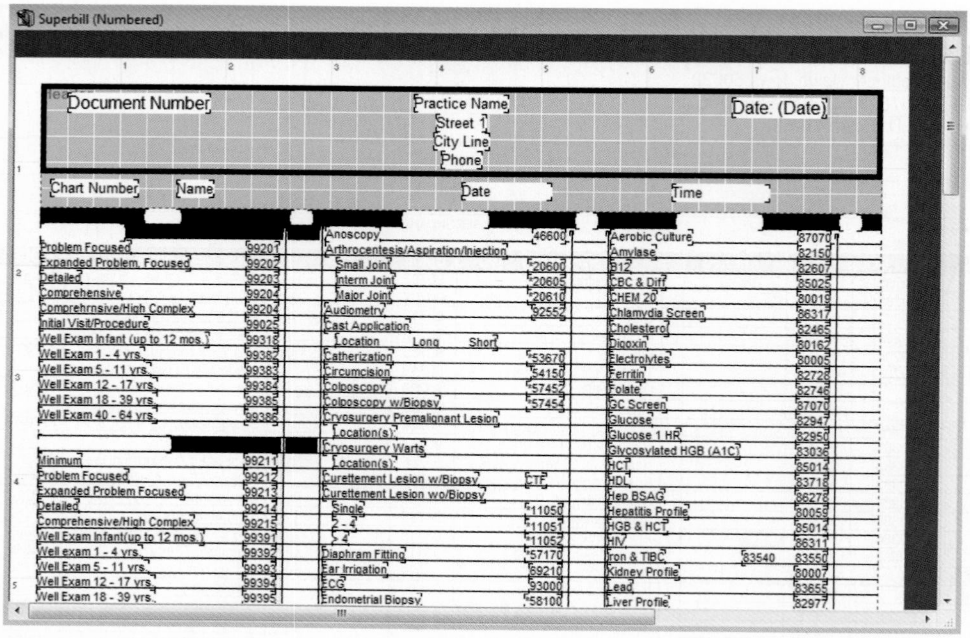

Fig. 5-7 Sample electronic encounter form. (Screenshot used by permission of MCKESSON Corporation. All Rights Reserved. ©MCKESSON Corporation 2012.)

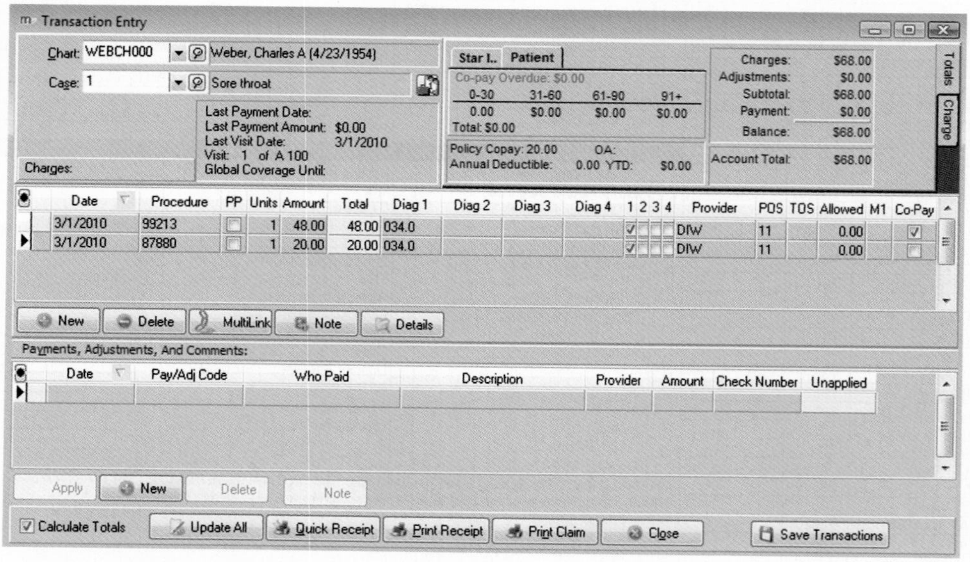

Fig. 5-8 Entering patient information into an electronic encounter form. (Screenshot used by permission of MCKESSON Corporation. All Rights Reserved. ©MCKESSON Corporation 2012.)

accounting and insurance audits. The original encounter form can be requested by auditors to verify services rendered to any patient or on any date of service. If practice management software is used, the information from the encounter form is entered into the computer and is computed automatically. A statement can immediately be printed for the patient showing the payment(s) and current balance, if any. Fig. 5-8 is an example of the screen where information from the encounter form is entered. Fig. 5-9 is a sample statement printout.

Patient Ledger Card

In offices that do not use practice management software, patient charges and payments are kept track of on a **patient ledger card** (Fig. 5-10). A ledger card is an accounting form on which professional service descriptions, charges, payments, adjustments, and current balance are posted chronologically. Although many medical offices are becoming computerized, there are still some that are not, so to become a well-rounded healthcare professional, you must be familiar with manual accounting methods.

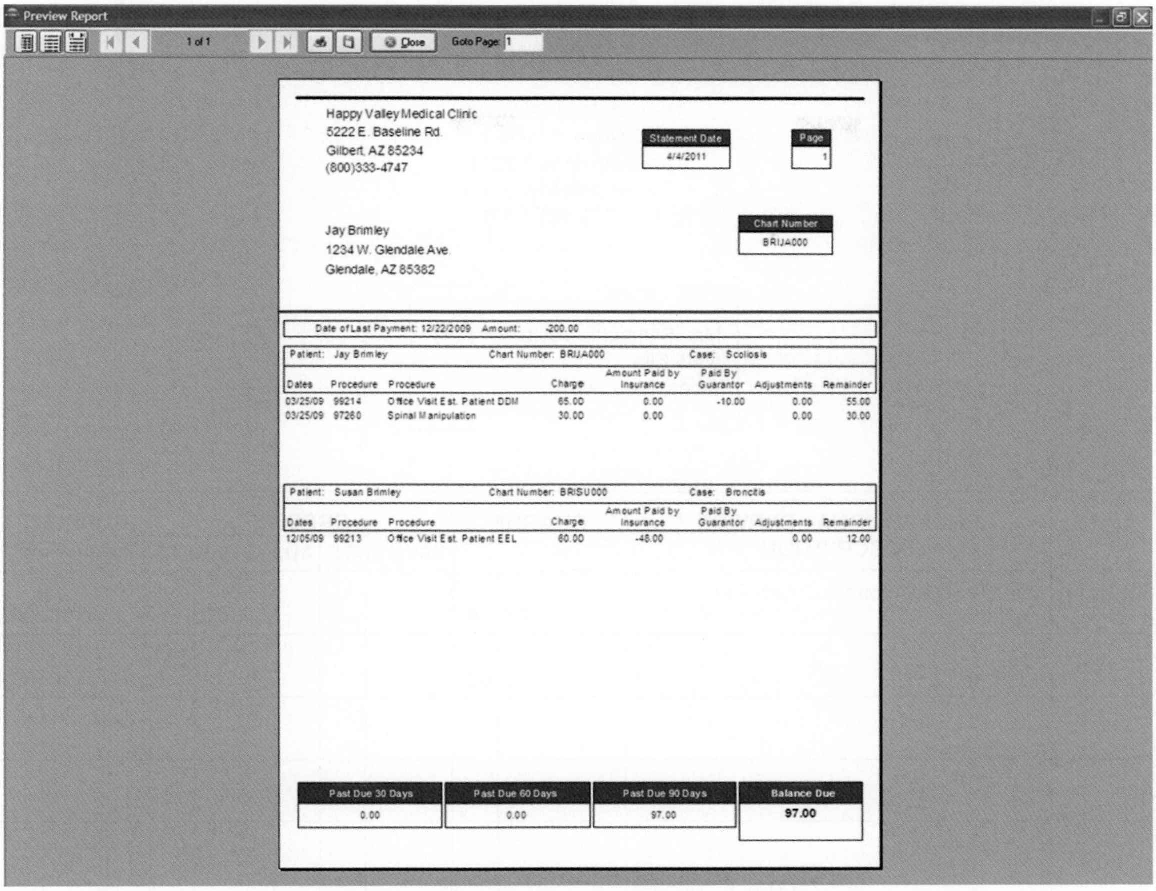

Preview Report

1 of 1 Close Goto Page: 1

Happy Valley Medical Clinic
5222 E. Baseline Rd.
Gilbert, AZ 85234
(800)333-4747

Statement Date: 4/4/2011
Page: 1

Jay Brimley
1234 W. Glendale Ave.
Glendale, AZ 85382

Chart Number: BRIJA000

Date of Last Payment: 12/22/2009 Amount: -200.00

Patient: Jay Brimley Chart Number: BRIJA000 Case: Scoliosis

Dates	Procedure	Procedure	Charge	Amount Paid by Insurance	Paid By Guarantor	Adjustments	Remainder
03/25/09	99214	Office Visit Est. Patient DDM	65.00	0.00	-10.00	0.00	55.00
03/25/09	97260	Spinal Manipulation	30.00	0.00		0.00	30.00

Patient: Susan Brimley Chart Number: BRISU000 Case: Broncitis

Dates	Procedure	Procedure	Charge	Amount Paid by Insurance	Paid By Guarantor	Adjustments	Remainder
12/05/09	99213	Office Visit Est. Patient EEL	60.00	-48.00		0.00	12.00

Past Due 30 Days	Past Due 60 Days	Past Due 90 Days	Balance Due
0.00	0.00	97.00	97.00

Fig. 5-9 Sample statement printout. (Screenshot used by permission of MCKESSON Corporation. All Rights Reserved. ©MCKESSON Corporation 2012.)

> **HIPAA Tip**
>
> A medical office can use sign-in sheets and announce names; however, reasonable safeguards still need to be used. This decision has been added to HIPAA's rules and regulations to address incidental disclosures of protected health information. Examples of safeguards used by some medical offices include the following:
>
> 1. Covering sign-in sheet with a separate, nontransparent sheet of paper
> 2. Using a heavy black marking pen to cross through names after the chart is verified, copay is collected (if applicable), and patient is seated

A patient ledger card is prepared for each new patient. In some medical offices, particularly family practice facilities, one ledger card is set up for the head of household and all dependent family members are included on it. This makes sense because it not only saves time and space in the ledger file but also addresses statements to parents and guardians of minor children, who are usually not responsible for their own bills. Caution must be used, however, in the case of divorced parents, because it is important that the parent who is financially responsible for the child is billed. More information is given on the maintenance of the patient ledger card as we proceed through the chapters on third-party payers and process insurance claims and reimbursements.

In offices that use practice management software, the ledger card is an integral part of the software program. All of the pertinent information—date, description of service(s), appropriate codes, charges, payments—is entered onto a screen, and the current balance is calculated (see Fig. 5-8).

Verifying Insurance with New Technology

Technology is constantly changing; therefore, the health insurance specialist should periodically check with each insurance payer to see what advancements are available. Examples of technological advancements in enrollee verification include the following:

Interactive Voice Response (IVR) systems, which offer solutions customized for explicit business needs. IVR systems typically utilize the telephone to interact directly with a database, and information can be passed to an existing personal computer or a Web application through customized software. IVR systems offer automated customer care and customer relationship management (CRM) applications, which make

STATEMENT

Tri-State Medical Group
400 North 4th Street
Anytown, Iowa 50622
Phone: 319-555-5734
Fax: 319-555-5758

Mrs. Samantha Taylor
6345 Elm
Ames, Iowa 50010

DATE	PROFESSIONAL SERVICE DESCRIPTION	CHARGE		CREDITS				CURRENT BALANCE	
				PAYMENTS		ADJUSTMENTS			
12-15-XX	Init OV, D hx/exam, LC decision making.	95	00					95	00
12-15-XX	EKG c̄ interpret & report.	55	00					150	00

Due and payable within 10 days.   **Pay last amount in balance column** ⇧

Key: PF: Problem-focused   SF: Straightforward   CON: Consultation   HCD: House call (day)
     EPF: Expanded problem-focused   LC: Low complexity   CPX: Complete phys exam HCN: House call (night)
     D: Detailed   MC: Moderate complexity   E: Emergency   HV: Hospital visit
     C: Comprehensive   HC: High complexity   ER: Emergency dept.   OV: Office visit

Fig. 5-10 Sample patient ledger card. (Modified from Fordney MT: *Insurance handbook for the medical office,* ed 11. St Louis, 2010, Saunders.)

verification of patient insurance eligibility easier and faster for medical practices. IVRs also can reduce collection time and enhance customer service. IVR systems can be purchased independently, and some insurance companies offer this technology; however, there is little uniformity among systems. It is recommended that healthcare providers take advantage of these services if and when they are available. It is simply good business practice to do whatever is necessary to verify a patient's insurance eligibility *before* services are rendered. Failure to confirm a patient's insurance coverage often creates a delay in payment that, in turn, affects the practice's cash flow.

Swipe terminals for enrollee health plan cards that work basically the same way credit card swipe terminals work in business establishments and provide a virtually instant response to an eligibility inquiry.

Internet-based eligibility check systems using software to connect providers' personal computers with the health plan's computers via the Internet. Internet inquiries provide real-time information about their patients' eligibility and benefit information.

Today's technology makes verification of a patient's healthcare coverage eligibility easier and faster but not all payers offer such services/devices. As mentioned, there is little uniformity among systems; however, medical practices are encouraged to use whatever technology is available. While enrollee verification may be time consuming, failure to do so could, in turn, harm the practice's cash flow.

What Did You Learn?

1. When does the insurance claims process begin?
2. List the information/documents essential for claims processing.
3. Explain why it is important to photocopy both back and front of the ID card.
4. What types of information are typically included on an encounter form?
5. Explain the rationale for verifying a patient's insurance coverage.

HIPAA Tip

Patients:

- must be told (in writing) how their protected healthcare information (PHI) may be used,
- have a right to see their medical records,
- have a right to amend incorrect/incomplete information in their record,
- must give authorization before PHI is released (with a few exceptions), and
- have a right to complain formally if they feel their privacy was not protected.

ADVANTAGES OF ELECTRONIC CLAIMS

Many practices submit their claims electronically because of the time and money savings that result. Experts tell practitioners that processing insurance claims electronically (1) improves cash flow, (2) reduces the expense of claims processing, and (3) streamlines internal processes, allowing them to focus more on patient care. On average, a paper insurance claim typically takes 30 to 45 days for reimbursement, whereas the average payment time for electronic claims is approximately 10 to 14 days. This reduction in insurance reimbursement time results in a significant increase in cash available for other practice expenses. As with everything, however, there is a tradeoff, because often the expense of setting up for an electronic process is not taken into account. First, the office has to purchase adequate equipment—computers, printers, and software programs. Additionally, everyone involved in the claim process must become computer literate. Depending on the size and needs of the practice, computer hardware and software can cost from $10,000 to $250,000. Also, an intensive training program may be necessary to teach staff how to use the equipment and become adept at operating the software.

TWO WAYS TO SUBMIT ELECTRONIC CLAIMS

There are basically two ways to submit claims electronically: through an electronic claims clearinghouse and directly to an insurance carrier. Many large practices can be set up to support both methods. Whether a practice chooses to use a clearinghouse or to submit claims directly to the carrier, it usually must go through an enrollment process before submitting electronic claims. The enrollment process is required so that the company the practice has hired can "set up" information about the practice on its computer system. Most government and many commercial carriers require such an enrollment. Some also require that the practice sign a contract with them. The enrollment process typically takes 6 to 7 weeks to complete. The biggest obstacle in getting set up for electronic claims processing is the time that it takes for approval from state, federal, and, in some cases, commercial/health maintenance organization carriers.

HIPAA Tip

For entities that choose to transmit claims electronically, practice management software or a clearinghouse is necessary to handle the conversion of data to meet HIPAA requirements.

Claims Clearinghouses

A **claims clearinghouse** is a company that receives claims from healthcare providers and specializes in consolidating the claims so that they can send one transmission containing batches of claims to each third-party payer.

A clearinghouse typically is an independent, centralized service available to healthcare providers for the purpose of simplifying medical insurance claims submission for multiple carriers. HIPAA defines a healthcare clearinghouse as "a public or private entity that processes or facilitates the processing of nonstandard data elements of health information into standard data elements." The clearinghouse acts as a simple point of entry for paper and electronic claims from providers. Clearinghouse personnel edit each claim for validity and accuracy before routing the edited claim on to the appropriate third-party carrier for payment. A medical practice can send all completed claims to one central location rather than to multiple payers. If the clearinghouse finds errors on the claim that would cause the claim to be rejected or denied, it sends the claim back to the provider for correction and resubmission.

Clearinghouses also are capable of translating data from one format to another (e.g., electronic to paper and vice versa). Many private clearinghouses that facilitate electronic and paper claims processing are available to healthcare providers and payers. Payers also can act as clearinghouses for claims of other payers.

Most clearinghouses have the ability to meet the requirements of each insurance company using the company's specific computer formats. They can submit electronic claims to any insurance company in a format that exactly matches that of the insurance company's computers. This clearinghouse task is essential for electronic claims because it is usually too complex and costly for independent billing services to perform on each claim. Clearinghouse services are not free, however. Charges for paper claims vary from 25 to 75 cents each, but some providers believe the advantages outweigh the disadvantages. Electronically submitted claims are less costly (some cost only 5 cents each), and many clearinghouses do not charge for claims submitted in certain standard electronic formats.

Here's how using a clearinghouse typically works: The medical practice subscribes to a clearinghouse. After this process is completed, the health insurance professional enters the practice's billing information in a preformatted template and a file that contains the practice's specific claim information is created from this template. This file is transmitted through the modem to the clearinghouse using the clearinghouse's specific built-in functionality.

As the clearinghouse receives claims from the medical practice, each claim is checked for completeness and accuracy. If an error has been made, the practice is notified that there is a problem with the claim. Ideally, the claim information is quickly corrected and the claim is resubmitted to the clearinghouse. This validation process normally takes just minutes, eliminating the costly delays associated with submitting "dirty" claims directly to the insurer. When submitted and validated for accuracy, claims are forwarded electronically (in most cases overnight) to the specific insurance carriers for reimbursement. More information on clearinghouses and electronic claims submission (ECS) is provided in Chapter 16.

Direct Claims

Submitting electronic claims directly to an insurance carrier is a little more complicated. As explained previously, the healthcare provider first must enroll with the carrier. Most government carriers and many commercial carriers require that providers enroll with them before submitting claims electronically to them. The provider also needs some additional software from each insurance carrier to which the practice will submit claims. Many carriers have their own software or can refer the health insurance professional to someone who supports direct transmissions in the area.

The most common **direct claim submission** method is done by creating a "print image" file of the claim and using the applicable direct claims software to send the claim to the proper insurance carrier. Printing claims to a file is as easy as printing claims to paper. The first step is to properly set up a printer that has the capability to designate "print to file." After completing the printer setup and entering the billing information, the health insurance professional can print claims to the carrier transmission file. He or she would select an option such as "print insurance claims" and select which claims to send to a particular insurance carrier. When prompted to select a printer to print claims, the professional simply selects the printer that has been set up to print to file. A prompt screen appears requesting entry of a filename. The professional enters the filename that was given by the direct claims software product. Then, using the direct claims software, he or she transmits the file to the carrier. Some carriers may "edit" claims; the health insurance professional needs to work with that particular insurance carrier to determine how to identify and resubmit claims that contain errors.

Clearinghouses Versus Direct

When deciding whether to send claims electronically through a clearinghouse or direct to the carrier, several things must be considered. Sending claims direct to the carrier is usually less expensive if the medical practice submits most claims to just one carrier. When multiple carriers are used, however, a clearinghouse is generally less expensive. With a clearinghouse, the health insurance professional needs to connect to, or dial into, only one location. If the decision is made to go direct to the carrier, there will be multiple **dial-ups**. (In this context, a "dial-up" occurs when a computer is programmed to automatically connect to another computer—e.g., that of a third-party payer—via the Internet using a modem and a telephone line [or other telecommunication device].) When a clearinghouse is used, all claims can be submitted in one transmission, and the convenience of sending all claims to one location should not be underestimated. Submitting claims to multiple insurance carriers requires members of the health insurance team to become experts in each of the claims submission software applications used. Because each one is unique, the health insurance professional must be adequately trained and available to submit all varieties of claims. Clearinghouses typically generate a separate confirmation report for each carrier to which claims are submitted directly.

Insofar as which method of electronic claims submission is better: If a medical practice submits insurance claims to multiple carriers and has someone who is well trained technically to handle the task of electronic claims submission, an electronic claims clearinghouse might be the better choice. If claims are sent primarily to one carrier, the practice should consider using direct submission to that carrier. Whichever method is selected, it is a proven fact that claims are processed much faster and reimbursement time is shortened with the use of electronic claims submission.

What Did You Learn?

1. What is a claims clearinghouse?
2. List two advantages of submitting claims electronically.
3. Explain the process for submitting direct claims.
4. Which of the two electronic submission processes (clearinghouse or direct) is better?

THE UNIVERSAL CLAIM FORM (CMS-1500)

The second way to submit a health insurance claim is with the CMS-1500 paper form. This form was considered a major innovation that made the process of health insurance claims submission simpler. As discussed earlier, before the emergence of this universal form, every insurance carrier had its own specialized type of paperwork for submitting claims.

The National Uniform Claim Committee (NUCC) and the National Uniform Billing Committee (NUBC) revised the CMS-1500 universal form. The original form, initiated in 1990, was referred to as CMS-1500 (12-90). The revised version is called the CMS-1500 (08-05). The 08-05 form is similar to the original form, but there are a few changes, for example, to accommodate a national provider identifier (NPI) and billing provider information. The front and back of the official CMS-1500 (08-05) are shown in Appendix A. Additional information regarding the revised form is available at the NUCC website, which is listed under "Websites to Explore" at the end of this chapter.

As previously mentioned, the NUCC's *1500 Health Insurance Claim Form Reference Instruction Manual* (for Form Version 08/05) provides detailed step-by-step claims completion instructions. The NUCC developed this general instruction manual for completing the CMS-1500 form, and it is intended to be a guide—not definitive instructions for this purpose. Users of this manual should refer to the most current federal, state, or individual payer for specific requirements applicable for using and completing the 1500 claim form. The link to this manual can be found on the Evolve site.

On June 28, 2010, the NUCC released its annual, updated version of the Instruction Manual. The updated manual (Version 6.0 7/10) is available on the NUCC website. Any interim changes, clarifications, or corrections to the instructions following this release will be posted on the NUCC website.

HIPAA Tip

Any person or organization that furnishes bills or is paid for healthcare electronically in the normal course of business is bound by HIPAA rules and regulations.

Format of the Form

The CMS-1500 form is an 8½ × 11–inch, two-sided document. The front is printed in **OCR scannable** red ink; the back of the form contains instructions for various government and private health programs. The CMS-1500 has two sections. The top portion is for the patient/insured information (Blocks 1-13), and the bottom portion is for the physician/supplier information (Blocks 14-33).

Optical Character Recognition

In most instances, when the paper CMS-1500 claim form is prepared for submission, **optical character recognition** (OCR) formatting guidelines should be used. OCR is the recognition of printed or written *text characters* by a computer. This involves photo scanning of the text character by character, analysis of the scanned-in image, and translation of the character image into character codes, such as **ASCII (American Standard Code for Information Interchange)**. ASCII is the most common *format* used for *text files* in computers and on the Internet.

In OCR processing, the scanned-in image is analyzed for light and dark areas to identify each alphabetical letter or numerical digit. When a character is recognized, it is converted into an ASCII code. Special circuit boards and computer chips designed expressly for OCR are used to speed up the recognition process. The CMS-1500 is printed in a special red ink to optimize this OCR process. When the form is scanned, everything in red "drops out" and the computer reads the information printed within the blocks.

Using OCR Format Rules

Because many third-party carriers use OCR scanning for reading health insurance claims, the health insurance professional should complete all paper CMS-1500 forms using the specific rules for preparing a document for OCR scanning. OCR works best with originals or very clear copies and **mono-spaced fonts** (in which each character takes up exactly the same amount of space); standard mono-spaced type fonts (such as Courier) in 12-point font size and black text are recommended. No special formatting, such as bold, italics, or underline, should be used, and extreme care should be taken in keying the information. Type should be lined up

Fig. 5-11 Section of the CMS-1500 form illustrating proper OCR format.

so that all entries and characters fall within the spaces provided on the form.

The following are specific guidelines for preparing OCR scannable claims:

- Use all uppercase (capital) letters.
- Omit all punctuation.
- Use the MM DD YYYY format (with a space—not a dash—between each set of digits) for date of birth.
- Use a *space* instead of the usual punctuation or symbols for each of the following situations:
  - dollar signs and decimal points in fee charges and ICD codes
  - dash preceding a procedure code modifier
  - parentheses around the telephone area code
  - hyphens in Social Security and employer identification numbers
- Omit titles and other designations, such as Sr., Jr., II, or III, unless they appear on the patient's identification (ID) card.
- Use two zeros in the cents column when the charge is expressed in whole dollars.
- Do not use lift-off tape, correction tape, or whiteout.
- Photocopied forms and forms printed from a color printer are not acceptable.

A section of the CMS-1500 form showing the proper OCR format is shown in Fig. 5-11.

When the health insurance professional has completed the claim form, it is important that the form is thoroughly examined for errors and omissions. A health insurance professional who is new to the profession should ask coworkers or supervisors to proofread forms before submission until he or she acquires the necessary proficiency in the claims process. The most important task the health insurance professional is responsible for is to obtain the maximum amount of reimbursement in the minimal amount of time that the medical record supports. Fig. 5-12 shows common CMS-1500 claim form errors and omissions.

If a claim is being resubmitted, most carriers require a new one using the original (red print) CMS-1500 form. Additional tips for submitting paper claims include the following:

- Improper identification of patient, either the insurance identification number or name
- Missing or invalid subscriber's name and/or birth date
- Missing or incomplete name, address, and identifier of an ordering provider, rendering, or referring provider (or others)
- Invalid provider NPI identifier (when needed) for rendering providers, referring providers, or others
- Missing "insurance type code" for secondary coverage (This information, such as a spouse's payer, is important for filing primary claims in addition to secondary claims.)
- Preauthorization codes missing
- Missing payer name and/or payer identifier, required for both primary and secondary payers
- Invalid diagnostic and/or procedure code(s)
- Missing or invalid admission date for inpatient services
- Missing or incomplete service facility name, address, and identification for services rendered outside the office or home, including invalid Zip Codes or two-letter state abbreviations
- Failing to include necessary documentation when needed
- Filing the claim after the deadline date

Fig. 5-12 List of common errors/omissions on the CMS-1500 claim form.

- Do not include any handwritten data (other than signatures) on the forms.
- Do not staple anything to the form.

Students can access the step-by-step instructions for filling out the CMS-1500 paper form on the Evolve site. It should be noted that these instructions are relatively "generic," and a particular payer may have more specific directives.

Completed CMS-1500 paper forms for various major payers, along with step-by-step completion instructions, can be viewed in Appendix B at the back of this textbook.

Who Uses the Paper Form?

To improve the efficiency and effectiveness of the healthcare system, HIPAA includes a series of administrative simplification provisions that require the HHS to adopt national standards for electronic healthcare transactions. By ensuring consistency throughout the industry, these national standards presumably make it easier for healthcare carriers, physicians, hospitals, and other healthcare providers to submit claims and other transactions electronically.

ASCA set the deadline for compliance with the HIPAA Electronic Healthcare Transactions and Code Set standards as October 2003, meaning that providers' offices must have been computerized and capable of submitting all claims electronically by that date. ASCA prohibited the HHS from paying Medicare claims that were not submitted electronically after this date, unless the Secretary of HHS (hereafter referred to as the Secretary) granted a **waiver** for this requirement. A waiver, in this case, would occur if the Secretary formally tells a provider (usually in writing) that he or she does not have to comply with this regulation. ASCA further stated that the Secretary must grant such a waiver if a provider had no method available for the submission of claims in electronic form or if the facility submitting the claim was a small provider of services or supplies. As noted earlier, a small provider or supplier is defined *as a provider of services with fewer than 25 full-time equivalent employees or a physician, practitioner, facility, or supplier (other than a provider of services) with fewer than 10 full-time equivalent employees.*

This provision does not prevent providers from submitting paper claims to other health plans, but if a provider transmits any claim electronically, it is subject to the HIPAA Administrative Simplification requirements, regardless of size. In other words, if a provider's office submits *any* claims electronically, ASCA says it must submit *all* claims electronically. It cannot submit some claims on paper and some electronically.

So, who uses the paper CMS-1500 form? If the provider falls into one of the following categories, the paper CMS-1500 form can be used—but it must be used exclusively with all carriers that have the capability of receiving electronic transmissions:

1. Providers who are not computerized and do not have the capability of submitting claims electronically can still use the paper version of the form.
2. "Small providers" who fit the previous description can still use the paper version of the form.
3. Other special situations listed in Box 5-1.

📁 HIPAA Tip

The "under 10" rule applies only to Medicare/Medicaid. If a medical facility has only one employee but is doing anything electronic, the office must be in compliance with HIPAA's privacy rules and regulations.

🕐 Stop and Think

We learned in this section that two categories of providers are exempt from the ASCA mandate that by October 2003, all claims must be submitted electronically. In your opinion, why are providers in these categories allowed to use the CMS-1500 paper form?

❓ What Did You Learn?

1. To whom do we credit the innovation of the "universal" claim form?
2. List the rules for OCR formatting.
3. Name the two categories of providers who can use the CMS-1500 paper form.

Proofreading

After the paper form has been completed according to the applicable payer guidelines, it should be meticulously proofread for accuracy. The goal is always to submit **clean claims**—claims that can be processed for payment quickly without being returned. Returned or rejected claims delay the payment process and cost the practice and the patient money. On average, nearly one-quarter of the claims submitted by medical practices to insurers are rejected because they contain some type of error. One national professional association estimates that resubmitting a paper claim could cost a medical practice between $24 and $42.

A claim that is rejected for missing or invalid information must be corrected and resubmitted by the provider. Common examples of claim rejections include the following:

- Incomplete/invalid patient diagnosis code
- Diagnosis code that does not justify the procedure code
- Missing or improper modifiers
- Omitted or inaccurately entered referring/ordering/supervising provider's name or NPI
- Performing physician/supplier is a member of a group practice but form does not show the full or accurate carrier-assigned PIN
- Insured's subscriber or group number missing or incorrect
- Charges not itemized
- Provider signature missing

When claims are submitted electronically, the health insurance professional should review all of the patient data that was entered into the practice management software to make sure there are no errors. Because the process is electronic and the claim is generated internally, there is normally no hard copy to proofread. This is why comparing the information on the form the patient fills out initially with what has been entered into the computer system is so important. If something has been entered into the practice software incorrectly, there is an original source document to compare it with.

Claim Attachments

Claim attachments are supplemental documents that provide additional medical information to the claims processor that cannot be included within the electronic claim format. These documents are necessary to support the services and procedures reported on the claim. Common attachments are Certificates of Medical Necessity (CMNs), discharge summaries, and operative reports. When a paper form is used, attachments are sent to the insurance carrier with the original claim.

Because HIPAA standards do not accommodate supplemental documents with electronic claims submission, it became necessary to develop standard claims attachment forms. In 1997, the American National Standards Institute (ANSI) attempted to develop standardized electronic claims attachments. In September 2005, HHS published a Notice of Proposed Rule Making for electronic claims attachments in the *Federal Register*, the daily journal of the U.S. government. The intent of this rule was to propose standards to implement some of the requirements of HIPAA. In January 2010, however, the HHS proposal was withdrawn after a survey found that only about 10% of claims require supplemental information and that pursuing this endeavor would be too costly.

So how do providers submit claim attachments for electronic claims when needed? Some carriers ask providers to send the attachments by mail using an attachment control number (ACN) that, on arrival, can be matched up with the appropriate claim. Alternatively, some providers use companies like National Electronic Attachment, Inc. (NEA), to send attachments electronically using software such as *FastAttach*. With this method, the healthcare office scans an image of the attachment into its computer (or captures an image already in the computer) through *FastAttach*. Then the image is transported to NEA's computer "storehouse." NEA immediately sends a report back to the provider's office with an NEA attachment number for each file. The healthcare office then submits the claim electronically with the NEA attachment number in the appropriate section of the claim form. This is done automatically for those users with access to the *FastAttach* Link. Some carriers' software programs allow providers to submit claims electronically with attachments using the Direct Data Entry (DDE) functionality through their online service center. An electronic copy of the attachment(s) can be uploaded with the claim, much like a document is attached to an email.

It is important to note that guidelines for electronic claim attachments claims vary from one carrier to the next; therefore, it is a good rule of thumb to contact the carrier in question for their specific guidelines for electronic claim attachments.

Tracking Claims

Many practices use some sort of claims follow-up system so that claims can be tracked and delinquent claims resolved before it is too late to resubmit them (as in the case of a lost claim). Most practice management software includes a claims tracking function that allows reports to be generated showing outstanding claims by date, by carrier, or by some other sorting function (Fig. 5-13). For medical offices that still use paper claims, an example of a claims follow-up system is an insurance log or insurance register. The insurance log or register should include various entries, such as the patient's name; insurance company's name; date claim filed; status of the claim (e.g., paid, pending, denied); date of explanation of benefits (EOB) or payment receipt; and resubmission date. A claims follow-up system can be set up manually or electronically. It is a helpful tool for the health insurance professional and the provider because it ultimately leads to an increase in payments to the practice. Insurance claims can be overlooked if a tracking system is not in place, leading to lost revenue. Fig. 5-14 shows an example of an insurance log. Fig. 5-15 is an example of a practice management software screen listing outstanding claims on a primary insurance aging report.

Claim Number	Chart Num	Carrier 1	Status 1	Media 1	Batch 1	Bill Date 1	EDI Receiver 1	Carrier 2	Status 2	Med
1	SIMTA000	AET00	Sent	Paper	1	12/3/2009				
2	AGADW000	MED01	Done	Paper	2	11/21/2009		AET00	Sent	Pap
3	BRIJA000	CIG00	Sent	Paper	4	3/25/2009		BLU01	Sent	Pap
4	BRISU000	CIG00	Done	Paper	5	12/5/2009		BLU00	Sent	Pap
5	WAGJE000	BLU00	Sent	EDI	0	6/1/2009	RM			
6	YOUMI000	US000	Ready To Send	Paper	0					
7	AGADW000	MED01	Sent	Paper	7	12/6/2009				

Fig. 5-13 Claims tracking function using practice management software. (Screenshot used by permission of MCKESSON Corporation. All Rights Reserved. ©MCKESSON Corporation 2012.)

Patient Name	Carrier Name	Date Filed	Claim Amount	Date of Payment/EOB	Payment Amount	Claim Status	Action Taken/Date
Anderson, Joseph L.	Metropolitan Life	01/12/XX	1450.00			Pending	Telephone call to Met Life 2/12/XX
Siverly, Penelope R.	Medicare	01/23/XX	125.00	02/13/XX	64.50		
Loper, Michael C.	Medicaid	01/25/XX	65.00			Denied	Appeal Letter to Medicaid 2/16/XX
Carpenter, Susan	BCBS	01/27/XX	255.00			Lost Claim	Resubmitted on 2/22/XX

Fig. 5-14 Sample insurance claim tracking form.

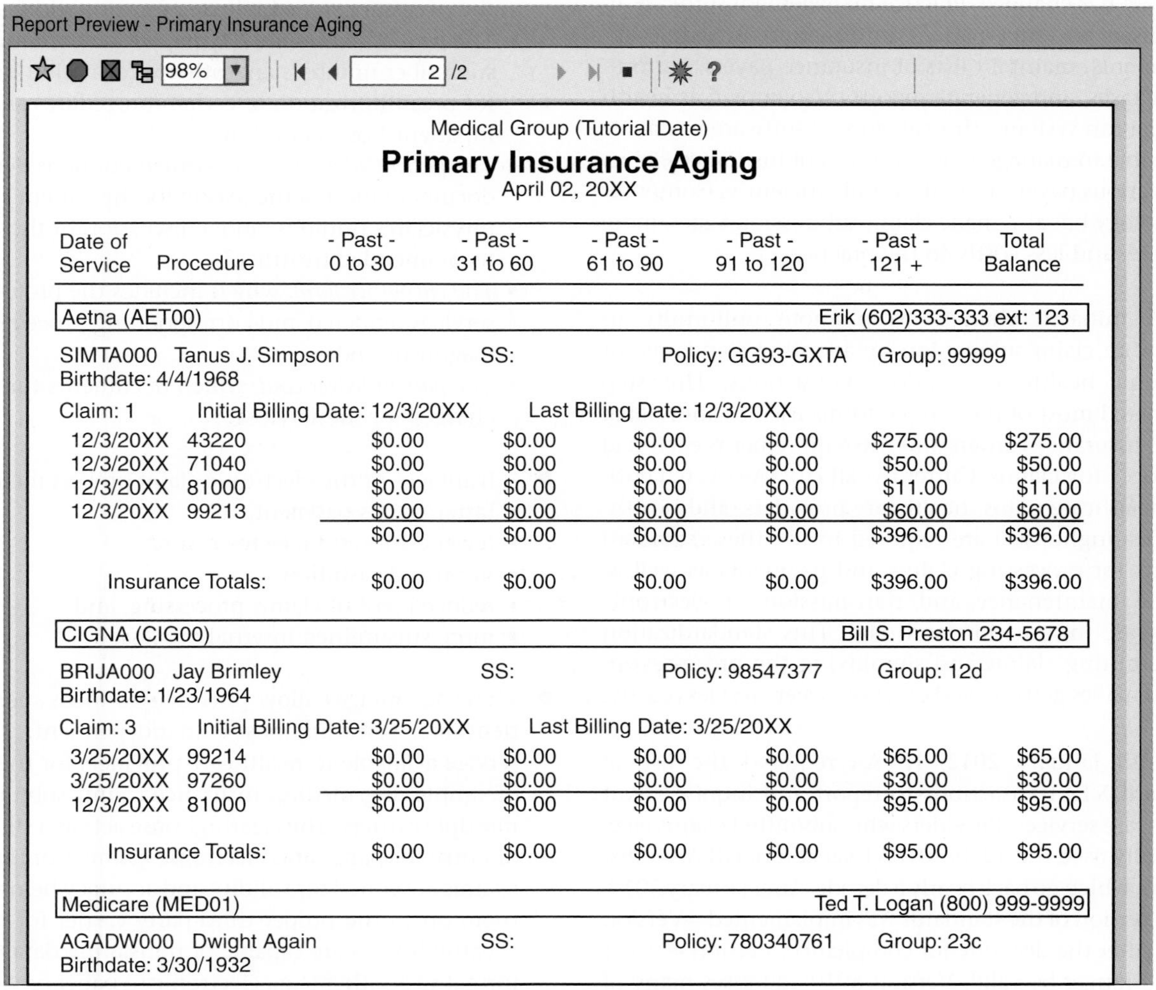

Report Preview - Primary Insurance Aging

☆ ● ☒ 📇 [98% ▼] ║ ◄ ◀ [2]/2   ► ► ■ ║ ✳ ?

Medical Group (Tutorial Date)

Primary Insurance Aging
April 02, 20XX

Date of Service	Procedure	- Past - 0 to 30	- Past - 31 to 60	- Past - 61 to 90	- Past - 91 to 120	- Past - 121 +	Total Balance
Aetna (AET00)						Erik (602)333-333 ext: 123	

SIMTA000   Tanus J. Simpson   SS: Policy: GG93-GXTA   Group: 99999
Birthdate: 4/4/1968

Claim: 1   Initial Billing Date: 12/3/20XX   Last Billing Date: 12/3/20XX

12/3/20XX	43220	$0.00	$0.00	$0.00	$0.00	$275.00	$275.00
12/3/20XX	71040	$0.00	$0.00	$0.00	$0.00	$50.00	$50.00
12/3/20XX	81000	$0.00	$0.00	$0.00	$0.00	$11.00	$11.00
12/3/20XX	99213	$0.00	$0.00	$0.00	$0.00	$60.00	$60.00
		$0.00	$0.00	$0.00	$0.00	$396.00	$396.00
Insurance Totals:		$0.00	$0.00	$0.00	$0.00	$396.00	$396.00

| CIGNA (CIG00) | | | | | | Bill S. Preston 234-5678 | |

BRIJA000   Jay Brimley   SS: Policy: 98547377   Group: 12d
Birthdate: 1/23/1964

Claim: 3   Initial Billing Date: 3/25/20XX   Last Billing Date: 3/25/20XX

3/25/20XX	99214	$0.00	$0.00	$0.00	$0.00	$65.00	$65.00
3/25/20XX	97260	$0.00	$0.00	$0.00	$0.00	$30.00	$30.00
12/3/20XX	81000	$0.00	$0.00	$0.00	$0.00	$95.00	$95.00
Insurance Totals:		$0.00	$0.00	$0.00	$0.00	$95.00	$95.00

| Medicare (MED01) | | | | | | Ted T. Logan (800) 999-9999 | |

AGADW000   Dwight Again   SS: Policy: 780340761   Group: 23c
Birthdate: 3/30/1932

Fig. 5-15 An electronic insurance aging report. (Screenshot used by permission of MCKESSON Corporation. All Rights Reserved. ©MCKESSON Corporation 2012.)

What Did You Learn?

1. What is a "clean" claim?
2. *True or False:* There is no way the health insurance professional can "proofread" an electronic claim prior to submission.
3. Discuss two methods that might be used if an electronic claim requires an "attachment."
4. Paper claims can be tracked using a follow-up system such as a/an _____ or _____.

SUMMARY CHECKPOINTS

▶ The two methods for submitting health insurance claims are electronic, using practice management software, and the paper CMS-1500 form.

▶ For several decades, medical billing, including insurance claims submission, was done almost entirely on paper. With the development and growth of computer technology and medical practice management software, this situation has changed. Practice management software allows users to enter patient information, schedule appointments, maintain lists of insurance payers, perform billing tasks, and generate reports. Also known as health information systems, this category of software has made it possible to manage large numbers of insurance claims with various payers accurately and efficiently. Computer technology has also made claims submission faster, more accurate, and less costly to the practice.

▶ HIPAA initiated changes to promote uniformity in healthcare claim submission by adopting standards for electronic health information transactions. This step eliminated most of the unique forms used by individual health insurance carriers and the requirements each had for processing claims. Currently, all HIPAA-covered entities (healthcare plans, healthcare providers, and healthcare clearinghouses) are required to use these standard formats for processing claims and payments as well as for the maintenance and transmission of electronic healthcare information and data. This standardization of submitting claims and simplifying the processes involved makes getting paid quicker, easier, and less costly.

▶ Up until January 2012, HIPAA required the use of Standard X12 transactions to report and inquire about healthcare services. Providers who submitted claims electronically used the 4010/4010A1 version of HIPAA transactions, which go back nearly a decade. After January 2010, a new version of the standards was implemented—Version 5010. After the deadline for compliance, Version 4010A1 will no longer be valid. Version 5010 addresses many of the limitations in the former version and supports the reporting of national provider identifiers (NPIs) and the new ICD-10 codes (see Chapter 12). Most healthcare entities are affected by the upgrade to Version 5010.

▶ The insurance claim process begins when a patient arrives at the medical facility, at which time he or she is given various forms to read and fill out. The front office staff enters the information into the medical facility's computer using the practice management software that meets electronic filing requirements as established by the HIPAA claim standards. It is from this information that the claim is generated through the internal functioning of the software. Once the patient visit is over, the health insurance professional transmits information from the record to the insurance company in the form of a claim. After the HIPAA legislation was passed in 1996, CMS directed insurers who submitted claims to Medicare to do so electronically, with few exceptions. However, some claims are still being submitted using the CMS-1500 paper form. The documents necessary for generating a claim are as follows:

- The *patient information form,* which supplies demographic and insurance information and provides the necessary signed release of information
- The *patient's insurance ID card,* which contains current subscriber numbers and other information necessary for preauthorization of certain procedures and inpatient hospitalization
- The *patient's health record,* which contains detailed documentation of the reason for the patient's visit, the physician's findings, and a discussion of the recommended treatment
- The *encounter form,* which includes the professional services rendered and corresponding procedure and diagnostic codes
- The *patient ledger card,* which documents the fees charged for the services

▶ Advantages of the electronic claim process include
- faster claims payment,
- fewer errors and rejected claims,
- improved cash flow,
- reduced cost of claims processing, and
- more streamlined internal processes.

▶ These advantages allow providers to focus more on patient care. A clearinghouse is an independent, centralized service available to healthcare providers for the purpose of simplifying medical insurance claims submission for multiple carriers. The clearinghouse acts as a single point of entry for paper and electronic claims from providers. Claims are edited for validity and accuracy before routing them on to the proper third-party carrier for payment. Clearinghouses are capable of translating data from one format to another (e.g., electronic to paper or vice versa). In contrast, when submitting electronic claims directly to an insurance carrier, the provider must first enroll with the carrier. Additional software is typically needed from each insurance carrier to whom claims are submitted directly.

▶ In the mid-1970s, the Health Care Financing Administration (HCFA, pronounced "hick-fa") created a new form for Medicare claims, called the *HCFA-1500*. The form was approved by the American Medical Association Council on Medical Services and was subsequently adopted by all government healthcare programs.

Although the HCFA-1500 originally was developed for submitting Medicare claims, it eventually was accepted by most commercial/private insurance carriers to assist the standardization of the claims process. Because HCFA is now called the Centers for Medicare and Medicaid Services (CMS), the name of the form has been changed to CMS-1500; however, it is basically the same document. The National Uniform Claim Committee (NUCC) and the National Uniform Billing Committee (NUBC) revised the CMS-1500 universal form to accommodate such things as national provider identifier (NPI) numbers.

CLOSING SCENARIO

Emilio and Latisha found studying the information in Chapter 5 one topic at a time and reviewing each main point to be helpful in comprehending the new material. The chapter contained a lot of information that could have proved difficult had they not adopted a structured method for studying.

Emilio and Latisha did a lot of research on the Internet to learn more about the electronic claims submission process. Supposing that the medical office where they would eventually find employment would be computerized, they believed they should be knowledgeable in the function and capabilities of medical practice management software programs. They are looking forward to the day when their instructor assigns them

to one of the local medical offices to "shadow" the health insurance professional to see how the process works from beginning to end in a real world environment—from the patient information entry screen continuing through each screen until the virtual insurance claim is transmitted to the payer.

Although they find the electronic claim process challenging but interesting, Emilio and Latisha realize they also need to learn how to complete the CMS-1500 paper form as well, because they may be employed in a small provider's office where the paper form is still used. Spending time on the Evolve site reviewing the step-by-step completion process proved a valuable use of their time outside of class.

WEBSITES TO EXPLORE

- For live links to the following websites, please visit the Evolve site at http://evolve.elsevier.com/Beik/today/
- To learn more about the electronic claims process, go to the CMS website at http://www.cms.gov/ and type "electronic claims" in the search window.
- To learn more about HIPAA's new 5010 Standards, log on to http://www.cms.gov/Versions5010andD0/ or go to the CMS website and type in "Version 5010" in the search window.
- For students who are interested in learning more about OCR technology, log on to the following website, key "OCR Technology" into the search block, and peruse articles of interest:
  http://www.eric.ed.gov/
- For tips on keeping up to date on CMS-1500 completion guidelines for Medicare and Medicaid, log on to the CMS website and type "CMS-1500 Guidelines" into the search block:
  http://www.cms.hhs.gov/
- For specific instructions on completing a new CMS-1500 form for Medicare, refer to the Medicare Claims Processing Manual, which is searchable if you visit
  http://www.cms.hhs.gov/

- For additional information on the revised CMS-1500 form, visit the NUCC website at
  http://www.nucc.org/
- More information on electronic claims and/or clearinghouses is available on the Federal Register. Use the following web address, then key applicable words, such as "claims clearinghouse" or "electronic claims":
  http://www.gpoaccess.gov/fr/index.html/
- Specific and detailed instructions for completing claims using the new CMS-1500 form are given in the National Uniform Claim Committee's instruction manual, which can be found at
  http://www.nucc.org/images/stories/PDF/claim_form_manual_v6-0_7-10.pdf/

Author's Note: Websites change frequently. If any of these URLs is unavailable, use applicable guide words in your Internet search to acquire additional information on the various subjects listed.

REFERENCES AND RESOURCES

Roediger JM: *Use every tool to verify patient eligibility,* Physician's News Digest, Narberth, PA, February 2000. http://www.obermayer.com/publications.php?action=view&id=38/.

CHAPTER 6

Traditional Fee-for-Service/Private Plans

Chapter Outline

I. Traditional Fee-for-Service/Indemnity Insurance
II. How a Fee-for-Service Plan Works
III. Healthcare Reform and Preexisting Conditions
   A. HIPAA and Credible Coverage
IV. Commercial or Private Health Insurance
   A. Who Pays for Commercial Insurance?
   B. High-Risk Pool
   C. Coverage Mandate 2014
   D. Health Insurance Exchange
   E. What Is Self-Insurance?
     1. Employee Retirement Income Security Act of 1974
     2. Third-Party Administrators/Administrative Service Organizations
     3. Single or Specialty Service Plans

V. Blue Cross and Blue Shield
   A. History of Blue Cross
   B. History of Blue Shield
   C. Blue Cross and Blue Shield Programs
     1. BlueCard and BlueCard Worldwide
     2. Federal Employees Health Benefits
     3. Federal Employee Program
     4. Medicare
     5. Healthcare Service Plans
     6. Medicare Supplement Plans
VI. Participating Versus Nonparticipating Providers
VII. Submitting BCBS and Commercial Claims
   A. Timely Filing
   B. Filing Electronic Claims
VIII. Commercial Claims Involving Secondary Coverage
   A. EOBs and ERAs

CHAPTER OBJECTIVES

After completing this chapter, the student should be able to:

1. Describe traditional fee-for-service (indemnity) insurance.
2. Explain how a fee-for-service plan works.
3. Discuss healthcare reform and preexisting conditions.
4. Define the components of commercial/private insurance.
5. Summarize the Blue Cross and Blue Shield health insurance program.
6. Differentiate between PARs and nonPARs.
7. Review submission guidelines for BCBS and commercial claims.
8. Outline the procedure for submitting claims involving secondary coverage.

CHAPTER TERMS

actuarial value
administrative services organization (ASO)
autonomy
basic health insurance
BlueCard Program
BlueCard Worldwide
Blue Cross and Blue Shield Federal Employee Program (FEP)
carrier
carve-out
coinsurance
commercial health insurance
comprehensive insurance
covered expenses
credible coverage
deductible
electronic remittance advice (ERA)
Employee Retirement Income Security Act (ERISA) of 1974
explanation of benefits (EOB)
ERISA plans
errata
Federal Employees Health Benefits (FEHB) Program
fee-for-service (FFS)/ indemnity plan
fiscal intermediary (FI)

OPENING SCENARIO

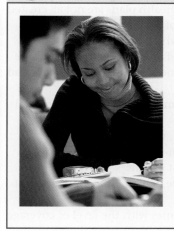

The subject matter of Chapter 6 is traditional fee-for-service insurance, sometimes referred to as indemnity, private, or commercial insurance. Traditional, indemnity, fee-for-service, private, commercial, self-insurance—Emilio and Latisha are amazed that so many different terms can be interrelated. Blue Cross and Blue Shield insurance is a type of insurance they are both familiar with.

As Emilio put it, "Who hasn't heard of 'The Blues'?" Emilio's parents currently have a Blue Cross and Blue Shield health insurance policy, and Emilio is still covered on it. Latisha's husband has a family plan with Liberty Value Insurance Company, a commercial carrier, through his employer. The term "commercial" did not have much meaning to Latisha until now, and she is looking forward to learning more about it.

grandfathered
group insurance
health savings account (HSA)
Healthcare Service Plans
health insurance exchange
health insurance policy
premium
health maintenance
organization (HMO)
insurance cap
lifetime maximum cap
major medical insurance
managed care plan
Medicare administrative
contractor (MAC)
Medicare supplement plan

minimum essential coverage
participating provider (PAR)
point-of-service (POS) plan
policyholder
preferred provider organization
(PPO)
premium
reasonable and customary fee
self-insured
single or specialty service plans
stop loss insurance
supplemental coverage
third-party administrator
(TPA)
third-party payer

TRADITIONAL FEE-FOR-SERVICE/INDEMNITY INSURANCE

Fee-for-service (FFS), or indemnity, insurance is a traditional type of healthcare policy. The insurance company pays fees for the services provided to the individuals covered by the policy. As discussed in an earlier chapter, this type of health insurance offers the most choices of physicians and hospitals. Typically, patients can choose any physician they want and can change physicians at any time. Additionally, they can go to any hospital in any part of the United States and still be covered. The "Blues"—Blue Cross and Blue Shield—are the best-known providers of fee-for-service health insurance, although they are not the only ones.

To review, we know why people need health insurance. Today's healthcare costs are continually rising, and individuals need to protect themselves from catastrophic financial losses that result from serious illnesses or injuries. If you have health insurance, a **third-party payer** covers a major portion of your medical expenses. A third-party payer is any organization (e.g., Blue Cross and Blue Shield, Medicare, Medicaid,

or commercial insurance company) that provides payment for specified coverages provided under the health insurance plan. Many Americans obtain health insurance through their employment, through what is referred to as **group insurance**. Group insurance is a contract between an insurance company and an employer (or other entity) that covers eligible employees or members. Group insurance is generally the least expensive kind. In many cases, the employer pays part or, in some cases, all of the cost.

If an employer does not offer group insurance or if the insurance offered is very limited, a wide variety of individual, private policies is available. Two basic categories are available in individual health insurance—a FFS plan and some type of **managed care plan**. A managed care plan typically involves the financing, managing, and delivery of healthcare services and is comprised of a group of providers who share the financial risk of the plan or who have an incentive to deliver cost-effective, but quality, service. It is important that people weigh the options carefully when choosing an individual healthcare plan because coverage and costs and how comprehensive the coverage is vary considerably from one insurance company to another.

HIPAA Tip

Although HIPAA makes it much easier for an individual to get health insurance from a new employer when switching jobs, it does not guarantee the same level of benefits, deductibles, and claim limits the individual might have had under the former employer's health plan.

Looking more closely at these two broad categories of insurance, we find four basic types of plans, as follows:
1. Traditional FFS/indemnity plans
2. Preferred provider organization (PPO) plans
3. Point-of-service (POS) plans
4. **Health maintenance organization (HMO) plans**

No one type of healthcare plan is universally better than the other. It depends on an individual's (or group's) needs and preferences. FFS health plans can cover everything, but the tradeoff is the cost. The **autonomy**, or the freedom to choose what medical expenses will be covered, offered by FFS plans is attractive to some, whereas others prefer the lower costs associated with most types of managed care.

Traditional FFS insurance is gradually becoming less popular as managed care moves to the forefront in healthcare. For individuals who value autonomy and flexibility of choices and can afford to spend a little extra money for the type of coverage they prefer, however, an individual health insurance policy may be the best plan.

FFS healthcare offers unlimited choices. The **policyholder** (the individual in whose name the policy is written) controls the choice of physician and facility, from primary caregiver to specialist, surgeon, and hospital. Flexible coverage offered by the FFS usually allows immediate treatment for medical emergencies or unexpected illness. FFS health plans do have restrictions, however. Often, they do not cover preventive medicine, so the costs of checkups, routine office visits, and injections (among a few other services) are likely to be the patient's responsibility. This can make FFS insurance impractical for a large family that requires many routine visits and a lot of preventive care. The Patient Protection and Affordable Care Act (March 2010), a part of the new Healthcare Reform legislation, has changed this situation. For those who purchased or joined a new plan on or after September 23, 2010, the insurance company must cover certain recommended preventive services without charging out-of-pocket costs. Under this act, services such as mammograms, colonoscopies, immunizations, prenatal and new baby care are also covered, and insurance companies will not be allowed to apply deductibles, copayments or coinsurance for these services.

⭐ Imagine This!

Maria Solaris is 52 years old and has worked out of her home as a self-employed health insurance professional for 10 years. In January 2011, Maria became employed at Mid-Prairie Health Clinic; she joined the clinic's group health plan, which had a $1000 deductible clause in the policy. Because of a family history of colon cancer, Maria decided to have a colonoscopy in February of that same year. In keeping with the rules of the new healthcare reform bill, even though she had not yet met her deductible, the clinic's policy paid for the procedure in full.

Choice does not come cheap. Although it is hard to predict the annual cost of healthcare under a FFS insurance plan, a few costs are relatively standard, as follows:

- A periodic payment (monthly or quarterly), called a **health insurance policy premium**
- A yearly deductible (out-of-pocket payment) before the health insurance carrier begins to contribute
- A per-visit **coinsurance**, or percentage of healthcare expenses

As a rule, healthcare services that are not covered by the health insurance policy (e.g., checkups) do not count toward satisfying the deductible. FFS health plans are not all created equal. There are three levels of coverage available:

1. **Basic health insurance,** which includes:
   - Hospital room and board and inpatient hospital care
   - Some hospital services and supplies, such as x-rays and medicine
   - Surgery, whether performed in or out of the hospital
   - Some physician visits
2. **Major medical insurance,** which includes:
   - Treatment for long, high-cost illnesses or injuries
   - Inpatient and outpatient expenses
3. **Comprehensive insurance,** which is a combination of the two.

The cost of the FFS plan varies with the level of coverage chosen—the better the coverage, the higher the premiums, and the higher the deductible, the lower the premium. Although indemnity health insurance plans offer choice and security, these advantages are reflected in the cost of the coverage.

❓ What Did You Learn?

1. Name the four basic types of insurance plans.
2. What main advantage does an individual (private) insurance plan offer?
3. What preventive services must be covered under the new Healthcare Reform legislation without the insurance company's applying deductibles, copayments, or coinsurance?
4. List the various levels of coverage available under an FFS plan.

HOW A FEE-FOR-SERVICE PLAN WORKS

With an FFS type of plan, the policyholder pays a periodic fee, or **premium**. In addition to the premium, an out-of-pocket amount must be paid before the insurance payments begin. This is called the **deductible**. In a typical plan, the deductible might be anywhere from $100 to $10,000. Most family plans require the deductible be paid on at least two people in the family. The deductible requirement applies each year of the policy, and not all healthcare expenses count toward the deductible—only the expenses specifically covered by the policy. After the deductible for the year has been met, the policyholder or dependents share the cost of services with the insurance carrier. The patient might pay 20% of **covered expenses** incurred that qualify for reimbursement under the terms of the policy contract, whereas the insurer pays 80%. This type of cost sharing is referred to as *coinsurance*.

Most FFS plans have an **insurance cap** (in some plans, it is called a "stop loss"), which limits the amount of money the policyholder has to pay out of pocket for any one incident or in any one year. The cap is reached when out-of-pocket expenses for deductibles and coinsurance total a certain amount. This amount may be $1000 or $5000. After the "cap" is reached, the insurance company pays the reasonable and customary amount in excess of the cap for the items the policy says it will cover and coinsurance provision does not apply. (The cap does not include the premiums.)

Prior to the Healthcare Reform Act, many FFS policies had a **lifetime maximum cap**, an amount after which the insurance company would not pay any more of the patient's medical bills. It could be a "per incident" cap or a "lifetime" cap, depending on the policy. These caps were typically quite high, ranging from $500,000 to $2 million. One of the provisions of healthcare reform was the removal of these lifetime caps on insurance.

Most insurance plans pay the **reasonable and customary fee** for a particular service. The term "reasonable and customary" is used to refer to the commonly charged or prevailing fees for health services within a geographic area. A fee is generally considered to be reasonable if it falls within the parameters of the average or commonly charged fee for the particular service within that specific community. If the healthcare provider charges $1000 for a specific procedure, but most other providers in the same geographic area charge only $600, the policyholder may be billed for the $400 difference. If the provider is a **participating provider (PAR)**, one who participates through a contractual arrangement with a healthcare service contractor in the type of health insurance in question, he or she agrees to accept the amount allowed by the carrier as payment in full. The policyholder does not have to pay the $400 difference—it is adjusted off, which means the provider absorbs this difference in cost.

⭐ Imagine This!

Jim Benson is seen in Dr. Mueller's office for the removal of a benign cyst of the right hand and is charged $125 for the procedure; however, his insurance carrier's allowed fee for this procedure is only $95. Jim has a 20/80 coverage plan and has met his yearly deductible. The difference between the two charges, or $30, is deducted from the original charged amount, resulting in an insurance payment of $76. If Dr. Mueller is a PAR with Jim's insurance carrier, the $30 difference between the original charge and the insurance carrier's allowed charge would have to be adjusted off of Jim's bill. If Dr. Mueller is nonPAR, he could bill Jim for this difference. Jim is still responsible for his 20% share of the allowed charge, or $19.

🕐 Stop and Think

Dr. Mueller, a family practitioner, asks you, his health insurance professional, for your opinion as to whether or not he should sign a contract and become a PAR for Western United Insurance. Olympia Products, a manufacturing plant employing 1350 people in the same city, has a group policy with Western United. What is your opinion?

💬 What Did You Learn?

1. What is an "insurance cap"?
2. How is a "lifetime maximum cap" different from an "insurance cap"?
3. With a PAR, what happens to any balance owing after the patient has paid his or her deductible and coinsurance and the insurer has paid the "allowable" fee?

HEALTH CARE REFORM AND PREEXISTING CONDITIONS

We talked about preexisting conditions in Chapter 4— physical or mental disorders that existed before a health insurance policy was issued for which the applicant (or one of his/her dependents) received treatment by a healthcare provider. Preexisting conditions are excluded from coverage under some policies, or a specified length of time must elapse before the condition is covered, typically anywhere from 30 days to 2 years. The Patient Protection and Affordable Care Act changed the preexisting condition requirements. Effective September 2010, children younger than 19 years with preexisting conditions may not be denied access to their parents' health plan because of a preexisting condition. In line with this change, insurers are no longer allowed to insure a child and, at the same time, exclude healthcare services for that child's preexisting condition. Beginning in 2014, this provision will apply to adults as well. Until 2014, however, the preexisting condition exclusion factor is still applicable for adults, and health plans may issue a policy conditionally by providing a preexisting condition exclusion period.

⭐ Imagine This!

Example 1: Eleanor R. is a 46-year-old woman who works as a medical biller/coder in a small, rural clinic that does not offer healthcare coverage for their employees. She has hypertension (high blood pressure), but it is well controlled by medication. She recently decided to purchase a private health insurance policy that included drug coverage. The only affordable plan she could find had a 12-month exclusion period for her preexisting condition— hypertension. For the first year of her policy, all of her claims (including visits to her doctor and her medication) related to her condition were denied. However, within that first year of coverage, she was diagnosed with a heart arrhythmia and type II diabetes. Both of these new conditions were covered completely, because they were not considered preexisting.

Example 2: Martin F., a 24-year-old man, was recently employed as a health insurance professional at

Mid-Prairie Health Clinic. Mid-Prairie allows employees to participate in its group health plan after a 90-day waiting period. Martin has back problems caused by an old sports injury; however, he had never seen a healthcare professional nor taken any prescription medications for this condition. He, therefore, was not subject to any exclusion period for his preexisting condition. Shortly after he started working at Mid-Prairie, his back problem worsened; he was fully covered for all of his back-related care.

> 📁 **HIPAA Tip**
>
> HIPAA limits the use of preexisting condition exclusions.

HIPAA and Credible Coverage

Prior to healthcare reform, HIPAA provided some protection when people needed to buy, change, or continue health insurance coverage, which includes:

- Limiting insurers on the use of preexisting condition exclusions.
- Preventing many health plans from denying coverage or charging more for coverage on the basis of the insured's (or a dependent's) health problems.
- Guaranteeing, under most circumstances, that when an individual loses a job along with coverage, he or she has the right to purchase new health insurance for himself or herself and the family.
- Guaranteeing, in most situations, that when health insurance is purchased, the policy can be renewed regardless of any of the policyholder's (or dependents') health conditions, as long as premiums are paid.

Although HIPAA does not apply in all situations, the law may decrease the chance that a person will lose existing coverage, makes it easier for people to switch health plans, and helps someone who has lost coverage through a job-related health plan to purchase new coverage.

An important feature of HIPAA is known as **credible coverage**. Credible coverage is health insurance coverage a person has before enrolling in a new health plan that has been in effect for a period of 63 or more days. In other words, if a person has had at least a full year of health coverage at a previous job and then enrolls in a new health plan without a break of 63 days or more, the new health plan cannot subject him or her to the preexisting condition exclusion.

> ❓ **What Did You Learn?**
>
> 1. How did the Patient Protection and Affordable Care Act affect the preexisting condition exclusion for children and adults?
> 2. What is meant by "credible coverage"?

COMMERCIAL OR PRIVATE HEALTH INSURANCE

Commercial health insurance (also called "private" health insurance) is any kind of health insurance paid for by someone other than the government. Medicare, Medicaid, TRICARE, and CHAMPVA are all government programs and do not fall into the category of commercial or private plans. There is one kind of commercial insurance, however, that the government does pay for—the **Federal Employees Health Benefits (FEHB)** Program, which is government health insurance coverage for its own civilian employees.

Government health insurance is standard for each program it sponsors, but commercial health insurance includes many variations in price and the kinds of benefits that the policy covers. The rules about a health insurance policy, such as what benefits are received and what rights the individuals covered under the policy have, depend on two things: the type of insurance (e.g., HMO, FFS) and who is paying for it.

> 📁 **HIPAA Tip**
>
> HIPAA protects millions of American workers by offering portability and continuity of health insurance coverage when they change jobs.

Who Pays for Commercial Insurance?

Commercial health insurance is usually paid for by an employer, a union, an employee and employer who share the cost, or an individual. When the cost of health insurance is shared, the cost to the patient is much less than if he or she is buying health insurance as an individual. Not all jobs come with health insurance, and sometimes individuals are between jobs and not eligible for coverage. In these situations, it may be necessary to consider a private insurance policy to maintain healthcare coverage.

> 📁 **HIPAA Tip**
>
> Under HIPAA, group health plans cannot deny an application for coverage solely on the basis of the individual's health status. It also limits exclusions for preexisting conditions.

High-Risk Pool

A high-risk health insurance pool is the most common way to provide individuals access to health insurance if the person has been denied coverage because of a preexisting condition and has been without coverage for a period of at least 6 months. Coverage options are very similar to those of traditional individual health insurance—generally a comprehensive major medical plan with a range of deductible dollar amounts. High-risk pools normally contract with a health insurance carrier or third-party administrator (TPA) to manage paperwork and claims. Once the individual is enrolled, benefits can be used just like in any other private insurance plan. High-risk pools are available in many states for those who are eligible for the federal health insurance tax credit provided by the Trade Adjustment Assistance Act of 2002. To research this Act further, visit the Evolve site.

Coverage Mandate 2014

In 2014, there will be changes in how health insurance is bought and paid for in the United States. As it stands now, people will be required to purchase health insurance with **minimum essential coverage** for themselves and their dependents or face financial penalties. The essential benefit package will provide a comprehensive set of benefits, which the Affordable Care Act says must

> include at least the following general categories and the items and services covered within the categories: ambulatory patient services; emergency services; hospitalization; maternity and newborn care; mental health and substance use disorder services, including behavioral health treatment; prescription drugs; rehabilitative and habilitative services and devices; laboratory services; preventive and wellness services and chronic disease management; and pediatric services, including oral and vision care.

Further, these services must be received from network providers. The package must cover 60% of the **actuarial value** (a method for comparing health plan benefits) of the covered benefits and limit annual cost-sharing to what is stated in the Act. Insurance policies must cover these benefits in order to be certified and offered in exchanges (see later). Additionally, all state Medicaid plans must cover these services by 2014.

Beginning on or after September 23, 2010, health plans may no longer impose a lifetime dollar limit on spending for these services. All plans, except **grandfathered** individual health insurance policies, must phase out annual dollar spending limits for these services by 2014. (The term grandfathered refers to an exception that allows an old rule to continue to apply to some existing situations.)

Health Insurance Exchange

A term you currently may be hearing is **health insurance exchanges.** Shortened to "exchanges," they are a set of state-regulated and standardized healthcare plans from which individuals may purchase coverage that is eligible for federal subsidies. Exchanges are one of the main focuses of the Patient Protection and Affordable Care Act and offer a variety of insurance coverage options for both individuals and small businesses. Exchanges allow people to shop and compare before enrolling in a healthcare plan. State-based health insurance exchanges are scheduled to become available in all states by 2014 and already are available in some states. In 2014, when the exchanges will be offered, federal assistance may also be available for some people, depending on their income level. To learn more about the Affordable Care Act and Health Insurance Exchanges, visit the Evolve site.

What Is Self-Insurance?

Some employers are **self-insured**, which means that when an employee needs healthcare, the employer, not an insurance company, is responsible for the cost of medical services. Most organizations that are self-insured are large entities, which can draw from hundreds or thousands of enrollees. Self-insured plans usually do not have to conform to traditional laws governing insurance, because they are technically not considered insurance companies.

Employee Retirement Income Security Act of 1974

Self-insured plans are sometimes called **ERISA plans.** The only law that governs self-insured plans is the federal law known as ERISA, an acronym for the **Employee Retirement Income Security Act of 1974.** ERISA sets minimum standards for pension plans in private industry, which are how most self-insured employers fund their programs.

Self-insured employers typically set up plans that provide benefits to employees in the form of life, disability, and health insurance, severance pay, and pensions. These benefits are funded through the purchase of insurance policies or through the establishment of trusts, paid for by the employer or by the employer and employee together. The trust money is then invested, and the employer takes a tax deduction for its contribution to the trust. If an employer maintains a pension plan, ERISA applies very specific provisions. Most ERISA provisions are effective for plan years beginning on or after January 1, 1975.

Third-Party Administrators/Administrative Services Organizations

Many self-insured groups hire **third-party administrators (TPAs)** or **administrative services organizations (ASOs)** to manage and pay their claims. A TPA is a person or organization that processes claims and performs other contractual administrative services. An ASO, similar to a TPA, provides a wide variety of health insurance administrative services for organizations that have chosen to self-fund their health benefits. TPAs and ASOs are neither health plans nor insurers but organizations that provide claims-paying functions for the clients they service. Although historically TPAs and ASOs only paid claims, their functions are expanding. They now typically perform additional functions, such as:
- General administrative tasks
- Planning
- Marketing
- Human resources management
- Financing and accounting

Many self-insured groups were pioneers in PPO development. As a result, a TPA or ASO may pay claims on the basis of discounted rates negotiated by a PPO on behalf of a self-insured group. A self-insured group may contract directly with providers, or it may use the services of a managed care organization.

Instead of paying premiums to insurance companies (which then charge enrollees premiums to pay for the healthcare services), self-insured groups assume the risk of providing such services on their own, usually with some kind of **stop loss insurance**. Stop loss insurance protects the insurer from the devastating effect of exorbitant medical claims by limiting what the insurer has to pay to a specified dollar amount. Examples are claims resulting from prolonged or intense medical services such as premature births, multiple trauma, transplant, and any other extended care that can result in catastrophic medical fees. At present, new healthcare reform laws eliminating the maximum lifetime cap do not apply to self-insured plans.

Single or Specialty Service Plans

Single or specialty service plans are health plans that provide services only in certain health specialties, such as mental health, vision, or dental plans. These specialty plans developed as people realized that eliminating a specific category of healthcare (e.g., mental health services) might slow the rate of increasing costs for healthcare in general and assist the management of care within these specialties. Eliminating a certain specialty of services from coverage under the healthcare policy is referred to as a **carve-out**. Employers wanting to include these special carved-out coverages for their employees can contract with one of these single or specialty service plans that focus on the desired specialty service.

Vision and dental plans and prescription drug coverage have often been add-on or **supplemental coverage** to health plans. Supplemental coverage varies greatly in the benefit services offered and represents another example of single or specialty service plans.

📁 HIPAA Tip

There is one major exception to the HIPAA rule on insurance portability: It provides no protection for switching from one individual health plan to another individual plan.

❓ What Did You Learn?

1. How can someone who has been denied coverage owing to a preexisting condition gain access to a healthcare plan?
2. List the services included in the minimum healthcare coverage mandate.
3. What is the intended purpose of a health insurance exchange?
4. Explain the difference between traditional insurance and self-insurance.
5. What is the function of TPAs and ASOs?
6. How might a "single or specialty service plan" benefit an employee?

BLUE CROSS AND BLUE SHIELD

Blue Cross and Blue Shield (BCBS) is probably the best-known commercial insurance company in the country. The Blue Cross and Blue Shield Association (BCBSA), created in 1982, is the result of a merger of the Blue Cross Association and National Association of Blue Shield Plans. The BCBSA is a national federation of 39 independent, community-based and locally operated BCBS companies that collectively provide healthcare coverage for nearly 98 million members—one-in-three Americans. BCBS plans, often referred to as "Blue Plans" as well as "the Blues," offer health insurance coverage in all 50 states, the District of Columbia, Puerto Rico, and Canada. These plans cover all sectors of the population, including large employer groups, small businesses, and individual consumers and their families. Most healthcare providers accept BCBS cards.

In addition to offering a variety of healthcare plans, BCBS insurers also provide group coverage to state government employees as well as the federal government under a nationwide option of the Federal Employees Health Benefits program established by the Association on their behalf.

BCBS offers both indemnity and managed care plans. One of their more popular types of managed care plans is referred to as a **preferred provider organization (PPO)**. Under this plan, members have the freedom to select any provider they choose, but they are encouraged to receive care from PPO network providers. The incentive to use PPO plan providers is that the out-of-pocket costs the member pays are typically less if they choose a provider within the network. Similar to Medicare, BCBS plans have provider identification (ID) numbers and participating provider (PAR) and nonparticipating provider (nonPAR) arrangements. Most plans pay participating providers directly, and the providers agree not to bill the patient for the difference between the plan's allowable charge and the actual fee charged. For more information on the BCBSA and its member companies, visit the Evolve site. ⊜

History of Blue Cross

In 1929 Justin Ford Kimball, an official at Baylor University in Dallas, introduced a plan to guarantee schoolteachers 21 days of hospital care for $6 a year. Other groups of employees in Dallas soon joined the plan, and the idea quickly attracted nationwide attention. By 1939, the Blue Cross symbol was officially adopted by a commission of the American Hospital Association as the national emblem for plans that met certain guidelines. In 1960 the commission was replaced with the Blue Cross Association, and all formal ties with the American Hospital Association were severed in 1972.

History of Blue Shield

The Blue Shield concept grew out of the lumber and mining camps of the Pacific Northwest early in the 20th century. Employers wanted to provide medical care for their workers, so they paid monthly fees to "medical service bureaus" composed of groups of physicians. These pioneer programs led to the first Blue Shield Plan, which was founded in California in 1939. The Blue Shield symbol was informally adopted in 1948 by a group of nine plans known as the Associated Medical Care Plans. This group eventually became the National Association of Blue Shield plans.

Blue Cross and Blue Shield Programs

Local chapters of the independent BCBS plans offer products and services uniquely tailored to meet community and individual consumer needs. At the same time, their membership in the BCBSA enables them to serve large regional and national employers effectively. Although healthcare coverage options differ from region to region, they typically include FFS, managed FFS, and PPO plans. The three-letter alpha prefix that precedes the subscriber number on the BCBS ID card identifies the plan to which the member belongs.

BlueCard and BlueCard Worldwide

The BlueCard Program and **BlueCard Worldwide** link independent Blue Plans so that members and their families can obtain healthcare services while traveling or working anywhere in the United States, receiving the same benefits they would receive if they were at home. The main identifiers for BlueCard members are the alpha prefix, a blank suitcase logo, and, for eligible PPO members, the "PPO in a suitcase" logo. BlueCard member ID numbers may also include alpha characters *within* the body of the number; however, these alpha characters should not be confused with the three-character alpha prefix that precedes the member number. If the member belongs to a BlueCard PPO, the initials PPO appear inside the suitcase logo (Fig. 6-1).

BlueCard Worldwide provides Blue Plan members inpatient and outpatient coverage at no additional cost in more than 200 foreign countries. Hospitals participating in BlueCard Worldwide are located in major travel destinations and business centers around the world. When plan members travel or live outside the United States and require inpatient hospital care, all they have to do is show their ID cards to any of these participating hospitals and their claims are handled just as if they were at home. Plan members have the choice of using a nonparticipating hospital; however, they may have to pay the hospital directly and then file a claim with BCBS

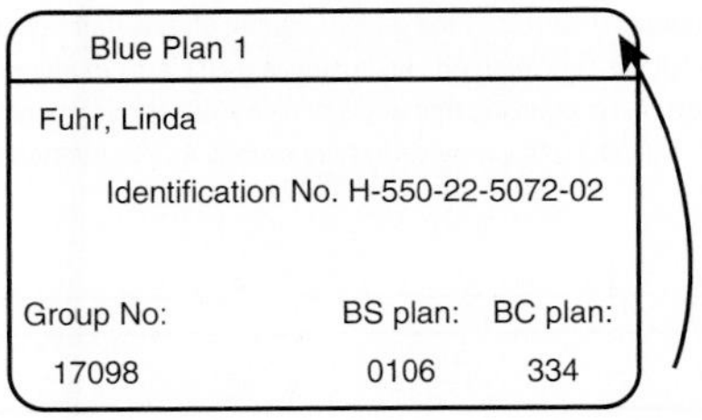

Fig. 6-1 Location on the health insurance card where the suitcase can be found.

for reimbursement of covered expenses. The preferred form to file for BlueCard Worldwide claims is shown in Fig. 6-2.

Federal Employees Health Benefits

Congress instituted the FEHB Program in 1960. FEHB is the largest employer-sponsored group health insurance program in the world, covering more than 9 million federal civilian employees, retirees, former employees, family members, and former spouses. Under this program, eligible members of the participating insurance companies (of which BCBS is one) have access to a wide variety of healthcare plans. Choices include various types of plans, as follows:

- FFS
- PPOs
- POS plans
- HMOs (if the individual works in an area serviced by an HMO plan)

Choices among healthcare plans are available to employees during an open enrollment period, after which the employee will be covered fully in any plan he or she chooses without limitations regarding pre-existing conditions. Premiums vary from plan to plan and are paid in part by the employer (the U.S. government agency that the employee works for), and the remainder is paid by the employee. In 2010 about 250 plans participated in the program.

Federal Employee Program

The BCBS government-wide Service Benefit Plan, also known as the **Blue Cross and Blue Shield Federal Employee Program (FEP)**, has been part of FEHB program since its beginning in 1960. FEP covers roughly 4.5 million federal employees, retirees, and their families out of the nearly 8 million people (enrollees as well as their dependents), amounting to about 57% of those receiving their benefits through the FEHB program. BCBSA works with the Office of Personnel Management to administer the Service Benefit Plan on behalf of the 39 independent BCBS companies. For more information on the FEP administered by BCBSA, visit the Evolve site.

Medicare

BCBS plans have partnered with the U.S. government in administering the Medicare program since its beginning in 1966. Blue Plans helped design the original platform for tracking and processing Medicare payments. Today, the Blue System is the largest single processor of Medicare claims, handling most Part A claims (from hospitals and institutions) and more than half of Part B claims (from physicians and other healthcare practitioners).

A commercial insurer or agent (e.g., Blue Cross) that contracts with the Centers for Medicare and Medicaid Services (CMS) through the Department of Health and Human Services (HHS) for the purpose of processing and administering Part A Medicare claims for reimbursement of healthcare coverage is referred to as a **fiscal intermediary (FI)**. Similar to a Medicare FI, a Medicare **carrier** is an organization that determines payment for Part B-covered items and provider

Please see the instructions on the reverse side of this form before completing. Please type or print.

1. Patient Information — 1A. Alpha prefix   Identification number *Copy this from your identification card.*

⎿ ⎿ ⎿   ⎿ ⎿ ⎿ ⎿ ⎿ ⎿ ⎿ ⎿ ⎿

1B. Patient's name (First, middle initial, last)	**1C. Patient's date of birth** MM/DD/YYYY / /	**1D. Patient's sex** ☐ Male ☐ Female
1E. Name of subscriber (First, middle initial, last)	**1F. Subscriber's date of birth** MM/DD/YYYY / /	**1G. Patient's relationship to subscriber** ☐ Self ☐ Spouse ☐ Child

1H. Subscriber's current mailing address (Street, city, state, and country or ZIP code)

2. Other Health Insurance — Is the patient covered under other health insurance, including Medicare A or B? ☐ Yes ☐ No
If yes, complete 2A through 2K below.

2A. Name and address of insuring company

2B. Type of policy ☐ Family ☐ Individual	**2C. Effective date** MM/DD/YYYY / /	**2D. Termination date** MM/DD/YYYY / /	**2E. Policy or identification number of other coverage**

2F. Type of coverage Hospital: ☐ Yes ☐ No Medical: ☐ Yes ☐ No Mental illness: ☐ Yes ☐ No	**2G. Name of subscriber**	**2H. Date of birth** MM/DD/YYYY / /

2I. Employer of subscriber	**2J. Employment status** ☐ Active employee ☐ Retired employee

2K. If patient is covered under Medicare, complete the following: Medicare Part A: ☐ Yes ☐ No Medicare Part B: ☐ Yes ☐ No
Effective date _____   Effective date_____

3. Diagnosis — 3A. Describe illness, injury, or symptoms requiring treatment	**3B. Was patient's treatment due to a work-related accident or condition?** ☐ Yes ☐ No

3C. Complete for care related to accidental injuries
Date of accident _____   Location: ☐ At home ☐ Auto ☐ Other _____
Time of accident _____   *If the accident was caused by someone else, attach a statement describing the accident.*

4. Charges — Use a separate line to list each type of service or provider and attach itemized bills for all services.

4A. Name and address of provider making charge	4B. Type of provider	4C. Description of service	4D. Dates of service or purchase	4E. Charges
_____	_____	_____	_____	____
_____	_____	_____	_____	____
_____	_____	_____	_____	____
_____	_____	_____	_____	____

5. Payee — Select one of the following payment options:
5A. ☐ Make payment to subscriber; provider has been paid.
1. Currency – Please check your preference for payment: ☐ Currency on itemized bill(s) ☐ U.S. dollars
2. Payment Method – Please select your preference for how to receive your payment: ☐ **Check** (Provide current telephone number) _____
☐ **Bank Wire.** If you want to receive a bank wire provide the following:

Subscriber name as it appears on bank account: _____   Bank name: _____

Bank's Physical Address: _____   Account #: _____

ABA# ⎿ ⎿ ⎿ ⎿ ⎿ ⎿ ⎿ ⎿ ⎿   *International Bank Account (IBAN) #: _____

*Bank Identifier Code (BIC/SWIFT) _____   *Required for bank wires to European Union countries.

5B. ☐ Make payment to provider (hospital, doctor). Please complete and sign to authorize assignment of benefits.
I, the undersigned, authorize and request my carrier to make payment for benefits due herein to:

Name of provider _____   Signature of subscriber or spouse_____   Date _____

6. Signature — I certify the above is complete and correct and that I am claiming benefits only for charges incurred by the patient named above. Authorization is hereby given to any provider of service, that participated in any way in the patient's care, to release to the subscriber's plan and its business associates in any country any medical or other personal information that they deem necessary to provide service or adjudicate this claim, recognizing that applicable law concerning personal information may differ among countries. Authorization is also given to the subscriber's plan and its business associates in any country to collect, use or release any medical or other personal information that they deem necessary to provide service or adjudicate a claim.

Signature of subscriber or patient _____   Date _____

Fig. 6-2 Sample international claim form.

Continued

General Information

The International Claim Form is to be used to submit institutional and professional claims for benefits for covered services received outside the United States, Puerto Rico, Jamaica and the U.S. Virgin Islands. For filing instructions for other claim types (e.g., dental, prescription drugs, etc.) contact your carrier.

The International Claim Form must be completed for each patient in full, and accompanied by fully itemized bills. It is not necessary for you to provide an English translation or convert currency.

Since the claim cannot be returned, please be sure to keep photocopies of all bills and supporting documentation for your personal records.

International Claim Form Instructions

Please complete all items on the claim form. If the information requested does not apply to the patient, indicate N/A (Not Applicable). Special care should be taken when completing the following items:

2. Other Health Insurance

If the patient holds other insurance coverage, please complete items A through K as completely as possible. It is especially important to indicate the name and address of the other insurance company and the policy or identification number of that coverage, as well as the name and birth date of the person who holds that policy.

In addition, if the patient is someone other than the subscriber and has received benefits from any other health insurance plan held by reason of law or employment, the Explanation of Benefits Form furnished by the other carrier pertaining to these charges must be included with the claim. A clear photocopy of the other carrier's Explanation of Benefits Form is acceptable in place of the original document.

4. Charges

Please list here the bills that are being included on this claim. Although itemized bills must also be submitted, your listing will enable us to process the claim more quickly and accurately. If additional space is needed for listing charges, please use a separate sheet of paper to list the following information.

4A. Name and Address of provider— as indicated on the bill. Multiple bills from the same provider may be included on the same line, as long as they are for the same type of service.
4B. Type of provider— for example: hospital, nurse, physician, clinic, physical therapist, etc.
4C. Description of service— for example: hospital admission, office visit, x-ray, laboratory test, surgery, etc.
4D. Date of service or purchase— inclusive dates may be indicated for bills containing multiple dates of service.
4E. Charge— bills must be itemized to show a separate charge for each service. If the bill has already been paid, please indicate the date it was paid.

5. Payee

5A. Make payment to subscriber, designation of currency and payment method — 1) Indicate whether you want to be paid in the currency reflected on the bill(s) or in U.S. dollars and if you want to receive payment via check or bank wire. Please note that not all forms of currency may be available for payment. In the event that you select payment in a currency that is not available, you will be paid in U.S. dollars. Banks will typically charge a flat fee or percentage-based fee to receive a wire. You may want to investigate fees charged by your bank prior to requesting a wire since you will be responsible for any such fees.

2) You must include the following information on this form: your full name (initials are not acceptable), your physical address (payments cannot be sent to a P.O. box). For wire payments, subscriber's name as it appears on the bank account, the bank's name and physical address (payments cannot be wired to a P.O. box), account number, ABA number. Please provide a copy of a voided check or deposit slip so that the bank information can be validated. Additionally, for wire payments to European Union countries, your must provide the International Bank Account Number (IBAN) and Bank Idenifier Code (BIC/SWIFT). For checks to be sent by express mail, you must provide a current telephone number.

5B. Authorization for assignment of benefits— complete item 5B if you prefer that benefits be paid directly to the provider of service.

6. Signature
The International Claim Form must be signed and dated by the subscriber, spouse, or the patient.

Itemized Bill Information

Each provider's original itemized bill must be attached and must contain:

- The letterhead indicating the name and address of the person or organization providing the service
- The full name of the patient receiving the service
- The date of each service
- A description of each service
- The charge for each service

This completed claim form, together with itemized bills and supporting documentation, should be submitted to:

Smith and Co. Insurance
113 Waverton
Springfield, XY 33142 USA

N13-04-086

Fig. 6-2—cont'd

services. FIs and carriers are now more commonly referred to **Medicare administrative contractors (MACs)**. CMS puts MAC contracts up for bidding at least once every five years. For related links to MACs visit the Evolve site.

In addition to handling financial matters, an FI and/or MAC may perform other functions, such as providing consultative services or serving as a center for communication with providers and making audits of providers' needs. It should be noted here that Blue Cross and Blue Shield is not the Medicare FI for all states.

Healthcare Service Plans

Healthcare service plans, typically operated by BCBS plans throughout the United States, have provided healthcare coverage for many years. Although they were initially involved in paying claims for indemnity carriers, many healthcare service plans have developed managed care products to compete with companies offering managed care plans.

Generally, healthcare service plans fall into four categories:
- Indemnity (fee-for-service),
- managed care (HMOs, PPOs)
- Point of Service (POS), and
- High-deductible health plans (HDHPs).

Each plan choice has certain advantages and disadvantages. It is important to understand the difference between the plans and what options each offer.

Indemnity plans allow an individual to use any healthcare provider in any healthcare location for almost any reason. The patient must pay a deductible, and after this deductible is met, the plan pays anywhere from 60% to 80% of the "allowable" costs.

Managed care plans are HMOs or PPOs. HMOs contract with various physicians and specific hospitals that make up the "network" of approved healthcare providers in that plan. There is typically no deductible to be met with a managed care plan; however, members must pay a monthly premium, and some services may require a relatively small copayment. Managed care patients choose a primary care physician (PCP) who coordinates all their care, and if a specialist is needed, the PCP arranges a referral. Prior approval is also required if the patient chooses to go outside the network for healthcare services or if the services are not covered. Even with prior approval, however, services outside the network are usually paid at a lower percentage.

Under PPO plans, patients can visit their PCP any time and receive full coverage. With a referral, patients can visit a specialist, but they typically pay a higher copayment and may receive only partial coverage, depending on whether the specialist is in the network.

A **point-of-service (POS) plan** combines characteristics of both the HMO and the PPO. Members of a POS plan do not make a choice about which system to use until the point at which the service is being used—hence the name. POS plans offer three service options. Patients can:
1. Visit an HMO provider where the service is covered in full.
2. Visit a provider in the PPO and make a copayment.

3. Visit a provider outside the network and pay a deductible; however, with this last option, only a portion of the cost is paid by the plan.

A high-deductible health plan (HDHP) requires individuals to make periodic deposits in a **Health Savings Account (HSA)**. An HSA is basically a savings and investment account that can be funded with pre-tax dollars to help pay for current or future *eligible* medical expenses not covered by the insurance plan. Deductibles, coinsurance, and in some cases health insurance premiums are some of the things that can be paid from HSA funds. It also allows earnings to grow in the account tax free. Because the HSA is used together with a high-deductible insurance plan, premiums are usually lower as well. (See Chapter 4 for more information on HSAs.) Enrollment in an HDHP allows freedom of choice of providers and/or hospitals.

Carriers that provide healthcare plans are regulated by state laws. The laws vary from state to state, but there are some general guidelines for these plans. For instance, they must
- provide coverage for emergency services without requiring prior approval;
- have a stated time frame in which to pay, contest, or deny any claim;
- be forthright in revealing medical information regarding service and treatment options;
- honor patients' right to a second opinion; and
- disclose procedures for settling grievances

Managed care plans are discussed at length in Chapter 7. For more information on healthcare service plans, visit the Evolve site.

Medicare Supplement Plans

In addition to indemnity and managed care plans, BCBS offers **Medicare supplement plans**. Medicare supplement insurance is designed specifically to provide coverage for some of the costs that Medicare does not pay, such as Medicare's deductible and coinsurance amounts. Also called *Medigap* plans, these supplement plans must meet the minimum standards set by state and federal law. If Medicare-eligible patients do not have supplemental coverage, they must pay the deductibles and coinsurance amounts themselves. Medicare Supplement Plans are discussed in more detail in Chapter 9.

❓ What Did You Learn?

1. What type of services does Blue Cross cover?
2. Explain the BlueCard program.
3. List the various programs offered under the Blue Cross and Blue Shield system.
4. What role do Blue Cross and Blue Shield play in the FEP program?
5. List the 4 healthcare service plan types.

PARTICIPATING VERSUS NONPARTICIPATING PROVIDERS

To review what we learned in Chapter 4, a participating provider (PAR) enters into a contractual agreement with a carrier and agrees to follow certain rules involving claims and payment in turn for advantages granted by the carrier. Not all insurance companies offer such contracts to healthcare providers, but BCBS does. A PAR with BCBS agrees to

- file claims (within the time limit stated in the contract) for all BCBS patients and
- accept the BCBS "allowed" fee as payment in full and write off (adjust) any differences between the fee charged and that which is allowed by BCBS.

In turn, under this contractual agreement, BCBS agrees to

- send payments directly to the provider,
- host periodic staff training seminars,
- offer guides and newsletters at no charge,
- provide assistance with claim problems, and
- publish the practice's information in the BCBS PAR directory.

Providers who are not a part of the previously described contractual agreement are referred to as *nonPARs*. NonPARs do not have to file patient claims and can balance bill the difference between their charges and BCBS-allowed charges. The downside is that in many cases, BCBS mails payments to the patient rather than the provider, however, and the health insurance professional must collect the fees directly from the patient unless the patient agrees to assign benefits (in writing). Benefits can be assigned by having the patient sign either Block 13 on the CMS-1500 form or a separate assignment of benefits form. Assigning benefits authorizes the third-party carrier to send the payment directly to the provider.

★ Imagine This!

Dr. Mueller is a nonPAR with Blue Cross and Blue Shield. The medical receptionist neglected to ask new patient Agnes Blank to assign benefits, so Blue Cross and Blue Shield sent the payment for Agnes' medical services directly to her. Agnes cashes the insurance check but fails to pay Dr. Mueller's bill. Statements mailed to Agnes are returned stamped "moved; no forwarding address."

❓ What Did You Learn?

1. Name two things a Blue Cross and Blue Shield PAR provider must agree to.
2. What special benefits do Blue Cross and Blue Shield extend to PAR providers?

SUBMITTING BCBS AND COMMERCIAL CLAIMS

Guidelines for submitting BCBS claims can be located using the website http://www.bcbs.com/, then clicking on "provider" and then "claims and payment." Step-by-step guidelines for completing commercial claims using the CMS-1500 claim form can be accessed on the Evolve site. It is important that the healthcare professional update the instructions for completing the CMS-1500 form periodically to ensure that any changes are noted. When a patient is covered by an insurance company with which the health information professional is unfamiliar, the carrier should be called and guidelines requested to assist in claim submission and to avoid claim delays and rejections.

Most BCBS member offices publish specialty-specific billing guides to help health insurance professionals code and bill specific services, such as physical medicine, eye care, and home medical equipment. These guides can be viewed online under "Provider Guides" on most member websites. Paper copies also are available on request. Keep in mind that claims completion requirements can differ from one commercial carrier to another—even from one BCBS member office to another. Refer to Fig. B-1 in Appendix B for an example of a completed claim for a patient with BCBS health insurance coverage.

Timely Filing

The time limit for filing claims varies among third-party payers. Normally, providers contracting with BCBS (PARs) must file claims within 365 days of the last date of service provided to the patient; however, the health insurance professional should be aware of the specific timely filing guidelines stated in the BCBS/provider contract, because claim filing deadlines may differ among BCBS payers. If a claim is not filed within the specified filing period, BCBS normally does not allow benefits for the claim. If payment on the claim is denied for this reason, the provider cannot collect payment from the patient. Unusual circumstances may allow the provider to request payment past the deadline. Situations such as these are handled on a case-by-case basis. If a claim is denied as "untimely" and the provider did submit it on time, an appeal should be filed, with proof of timely filing attached to the appeal documents and forwarded to the payer.

Filing Electronic Claims

If the provider's office is set up for electronic claims filing, the health insurance professional should contact the carrier before submitting the claims directly to find out what format will be compatible. If the provider uses a claims clearinghouse, the clearinghouse manages this process. The Health Insurance Portability and Accountability Act–Administrative Simplification (HIPAA-AS), passed by Congress in 1996, set standards for the electronic transmission of healthcare data and to protect the privacy of individually identifiable healthcare information. It is important that these standards be adhered to.

To make sure electronic claims have been received by the payer (or clearinghouse) for processing within the timely filing limits, the health insurance professional should review the electronic claims receipt, a report that the carrier normally sends after each electronic transmission. This report is usually available to review within 24 to 48 hours after transmission and confirms timely filing. It also provides a summary of all claims that are accepted, are rejected, and/or contain errors. Accepted claims are passed on to the insurer's internal claims processing system(s) for consideration. Rejected claims appear individually on the report with the reason for rejection. To be considered for further processing, claims with errors must first be corrected and then resubmitted electronically. To review an example of an electronic claims receipt report, visit the Evolve site.

? What Did You Learn?

1. What is the filing deadline for submitting Blue Cross and Blue Shield claims?
2. If the provider's office is set up for electronic claims filing, how can the health insurance professional find out whether his or her facility is compatible with the carrier's electronic standards?
3. What federal legislation set standards for the electronic transmission of healthcare data and to protect the privacy of individually identifiable healthcare information?
4. Name the document that guarantees that claims reached the payer/clearinghouse on time?

COMMERCIAL CLAIMS INVOLVING SECONDARY COVERAGE

It is not unusual for a patient to be covered under a second insurance policy. A typical situation would be when a husband and wife are employed with companies who offer paid, or partially paid, group insurance plans. Because of the rising costs of health insurance, however, dual coverage is becoming less common. When a situation such as this arises, it is important to find out which policy is primary and to submit the claim to that carrier first. Usually, the best way to determine primary coverage is to ask the patient. Normally, when a husband and wife are covered under separate policies, primary coverage follows the patient. If the patient is unsure, the health insurance professional should

call his or her employer or contact the third-party payer directly.

When the primary carrier has processed the claim and payment is determined, a new claim is sent to the secondary carrier with the **explanation of benefits** (EOB) from the primary carrier attached. An EOB, also called a *remittance notice* or *remittance advice (RA),* is a document prepared by the carrier that gives details of how the claim was adjudicated. It typically includes a comprehensive listing of patient information, dates of service, payments, or reasons for nonpayment (Fig. 6-3). In some situations, as with patients who have both Medicare and Medicaid, there is what is called a "crossover," that is, the claim is filed first with Medicare, during which any deductible and/or coinsurance is applied, then it is automatically forwarded to Medicaid. Providers do not bill Medicaid separately. This automatic crossover process is the same for patients with both Medicare and Medigap policies.

⏱ Stop and Think

Carol Bolton is a computer programmer for American Commuter Services, Inc (ACS). She and her dependents are covered under an employer-sponsored group policy, and ACS pays the entire premium. Jim Bolton, her husband, is employed by ESI Repairs and is covered under a similar family plan through his employer. How might it be determined which policy is primary when Carol is seen in the office for her yearly physical?

Electronic Remittance Advice (ERA)

In January 2011, CMS began the implementation process to convert from ANSI version 4010A1 to ANSI version 5010 base and **errata**—revisions to the published document to correct minor errors. This conversion process will affect the Health Care Claim Payment/Advice 835 electronic remittance transaction. Visit the Evolve site to view a side-by-side comparison of the old **electronic remittance advice (ERA)** and the new 5010 ERA. More information on the electronic ERA is provided in Chapter 16.

? What Did You Learn?

1. What is the best way to determine primary coverage for a patient who has two insurance policies?
2. What is the purpose of an EOB?

Explanation of Health Care Benefits
THIS IS NOT A BILL

Page Number
1

MURRAY L. WHITE
3434 West Covington Place
Somewhere, XY 12345

Identification No.:	111-23-4567
Patient Name:	Sarah M. White
Provider Name:	Dean P. Locks, MD

Benefits Summary

Billed Charges	Provider Savings	Other Insurance Settlement	Blue Cross Blue Shield Settlement	Amount You Owe
136.00				136.00

Claim Details

Place of Service	OFFICE	OFFICE	OFFICE	OFFICE
Description of Service	MEDICAL CARE	LABORATORY	LABORATORY	LABORATORY
Service Date: From/To	12/11 12/11/03	12/11 12/11/03	12/11 12/11/03	12/11 12/11/03
Billed Charge	90.00	18.00	18.00	10.00
Provider Savings (-)				
Contract Limitations (-)		11.00	11.00	6.25
Copayment (-)				
Deductible (-)	90.00	7.00	7.00	3.75
Sub-Total		1	1	1
Coinsurance				

Please see the back of this form for the "Definition of Terms."

Group Number	Claim Number	Account Number	Provider Number	Date Received	Date Processed
000059999–2104	05040190981500	A–0000960	17437	01–19–04	01–20–04

NOTES

1–YOU MAY BE MISSING OUT ON SAVINGS THAT YOU WOULD RECEIVE IF SERVICES HAD BEEN PERFORMED BY A BLUE CROSS AND BLUE SHIELD PARTICIPATING PROVIDER. (Z183)

$107.75 OF THIS CLAIM HAS BEEN APPLIED TO YOUR BASIC BLUE CROSS AND BLUE SHIELD DEDUCTIBLE. FOR THE PERIOD BEGINNING ON 10/01/02 THROUGH 12/31/03, THIS PATIENT HAS SATISFIED $2969.42 OF THE $5000.00 DEDUCTIBLE. (Z551)

530-409 C-5356 (MD) 7/02

Fig. 6-3 Sample explanation of benefits.

Continued

NOTES KEY

A. Your benefit plan covers accidental injury, medical emergency and surgical care. Other medical care received in the hospital's outpatient department or practitioner's office is not covered by your benefit plan.

B. The services identified on this claim do not meet the criteria of a medical emergency as defined in your benefit plan.

C. These services and/or supplies are not a benefit for the diagnosis, symptom or condition given on the claim.

D. These services are not covered by your benefit plan as described in the **Services Not Covered** section.

E. Routine physical exams and related services are not covered by your benefit plan as described in the **Services Not Covered** section.

F. These services were not performed within the time limit for treatment of accidental injury.

G. Routine vision examinations, eyeglasses, or examinations for their prescription or fittings are not covered by your benefit plan as described in the **Services Not Covered** section.

H. The services of this provider are not covered by your benefit plan.

I. These services exceed the maximum allowed by your benefit plan as described in the **Summary of Payment** section.

J. These services were received before you satisfied the waiting period required by your benefit plan as described in **Your Payment Obligations** section.

K. These services were not submitted within timely filing limits. Timely filing requires that we receive claims within 365 days after the end of the calendar year you receive services.

L. Using the identification number provided, we are unable to identify you as a member.

M. These services were performed before your benefit plan became effective.

N. These services were performed after your benefit plan was cancelled.

O. This individual is not covered by your benefit plan.

P. This individual may be eligible for Medicare. File this claim first with Medicare, if the individual has no other group health coverage as primary.

Q. The Plan in the state where these services were received will process this claim. Your claim has been sent to that Plan for processing.

R. These services have been billed to the wrong plan. Please forward your claim to the plan named on your identification card for processing.

S. These services are a duplication of a previously considered claim.

T. All or part of these services were paid by another insurance company or Medicare.

U. We have received no response to our request for additional information. Until this information is received, the claim is denied.

V. Personal convenience items or hospital-billed non-covered services are not covered by your benefit plan as described in the **Services Not Covered** section.

W. Services covered by Worker's Compensation are not covered by your benefit plan as described in the **Services Not Covered** section.

X. These services should be billed to the carrier that provides your hospital or medical coverage.

DEFINITION OF TERMS

Billed Charge: The total amount billed by your provider. *(If your coverage is Select and you receive covered services in the office of a Select provider, your coinsurance is based on this amount).*

Coinsurance: The amount, calculated using a fixed percentage, you pay each time you receive certain covered services.

Copayment: The fixed dollar amount you pay for certain covered services.

Deductible: The fixed dollar amount you pay for covered services before benefits are available.

Sub-Total: The amount reached by subtracting from the billed charge the following applicable amounts: provider savings; contract limitations; copayment and deductible. Your coinsurance is calculated on this amount *(unless your coverage is Select and you receive covered services in the office of a Select provider. In this case, your coinsurance is based on billed charge).*

Settlement: The total amount fulfilled by us as a result of our agreement with the provider; or the amount we pay directly to you.

Other Insurance Settlement: The total amount settled by another carrier (or us) because you are covered by more than one health plan.

Provider Savings: The amount saved because of our contracts with providers. For some inpatient hospital services, this amount may be an estimate. See explanation of payment arrangements in your benefits certificate.

Contract Limitations: Amounts for which you are responsible based on your contractual obligations with us. Examples of contract limitations include all of the following:
• Amounts for services that are not medically necessary.
• Amounts for services that are not covered by this certificate.
• Amounts for services that have reached contract maximums.
• If you receive services from a nonparticipating provider, any difference between the billed charge and usual, customary, and reasonable (UCR) amount.
• Penalty amounts for services that are not properly precertified.
• Penalty amounts for receiving inpatient hospital services from a nonparticipating hospital.

NOTICE OF RIGHT TO APPEAL AND ERISA RIGHTS

If you disagree with the denial, or partial denial of a claim, you are entitled to a full and fair review.

1. Submit a WRITTEN request for a review within 180 days OF THE DATE OF THIS NOTICE. Your request should include:

   • Date of your request;
   • Your printed name and address (and name and address of authorized representative if you have designated one);
   • The identification number and claim number from your Explanation of Health Care Benefits;
   • The date of service in question.

2. Send your request to:

Fig. 6-3—cont'd

SUMMARY CHECKPOINTS

▶ FFS, or indemnity, insurance is a traditional kind of healthcare policy. The insurance company pays a specific percentage of the fees for the services provided to the insured individuals covered by the policy. FFS health insurance offers the most choices of physicians and hospitals. Typically, patients can choose any physician they want and can change physicians at any time. Additionally, they can go to any hospital in any part of the United States and still be covered.

▶ With an FFS plan, the policyholder pays a periodic fee, or premium. In addition to the premium, a specific amount of money, called the deductible, must be paid out of pocket each year as costs are incurred before the insurance payments begin. (The deductible might be anywhere from $100 to $10,000.) Not all healthcare expenses count toward the deductible—only those specifically covered by the policy. After the deductible has been met, the policyholder or dependents share the cost of services with the insurance carrier. For example, the patient might pay 20% of covered expenses and the insurer 80%. This type of cost sharing is referred to as coinsurance.

▶ FFS insurance offers three levels of coverage:
1. *Basic health insurance* coverage includes
   • hospital room and board and inpatient hospital care;
   • some hospital services and supplies, such as x-rays and medicine;
   • surgery, whether performed in or out of the hospital; and
   • some physician visits.
2. Major medical insurance coverage includes
   • treatment for long, high-cost illnesses or injuries and
   • inpatient and outpatient expenses.
3. *Comprehensive* is a combination of the two.

▶ Preexisting conditions—physical or mental disorders that existed before a health insurance policy was issued and for which the individual received treatment—are frequently excluded from coverage under some insurance policies, or a specified time must elapse before the condition is covered, typically anywhere from 30 days to 2 years. The Patient Protection and Affordable Care Act, part of the Healthcare Reform legislation, changed the preexisting condition requirements. Effective September 2010, children younger than 19 years with preexisting conditions may not be denied access to their parents' health plan because of a preexisting condition. Until 2014, however, the preexisting condition exclusion factor for adults is still applicable, and health plans may issue a policy conditionally by providing a preexisting condition exclusion period.

▶ A self-insured health plan is one in which an employer or other group sponsor, rather than an insurance company, is financially responsible for paying plan expenses, including claims made by group plan members.

▶ The national Blue Cross and Blue Shield Association was formed in the 1982 merger of the Blue Cross Association and the National Association of Blue Shield Plans. BCBS insurers also act as Medicare administrators in many states or regions of the United States. They also provide group coverage to state government employees, as well as the federal government, under a nationwide option of the Federal Employees Health Benefit Plan (FEHBP) established by the Association on their behalf. Plan choices include
• FFS plans,
• PPO plans,
• POS plans, and
• HMO plans.

▶ More than 80% of healthcare providers in the United States accept BCBS patients.

▶ BCBS underwrites or administers many plans, including
• BlueCard and BlueCard Worldwide Programs,
• FEHB Program,
• FEP,
• Healthcare service plans, and
• Medicare supplemental plans.

▶ PARs enter into a contractual agreement with the carrier and agree to follow the payer's specific guidelines for claims and payment in turn for certain advantages granted by the payer. Providers who do not enter into such a contractual agreement with the payer are referred to as *nonPARs*.

▶ BCBS claims usually must be filed within 365 days after the last date of service provided to the patient; however, the timely filing deadline can vary among payers. Health insurance professionals should follow provider/payer contract guidelines.

▶ For people who are covered by two different commercial insurance policies, the claim is sent to the primary carrier first. After it has been processed and payment is determined, an explanation of benefits (EOB), along with a payment (if any), is sent to the provider. A new claim is sent to the secondary carrier with the EOB from the primary carrier attached. In some situations, as with patients who have both Medicare and Medicaid, there is what is called a "crossover," that is, the claim is filed first with Medicare, for which any deductible and/or coinsurance is applied, then it is automatically forwarded to Medicaid. Providers do not bill Medicaid separately. This automatic crossover process is the same for patients with both Medicare and Medigap policies.

⟳ CLOSING SCENARIO

Some of the topics in this chapter turned out to be a little more challenging than Emilio and Latisha had anticipated, especially the concepts of self-insurance and exchanges. Both students found the information on Blue Cross AND Blue Shield particularly interesting, and they were already aware that it was a large and well-known organization. They had seen TV commercials on "The Blues," but they were unaware of how the organization got its start. Compared with today's costs, the idea of a plan providing 21 days of hospital care for only $6 a year was difficult to comprehend.

Emilio recalls changing physicians 2 years ago because the practice from which his family received most of their medical care discontinued its PAR contract with Blue Cross and Blue Shield. He was unaware at the time, however, of the ramifications of a provider's being either PAR or nonPAR. Now, he realizes how this difference can affect the patient directly.

Latisha is focusing her attention on the Blue Cross and Blue Shield guidelines for completing the CMS-1500 paper claim form and comparing it with the process of generating a claim on the practice management software program available in the computer lab. Many of the patients in the healthcare facility where she previously worked were covered under a Blue Cross and Blue Shield preferred provider plan, and she was familiar with how that plan functioned.

⊖ WEBSITES TO EXPLORE

- For live links to the following websites, please visit the Evolve site at
  http://evolve.elsevier.com/Beik/today/
- A wealth of information about BCBS can be found on their website:
  http://www.bluecares.com/
- For more information on HIPAA-AS, log on to
  http://www.hipaadvisory.com/
- To learn about the changes happening to healthcare, go to
  http://askbluereform.com/

- BCBS has developed an interactive tool to help people learn about the new healthcare reform laws at
  http://www.bcbs.com/news/bcbsa/bcbsa-introduces-askblue-healthcare-reform.html/
- New claim form for Blue Card Worldwide:
  http://www.bcbstx.com/ut/pdf/tx_international.pdf/

Author's Note: Websites change frequently. If any of these URLs is unavailable, use applicable guide words in your Internet search to acquire additional information on the various subjects listed.

CHAPTER 7

Unraveling the Mysteries of Managed Care

Chapter Outline

I. What Is Managed Care?
II. Common Types of Managed Care Organizations
   A. Preferred Provider Organization
   B. Health Maintenance Organization
      1. Staff Model
      2. Group Model
      3. Network Model
      4. Mixed Model
      5. Direct Contract Model
      6. Individual Practice Association
   C. Other Types of MCOs
      1. Point of Service
      2. Provider-Sponsored Organization (PSO)
III. Advantages and Disadvantages of Managed Care
   A. Advantages
   B. Disadvantages
IV. Managed Care Certification and Regulation
   A. National Committee on Quality Assurance
   B. National Committee on Quality Assurance; Health Insurance Portability and Accountability Act
C. The Joint Commission
D. URAC
E. Utilization Review
F. Complaint Management
V. Preauthorization, Precertification, Predetermination, and Referrals
   A. Preauthorization
   B. Precertification
   C. Predetermination
   D. Referrals
      1. How a Patient Obtains a Referral
      2. Referrals Versus Consultations
VI. Health Insurance Portability and Accountability Act and Managed Care
VII. Impact of managed care
   A. Impact of Managed Care on the Physician-Patient Relationship
   B. Impact of Managed Care on Healthcare Providers
VIII. Healthcare Reform's Impact on MCOs
IX. Future of Managed Care

CHAPTER OBJECTIVES

After completion of this chapter, the student should be able to:

1. Explain the concept of managed care.
2. List and briefly explain the common types of managed care organizations.
3. Evaluate the advantages and disadvantages of managed care.
4. Identify and explain the role of managed care accrediting organizations.
5. Explain the function of preauthorization, precertification, and referral.
6. Discuss HIPAA's influence on managed care.
7. Describe the impact of Managed Care on the Patient/Provider relationship.
8. Determine Healthcare Reform's effect on Managed Care Organizations.
9. Analyze the future predictions of managed care.

CHAPTER TERMS

capitation
closed-panel
consultation
copayment
direct contract model

enrollees
grievance
group model
health maintenance organization (HMO)

OPENING SCENARIO

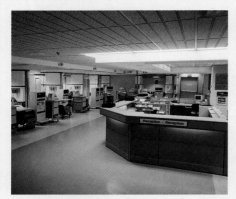

Emilio and Latisha had heard a lot about managed care before they enrolled in the course, but they did not think they fully understood the term and its effect on healthcare in general. Both students remember hearing stories on the news of medical cases gone wrong because of an HMO's refusal to pay for certain services; however, they are determined to remain open-minded regarding these controversial issues. They are prepared to learn the pros and cons of all facets of medical insurance and realize that there is a lot to learn in this particular area of healthcare.

Latisha has gotten a part-time job at Isis Healthcare. She is certain her new job will offer a great deal of insight into managed care because many of the patients visiting the facility are enrolled in a preferred provider organization. She admits that she does not fully understand the ramifications of this type of managed care.

Emilio has decided to volunteer at the free clinic in his neighborhood, which he hopes will foster his understanding of health insurance and what it means to be a health insurance professional. His mentor at the clinic has explained how its HMO functions. Like Latisha, Emilio still has a lot of unanswered questions. Both students are anticipating the information this chapter offers and are confident their questions will be answered and their uncertainty put to rest.

iatrogenic effects
individual practice association (IPA)
managed care
network
network model
open-panel plan
point-of-service (POS)
preauthorization
precertification

predetermination
preferred provider organization (PPO)
primary care physician (PCP)
referral
specialist
staff model
utilization review

WHAT IS MANAGED CARE?

No doubt you have heard the term *managed care*. It became the "buzz word" in healthcare after the enactment of the Health Maintenance Organization Act of 1973. But what exactly is managed care, and why do some find the term so mysterious? According to the United States National Library of Medicine, the term managed care encompasses programs that are intended to reduce unnecessary health care costs through a variety of mechanisms, including: economic incentives for physicians and patients to select less costly forms of care; programs for reviewing the medical necessity of specific services; increased beneficiary cost sharing; controls on inpatient admissions and lengths of stay; the establishment of cost-sharing incentives for outpatient surgery; selective contracting with health care providers; and the intensive management of high-cost health care cases. The programs may be provided in a variety of settings, such as Health Maintenance Organizations and Preferred Provider Organizations.

We learned what traditional fee-for-service (indemnity) insurance was in Chapter 6. In this chapter, we will attempt to unravel the mysteries of **managed care**.

The cost of healthcare is increasing rapidly. In the 1970s, there was a growing concern within the general population about how much individuals in the United States had to pay for good healthcare. Experts came up with some ideas for controlling, or "managing," these costs. Managed care has changed the face of healthcare in the United States today, and it looks as if it is here to stay.

Managed care is a complex healthcare system in which physicians, hospitals, and other healthcare professionals organize an interrelated system of people and facilities that communicate with one another and work together as a unit, commonly referred to as a **network**. This network coordinates and arranges healthcare services and benefits for a specific group of individuals, referred to as **enrollees**, for the purpose of managing cost, quality, and access to healthcare. Managed care organizations (MCOs) typically perform three main functions:

- Set up the contracts and organizations of the healthcare providers who furnish medical care to the enrollees.
- Establish the list of covered benefits tied to managed care rules.
- Oversee the healthcare they provide.

Managed care has strongly influenced the practice of medicine. The principles of managed healthcare shown in Fig. 7-1 represent key components in promoting effective managed care techniques that are fair and equitable to physicians in ensuring that high-quality healthcare services are delivered to patients. MCOs and third-party payers are strongly encouraged to use these guidelines in developing their own policies and procedures. In addition, any public or private entities that evaluate managed care organizations or their contracted entities for purposes of certification or accreditation are encouraged to use these principles in conducting their evaluations.

1. Managed care organizations should encourage access to health coverage—including those individuals with the greatest health risk.
2. Managed care organizations must recognize physicians' principal role in making medical decisions and guarantee strong physician leadership.
3. Managed care organizations should promote members' health by ascertaining that health plans and providers have incentives to provide high quality medical care.
4. Managed care organizations should be accountable for the health of members by preventing, as well as managing, diseases and illnesses.
5. Managed care organizations are ultimately accountable for the health of the enrollees, and for the outcomes of the treatment they receive.
6. Managed care organizations should communicate the outcomes of their services based on valid measures of medical quality.
7. To fulfill their responsibility to society and the communities they serve, managed care organizations should work together with public sector agencies to resolve gaps between commercial insurance and "safety net" programs.
8. Managed care organizations can help the government fulfill its responsibility to ensure healthcare for all through the provision of a more cost-effective and comprehensive system of care.

Fig. 7-1 Principles of managed healthcare.

⭐ Imagine This!

Managed care is not a new idea or even a recent one. Its origins can be traced back to the 1880s, when German Chancellor Otto von Bismarck developed a form of pre-paid health insurance for his workers as a means of warding off plans for a government-run insurance program in Germany. Here in the United States, the original form of managed care dates back to 1933, when a young California surgeon accepted the invitation of Henry Kaiser to provide his workers healthcare on a prepaid basis. The Permanente Foundation Hospital was established. The hospital was named after the Permanente River, which never ran dry (*permanente* means "everlasting" in Spanish.) Today, Kaiser Permanente is the largest HMO in the United States.

💬 What Did You Learn?

1. Explain the concept of managed care.
2. How did managed healthcare get started in the United States?
3. What main functions do MCOs perform?

COMMON TYPES OF MANAGED CARE ORGANIZATIONS

Although there are many forms of managed healthcare, we are going to concentrate on the two most common types:
- Preferred provider organization (PPO)
- Health maintenance organization (HMO)

These two common types of MCOs are compared with traditional (fee-for-service) insurance in Fig. 7-2.

Table 7-1 summarizes the types of Medicare managed care organizations.

PLAN COST	PROVIDER SELECTION	CONSULTS/SPECIALIST	MEMBER OUT-OF-POCKET COSTS
Traditional Insurance	Patient can select any physician, hospital, or healthcare provider (HCP).	Patient can use any specialist. However, some plans require preapproval for certain procedures performed by specialists.	Patients may have to pay an annual deductible usually ranging from $250 to $1000 (depending on what they choose). Patients may also be responsible for coinsurance payments (typically 20%). Coverage for routine care and drugs varies with the policy.
PPO	Patients may select any HCP in the network. If they use a provider outside of the network, they pay a larger portion (up to 50%) of the fee.	Patients may use any specialist in the network, but if they use a provider outside of the network, they will pay a larger portion of the fee.	Patients may have to pay copayments for network doctor visits and drugs. When using a provider outside the network, there may be a deductible and then the plan will reimburse at 70% of the costs.
HMO	Patients may only select providers in the network. If they select a provider outside the network without the HMO approval, they will pay the entire bill.	The PCP determines the need for a specialist—if approval is not received the patient is responsible for the entire bill.	Patients may have to pay copayments for doctor visits and drugs. May be charged copayments for hospital stays and ER visits. Usually there are no deductibles.

Fig. 7-2 Comparison of types of healthcare plans, providers, consultants, and costs.

TABLE 7-1	Summary Charts of Types of Medicare Managed Care Organizations
TYPE OF MANAGED CARE ORGANIZATION (MCO)	**DESCRIPTION**
Health maintenance organization (HMO)	Insurers contract with groups of physicians, hospitals, and other providers to provide medical care to its members. Members must use only network providers and are required to select a primary care physician (PCP). Access to specialists requires referral from the PCP. Most services require small or no copayments.
Preferred provider organization (PPO)	Insurers contract with groups of physicians, hospitals, and other providers to provide medical care to its members. Members are not required to select a PCP. Plan's permission is not required for a member to see a specialist for a Medicare-covered service. A small co-payment is associated with use of a network provider. Costs are higher for use of a non-network provider.
Point-of-service (POS) plan	Allows members to use medical providers at an additional fee that are not part of the managed care plan's provider network. Plan will pay a percentage of cost for use of services of a health care provider outside the network. Member may need plan's approval to receive out-of-network services.
Provider-sponsored organization (PSO)	A plan owned by physicians and hospital(s). Physicians and hospital(s) agree to provide the majority of Medicare-covered services. If unable to provide services directly, they must arrange with other medical providers to furnish needed care.
Private fee-for-service plan	Private insurance companies, approved by CMS, to offer their fee-for-service plans to Medicare beneficiaries. Members may use any provider who agrees to the payment terms of the plan or may use other providers and pay the difference between the provider charges and the plan fees.
Medicare Medical Savings Accounts (MSAs)	Two parts: High-deductible health insurance plan. Members must satisfy the annual deductible through the MSA or personal savings before the health plan pays for medical expenses. CMS will contribute money to the savings account every year. The funds collect interest and carry over each year. The money may be used to pay for medical expenses to satisfy the annual deductible or to cover medical expenses not covered by original Medicare, such as prescription drugs. Either a managed care plan or a fee-for-service plan. Members may not end enrollment until December 31st of each year.

Preferred Provider Organization

Preferred provider organizations (PPOs) are popular throughout the United States. PPOs typically provide a high level of healthcare and offer a variety of medical facilities to everyone who chooses to participate in them.

Here's how a PPO functions: A group of healthcare providers works under one umbrella, the PPO, to provide medical services at a discount to the individuals who participate in the PPO. The PPO contracts with this network of providers, who agree to offer medical services to the PPO members at lower rates (smaller and lower coinsurance limits) in exchange for being part of the network. This agreement allows the PPO to reduce overall healthcare costs. Two things about PPOs make them popular:

- Members do not have to choose a **primary care physician (PCP)**, a specific provider who oversees the member's total healthcare treatment.
- Participants do not need authorization from the PCP, commonly called a **referral**, to visit any physician, hospital, or other healthcare provider who belongs to the network.

Plan members can visit physicians and hospitals outside the network. Visits to healthcare providers who do not belong to the PPO network do not have the same coverage,

however, as visits to providers within the network, and the amount of money the patient has to pay out of his or her own pocket, the **copayment**, is higher. The deductible normally does not change if and when a PPO member sees a provider outside the network.

Other advantages of PPOs include the following:
- PPO networks are not as tightly controlled by laws and regulations as HMOs.
- Many PPOs offer a wider choice of treatments to members with fewer restrictions than HMOs.

Disadvantages include the following:
- Loosely controlled PPOs are often not much better at controlling costs than traditional fee-for-service (indemnity) health insurance, resulting in higher premiums over time.
- More tightly controlled PPOs come at the expense of the patients' ability to manage their own healthcare treatments.
- The fact that an individual belongs to a PPO may lead the individual to believe that he or she is paying lower premiums than he or she would for traditional healthcare, when this may not be the case at all.

Stop and Think

Ellen Comstock's health insurance carrier is a PPO. Soon after her second child is born, Ellen learns that Dr. Wallingford, her obstetrician, has severed her contractual affiliation with the PPO network. Ellen wants to continue seeing Dr. Wallingford. What ramifications should Ellen consider in seeing a provider outside her PPO network?

Health Maintenance Organization

Under the federal HMO Act, an entity must have the following three characteristics to call itself a **health maintenance organization (HMO):**

- An organized system for providing healthcare or otherwise ensuring healthcare delivery in a geographic area
- An agreed-on set of basic and supplemental health maintenance and treatment services
- A voluntarily enrolled group of people

HMOs provide members with basic healthcare services for a fixed price and for a given period. In return, the participant receives medical services, including physician visits, hospitalization, and surgery, at no additional cost other than a small per-encounter copayment, which is typically less than $25 per visit and sometimes only $5.

Each HMO has a network of physicians who participate in the HMO system. When an individual first enrolls in the HMO, he or she chooses a PCP from the HMO network. This PCP serves as caretaker for the enrollee's future medical needs and is the first person the patient calls when he or she needs medical care. PCPs are usually physicians who practice family medicine, internal medicine, or pediatrics. The PCP determines whether or not the patient's problem warrants a referral to a **specialist,** a physician who is trained in a certain area of medicine (e.g., a cardiologist, who specializes in diseases and conditions of the heart). If an enrollee sees a specialist without the PCP's approval, the HMO normally does not pay the specialist's fees, even if the specialist practices within the network.

HMOs are more tightly controlled by government regulations than PPOs. Members must use the HMO's healthcare providers and facilities, and medical care outside the system usually is not covered except in emergencies. HMOs typically have no deductibles or plan limits. As mentioned earlier, the member pays only a small fee, called a *copayment,* for each visit or sometimes nothing at all. Because the HMO provides all of a member's healthcare for one set monthly premium, it is considered in everyone's best interest to emphasize preventive healthcare.

Some HMOs operate their own facilities, staffed with salaried physicians; others contract with individual physicians and hospitals to be part of the HMO. A few do both. An HMO can be a good choice for some individuals; however, there are many restrictions. If its facilities are convenient and the individual wants to avoid most out-of-pocket expenses and paperwork, an HMO might be a good healthcare option.

One problem exists, however. Some states, especially those that are predominantly rural, offer few HMO choices. Iowa, for instance, had only 37 functioning HMOs in 2009, compared with 101 in California. At that time, there were a total of 441 HMOs in the entire United States.

Several types of managed care come under the HMO umbrella. We'll look at some of the more common types in the following paragraphs.

Staff Model

A **staff model** HMO is a multispecialty group practice in which all healthcare services are provided within the buildings owned by the HMO. The staff model is a **closed-panel** HMO, meaning that other healthcare providers in the community generally cannot participate. Participating providers are salaried employees of the HMO who spend their time providing services only to the HMO enrollees. All routine medical care is furnished, or authorized, by a member's PCP. Preauthorization is necessary for referrals to specialists. In a staff model HMO, the HMO bears the financial risk for the entire cost of healthcare services furnished to the HMO's members.

Group Model

In a **group model,** the HMO contracts with independent, multispecialty physician groups who provide all healthcare services to its members. Physician groups usually share the same facility, support staff, medical records, and equipment. Providers within a group model do not see patients outside the HMO. Group physicians receive reimbursement in the form of **capitation,** a reimbursement system in which healthcare providers receive a fixed fee for every patient enrolled in the plan, regardless of how many or few services the patient uses. (The word "capitation" comes from the Latin phrase *per capita,* meaning "each head.") For example, the managed care insurer negotiates with the provider and agrees to pay him or her $100 a month to care for each of its subscribers, regardless of the amount of services each subscriber uses. The HMO pays the group, which in turn decides how to distribute the money among each of its members.

Network Model

The **network model** HMO allows multiple provider arrangements, including staff, group, and IPA structures. It is similar to the group model HMO, but services are provided at multiple sites by multiple groups so that a wider geographic area is served.

This model usually allows the healthcare provider to be paid on a fee-for-service basis, whereas the group practices in the network might receive a capitation payment from the healthcare plan.

Mixed Model

"Mixed model" describes certain HMO plans in which the provider network is a combination of delivery systems. In general, a mixed model HMO offers the widest variety of choices and the broadest geographic coverage to its members. Patients often have choices of clinics, laboratories, pharmacies, and hospitals as their providers of care.

Direct Contract Model

The **direct contract model** HMO is similar to an individual practice association (see later) except the HMO contracts directly with the individual physicians. The HMO recruits a variety of community healthcare providers, including PCPs and specialists.

Individual Practice Association

In an **individual practice association (IPA)**, services are provided by outpatient networks composed of individual healthcare providers (the IPA) who provide all the needed healthcare services for the HMO. The providers maintain their own offices and identities and see both patients who belong to the HMO and patients who do not. This is an **open-panel plan** because healthcare providers in the community may participate, if they meet certain HMO/IPA standards. IPA reimbursement methods vary from plan to plan.

Other Types of MCOs

Point of Service

The **point-of-service (POS)** model is a "hybrid" type of managed care (also referred to as an *open-ended HMO*) that allows patients to use the HMO provider or go outside the plan and use any provider they choose. When individuals enroll in a POS plan, they are required to choose a PCP to monitor their healthcare. This PCP must be chosen from within the healthcare network and becomes the person's "point of service." The primary POS physician may make referrals outside the network; however, this practice is discouraged because copayments and deductibles are higher for the patients.

Provider-Sponsored Organization (PSO)

A PSO is a type of managed care organization that falls under the Medicare Part C (formerly Medicare + Choice) provision of the Balanced Budget Act of 1997. Now referred to as Medicare Advantage plans, PSOs provide Medicare beneficiaries with alternatives to original Medicare. The PSO receives a fixed monthly payment from the federal government to provide care for Medicare beneficiaries enrolled in the plan and accepts full risk for the lives of these patients. PSOs may be developed as for-profit or not-for-profit entities, of which at least 51% must be owned and governed by healthcare providers (physicians, hospitals, or allied health professionals), and may be organized as either public or private companies. A PSO must supply at least 70% of all medical services required by Medicare law and must do so primarily through its network. The remaining services may come from contracts with other providers if necessary.

To read more about the different types of HMOs, visit the Evolve site.

? What Did You Learn?

1. Name the two most common types of managed care.
2. Explain how a PPO works.
3. List the main differences between PPOs and HMOs.
4. What is the function of a PCP?
5. List four types of managed care.

ADVANTAGES AND DISADVANTAGES OF MANAGED CARE

Managed care has advantages and disadvantages.

Advantages

Preventive care: HMOs pay for programs aimed at keeping their members healthy (e.g., yearly wellness checkups) to avoid paying for more costly services if and when they get sick.

Lower premiums: Because they limit which physicians their members can see and when they can see them, HMOs are able to charge lower premiums.

Prescriptions: As part of their preventive approach, HMOs typically cover most prescriptions for a low copayment (e.g., $2).

Fewer unnecessary procedures: HMOs give physicians financial incentives to provide only necessary care, so physicians are less likely to order tests or operations their patients might not need.

Limited paperwork: Although physicians and hospitals have more paperwork under some types of managed care, HMO members usually only have to show their membership card and pay a relatively low copayment.

Disadvantages

Limited provider pool: To keep costs down, many HMO models tell their members which physicians they can see, including specialists.

Restricted coverage: Often, members cannot expect treatment on demand because the PCP first must justify the need on the basis of what benefits the plan covers.

Prior approval needed: If a member wants to see a specialist, authorization from the PCP is necessary.

Possibility of undertreatment: Because HMOs typically give physicians financial incentives to limit care, some physicians have been known to hold back on the treatment they give their patients.

Compromised privacy: HMOs use patient records to monitor physicians' performance and efficiency, so details of members' medical histories are seen by other people, possibly breaching their right to privacy.

⏱ Stop and Think

Imagine you are employed as a health insurance professional with a multispecialty medical group. Mr. Washburn, a new patient, says to you, "I hear a lot of bad things about HMOs. Are they all true?" What would you tell him?

MANAGED CARE CERTIFICATION AND REGULATION

HMOs receive their accreditation from several organizations: The National Committee on Quality Assurance (NCQA), the Joint Commission, and URAC.

National Committee on Quality Assurance

NCQA, a private, nonprofit organization, accredits healthcare plans on the basis of careful evaluation of the quality of care members receive and of member satisfaction rates. Its membership includes about 90% of all MCOs nationwide. NCQA is committed to improving the quality of healthcare throughout the United States. NCQA provides healthcare information through the Internet and the media to help consumers and employers make more informed healthcare choices.

In addition to accrediting and certifying a wide range of healthcare organizations, NCQA manages the development of the Health Plan Employer Data and Information Set (HEDIS), the performance measurement tool used by most health plans in the United States. MCOs must collect and report HEDIS data to earn NCQA accreditation.

For a particular managed healthcare plan to become accredited by NCQA, it must first undergo a survey and meet certain standards designed to evaluate the facility's clinical and administrative systems. These standards fall into five broad categories, as follows:
- Access and service
- Qualified providers
- Staying healthy
- Getting better
- Living with illness

To evaluate these five categories, NCQA reviews health plan records and providers' credentials, conducts surveys, and interviews health plan staff. A national committee of physicians assigns one of five possible accreditation levels (excellent, commendable, accredited, provisional, or denied) on the basis of the plan's level of compliance with NCQA standards.

National Committee on Quality Assurance; Health Insurance Portability and Accountability Act

The Standards and Guidelines for the Accreditation of Managed Care Organizations, which went into effect in July 2003, also make NCQA's privacy and confidentiality requirements reflect key elements of the Health Insurance Portability and Accountability Act (HIPAA). In particular, NCQA has strengthened standards requiring members to be notified at the time of enrollment of their MCO's policies on the use of their personal health information (e.g., treatment records, claims data). According to the new standards, an organization must inform members about its privacy policies, along with the members' rights and options for accessing their own medical information. The 2003 standards have been made available as printed or electronic publications.

The Joint Commission

The Joint Commission also evaluates and accredits healthcare organizations. Like NCQA, The Joint Commission is an independent, not-for-profit organization and is considered the predominant standards-setting and accrediting body in healthcare in the United States. The Joint Commission is governed by a Board of Commissioners that includes nurses, physicians, consumers, medical directors, administrators, providers, employers, a labor representative, health plan leaders, quality experts, ethicists, a health insurance administrator, and educators. Their mission is "To continuously improve health care for the public, in collaboration with other stakeholders, by evaluating health care organizations and inspiring them to excel in providing safe and effective care of the highest quality and value."

The Joint Commission's accreditation is nationally recognized as a symbol of quality that reflects an organization's commitment to meeting quality performance standards. To earn and maintain accreditation, an organization must undergo an on-site survey by a Joint Commission survey team every 2 to 3 years, depending on the type of facility.

The Joint Commission's standards outline performance expectations for activities that affect the safety and quality of patient care. These standards include
- the rights of patients,
- the assessment and treatment of patients,
- a safe environment for patients and healthcare employees,
- the quality of patient care,
- the management of patients' records, and
- the organizational responsibilities of leadership and staff.

Both The Joint Commission and the NCQA have incorporated the HIPAA standards into their own accreditation criteria.

URAC

Formerly known as the Utilization Review Accreditation Commission, URAC is a nonprofit organization promoting healthcare quality by accrediting many types of healthcare organizations, depending on the functions they carry out. Any organization that meets the URAC standards, including hospitals, HMOs, PPOs, third-party administrator (TPAs), and provider groups, can seek accreditation. Accreditation adds value to these programs by providing an external seal of approval and by promoting quality improvement within the organization as part of the accreditation process.

Utilization Review

Utilization review, sometimes referred to as *utilization management,* is a system designed to determine the medical necessity and appropriateness of a requested medical service, procedure, or hospital admission prior to, during, or after the event. A utilization review may include ambulatory review, case management, certification, concurrent review, discharge planning, prospective review, retrospective review, or second opinions. The utilization review is generally done by the third-party payer's professional staff (nurses and physicians) using standardized medical research data from across the United States and reviewing patient health records in an attempt to make fair and reasonable decisions on behalf of the patients and the third-party payers. Deciding whether or not a service, procedure, or hospital admission is "appropriate" can also be influenced by what is covered in the individual's health insurance plan.

Utilization review is used in managed care plans to reduce unnecessary medical inpatient or outpatient services. One or more individuals within the plan or a separate organization on behalf of the insurer reviews the necessity, use, appropriateness, effectiveness, or efficiency of healthcare services, procedures, providers, or facilities.

Complaint Management

If a particular medical service or procedure is determined not to be medically necessary by the payer or by an independent utilization review organization, it will not be paid for by the insurer. If the patient disagrees, he or she may file a grievance protesting the decision. A **grievance** is a written complaint submitted by an individual covered by the plan concerning any of the following:

1. An insurer's decisions, policies, or actions related to availability, delivery, or quality of healthcare services
2. Claims payment or handling of reimbursement for services
3. The contractual relationship between a covered individual and an insurer
4. The outcome of an appeal

Some states have enacted laws that allow residents to air their complaints to the state insurance commissioner's office when certain medical payments are denied by their health insurer. If a complaint is accepted, an independent review organization (IRO) looks into the situation and determines whether or not the claim should have been paid under the guidelines of the medical policy. The IRO decision is generally final, and if the IRO sides with the insurer, the individual's only remaining alternative is to pursue remediation through the court system. Fig. 7-3 shows an example of one state's insurance complaint system.

The insurance company consumer complaint comparison guide provides helpful information to assess complaints filed against a particular health insurance company and compares it with other companies. The consumer complaint index measures the number of complaints for one company in relation to others in the same market. A company with a complaint index of 1 has an average number of complaints,

---

A Review of Michigan's Insurance Complaint System

Michigan's Office of Financial and Insurance Services (OFIS) contracted with two organizations to act as independent review organizations to review residents' complaints. The system was put into effect in May of 2002. The external review process followed strict policies and procedures; the independent review organizations had 14 days to process the review request. The independent review panel was staffed with qualified, trained, and licensed clinicians as well as other health professionals who were experts in the treatment of the medical condition that is the subject of the external review.

Findings: During the first 16 months of the insurance complaint program, 418 requests for claim reviews were filed with Michigan's OFIS. From the initial 418 requests, there were 309 cases that went to internal review organizations for adjudication. Of these 309 cases, 143 cases were resolved in favor of the patient. A total of 36 cases were dismissed, resulted in a split decision, or have yet to be decided. The OFIS staff resolved the remaining 72 cases internally, thus avoiding the need for external review. One request for external review was withdrawn.

Fig. 7-3 A review of Michigan's insurance complaint system.

whereas a company with a complaint index higher than 1 has more complaints than average. Visit the Evolve site to study this index.

⭐ Imagine This!

Texas is the first state to post information about complaints filed against HMOs and other insurers on the Internet. The Internet Complaint Information System, launched by the state's Department of Insurance, also includes complaints against auto and property insurers. The information is updated quarterly, and only complaints that have been investigated and resolved are included. The most common complaints from members concerned prescription coverage, reimbursement, and denial or nonpayment for emergency care. Most provider complaints were related to denial or delay of payment.

💬 What Did You Learn?

1. Name the organizations from which MCOs receive their accreditation.
2. List NCQA's five evaluative categories.
3. Identify The Joint Commission's standards for activities that affect the safety and quality of patient care. What is a utilization review?

PREAUTHORIZATION, PRECERTIFICATION, PREDETERMINATION, AND REFERRALS

A common method many healthcare payers use to monitor and control healthcare costs is evaluating the need for a medical service before it is performed. Most commercial healthcare organizations and MCOs now request that they be made aware of and consent to certain procedures or services before their enrollees undergo or receive them. Preauthorization and precertification are two cost-containment features whereby the insured must contact the insurer before a hospitalization or surgery and must receive prior approval for the service.

Preauthorization

Preauthorization is a procedure required by most managed healthcare and indemnity plans before a provider carries out specific procedures or treatments for a patient, typically, inpatient hospitalization and certain diagnostic tests. Preauthorization usually works as follows: The healthcare provider or a member of his or her staff contacts the healthcare plan by phone, by fax, or in writing and requests permission to perform the treatment or service proposed. The plan's representative authorizes the service or procedure or not, depending on what the plan covers and whether the procedure or service is considered medically necessary and appropriate. Often, when a procedure or service is authorized, the MCO or carrier assigns a specific identifying number or code.

📁 HIPAA Tip

Before faxing any patient information, the health insurance professional must make sure that the individual on the receiving end of the transmission has a "medical right to know" and that the destination location has a security system in place. HIPAA requires a "confidentiality statement" at the bottom of each fax cover sheet.

Preauthorization pertains to medical necessity and appropriateness only and does not, in all instances, guarantee payment. It is not a treatment recommendation or a guarantee that the patient will be insured or eligible for benefits when the procedure or service is performed.

Preauthorization is also used to identify members for case management or disease management programs. Approval or denial of requests for services is determined by review of all available related medical information and possibly a discussion with the requesting physician (Fig. 7-4).

🕐 Stop and Think

You overhear a patient telling another that she is going to be admitted to the hospital for an operation. "They have to get permission from my HMO before I can be admitted," the woman says. "If my HMO says it's okay," she continues, "they'll pay all of my hospital bills." Should you, as a health insurance professional, interrupt the conversation to clarify what impact a preauthorization has on her hospitalization? If so, what would you say?

Precertification

Precertification is a process used by health insurance companies to control healthcare costs and is similar to preauthorization. Precertification can be defined as "a formal assessment of the medical necessity, efficiency, or appropriateness of a medical provider's treatment plan for a specific illness or injury." The treatment plan needs to be consistent with the diagnosis or condition; rendered in a cost-effective manner; and in line with national medical practice guidelines regarding type, frequency, and duration of treatment.

Precertification involves collecting information before inpatient admissions or performance of selected ambulatory procedures and services (Fig. 7-5). The process permits advance eligibility verification, determination of coverage, and communication with the physician or plan member or both. It also allows the insurance company to coordinate the patient's transition from the inpatient setting to the next level of care (discharge planning) or to register patients for specialized programs, such as disease management, case management, or a prenatal program.

In some instances, precertification is used to inform physicians, members, and other healthcare providers about cost-effective programs and alternative therapies and treatments. Typically, the plan's representative takes the following into consideration when precertifying a service or procedure:

- Verifying the member's eligibility and benefits in accordance with applicable plan documents
- Determining coverage for inpatient admissions and selected ambulatory services
- Assessing appropriateness of the proposed site of service
- Identifying alternatives to proposed care or site of service when appropriate
- Identifying and referring to case management programs when appropriate
- Identifying any quality-of-care issues and referring for review
- Identifying and documenting potential coordination of benefits, subrogation, or workers' compensation information.

Predetermination

Predetermination occurs when the provider notifies the insurance company of the recommended treatment before it begins. The insurance company estimates the benefit amount that is normally paid for this, or like, treatment; however, as with preauthorization, predetermination is not always a guarantee of payment.

Referrals

A *referral* is a request by a healthcare provider for a patient under his or her care to be evaluated or treated by another provider, usually a specialist. The purpose of a referral by a PCP to a specialist is to

- inform a specialist that the patient needs to be seen for care (or second opinion) in his or her field of specialty and

Tri-State Medical Group

PREAUTHORIZATION REQUEST FORM

PATIENT INFORMATION

Last Name: _____ First Name: _____

DOB: _____ Member #: **R** _____ Group #: _____

PREAUTHORIZATION REQUEST INFORMATION

Please list *both* procedure/product code <u>and</u> narrative description:

CPT / HCPCS Code(s): _____ Durable Medical Equipment: ☐ Rental ☐ Purchase

Description: _____

_____

Date of Service: _____ Length of Stay (if applicable): _____

Place of Service or Vendor Name: _____

Assistant Surgeon Requested? ☐ Yes ☐ No **Please list *both* diagnosis(es) code <u>and</u> narrative description:**

1. ICD-9 Code: _____

   Description: _____

2. ICD-9 Code: _____

   Description: _____

Ordering Physician/Provider: _____ Office Location: _____
FIRST <u>AND</u> LAST NAMES PLEASE

Referring Physician/Provider: _____
FIRST <u>AND</u> LAST NAMES PLEASE; REQUIRED FOR PRIME PLANS

Date: _____ Contact Person: _____ Phone: _____

> **Please Note: <u>Incomplete forms will delay the preauthorization process.</u>**
> **Requests received after 3:00 PM are processed the next working day.**
>
> **PacificSource responds to preauthorization requests within 2 working days.**
> **A determination notice will be mailed to the requesting provider, facility, and patient.**
>
> **Please attach pertinent chart notes as appropriate.**

FOR INTERNAL OFFICE USE ONLY:

STATUS: APPROVED / DENIED / PENDING / EXPLANATION

DATE: _____ ACUITY: _____ INITIALS: _____

Reason/Status _____

_____

Field 11 Notes _____ LOS Approved _____

☐ Chart notes filed with preauthorization

Notes _____

Field 10 Facility Copy _____

PO Box 5555 • Somewhere OR 00908 • (541) 555-5584 • (800) 555-6052 x 2584

MEDICAL AFFAIRS DEPARTMENT CONFIDENTIAL FAX: (541) 555-2051

9/8/2003

Fig. 7-4 Generic preauthorization form.

Tri-State Medical Group

FAX Request Form for Precertification Review

To:_____ Date:_____

(Area Code) Fax:_____

(Area Code) Phone:_____

Attn:_____

From:_____ Fax:_____

Number of Pages (Including Cover Sheet):_____
If there is problem with the receipt of this fax, please call _____.Thank you.

Recipient/Patient Name:_____
Complete Recipient
Address _____

_____

ID Number:_____ CAMA ☐ Yes   ☐ No

Requested Admit Date:_____ Diagnosis Code(s):_____

Procedure Date(s): _____

Days Requested: _____ Procedure Code(s):_____

New Admit? ( ) Transfer ( )

Recertification Review? Y( ) If So, Par/Reference #_____

Setting: ☐ Inpatient   ☐ Physician Office
                     ☐ Outpatient   ☐ Out of State

Admit Type: ☐ Non-urgent/Emergent   ☐ Urgent/Emergent

Physician Name:_____ Phone:_____
                                        Fax:_____

Facility:_____ Phone:_____
                                        Fax:_____

Clinical Information:_____
_____
_____
_____
_____

Fig. 7-5 Generic precertification form.

- inform the insurance company that the PCP has approved the visit to a specialist because most managed care companies would not pay for care that has not been authorized with a referral.

How a Patient Obtains a Referral

The patient schedules a visit with the PCP, who evaluates the problem. If the PCP decides that the patient's condition or symptoms warrant a specialist's opinion, a referral form is completed (Fig. 7-6). In most managed care situations, for the insurance company to recognize the referral, it must come from the patient's designated PCP or a provider who is covering for the PCP. If an orthopedic physician refers a patient to a physical therapist, the patient must also obtain a referral from his or her PCP to process through the insurance company.

Referrals versus Consultations

There is a significant difference between a referral and a **consultation**. A consultation occurs when the PCP sends a patient to another healthcare provider, usually a specialist, so that the consulting physician may render his or her expert opinion regarding the patient's condition. The intent of a consultation is usually for the purpose of an expert opinion only, and the PCP does not relinquish the care of the patient to the consulting provider. In the case of a referral, the PCP typically relinquishes care of the patient, or at least a specific portion of care, to the specialist. The insurance professional must determine whether the visit is a consultation or a referral, because this status will affect accurate Current Procedural Terminology (CPT) code selection for the visit.

⭐ Imagine This!

Daniel Bowers visited Dr. Adler, his PCP, with complaints of back pain and numbness in his left leg radiating down to his left foot. Dr. Adler x-rayed Daniel's spinal column and discovered a degenerative disk condition and subsequently referred him to Dr. Langford, who specialized in degenerative disk disease.

Susan Lane, another patient of Dr. Bowers, complained of heart palpitations during an office visit for treatment of a severe case of poison ivy. After performing an electrocardiogram, Dr. Bowers informed Susan he was sending her to Dr. Woodley for a stress electrocardiogram and an echocardiogram to determine whether her palpitations represented a serious cardiac problem.

While in the hospital for a hip replacement, Evelyn Conner was diagnosed with diabetes. Dr. Blake, her surgeon, asked Dr. Martin, a specialist in endocrinology, to manage Mrs. Conner's diabetic condition.

🕐 Stop and Think

Study the three cases in Imagine This! Decide whether each one is a consultation or a referral.

💬 What Did You Learn?

1. Explain the difference between preauthorization and precertification.
2. List some of the typical things that a plan's representative takes into consideration when precertifying a procedure or service.
3. What is a referral?

HEALTH INSURANCE PORTABILITY AND ACCOUNTABILITY ACT AND MANAGED CARE

The Health Insurance Portability and Accountability Act of 1996 was intended to improve the efficiency of healthcare delivery, reduce administrative costs, and protect patient privacy. In general, the law required covered entities (most health plans, healthcare clearinghouses, and healthcare providers who engage in certain electronic transactions) to come into compliance with each set of HIPAA standards within 2 years following adoption, except for small health plans, which had 3 years to come into compliance. For the electronic transaction and code sets rule only, Congress in 2001 enacted legislation extending the deadline to October 16, 2003, for all covered entities, including small health plans. The legislative extension did not affect the compliance dates for the health information privacy rule, which was April 14, 2003, for most covered entities (and April 14, 2004, for small health plans).

Previously, we discussed the fact that if an insured person lost insurance coverage for some reason (e.g., losing a job), he or she could be required to prove insurability before obtaining new coverage. For most individuals, this was not a problem; however, for individuals with chronic or preexisting health problems or whose health deteriorated while they were covered, it was a serious problem. One of the most important protections under HIPAA is that it helps those with preexisting conditions get health coverage. In the past, some employers' group health plans limited, or even denied, coverage if a new employee had such a condition before enrolling in the plan. Under HIPAA, that is not allowed. If the plan generally provides coverage but denies benefits to an individual because he or she had a condition before coverage began, then HIPAA applies.

Under HIPAA, a plan is allowed to look back only 6 months for a condition that was present before the start

Broadmoor Medical Center

Date Referred: _____

Referred By: _____ Supervising MD _____ Phone: _____ Fax: _____

Referred To: _____ Fax #: _____

Office Address: _____ Phone #: _____

Patient Name: _____ DOB: _____ Gender: F / M

Parent's Name (if patient is a minor): _____

Home Phone: _____ Work Phone: _____ Cell Phone: _____

Patient's Address: _____

Authorization: ☐ Not Required   ☐ Requested/Pending   ☐ Requested/Obtained Auth # _____

Primary Medical Insurance: _____ Subscriber ID#: _____

Secondary Medical Insurance: _____ Subscriber ID#: _____

Worker's Comp Insurance (if any): _____ Employer: _____

Adjustor: _____ Claim #: _____ Date of Injury: _____

Comp Address: _____ Comp Telephone: _____

For Urgent Referrals (need to be seen within a week), **the referring clinician should call the specialist.**

☐ **Reason for Referral (Symptoms of Concern)** (also send related medical records or dictated summary)

    ☐ Please advise on the patient's care   ☐ Please assume care of this patient
    Please ask patient to provide related records from other specialists, if any.

☐ **Relevant lab test and imaging results** (also send related medical records)

☐ **Medications and Dosages tried and outcomes** (if not specifically noted in medical records sent with referral)
    Please ask patient to bring his/her complete medication list with dosages (or bring the meds themselves) to their appointment.

Appointment is scheduled with: _____ on _____ at _____ arrival time

Prior to appointment please obtain the following information, tests, etc: Date faxed to referring clinician: _____

☐ We will contact patient to schedule   ☐ Please have patient call to schedule   ☐ Please call patient to schedule

CONFIDENTIAL NOTICE: This facsimile, including any attachments, is for the sole use of the intended recipient(s) and may contain confidential and privileged information or otherwise protected by law. Any unauthorized review, use, disclosure or distribution is prohibited. If you are not the intended recipient, please contact the sender and destroy all copies of the original facsimile.   Rev 10/10/06

Fig. 7-6 Universal referral form.

of coverage in a group health plan. Specifically, the law says that preexisting condition exclusion can be imposed on a condition only if medical advice, diagnosis, care, or treatment was recommended or received during the 6 months prior to the individual's enrollment date in the plan.

★ Imagine This!

Elwood Freitag had arthritis for many years before he began working at Festival Specialty Tools. He did not receive medical advice, diagnosis, care, or treatment, nor was any recommended, in the 6 months prior to his enrolling in the Festival's group health plan. As a result, his prior disorder cannot be subject to a preexisting condition exclusion. If he had received medical advice, diagnosis, care, or treatment within the 6 months before enrolling, then the plan could have imposed a preexisting condition exclusion for that condition (arthritis).

📁 HIPAA Tip

HIPAA prohibits plans from applying a preexisting condition exclusion to pregnancy, genetic information, and certain children.

Going back to the example in the preceding Imagine This!, if Elwood had a preexisting condition that could have been excluded from Festival's plan coverage, then there is a limit to the preexisting condition exclusion period that can be applied. HIPAA limits the preexisting condition exclusion period for most people to 12 months (18 months for people who enroll late), although some plans may have a shorter period or none at all. In addition, some people with a history of prior health coverage will be able to reduce the exclusion period even further using credible coverage. (Review the topic "HIPAA and Credible Coverage" in Chapter 6.) It is important to remember that a preexisting condition exclusion relates only to benefits for the employees' (and dependents') preexisting conditions. After enrollment, coverage will be effective for the plan's other benefits during that time.

Although HIPAA adds protections and makes it easier to switch jobs without fear of losing health coverage for a preexisting condition, the law has limitations. For instance, HIPAA

- does not require that employers offer health coverage;
- does not guarantee that any condition an individual now has (or has had in the past) is covered by a new employer's health plan; and
- does not prohibit an employer from imposing a preexisting condition exclusion period if an employee has been treated for a condition during the past 6 months. (But see Chapter 6 on credible coverage to reduce or eliminate the exclusion.)

HIPAA regulations affect other areas of healthcare, too, including

- maintaining patient confidentiality,
- implementing standards for electronic transmission of transactions and code sets,
- establishing national provider and employer identifiers, and
- resolving security and privacy issues arising from the storage and transmission of healthcare data.

How do these regulations affect managed healthcare? Some experts claim that the cost of complying with HIPAA exceeds $9 billion. The repercussions of this added cost likely affects all healthcare, not just managed care. Large medical facilities for the most part were able to shoulder the expense of becoming HIPAA compliant; however, many small, one- or two-physician practices found it very difficult. HIPAA zeros in on electronic health information. Even if a solo practitioner has all paper records, as soon as he or she starts dealing electronically with billing of third-party payers, he or she encounters HIPAA's strict regulations.

★ Imagine This!

Elliot Larson was the sole proprietor of a small podiatry practice in south-central Iowa. He employed two full-time staff members, a receptionist and an assistant who was a licensed practical nurse. When the HIPAA law was enacted, his office was already computerized and submitting claims electronically to a certain major carrier. Dr. Larson's financial advisor calculated that it would cost approximately $50,000 to upgrade his office to HIPAA compliance. Dr. Larson did not want to revert to a manual accounting system, plus he was under contract to submit claims electronically to the major carrier under which most of his patients had coverage. To justify the cost to upgrade to HIPAA's regulations, he would have to raise his fees. The socioeconomic area where he practiced was predominantly agricultural, where the farmers and rural people could not afford increased charges. Dr. Larson closed his practice in the small, rural town where he'd been practicing for 10 years and joined a multispecialty group in Des Moines.

The consequences of noncompliance are the legal penalties HIPAA provides for failure to adopt its standards. Fines range from $100 for violating a general requirement to $50,000 or more for more serious offenses, such as wrongful disclosure of individually identifiable health information.

📁 HIPAA Tip

HIPAA's impact on MCOs is the same as that on fee-for-service-type structures. HIPAA does not have a separate set of rules and regulations for MCOs.

What Did You Learn?

1. List four areas of healthcare affected by HIPAA regulations.
2. Under HIPAA, how many months is a plan allowed to look back for a condition that was present before the start of coverage in a group health plan?
3. True or False: HIPPA requires that employers offer health coverage.
4. What are the consequences of HIPAA noncompliance?

Imagine This!

Arnold Talbott is a fabrication specialist with Jones Implement. Employees were covered under a group health insurance contract with Superior Healthcare Systems, an HMO, when Arnold first started working for Jones Implement in 1993. Over the years, Arnold and his family established a mutually satisfying patient-provider relationship with Dr. VanHorn, their PCP. In 2004, Jones changed carriers and switched their group coverage to Ideal Health Maintenance Group. Because Dr. VanHorn was not a part of Ideal's network, Arnold and his family had to choose a new PCP and have all of their health records transferred.

IMPACT OF MANAGED CARE

Since the 1990s, the United States has witnessed a transformation in all phases of the healthcare system, from financing to the way healthcare services are organized and delivered. The driving force in this transformation, experts say, is the shift from traditional fee-for-service systems to managed care networks. These changes in the U.S. healthcare system came in response to market forces for cost control, to regulatory initiatives on cost and quality, and to consumer demands for quality care and greater flexibility in provider choice. Because these changes occurred so rapidly and extensively, little is known about the long-term effects of managed care on access to care, cost, and quality of care.

The Agency for Healthcare Policy and Research (AHCPR) is the leading federal agency charged with supporting and conducting health services research. The AHCPR's studies are designed to produce information that ultimately will improve consumer choice, improve the quality and value of healthcare services, and support and improve the healthcare marketplace. Most research on managed care has been conducted in HMOs.

Impact of Managed Care on the Physician-Patient Relationship

Managed care can affect relationships between physicians and patients in a variety of ways. First, it may change the way in which such relationships begin and end. The typical HMO pays only for care provided by its own physicians. Preferred provider groups restrict access to physicians by paying a smaller percentage of the cost of care when patients go for care outside the network. These restrictions can limit patients' ability to establish a relationship with the physician of their choice. Termination of physician-patient relationships can also occur without patients' choosing. When employers shift managed care health plans that mandate the determination of PCPs, employees may have no choice but to sever ties with the PCP of the previous plan and establish a relationship with a new one.

Managed care arrangements often control patients' access to medical specialists, restricting patients' freedom to choose providers and obtain the medical services they desire. In HMOs, PCPs function as "gatekeepers" who authorize patient referrals to medical specialists. Critics of managed care claim that this gatekeeping lowers the quality of care, whereas supporters believe that gatekeeping yields benefits such as reducing **iatrogenic effects** (a symptom or illness brought on unintentionally by something that a physician does or says), promoting rigorous review of standards of care, and emphasizing low-technology, care-oriented services.

Seeing a physician and the practice as a whole is the main experience of the managed care plan for most patients. If that experience is difficult or substandard, the patient is likely to blame the practice. Whatever help a practice can give its patients in navigating the waters of managed care can reduce problems for everybody.

Impact of Managed Care on Healthcare Providers

Most healthcare providers believe that the shift within the healthcare industry from fee-for-service toward managed care is requiring providers to

1. become participants in larger provider practice structures (e.g., single-specialty or, preferably, multispecialty group practices, or independent practice associations);
2. become participants in integrated delivery systems, which may include acquisition of physician practices by a hospital system; or
3. become employees and service providers for large insurance organizations or HMOs or both.

With the establishment of managed care, such acquisitions are being considered necessary more often by smaller-scale healthcare providers (e.g., sole practitioners and small partnerships and group practices) to satisfy the increasing demands of managed care contracting. Large employers, insurance organizations, and HMOs view as appealing and seek to contract with healthcare providers who can offer a complete package of "seamless" healthcare services, which satisfies most medical needs within a single integrated delivery system. Providers within these more integrated medical organizations are likely to experience greater economic viability as managed care continues to transform the medical environment.

The PCP is considered by most within the medical sector of the healthcare industry to be the future controller of patient flow and revenue-generating potential for fellow practitioners. Functioning in the role of gatekeeper, the PCP is likely to be required to perform a higher level of services that formerly were referred to specialists in order to control healthcare costs in capitation model healthcare plans.

On a more positive note, in a study of 20,000 subjects that examined variations in healthcare delivery systems, AHCPR-supported research indicated the following:

- *HMO physicians spent more time* with their patients than fee-for-service physicians, and their patients received more preventive care, asked more questions, and were more involved in treatment planning.
- *Managed care patients spent 2 fewer days* in an intensive care unit (ICU) than patients with fee-for-service health insurance, with the average stay for managed care patients costing less. (There was no difference, however, in rates of mortality or ICU readmission between the two groups.)
- *HMO patients were hospitalized 40% less* than patients with fee-for-service plans and treated in solo practices. Group practice outpatient clinic patients had shorter stays and incurred lower costs at a hospital in the study but received the same quality of care as traditional clinic patients at the hospital.
- *Chronically ill patients in managed care plans had better access to care* than patients in fee-for-service plans, but (in a study of 1200 patients in three cities) their care was not as comprehensive, they waited longer for care, and physician-patient continuity was less.

Most patients and healthcare providers agree that the theory of managed care is a good one: Patients receive care through a single, "seamless" system as they move from wellness to sickness back to wellness again. Continuity of care, prevention, and early intervention are stressed.

What Did You Learn?

1. What is AHCPR, and how does it relate to managed care?
2. How does managed care affect the patient-physician relationship?
3. List ways that managed care affects healthcare providers.

HEALTHCARE REFORM'S IMPACT ON MCOs

The new healthcare reform bill promotes wellness—prevention of disease and early intervention. Because wellness and prevention are the mission of most managed care organizations, experts believe that healthcare reform will ultimately lead to some form of a managed care model with limits on spending, and highly integrated healthcare systems will be in the best position to produce more efficient care that provides value and to address three dominant healthcare issues: access, cost, and quality.

HIPAA Tip

The new health reform law adds to the rights and protections under HIPAA, but the most significant ones won't take effect until 2014.

FUTURE OF MANAGED CARE

Many changes are expected to occur as the new healthcare reform laws take effect, and managed care programs will certainly be affected. It is predicted that they will begin competing among themselves and with new types of plans. Cost and efficiency may no longer be the main selling points, being replaced by quality of services. One expert has gone so far as to suggest that along with new systems of managed care and continuing systems of indemnity plans, healthcare providers may even organize and offer services directly to employers, thus eliminating the middlemen. This development may be beneficial to all involved: employers would pay less; providers would be better compensated; and patients would receive better care. Managed care is still evolving and is very much a work in progress. It will be interesting to see what the future brings.

What Did You Learn?

1. Name some of the changes predicted for managed care.
2. What do you think is meant by the statement "Managed care is still evolving and is very much a work in progress"?

SUMMARY CHECKPOINTS

▶ Managed care is a healthcare system in which insurance companies attempt to control the cost, quality, and access of medical care to individuals enrolled in their plan by limiting the reimbursement levels paid to providers, by reducing utilization, or both.

▶ A PPO is a group of hospitals and physicians that agree to render particular services to a group of people, generally under contract with a private insurer. These services may be furnished at discounted rates if the members receive their healthcare from member providers. Services received from providers outside the organization may result in higher out-of-pocket expenses.

▶ In HMOs, enrollees receive comprehensive preventive and hospital and medical care from specific medical providers who receive a prepaid fee. Members select a PCP or medical group from the HMO's list of affiliated physicians. A PCP coordinates the patient's total care, which is normally free from hassles involving deductibles or claim forms. When using medical services, members pay a small copayment, usually between $5 and $25. There are several types of plans under the HMO umbrella, as follows:

- *Staff model:* A closed-panel HMO in which a multispecialty group of physicians is contracted to provide healthcare to HMO members and is compensated by the contractor via salary and incentive programs.
- *Group model:* A managed healthcare model involving contracts with physicians organized as a partnership, professional corporation, or other association. The healthcare plan compensates the medical group for contracted services at a negotiated rate, and that group is responsible for compensating its physicians and contracting with hospitals for care of their patients.
- *IPA:* A type of HMO in which enrollees' healthcare is arranged through contracting physicians in the community who practice in their own offices and may see patients from other HMOs or non-HMO patients on a fee-for-service basis. Physicians may be paid on a capitated or discounted fee-for-service basis.
- *Network model:* A type of HMO that contracts with two or more independent group practices to care for members. Compensation is specific to the contract between the medical groups and the physicians. Participating groups maintain their independent practices and serve their own patients and HMO patients.
- *Direct contract model:* Similar to an independent practice association, except that the HMO contracts directly with individual physicians.
- *POS:* a managed care plan (also called an open-ended HMO) that allows enrollees to use the HMO providers or to go outside the plan and use a provider of their choice; however, when non-HMO providers are used, enrollees typically pay higher out-of-pocket expenses.

▶ Advantages of managed care include
- preventive care,
- lower premiums,
- prescription coverage,
- fewer unnecessary procedures, and
- limited paperwork.

▶ Disadvantages of managed care include
- limited physician pool,
- restricted coverage,
- prior approval needed for specialists,
- possibility of undertreatment, and
- compromised privacy.

▶ Managed care organizations (MCOs) receive their accreditation from several organizations: NCQA, The Joint Commission, and URAC.

- NCQA is a private, not-for-profit organization dedicated to improving healthcare quality and is frequently referred to as a watchdog for the managed care industry. NCQA has been accrediting MCOs since 1991 in response to the need for standardized, objective information about the quality of these organizations. Although the MCO accreditation program is voluntary, it has been well received by the managed care industry. For an organization to become accredited by NCQA, it must undergo a rigorous survey and meet certain standards designed to evaluate the health plan's clinical and administrative systems. In particular, NCQA evaluates health plans in the areas of patient safety, confidentiality, consumer protection, access, service, and continuous improvement.
- The Joint Commission is a private, independent, nonprofit organization that evaluates medical facility compliance on the basis of a focused set of standards that are long known as essential to the delivery of good patient care. The Joint Commission standards are guidelines for achieving "quality" patient care. These standards include
  - the rights of patients,
  - the assessment and treatment of patients,
  - a safe environment for patients and healthcare employees,
  - the quality of patient care,
  - the management of patients' records, and
  - the organizational responsibilities of leadership and staff.
- URAC, another nonprofit organization, also promotes healthcare quality by accrediting many types of healthcare organizations, depending on the functions they carry out. Any organization that meets the URAC standards, including hospitals, HMOs, PPOs, TPAs and provider groups, can seek accreditation.

  Accreditation adds value to these programs by providing an external seal of approval and by promoting quality improvement within the organization as part of the accreditation process.

▶ The *utilization review* process is a method of tracking, reviewing, and giving opinions regarding care provided to patients. Utilization review evaluates the necessity, appropriateness, and efficiency of the use of healthcare services, procedures, and facilities to control costs and manage care. It is one of the primary tools used by MCOs and other health plans.

▶ *Preauthorization* is the process whereby certain tests, procedures, or inpatient hospitalizations are ascertained as "medically necessary" before a service or procedure is performed. Preauthorization does not guarantee payment.

▶ *Precertification* is a process whereby the provider (or a member of his or her staff) contacts the patient's managed care plan before inpatient admissions and performance of certain planned procedures and services to verify the patient's eligibility and coverage for them.

▶ A *referral* occurs when the PCP requests another provider (usually a specialist) to render a second opinion or to perform a more extensive evaluation or treatment of a patient's problem.

▶ HIPAA impacted managed care organizations much the same as it did fee-for-service plans. One of the most important protections under HIPAA is for those with pre-existing conditions to get healthcare coverage. HIPAA's regulations affect other areas of healthcare—both traditional healthcare plans—as well as managed care organizations. These regulations include
- maintaining patient confidentiality,
- implementing standards for electronic transmission of transactions and code sets,
- establishing national provider and employer identifiers, and
- resolving security and privacy issues arising from the storage and transmission of healthcare data.

▶ Managed care can affect relationships between physicians and patients in a variety of ways. The typical HMO pays only for care provided by its own physicians. PPOs restrict access to physicians by paying a smaller percentage of the cost of care when patients go outside the network for care. Managed care arrangements often control patients' access to medical specialists, restricting

patients' freedom to choose providers and obtain the medical services they desire. In HMOs, PCPs function as "gatekeepers" who authorize patient referrals to medical specialists. Critics claim that this gatekeeping lowers the quality of care, whereas supporters believe that gatekeeping yields benefits such as reducing iatrogenic effects, promoting rigorous review of standards of care, and emphasizing low-technology, care-oriented services.

▶ Healthcare reform has also had an effect on managed care organizations. The new healthcare reform bill promotes wellness—prevention of disease and early intervention. Because wellness and prevention are the mission of most managed care organizations, experts believe that healthcare reform will ultimately lead to some form of a managed care model with limits on spending, and highly integrated healthcare systems will be in the best position to produce more efficient care that provides value and addresses three dominant healthcare issues: access, cost, and quality.

▶ The future of managed care is not clear-cut, but the movement from fee-for-service systems to managed care has slowed, and managed care choices tend to be moving away from the more tightly controlled staff model HMOs toward less centralized systems, such as PPOs and POS plans. Experts predict, however, that managed healthcare will overcome its problems and will have a prominent place in the future of healthcare.

CLOSING SCENARIO

There was a lot of information to assimilate in this chapter regarding managed care, especially because Emilio and Latisha knew so little about it before they began the course. They now think they understand the concepts much better, however. Latisha was surprised to learn that there were so many different types of HMOs—she thought an HMO was an HMO. She and Emilio, like so many others, had heard a lot of negative reports about managed care, and they assumed it was inferior healthcare. They now realize that not all MCOs are bad; there are many good ones and a few inferior ones, as is true of fee-for-service carriers.

At the free health clinic where Emilio volunteers, he has developed an information sheet for patients explaining managed care in simple terms, comparing it with the more familiar

fee-for-service structure and including the pros and cons of both. Equipped now with a better understanding of the various structures of health insurance, he is beginning to feel more comfortable in his volunteer work at the free clinic. What it means to be a health insurance professional has taken on a new meaning: It's not just knowing how to complete an insurance form and submitting it; it's also knowing how to build positive relationships with all members of the healthcare team and the patients. Knowing that all the jobs at the clinic are interrelated and that everyone has to work together for the entire system to work efficiently was an important learning experience for Emilio. An appreciation and understanding of the profession are growing as the students continue their lifelong learning experiences in class and in the workplace.

WEBSITES TO EXPLORE

- For a live link to the following website, please visit the Evolve site at
  http://evolve.elsevier.com/Beik/today/
- To learn more about managed care, visit the websites of the groups that evaluate MCOs in the United States, the National Committee for Quality Assurance (NCQA), at
  http://www.ncqa.org/;

The Joint Commission, at
  http://www.jointcommission.org/;
  and URAC, at http://www.urac.org/about/
Author's Note: Websites change frequently. If any of these URLs is unavailable, use applicable guide words in your Internet search to acquire additional information on the various subjects listed.

CHAPTER 8

Understanding Medicaid

Chapter Outline

I. What is Medicaid?

II. Evolution of Medicaid
   A. Temporary Assistance for Needy Families (TANF)
   B. Supplemental Security Income (SSI)
      1. Eligibility
      2. Eligibility Expansion
   C. Medicaid and Healthcare Reform

III. Structure of Medicaid
   A. Federal Government's Role
   B. Mandated Services
   C. States' Options
      1. Categorically Needy
      2. Medically Needy
   D. Community First Choice Option
   E. State Children's Health Insurance Program
   F. Fiscal Intermediaries/Medicaid Contractors
   G. Medical Integrity Contractors

IV. Other Medicaid Programs
   A. Maternal and Child Health Services
   B. Early and Periodic Screening, Diagnosis and Treatment Program
   C. Program of All-Inclusive Care for the Elderly
   D. Medicaid Home and Community-Based Services Waivers

V. Premiums and Cost Sharing
   A. Non-Emergency Use of the Emergency Department
      1. Enforcement

VI. Payment for Medicaid Services
   A. Medically Necessary
   B. Prescription Drug Coverage
   C. Dual Eligibles

D. Accepting Medicaid Patients
E. Participating Providers

VII. Verifying Medicaid Eligibility
   A. Medicaid Identification Card
   B. Electronic Data Interchange
   C. Point-of-Sale Device
   D. Computer Software Program
   E. Benefits of Eligibility Verification Systems

VIII. Medicare/Medicaid Relationship
   A. Special Medicare/Medicaid Programs
   B. Medicare and Medicaid Differences Explained

IX. Medicaid Managed Care

X. Medicaid Claims
   A. Completing the CMS-1500 Using Medicaid Guidelines
   B. Medicaid Secondary Claims
   C. Resubmission of Medicaid Claims
   D. Reciprocity

XI. Medicaid and Third-Party Liability

XII. Common Medicaid Billing Errors

XIII. Medicaid Remittance Advice

XIV. Special Billing Notes
   A. Time Limit for Filing Medicaid Claims
   B. Copayments
   C. Accepting Assignment
   D. Services Requiring Prior Approval
   E. Preauthorization
   F. Retention, Storage and Disposal of Records

XV. Fraud and Abuse in the Medicaid System
   A. What is Medicaid Fraud?
   B. Patient Abuse and Neglect

XVI. Medicaid Quality Practices

CHAPTER OBJECTIVES

After completion of this chapter, the student should be able to:

1. Explain Medicaid in general.
2. Summarize the evolution of Medicaid.
3. Describe the structure of Medicaid and identify federal and states' roles.
4. List and briefly discuss key Medicaid programs (CHIP, EPSDT, PACE).
5. Identify Medicaid groups that are impacted by cost sharing.
6. Discuss circumstances that impact Medicaid payments to providers.
7. Explain the various methods for verifying Medicaid eligibility.
8. Describe the relationship between Medicare and Medicaid.
9. Discuss the role of managed care in Medicaid.
10. Outline the Medicaid claim process.
11. Interpret third-party liability as it relates to Medicaid.
12. List common Medicaid billing errors.
13. Demonstrate an understanding of the Medicaid standard remittance advice.
14. Define fraud and abuse and how it affects the Medicaid program.
15. Discuss Medicaid Quality Practices.

CHAPTER TERMS

abuse
adjudicated
balance billing
budget period
capitation
categorically needy
Children's Health Insurance Program (CHIP)
cost avoid(ance)
cost sharing (share of cost)
countable income
disproportionate share hospitals
dual coverage (Medi-Medi)
dual eligibles
Early Periodic Screening Diagnosis and Treatment (EPSDT)
federal poverty level (FPL)
fraud
"in-kind" income
mandated services
Maternal and Child Health Services
Medi-Medi
Medicaid

Medicaid contractor
Medicaid integrity contractors
Medicaid secondary claim
Medicaid "simple" claim
medically necessary
medically needy
Medicare hospital insurance (Medicare HI)
Medicare-Medicaid crossover claims
optional services
payer of last resort
pay and chase claims
Program of All-Inclusive Care for the Elderly (PACE)
Qualified Disabled and Working Individuals
Qualified Medicare Beneficiaries
reciprocity
remittance advice (RA)
safety-net providers
share of cost
Specified Low-Income Medicare Beneficiaries (SLMBs)

spend down
State Children's Health Insurance Program (SCHIP)
supplemental medical insurance (SMI)

Supplemental Security Income (SSI)
Temporary Assistance for Needy Families (TANF)
third-party liability

WHAT IS MEDICAID?

Medicaid is a combination federal and state medical assistance program designed to provide comprehensive and quality medical care for low-income families, with special emphasis on children, pregnant women, the elderly, the disabled, and parents with dependent children who have no other way to pay for healthcare. Congress established the Medicaid program under Title XIX (19) of the Social Security Act of 1965. Medicaid is the largest source of funding for **safety-net providers** (community health centers and public hospitals) that serve the poor and uninsured. In January of 2011, 60 million low-income Americans received healthcare coverage under Medicaid.

According to the national Medicaid guidelines, federal and state governments must each contribute a specified percentage of total healthcare expenditures. The federal contribution in 2011 was approximately 57%, with the states paying the remaining costs. The federal government establishes general guidelines for eligibility and mandatory services, and each state then is allowed to expand its own guidelines regarding eligibility, services, benefits package, payment rates, and program administration within the broad federal guidelines. Flexibility to set eligibility levels has been limited over time by increases in federal minimum levels for children and pregnant women and more recently by eligibility protections established under the American Recovery and Reinvestment Act (ARRA) and the Patient Protection and Affordable Care Act (ACA). Medicaid benefits vary from state to state, and although state participation in Medicaid is optional, all states have Medicaid programs. As a result, there are essentially 56 different Medicaid programs—one for each state, each territory, and the District of Columbia. Not all states call their programs Medicaid. For example, in California the program is called Medi-Cal, in Massachusetts it's MassHealth, in Oregon it's Oregon Health Plan, and in Tennessee it's TennCare. States may combine the administration of Medicaid with that of other programs, such as the Children's Health Insurance Program (CHIP), so the same organization that manages Medicaid may also manage other programs. For general information on the Medicaid program, visit the Evolve site.

What Did You Learn?

1. What is Medicaid?
2. When was the Medicaid program established?
3. Under what major act does the Medicaid program fall?

OPENING SCENARIO

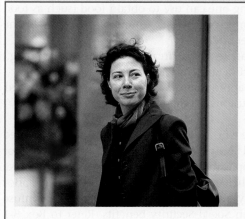

Nela Karnama has been employed as a medical receptionist in a multispecialty medical practice for 9 years. She had heard that there was soon going to be an opening in the billing department, which would be a promotion for Nela if she qualified for the position. She had always wanted to specialize in this area but did not feel qualified, so she enrolled in an evening course at a community college satellite center in a nearby town. Nela thought she knew quite a lot about Medicaid because after her husband was killed in an automobile accident, she and her children became eligible for benefits. After reading Chapter 8, it was obvious to her, however, that what she did know about it was limited to the program that provided benefits for her and her children, and that there was a lot more to learn.

Nela carpooled with Berta Kazinski, a neighbor who also had enrolled in the course. Berta, a nontraditional student, was basically unfamiliar with the program. She recalled that Medicaid had begun paying for part of her mother-in-law's expenses after she had been in a nursing home for several years, but Berta was unaware of the financial developments that led to her mother-in-law's eligibility for this care.

The discussion concerning Medicaid broadened during their commute to the class, and it was obvious that there was more to the Medicaid program than either of the women realized. Using the time study schedule they created in Chapter 2, they laid out their study plans for the next learning phase of their health insurance career.

EVOLUTION OF MEDICAID

Medicaid originally was created to give low-income Americans access to healthcare. Since its beginning, Medicaid has evolved from a narrowly defined program available only to individuals eligible for cash assistance (welfare) into a large insurance program with complex eligibility rules. Today, Medicaid is a major social welfare program and is administered by the Centers for Medicare and Medicaid Services (CMS), formerly called the Healthcare Financing Administration (HCFA).

Temporary Assistance for Needy Families

The Medicaid program, referred to in the past as Aid to Families with Dependent Children (AFDC), is now called **Temporary Assistance for Needy Families (TANF)**. TANF was created through a block grant by the Personal Responsibility and Work Opportunity Reconciliation Act of 1996. The TANF block grant replaced the AFDC program, which had provided cash welfare to poor families with children since 1935. TANF is a federal-state cash assistance program for poor families typically headed by a single parent. Each state sets its own income eligibility guidelines for TANF, and individuals who are eligible for TANF automatically qualify for Medicaid.

Not all states refer to this program as TANF. Many states have coined their own names. Vermont calls it ANFC/RU (Aid to Needy Families with Children/Reach Up); New York calls it simply the Family Assistance (FA) Program; and Kentucky's program is called K-TAP (Kentucky Transitional Assistance Program). To learn about the TANF program in your state, type the name of your state along with TANF in your Internet search engine.

Supplemental Security Income

In 1972 federal law established the **Supplemental Security Income (SSI)** program, which provides federally funded cash assistance to qualifying elderly and disabled poor. Under the SSI program, the Social Security Administration determines eligibility criteria and sets the cash benefit amounts for SSI. SSI is a cash benefit program controlled by the Social Security Administration; however, it is not related to the Social Security Program. States may choose to supplement federal SSI payments with state funds.

Eligibility

To be eligible for SSI, an individual must be at least 65 years old or blind or disabled and must have limited assets (or resources). Income is determined by the standards set forth in the **federal poverty level (FPL)** guidelines, shown in Table 8-1. The figures in this table represent the income of the individual or family. The U.S. Department of Health and Human Services (HHS) issues new FPL guidelines in January or February each year. These guidelines serve as one of the indicators for determining eligibility in a wide variety of federal and state programs. The income benefits limit for SSI eligibility is $674 per month for an individual and $1011 for a couple (2011 figures). In most states, SSI beneficiaries also can get medical assistance (Medicaid) to pay for hospital stays, doctor bills, prescription drugs, and other health costs. In addition, to receive SSI, a person must:

- be a resident of the United States,
- not be absent from the country for more than 30 days, and
- be either a U.S. citizen or national, or in one of certain categories of eligible noncitizens.

TABLE 8-1	2011 Department of Health and Human Services Poverty Guidelines		
NO. PERSONS IN FAMILY	48 CONTIGUOUS STATES & WASHINGTON, D.C.	ALASKA	HAWAII
1	$10,890	$13,600	$12,540
2	$14,710	$18,380	$16,930
3	$18,530	$23,160	$21,320
4	$22,350	$27,940	$25,710
5	$26,170	$32,720	$30,100
6	$29,990	$37,500	$34,490
7	$33,810	$42,280	$38,880
8	$37,630	$47,060	$43,270
For each additional person, add	$3,820	$4,780	$4,390

From *Federal Register*, Vol. 76, No. 13, January 20, 2011, pp 3637-3638.

(For SSI updates, see Websites to Explore at the end of this chapter).

The amount of the SSI payment is the difference between the individual's **countable income** and the Federal Benefit Rate (FBR). *Income* is anything a person receives during a calendar month and uses to meet his or her needs for food, clothing, or shelter. It may be in cash income or "**in-kind**" **income**. In-kind income is not cash; it is food, clothing, shelter, or something one can use to obtain food (such as food stamps), clothing, or shelter. Countable income is the amount left over after

1. eliminating all items that are not considered income (e.g., child support or student loans) and
2. applying all appropriate exclusions (earned or unearned income exclusions) to the items that are considered income.

Many people who are eligible for SSI may also be entitled to receive Social Security benefits. In fact, the application for SSI is also an application for Social Security benefits. Unlike Social Security benefits, SSI benefits are not based on prior work or a family member's prior work. It is easy to confuse SSI benefits with Social Security benefits. Refer to Box 8-1 for a comparison of the two programs.

Eligibility Expansion

During the late 1980s and early 1990s, Congress expanded Medicaid eligibility to include more categories of people—the poor elderly, individuals with disabilities, children, and certain categories of pregnant women. In addition to expansion of eligibility parameters, Medicaid programs were broadened as a result of federal mandates. These program expansions include the following:

- Payments to hospitals that serve large numbers of poor, uninsured, or Medicaid recipients
- Coverage of prenatal and delivery services for qualifying pregnant women and their infants who have no other insurance

---

Box 8-1

SSI and Social Security Benefits

How is SSI Different from Social Security Benefits?
Many people who are eligible for SSI may also be entitled to receive Social Security Benefits. In fact, the application for SSI is also an application for Social Security benefits.

- Unlike Social Security benefits SSI benefits are not based on a person's (or a family member's) prior work.
- SSI is financed by general funds of the U.S. Treasury—from personal income taxes, corporate taxes, and other taxes. Social Security taxes are withheld under the Federal Insurance Contributions Act (FICA) or the Self Employment Contributions Act (SECA) and do not fund the SSI program.
- In most states, SSI beneficiaries also can get medical assistance (Medicaid) to pay for hospital stays, doctor bills, prescription drugs, and other healthcare costs.
- SSI beneficiaries may also be eligible for food assistance (except in California). In some states, an application for SSI benefits also serves as an application for food assistance.

- To receive SSI benefits, a person must be disabled, blind, or at least 65 years old and must have "limited" income and resources.
- In addition, to receive SSI benefits, an individual must
  o be a resident of the United States,
  o not be absent from the country for more than 30 days, and
  o be either a U.S. citizen or national, or in one of certain categories of eligible noncitizens.

How is SSI Like Social Security Benefits?
- Both programs pay monthly benefits.
- The medical standards for disability are the same in the two programs for individuals age 18 or older. There is a separate definition of disability under SSI for children from birth to age 18.
- SSA administers both programs.

Source: http://www.ssa.gov/ssi/text-over-ussi.htm

- Expansion of services to many children in low-income families who do not receive cash assistance (TANF)
- Expansion of Medicaid to fill gaps in Medicare services to the poor elderly or disabled individuals
- Coverage of the full range of federally allowable Medicaid services as medically necessary and appropriate for all children receiving Medicaid

As a result of these and other federal law changes, the eligibility determination process is more complex today than in the past. Computer systems designed for a smaller and simpler program now manage information for millions of people in dozens of different eligibility groups.

Medicaid and Healthcare Reform

Unless the new healthcare reform laws are repealed, beginning in 2014, nearly everyone younger than 65 years with income up to 133% of the FPL will be eligible for Medicaid. Former categorical restrictions will be eliminated for those who fall into this group. These changes establish Medicaid as a way for low-income Americans to acquire near-universal coverage as approved in the healthcare reform law. Medicaid eligibility rules for the elderly and disabled will not change under health reform. For more information on how healthcare reform will affect the Medicaid program, type "Medicaid and Healthcare Reform" in your Internet search engine.

📁 HIPAA Tip

Medicaid HIPAA Compliant Concept Model (MHCCM) shows how HIPAA affects Medicaid and provides practical tools to help a state determine the best course of action for analyzing HIPAA's impact, determine implementation strategies, determine best practices, and validate what a state has accomplished.

❓ What Did You Learn?

1. As it was originally created, what was the only group Medicaid covered?
2. What is TANF?
3. What does SSI provide?
4. What additional group was added to the Medicaid program in 1972?
5. Who administers Medicaid?
6. Why is it difficult to determine Medicaid eligibility in today's healthcare environment?

STRUCTURE OF MEDICAID

As discussed in the beginning of this chapter, Medicaid is a combination federal and state public assistance program that pays for certain healthcare costs of individuals who

qualify. The program is administered by CMS under the general direction of the Department of Health and Human Services (HHS). Eligibility is based on need, which is determined by whether the patient meets certain income and resource limits. The federal government has established broad requirements for eligibility, and the individual states refine eligibility requirements and coverage to the needs of their populations.

Federal Government's Role

Within the guidelines set forth by the federal government, each state establishes its own eligibility standards; determines the type, amount, duration, and scope of services; sets the rate of payment for services; and administers its own program. Under the provisions of the federal statute, individuals, no matter what their financial status, must fall into a designated group before they are eligible for Medicaid. These groups are shown in Fig. 8-1.

Mandated Services

Title XIX of the Social Security Act requires that for a state to receive federal matching funds for their Medicaid programs, certain basic services (referred to as **mandated [or mandatory] services**) must be offered to the categorically needy population in the state's program. These services are listed

---

CATEGORICALLY NEEDY

Families, pregnant women, and children
- Persons meeting Family Medical criteria (including TANF recipients)
- Children under the age of 1 and pregnant women whose countable income does not exceed 150% of the FPL
- Children ages 1-5 whose countable income does not exceed 133% of the FPL
- Children ages 6-18 whose countable income does not exceed 100% of the FPL

Aged and Disabled Individuals
- SSI recipients
- Qualified Medicare Beneficiaries (QMBs)
- Individuals residing in intermediate or long-term care facilities
- Medicaid beneficiaries
- Dual coverage (Medi-Medi) beneficiaries

MEDICALLY NEEDY

Individuals who do not qualify for Medicaid benefits under the categorically needy programs because of income or resources exceeding the level of qualifying criteria but are medically indigent
- Pregnant women
- Children up to age 18 (or age 18 working toward a high school diploma or its equivalent)
- Persons 65 years of age and older
- Persons who are disabled or blind under SSA standards

Fig. 8-1 Who is eligible for Medicaid.

in Table 8-2. To see a timeline of Medicaid's key developments, visit the Evolve site.

States' Options

States may also receive federal funding if they elect to provide certain **optional services** in addition to the mandatory services that each Medicaid program must provide under federal statute. A state may choose from more than 30 optional services. Once an optional service is identified in the state plan, however, that service must be provided within federal requirements. The optional services authorized by the Medicaid Act include those listed in Table 8-2.

To be eligible for federal funds, states are required to provide Medicaid coverage for certain individuals who receive federally assisted income-maintenance payments and for related groups not receiving cash payments. In addition to their Medicaid programs, most states have other "state-only" programs to provide medical assistance for specified poor individuals who do not qualify for Medicaid. Federal funds are not provided for state-only programs.

Categorically Needy

States must cover **categorically needy** individuals, but they have options as to how to define categorically needy. Individuals falling into this group typically include those listed under the heading "Categorically Needy" in Fig. 8-1. Who qualifies for Medicaid benefits in a particular state varies according to the options that state has elected to include in the program. States that include the SSI program cover everyone who qualifies for the SSI (aged, blind, and disabled). These states cannot have rules, however, that are more restrictive than the federal government rules for SSI.

Medically Needy

More than 40 states plus the District of Columbia operate **medically needy** programs, which allow them to provide Medicaid to certain groups of individuals who are not otherwise eligible for Medicaid. People who have been denied Medicaid coverage because their income is too high might qualify as medically needy individuals on the basis of income and health status.

States that offer a medically needy program must cover pregnant women and children younger than 18 years. States also have the option to cover children up to age 21, parents and other caretaker relatives, elderly individuals, and individuals with disabilities. A state's medically needy program may also expand coverage to people who **spend down** their income by accumulating medical expenses so that their income falls below a state-established medically needy income limit. A spend-down occurs when private or family finances are depleted to the point at which the individual or family becomes eligible for Medicaid assistance. Almost any medical bills that the applicant or the applicant's family still owes or that were paid in the months for which Medicaid is requested (called the **budget period**)

TABLE 8-2	Medicaid Mandatory and Optional Services
Mandatory services	Inpatient hospital care Outpatient hospital care Physician's services Nurse midwife services Pediatric and family nurse practitioner services Federally qualified health center ("FQHC") Laboratories and x-ray services Rural health clinic services Prenatal care Family planning services Skilled nursing facility services for persons over age 21 Home health care services for persons over age 21 who are eligible for skilled nursing services (includes medical supplies and equipment) Early periodic screening, diagnosis, and treatment (EPSDT) for persons under age 21 Vaccines for children
States' optional services*	Podiatrists' services Optometrists' services and eyeglasses Chiropractic services Private duty nurses Clinic services Dental services Physical therapy Occupational therapy Speech, hearing, and language therapy Prescribed drugs Dentures Prosthetic devices Diagnostic services Screening services Preventive services Rehabilitative services Transportation services Services for persons age 65 or older in mental institutions Intermediate care facility services Intermediate care facility services for persons with MR/DD and related conditions Inpatient psychiatric services for persons under age 22 Christian Science schools Nursing facility services for persons under age 21 Emergency hospital services Personal care services Hospice care Case management services Respiratory care services Home- and community-based services for those with disabilities and chronic medical conditions

Note: Medicaid's EPSDT program requires that states offer all these services to children up to age 21.

can be used to meet the spend down requirement. The opportunity to spend down may be particularly important to elderly residents in a nursing home. Also, children and adults with disabilities who may have high prescription drug, medical equipment, or other health care expenses may qualify for a spend down.

It is important to note, however, that Medicaid does not provide medical assistance for all poor persons. Even under the broadest provisions of the federal statute (except for emergency services for those who qualify), the Medicaid program does not provide healthcare services unless the individuals fall into one of the designated eligibility groups. Low income is only one test for Medicaid eligibility; assets and resources are also tested against established limits. As noted earlier, categorically needy persons who are eligible for Medicaid may or may not also receive cash assistance from the TANF program or from the SSI program. Medically needy persons who would be categorically eligible except for income or assets may become eligible for Medicaid solely as a result of excessive medical expenses.

The Affordable Care Act, passed in March 2010, will significantly expand the number of people in the country who are eligible for Medicaid. This expansion may cover many of the people who currently are in a medically needy program. Fig. 8-2 shows pie charts illustrating Medicaid enrollment and Medicaid spending. To learn more about the Affordable Care Act, visit the Evolve site.

The health insurance professional must learn the specific guidelines for the Medicaid programs offered in the state in which he or she is employed in order to perform his or her job judiciously. The health insurance professional should contact the **Medicaid contractor** (a commercial insurer contracted by the HHS for the purpose of processing and administering claims) in his or her state to obtain a guide as to what programs are available and what each one covers in that state. An alternative resource for this information is listed in Websites to Explore at the end of this chapter. For a more in-depth discussion of Medicaid, visit the websites listed at the end of the chapter.

Community First Choice Option

The Community First Choice (CFC) Option is a relatively new state option that gives individuals with disabilities who are eligible for nursing homes and other institutional settings options to receive community-based services. CFC provides qualifying Medicaid beneficiaries the choice to leave facilities and institutions (e.g., nursing homes) for care in their own homes and communities with appropriate, cost-effective services and supports. CFC also helps address state waiting lists for services by providing qualified individuals access to a community-based benefit within Medicaid. The option does not allow caps on the number of individuals served, nor allow waiting lists for these services. For more information on Community First Choice Option, visit the Evolve site.

State Children's Health Insurance Program

Enacted as part of the Balanced Budget Act of 1997, the **State Children's Health Insurance Program (SCHIP)**—later known more simply as the **Children's Health Insurance Program (CHIP)**—provides federal matching funds for states to implement health insurance programs for children in families that earn too much to qualify for Medicaid but too little to reasonably afford private health coverage.

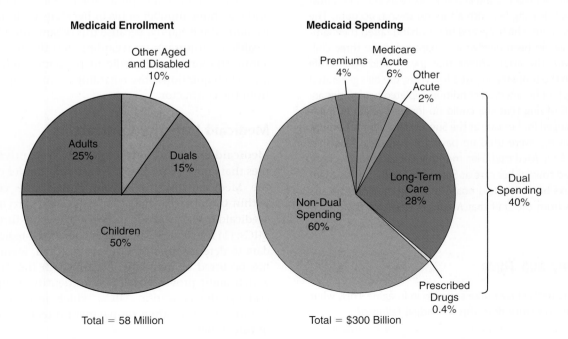

Fig. 8-2 Medicaid Enrollment versus Medicaid Spending. (From Urban Institute estimates based on data from MSIS and CMS Form 64, prepared for the Kaiser Commission on Medicaid and the Uninsured, 2010.)

With CHIP, states can provide coverage through two different options:

- creation of a separate children's health program that meets the requirements specified under Section 2103 of the act, an option known as "separate" or "stand alone" CHIP, or
- expansion of eligibility for benefits under the state's Medicaid plan under Title XIX of the act, an option known as "Medicaid expansion" CHIP.

States can operate either of these options, alone or in combination.

Within federal guidelines, each state determines the design of its CHIP program, eligibility groups, benefit packages, payment levels for coverage, and administrative and operating procedures. Eligibility levels range from 133% of the FPL in Wyoming to 350% of the FPL in New Jersey, with most states at 200% of FPL.

CHIP health benefits typically cover physician, hospital, well-baby, and well-child care; prescription drugs; and limited behavioral and personal care services. In contrast with Medicaid, private-duty nursing, personal care, and orthodontia are usually not covered by CHIP.

Many CHIP programs require small premiums and copayments, but federal law prohibits cost sharing from exceeding 5% of a family's income. Most have a multilevel cost-sharing approach, with greater cost sharing for families with higher incomes (that is, above 150% of the FPL). Copayments range from $1 for a generic drug prescription to $100 for an inpatient hospital stay.

To learn more about the CHIP program, visit the Evolve site.

⭐ Imagine This!

Inez Burke, a widow, resides in a nursing home and has complications of diabetes and cellulitis. Six years ago, Inez's husband died, leaving her with a modest savings account. The homestead on which she and her husband raised their family had earlier been divided into parcels for the three children, with the arrangement that Inez would receive life estate in the property. In just a few years, the bills generated as a result of her medical condition depleted her savings account. Realizing that she could no longer live alone, Inez's son arranged for her care at the Sunset Care Center. Because Inez's savings were used up paying her medical bills, Inez qualified for Medicaid. Her monthly Social Security check is applied toward her care at Sunset; other than that, Medicaid pays her room and board plus any medical care she receives from the staff that Medicare does not pay.

🕐 Stop and Think

Referring to the Inez Burke scenario in Imagine This!, what Medicaid category does this individual fall into?

⭐ Imagine This!

Jim Norton has monthly income of $723. If the Medicaid income limit is $623, then Jim is over the limit by $100. If Jim has monthly medical expenses of more than $100, he can be eligible for Medicaid with a spend-down of $100. (He then must spend $100 per month on his medical expenses before Medicaid will begin paying).

Fiscal Intermediaries/Medicaid Contractors

Medicaid does not, as a rule, process claims. Instead, individual states contract with an organization specializing in administering government healthcare programs. These contracting organizations, formerly called fiscal intermediaries (FIs), are now more commonly referred to as contractors. Medicaid contractors process all healthcare claims on behalf of the Medicaid program. Some states have more than one contractor, one for fee-for-service claims and a second one for managed care claims. Before a contractor is selected by the state, there is a bidding process similar to the bidding by construction contractors for the job of building a bridge or road.

Responsibilities of a Medicaid contractor may differ from state to state; however, more common responsibilities are as follows:

- Process claims
- Provide information for healthcare providers for the particular government program involved
- Generate guidelines for providers to facilitate the claims process
- Answer beneficiary questions about benefits, claims processing, appeals, and the explanation of benefits (remittance advice [RA]) document.

The health insurance professional should know the name and telephone number of his or her state Medicaid contractor and keep it handy, because this organization can offer a wealth of information regarding healthcare claims and administration of the Medicaid program. Additionally, if and when questions arise regarding claims, help is available from the contractor.

Medicaid Integrity Contractors

Medicaid integrity contractors (MICs) are private companies that conduct audit-related activities under contract to the Medicaid Integrity Group (MIG), the component within CMS that is charged by HHS with carrying out the Medicaid Integrity Program (MIP). There are three primary MICs: (1) the Review MICs, which analyze Medicaid claims data to determine whether provider fraud, waste, or abuse has occurred or may have occurred; (2) the Audit MICs, which audit provider claims and identify overpayments; and (3) the Education MICs, which provide education to providers and others on payment integrity and quality-of-care issues.

What Did You Learn?

1. What is the federal government's role in Medicaid?
2. Explain the state's role in Medicaid.
3. Name the major category of Medicaid eligibles that states must cover under federal mandates.
4. Identify the major categorical group a state might "elect" to cover.
5. Define the term "mandated service."

OTHER MEDICAID PROGRAMS

We already have learned that the Medicaid program is divided into two major groups—the categorically needy and the medically needy—and who may qualify for these two groups. We discussed the CHIP program. This section provides information for other groups qualifying for assistance through various Medicaid programs.

Maternal and Child Health Services

Maternal and Child Health Services has operated as a federal-state partnership for more than 65 years. When the Social Security Act was passed in 1935, the federal government, through Title V, promised to support state efforts to improve the health of all mothers and children consistent with the health status goals and objectives established by the Secretary of the HHS.

States and jurisdictions use Title V funds to design and implement a wide range of maternal and child health programs that meet national and state needs. Although specific initiatives may vary among the 59 states and jurisdictions utilizing Title V funds, all programs work to do the following:

- Reduce infant mortality and incidence of handicapping conditions among children
- Increase the number of children appropriately immunized against disease
- Increase the number of children in low-income households who receive assessments and follow-up diagnostic and treatment services
- Provide and ensure access to comprehensive perinatal care for women; preventive and child care services; comprehensive care, including long-term care services, for children with special health care needs; and

rehabilitation services for blind and disabled children under 16 years of age who are eligible for SSI
- Facilitate the development of comprehensive, family-centered, community-based, culturally competent, coordinated systems of care for children with special health care needs.

Early and Periodic Screening, Diagnosis, and Treatment Program

Medicaid's child health component, known as the **Early Periodic Screening, Diagnosis, and Treatment (EPSDT)** program, was developed to fit the standards of pediatric care and to meet the special physical, emotional, and developmental needs of low-income children. Federal law, including statutes, regulations, and guidelines, requires that Medicaid cover a comprehensive set of benefits and services for children different from adult benefits. EPSDT offers an important way to ensure that young children receive appropriate health, mental health, and developmental services.

Program of All-Inclusive Care for the Elderly

In addition to mandatory and optional services, there are other program options, such as the **Program of All-Inclusive Care for the Elderly (PACE)**. This program provides comprehensive alternative care for noninstitutionalized elderly people who otherwise would be in a nursing home. PACE is centered on the belief that it is better for the well-being of elderly with long-term care needs and their families to be served in the community where they live whenever possible. PACE serves individuals who are age 55 or older, certified by their state to need nursing home care, able to live safely in the community at the time of enrollment, and live in a PACE service area. Although all PACE participants must be certified to need nursing home care in order to enroll in PACE, only a small percentage of PACE participants reside in nursing homes nationally. If a PACE enrollee does need nursing home care, the PACE program pays for it and continues to coordinate his or her care. To see a PACE "Fact Sheet," visit the Evolve site.

Medicaid Home and Community-Based Services Waivers

Medicaid Home and Community-Based Services (HCBS) waivers (also known as 1915[c] waivers) allow states the flexibility to develop and implement creative alternatives to placing Medicaid-eligible individuals in hospitals, nursing homes, or intermediate care facilities for persons with mental retardation. The HCBS waiver program recognizes that many people at risk of being placed in these facilities can be cared for in their homes and communities, preserving their independence and ties to family and friends at a cost no higher than that of institutional care.

Under section 1915(c) of the Social Security Act, states may request waivers of certain federal requirements in order to develop Medicaid-financed, community-based treatment alternatives. The requirements that may be waived deal with statewideness, comparability of services, and community income and resource rules for the medically needy. (Statewideness means that state Medicaid programs may not vary the mandatory or optional benefits they offer based on where people live in the state.) The following services are explicitly included in the HCBS waiver program, and states can choose to include or exclude them:

1. case management,
2. homemaker services,
3. home health aide services,
4. personal care services,
5. adult day health services,
6. psychosocial rehabilitation services, and
7. clinic services for individuals with chronic mental illness.

To receive approval to implement HCBS waiver programs, state Medicaid agencies must assure CMS that the cost of providing home- and community-based services will not exceed the cost of care for that same individual in an institution. The Medicaid agency must also document that there are safeguards in place to protect the health and welfare of beneficiaries.

To view the latest summary report of all regular approved home- and community-based services waivers, visit the Evolve site.

HCBS State Plan Option Expansion

The health reform law provides states with new flexibility under the Medicaid HCBS state plan option that was created in the 2005 Deficit Reduction Act (DRA). The new law, which took effect in April 2010, expands the scope of services covered under the option beyond the services that were originally listed under the state plan benefit option. Other changes to the option include the elimination of the states' ability to cap enrollment, the requirement of statewide coverage, the ability to offer the benefit to individuals with a higher level of need, and the ability to target the HCBS option to specific populations (e.g., individuals with specific conditions). The law also creates a new optional eligibility category within Medicaid, thereby extending full Medicaid benefits to individuals with incomes up to 150% of the FPL who meet the states' HCBS state plan benefit needs-based criteria.

? What Did You Learn?

1. Name three things that the Maternal and Child Health Services work to accomplish.
2. What is the name of the program that was developed to fit the standards of pediatric care and to meet the special physical, emotional, and developmental needs of low-income children?
3. Name the program that is centered on the belief that it is better for the well-being of elderly with long-term care needs and their families to be served in the community where they live whenever possible.
4. List at least 5 of the services that are included in the HCBS waiver program.

PREMIUMS AND COST SHARING

The Deficit Reduction Act (DRA) of 2005 (introduced and clarified in the Tax Relief and Health Care Act of 2006) allows states to impose cost sharing charges and premiums on certain categories of Medicaid recipients. (In **cost sharing**, Medicaid beneficiaries pay a portion of their health costs, such as deductibles, coinsurance, or copayment amounts.) Basically, this change applies to people who do not meet the income/assets requirements (medically needy) of Medicaid but may qualify for assistance if they use their medical expenses to spend down their income before Medicaid considers their eligibility. Qualifying patients are then allowed to pay Medicaid the amount of money that is still over the Medicaid income allowance. This practice is referred to as **share of cost** or Payment Error Rate Measurement (PERM). Once this amount is paid, the patient becomes eligible for Medicaid services. It should be noted here that although the DRA sets federal guidelines for this program, cost-sharing amounts and premiums may vary from state to state.

Groups exempt from paying premiums and cost sharing include, but are not limited to, children, pregnant women, and people receiving hospice care. Services excluded from cost-sharing charges include, but are not limited to, emergency, family planning, and qualifying preventive services. A complete list of populations and services exempt from premiums and cost sharing can be found in the State Medicaid Directors letters addressing sections 6041 through 6043 of the DRA.

The amount a state may charge for premiums and/or cost sharing is based on the individual's family income. For all recipients, the total amount of premiums and cost-sharing charges cannot exceed 5% of a family's income. Qualifying "poor" recipients cannot be required to pay any premiums or cost sharing that exceeds a nominal amount. Premium amounts are determined on a sliding scale, and cost-sharing charges can range from a few dollars up to 10% or 20% of the cost of the service, depending on the individual's family income.

The DRA allows states to apply separate cost-sharing rules to prescription drugs and may vary cost-sharing amounts on the basis of whether the drug is considered "preferred" or "nonpreferred" and on the income level of the recipient. Only nominal amounts can be charged for nonpreferred drugs to individuals who are otherwise exempt from cost sharing.

Nonemergency Use of the Emergency Department

Under the DRA, states may permit hospitals to charge a fee (cost sharing) for use of a hospital emergency department for nonemergency care if the recipient has access to an alternative provider. In such cases, the hospital must provide the name of the alternative provider along with a referral to coordinate scheduling of an appointment. As with other professional service costs, the amount the state may charge depends on the individual's family income.

Enforcement

Under DRA rules, states are permitted to allow providers to withhold care or services from individuals who do not meet their cost-sharing obligations, except for individuals whose income is at or below 100% of the FPL. Additionally, states have the option to terminate coverage if a recipient fails to make premium payments for periods longer than 60 days. States may waive this penalty in cases in which it would impose "undue hardship."

Emergency Medical Treatment & Labor Act

Congress enacted the Emergency Medical Treatment & Labor Act (EMTALA) in 1996 to make sure that the public has access to emergency services regardless of ability to pay. Section 1867 of the Social Security Act states that Medicare-participating hospitals that offer emergency services must provide a medical screening examination and/or treatment for an emergency medical condition, including active labor, regardless of an individual's ability to pay. Hospitals are then required to stabilize patients with emergency medical conditions. If a hospital is unable to stabilize a patient within its capability, or if the patient requests it, he or she should be transported to an appropriate alternative facility.

What Did You Learn?

1. Name the categorically needy groups that are mandated by federal law.
2. What groups make up the "medically needy" classification?
3. What does the PACE program provide?
4. Premiums and cost sharing apply to what class of Medicaid beneficiaries?

PAYMENT FOR MEDICAID SERVICES

Medicaid payments are made directly to the healthcare provider. Providers participating in Medicaid (PARs) must accept the Medicaid reimbursement as payment in full. Each state is free to determine (within certain federal restrictions)

how reimbursements are calculated and the resulting rates for services, with three exceptions:

1. For institutional (e.g., hospital) services, payment may not be more than would be paid under Medicare payment rates.
2. For **disproportionate share hospitals**, different limits apply. (Disproportionate share hospitals are facilities that receive additional payments to ensure that communities have access to certain high-cost services, such as trauma and emergency care and burn services.)
3. For hospice care.

States may impose nominal deductibles, coinsurance, or copayments on some Medicaid recipients for certain services, such as dental and podiatry care. Emergency services and family planning services must be exempt from such copayments. Certain Medicaid recipients must be excluded from this cost sharing, including pregnant women, children younger than 18 years, hospital or nursing home patients who are expected to contribute most of their income to institutional care, and categorically needy HMO enrollees.

Medically Necessary

As a general rule, Medicaid pays only for services that are determined to be **medically necessary**. For a procedure or service to be considered medically necessary, it typically must be consistent with the diagnosis and in accordance with the standards of good medical practice, performed at the proper level, and provided in the most appropriate setting. If the health insurance professional questions whether a service or procedure is medically necessary, he or she should consult the current Medicaid provider handbook provided by the state in which he or she is employed or should telephone the contractor that administers local Medicaid programs. This action should be taken before the service or procedure is performed to avoid problems with collecting payment from Medicaid or the patient after the fact.

Prescription Drug Coverage

Recognizing that prescription drugs are an increasingly important element of comprehensive healthcare, all states have chosen the option of providing prescription drug coverage for their categorically needy populations and most cover some or all of the other groups. To find out which prescription drugs are covered for the categorically needy group in a particular state, the health insurance professional should contact the local Medicaid contractor or consult the provider's manual for that state.

Dual Eligibles

Medicaid previously provided drug coverage for more than 6 million Medicare beneficiaries, known as **dual eligibles**. Dual eligibles have both Medicare and Medicaid coverage. Beginning January 1, 2006, full-benefit dual-eligible individuals began receiving drug coverage through the Medicare Prescription Drug Benefit (Part D) of the Medicare Prescription Drug, Improvement, and Modernization Act of 2003 rather than through their state Medicaid programs. Certain drugs are excluded from coverage under the Medicare Prescription Drug Benefit, however. The Secretary of HHS is responsible for automatically enrolling dual-eligible individuals into Part D plans if they do not sign up on their own.

To the extent that state Medicaid programs cover the excluded drugs for Medicaid recipients who are not full-benefit dual eligibles, states are required to cover the excluded drugs for full-benefit dual eligibles with federal financial participation. More information on the Medicare Prescription Drug Plan (Medicare Part D) can be found in Chapter 9. Also, visit the Evolve site for a link that provides more details about dual eligibles.

Accepting Medicaid Patients

Physicians have the choice of whether or not to accept Medicaid patients—patients with Medicaid coverage only or with coverage by any combination of Medicaid and another insurance company, whether it is a primary or secondary payer. In an emergency, or if it cannot be determined whether the patient has Medicaid at the time of treatment, the patient must be informed as soon as possible after Medicaid coverage has been identified whether the practice will accept him or her as a Medicaid patient.

In most states, physicians can limit the number of Medicaid patients they accept, as long as there is no discrimination by age, sex, race, religious preference, or national origin, in addition to the limits of their scope of practice. If a practice sees only children, refusing to accept adult patients is not considered discrimination. If a patient has Medicare and Medicaid coverage, however, and the practice does not accept the Medicaid coverage, the health insurance professional must make sure the patient understands this before treatment. The patient then has the opportunity to find a physician who would accept the patient's Medicaid coverage. If a Medicaid recipient insists on being treated by a nonparticipating healthcare provider (one who does not accept Medicaid), it is recommended that the health insurance professional ask the patient to sign a form verifying his or her understanding that the practice does not accept Medicaid and that he or she will be responsible for paying the deductible and coinsurance amounts.

Participating Providers

The healthcare provider can elect to accept or refuse Medicaid patients; however, many state regulations say that if a Medicaid-participating provider elects to treat one Medicaid patient, the provider must accept all Medicaid patients; the provider cannot single out which ones to treat. Providers can put a cap, however, on the total number of new patients, including Medicaid patients, that they will accept. Additionally, providers must agree to accept what Medicaid pays as payment in full for covered services (with the exception of any cost-sharing obligations on the part of the patient) and are prohibited by law to balance bill Medicaid patients for these services. The healthcare professional should know beforehand whether or not a particular service or procedure is covered by Medicaid. If the patient insists on being treated for a particular noncovered service, it is recommended that he or she sign a waiver that spells out the fact that the service is not covered by Medicaid and that the patient acknowledges responsibility for payment. Some practices even ask the patient to pay for noncovered services in advance.

⏱ Stop and Think

As a general rule, Dr. Vandenberg accepts Medicaid patients in her family practice. After seeing Harold Apple, a patient with an unpleasant personality, Dr. Vandenberg advises the medical receptionist not to schedule any further follow-up appointments for Mr. Apple. Is Dr. Vandenberg violating any Medicaid principles?

❓ What Did You Learn?

1. Explain the term "cost sharing."
2. What criteria does a procedure or service have to meet to be considered "medically necessary"?
3. Explain the recommended procedure a health insurance professional should follow if a Medicaid recipient insists on being treated in a medical facility that does not accept Medicaid patients.

VERIFYING MEDICAID ELIGIBILITY

Before providing services, Medicaid providers always should make sure that Medicaid will pay for patients' medical care, to determine eligibility for the current date and to discover any limitations to the recipient's coverage. Because most states grant eligibility a month at a time for most Medicaid-eligible patients, eligibility should be verified every month in which the patient visits the practice. If a patient is being seen more often, such as for weekly allergy injections or frequent monitoring for some other condition, verifying eligibility on a monthly basis is probably often enough; however, the health insurance professional might want to check with the local Medicaid contractor. Several methods of verification are available in most states; the health insurance professional may be able to verify eligibility by using:

- the patient's Medicaid identification (ID) card
- an automated voice response (AVR) system
- electronic data interchange (EDI)
- a point-of-sale device
- a computer software program

THIS DOCUMENT CONTAINS FLUORESCENT FIBERS, FLUORESCENT ARTIFICIAL WATERMARK AND IS PRINTED ON CHEMICAL REACTIVE PAPER

07-01-06 to 07-31-06

P.O. Box 111
Any City, NC
Zip=12345

CASE ID   10847667
CASEHEAD   Jane Recipient

Eligible Members

Jane Recipient

123-45-6789K

MEDICAID IDENTIFICATION CARD

N.C. DEPT. OF HEALTH AND HUMAN SERVICES DIVISION OF MEDICAL ASSISTANCE

CAP	COUNTY CASE NO	ISSUANCE	PROGRAM	CLASS
	123456	06181 S	AAF	N

VALID

FROM	THRU
07-01-06	07-31-06

RECIPIENT ID	ELIGIBLES FOR MEDICAID	INS NO	BIRTHDATE	SEX
123-45-6789K	Jane Recipient	1	12-17-73	F
	Dr Joe PCP Provider 123 Any Street Any City, NC 12345			
	555-5555 555-55555			

INS NO	NAME CODE	POLICY NUMBER	TYPE
1	091	Y23684219	00

Carolina ACCESS Enrollee
JUL 2006 AAF11   10847667 101
456 That Street
That City, NC 45678

RECIPIENT   (Not valid unless signed)
(Signature) _Jane Recipient_____

MISUSE MAY RESULT IN FRAUD PROSECUTION

Fig. 8-3 Medicaid ID card. (Source: North Carolina Department of Health and Human Services.)

Medicaid Identification Card

A common method for verifying the patient's Medicaid eligibility is the ID card. This card provides important information regarding eligibility date and type, which are shown on the card. The following steps are suggested for eligibility verification with the ID card. The health insurance professional should keep in mind, however, that Medicaid ID cards and the method for verifying eligibility varies from state to state.

- Ensure that the patient's name is on the ID card. (Typically, the patient's birth date and sex also are listed.)
- Unless the professional knows the patient personally, he or she should ask to see another form of identification to confirm the patient's identity.
- Check the eligibility period. There should be "from" and "through" dates that tell the time period in which the patient is Medicaid eligible. Medicaid pays only for dates of service during this eligibility period.
- Look for insurance information. In the example shown in Fig. 8-3, there is a "1" under the "Ins. No." column. The "Insurance Data" block shows details of the patient's insurance coverage.
- Ask the patient whether he or she has any other insurance coverage.
- Photocopy the Medicaid ID card, and enter any new information in the patient's record.

Many states color-code the ID cards, and the color of the card tells the health insurance professional which type of Medicaid program the recipient is enrolled in. Also, the card should be examined closely to see whether the patient is in a special program or has special coverage. It is important for the health insurance professional to obtain a provider's guide from the Medicaid contractor in his or her state for assistance in interpreting the codes on the Medicaid ID card. Fig. 8-4 shows an example of Michigan's Medicaid (mihealth) ID card that shows the beneficiary name and ID number.

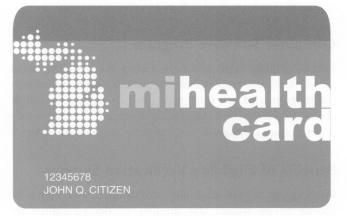

12345678
JOHN Q. CITIZEN

Fig. 8-4 Michigan's Medicaid ID card, showing the beneficiary name and ID number. (Source: Michigan Department of Community Health.)

Automated Voice Response System

The automated voice response (AVR) system allows a touch-tone phone call to be used to obtain eligibility information. For this method of verification, the health insurance professional needs to know the patient's Medicaid ID number or Social Security number and date of birth. The AVR system can provide a variety of eligibility information, including the following:

- Eligibility for specific dates of service
- The type of coverage or special programs in which the patient is enrolled
- Whether the patient is covered under Medicare Part A and Part B
- Information known by Medicaid concerning other insurance coverage

If the medical practice has access to this type of eligibility verification, the health insurance professional should know how to use it correctly and should keep current by requesting and reading periodic updates.

Electronic Data Interchange

Providers may obtain Medicaid eligibility information electronically. Online, interactive eligibility verification is available from Electronic Data Interchange (EDI) vendors (sometimes referred to as clearinghouses). Use of an EDI vendor is voluntary to providers. EDI vendors interface directly with the Medicaid recipient database maintained by an electronic data service (EDS) for claims processing. The database is updated every day from the state's master eligibility file. This service is available 24 hours a day, 7 days a week, except for periods when it is down for system maintenance. EDI vendors normally charge a fee for their services, and providers might be required to pay a transaction fee to the state's Medicaid contractor.

Point-of-Sale Device

With a point-of-sale device, the patient is issued an ID card that is similar in size and design to a credit card. Through the information on the magnetic strip, the provider can swipe the card through the card reader device and receive an accurate return of eligibility information within a matter of seconds.

Computer Software Program

With eligibility verification through a computer software program, the provider can key the patient's information into the program and in a short time have an accurate return of eligibility information. Most state Medicaid offices provide the necessary software at no charge to enrolled providers.

Benefits of Eligibility Verification Systems

By using one of these eligibility verification system methods, providers can reduce the number of denied claims by verifying recipient eligibility and insurance information before services are provided. Up-front verification using an eligibility verification system results in the submission of more accurate claims and decreases eligibility-related claims denials.

📁 HIPAA Tip

Medicaid providers and their vendors who bill electronically need to verify that their systems accept HIPAA-compliant Medicaid transactions.

❔ What Did You Learn?

1. Why is it important for the health insurance professional to verify eligibility?
2. What should the health insurance professional do if a patient insists on receiving services that are not covered by Medicaid?
3. What are the benefits of the eligibility verification system?

MEDICARE/MEDICAID RELATIONSHIP

Most elderly or disabled individuals who are very poor are covered under Medicaid and Medicare, commonly referred to as **dual coverage**, dual eligibility, or **Medi-Medi**. These individuals may receive Medicare services for which they are entitled and other services available under that state's Medicaid program. Because each state sets up its Medicaid plan, certain services typically not covered by Medicare (e.g., hearing aids, eyeglasses, and nursing facility care beyond the 100 days covered by Medicare) may be provided to these individuals by the state's Medicaid program. In addition, the Medicaid program pays all of the cost-sharing portions (deductibles and coinsurance) of Medicare Part A and Part B for these dually eligible beneficiaries.

Special Medicare/Medicaid Programs

Other Medicare beneficiaries who are not fully eligible for Medicaid can receive some help through the state's Medicaid program for part or all of the individual's Medicare premiums and cost-sharing expenses. Individuals identified as **Qualified Disabled and Working Individuals (QDWIs)**, who lose their Medicare benefits because they returned to work, are allowed to purchase **Medicare hospital insurance (Medicare HI)**. Premiums for such coverage must be paid by the state Medicaid program if the individual qualifies as a QDWI and his or her income falls below 200% of the FPL. **Supplemental medical insurance (SMI)** coverage also is available to qualifying beneficiaries; however, premiums for SMI coverage are not paid by Medicaid.

Other Medicare beneficiaries who may receive some Medicaid assistance are referred to as **Qualified Medicare Beneficiaries (QMBs)**. These Medicare beneficiaries qualify only if they have incomes below the FPL and resources at or below twice the standard allowed under the SSI program. In this case, the state pays all the Medicare cost-sharing expenses and premiums for Medicare hospital insurance and SMI.

The Medicaid program pays SMI premiums of another classification, known as **Specified Low-Income Medicare Beneficiaries (SLMBs)**, who are beneficiaries with resources similar to those of Qualified Medicare Beneficiaries but with slightly higher incomes. Medicaid does not pay for the Medicare hospital insurance premium for this group. The Qualified Individuals (QIs) program, which is also known as the Additional Low-Income Medicare Beneficiary (ALMB) Program, is a limited expansion of the SLMB Program. The QI Program requires state Medicaid programs to pay the Medicare Part B premium for individuals who are not otherwise eligible for Medicaid and who have incomes between 120% and 135% of the FPL and limited resources. There is currently no asset limit. Applications and information about these programs are available at local Department of Social Services offices.

In all cases, Medicaid is always the **payer of last resort**, meaning that all other available third-party resources must meet their legal obligations to pay claims before the Medicaid program pays for the care of an individual eligible for Medicaid. If an individual is a Medicare beneficiary, payments for any services covered by Medicare are made by the Medicare program before any payments are made by the Medicaid program. The bottom line: Medicaid pays last.

Medicare and Medicaid Differences Explained

People are often confused about the differences between Medicare and Medicaid. Eligibility for Medicare is not tied to individual need. Rather, it is an *entitlement* program. Individuals are entitled to it because they or their spouses paid for it through Social Security taxes withheld from their wages. Medicaid is a federal *assistance* program for low-income, financially needy individuals, set up by the federal government and administered differently in each state. Although an individual may qualify and receive coverage from Medicare and Medicaid, there are separate eligibility requirements for each program, and being eligible for one program does not mean an individual is eligible for the other.

The following lists describe the differences between the two programs:

Medicare:
- Provision of healthcare insurance for disabled individuals, individuals 65 years and older, and any age individual with end-stage renal disease (ESRD).
- Individuals must have contributed to Medicare system (deductions from wages) to be eligible.
- Payment for primary hospital care and related medically necessary services.
- Generally, individuals must be older than 65 to be eligible.
- There may be a copay provision, depending on the services received.
- Is a federally controlled, uniform application across the United States.

Medicaid:
- Needs-based healthcare program.
- Payment for long-term care for qualifying individuals.
- Individuals must meet income and financial limitations to be eligible for certain programs.
- Individuals must be 65 years of age or older, or disabled, or blind to qualify for coverage.
- Requires mandatory contribution of *all* of a recipient's income in certain programs.
- Individual state-by-state plan options create a different program in each state (generally similar but may be different in specific application).

Table 8-3 provides a brief summary of the major differences between the two programs.

TABLE 8-3	Medicare and Medicaid: Two Different Programs	
MEDICARE	**MEDICAID**
Title 18	Title 19
Federal administration	State administration with federal oversight
Work history affects eligibility	Eligibility based on need
Public insurance	Public assistance
For aged, blind, disabled	For aged, blind, disabled, pregnant women, children, and caretaker relatives
Funded by Social Security and Medicare payroll tax deductions	Funded by federal general fund appropriations combined with individual state funds

What Did You Learn?

1. If an individual has dual coverage under Medicaid and Medicare, which claim is filed first?
2. Name two categories of Medicare beneficiaries (other than full dual eligibles) who are eligible for partial Medicaid coverage.
3. What are the major differences between Medicaid and Medicare?

MEDICAID MANAGED CARE

We learned previously (see Chapter 7) that managed care organizations (MCOs) are designed to improve access to healthcare and reduce costs by eliminating inappropriate and unnecessary services, emphasizing primary care and coordination of care. Managed care delivery systems grew rapidly in the Medicaid program during the 1990s, and now they are the most common method of delivering healthcare in the Medicaid program. A variety of health plans serve Medicaid MCOs, including for-profit and not-for-profit plans that provide health benefits and additional services through an arrangement between a state Medicaid agency and MCOs that accept a set payment, or **capitation**, for these services. Approximately two-thirds of Medicaid beneficiaries are enrolled in some form of managed care, mostly in health maintenance organization (HMO) and primary care case management (PCCM) arrangements.

The Balanced Budget Act (BBA) of 1997 gave states authority to require enrollment in managed care organizations (MCOs) without obtaining a federal waiver (except for special needs children, Medicare beneficiaries, and Native Americans). Most states have all, or a portion of, their Medicaid population enrolled in MCOs. If a state provides a choice of at least two plans, it can make enrollment in managed care mandatory.

Healthy children and families make up the majority of Medicaid managed care enrollees, but a growing number of states are expanding managed care to previously excluded groups, such as people with disabilities, pregnant women, and children in foster care.

The future success of Medicaid managed care depends on the adequacy of the capitation rates and the ability of state and federal governments to monitor access and quality.

What Did You Learn?

1. Medicaid MCOs provide health benefits through an arrangement between a state Medicaid agency and MCOs that accept a set amount for these services, called _____.
2. Name the act that gave states authority to require enrollment in managed MCOs without obtaining a federal waiver.
3. What does the future success of Medicaid MCOs depend on?

MEDICAID CLAIMS

The universal CMS-1500 claim is accepted by Medicaid contractors in most states. Some states have their own form, however, that is used for submitting claims for Medicaid recipients. The health insurance professional must check with the local Medicaid contractor to make sure to use the correct claim form. Most states require every provider who submits Medicaid claims electronically to sign an annual certification agreement that binds the provider to the requirements stated in the agreement. This certification process helps prevent providers from submitting fraudulent claims. For an example of an electronic data interchange agreement, visit the Evolve site.

There is no one specific computer program or universal requirement for submitting Medicaid claims except for the prerequisite of following HIPAA standards for electronic data submission. All states have their own software and guidelines, and most will provide this software to enrolled providers at no charge after providers complete an enrollment form and submit it to the appropriate Medicaid contractor. As with all third-party payers, the health insurance professional should contact the Medicaid contractor in his or her state for guidelines and should make sure to have the current guidelines on hand.

Completing the CMS-1500 Using Medicaid Guidelines

The guidelines for completing a **Medicaid "simple" claim**—that is, the patient has Medicaid coverage only and no secondary insurance—can be found in Appendix B along with

an example of a completed Medicaid simple claim. Keep in mind that these guidelines are generic, and the health insurance professional must follow the exact guidelines for completing the CMS-1500 form issued by the Medicaid contractor in his or her state.

Medicaid Secondary Claims

A **Medicaid secondary claim** occurs when the beneficiary has two types of healthcare coverage, Medicare and medical insurance coverage (such as commercial or group policies) or dual coverage with traditional (original) Medicare enrollment. It is important that the health insurance professional determine which type of claim is being submitted, because Medicaid simple and crossover claims are sent to different addresses and are processed differently. A claim that is submitted to the wrong address will be processed incorrectly or denied. Fig. B-4 in Appendix B shows a CMS-1500 claim form for a patient with both Medicare and Medicaid coverage. *Remember ... Medicaid is always paid last.*

Resubmission of Medicaid Claims

When errors/omissions are detected on a Medicaid claim, it is typically rejected and returned to the provider for correction and resubmission. Although every Medicaid contractor may have different guidelines for correcting and resubmitting claims, most require a resubmission code and/or reference number, which is reported in Block 22 of the CMS-1500 claim form. In some states, Medicaid contractors offer online, real-time claims processing and resubmission capabilities. Every health insurance professional should be aware of the Medicaid resubmission rules applicable in his or her state.

Reciprocity

A simple dictionary definition of **reciprocity** is the occurrence of a situation in which individuals or entities offer certain rights to each other in return for the rights being given to them. In the field of healthcare insurance and coverage, when one state allows Medicaid beneficiaries from other states (usually states that are adjacent) to be treated in its medical facilities, this exchange of privileges is referred to as reciprocity. Health insurance professionals should be aware of which states, if any, offer reciprocity for Medicaid claims in their states.

What Did You Learn?

1. What is a Medicaid "simple" claim?
2. Define a Medicaid secondary claim.
3. Explain what is meant by "reciprocity"?

Imagine This!

Ellen Statler is a single mother of two dependent children living in a small Illinois town along the Mississippi River. Ellen is covered under Illinois Medicaid; however, because the nearest Illinois town where there is a healthcare provider who accepts Medicaid patients is 35 miles away, Ellen travels across the bridge into Iowa and receives care from a family practice clinic there, 2 miles from her home. This arrangement works out much more favorably for Ellen because both of her children have acute asthma, and periodic emergency visits are common.

MEDICAID AND THIRD-PARTY LIABILITY

Third-party liability refers to the legal obligation of third parties to pay all or part of the expenditures for medical assistance furnished under a state plan. Earlier in this chapter, we discussed the fact that the Medicaid program, by law, is intended to be the payer of last resort. Examples of third parties that may be liable to pay for services before Medicaid include the following:
- Employment-related health insurance
- Court-ordered health insurance by a noncustodial parent
- Workers' compensation
- Long-term care insurance
- Other state and federal programs (unless specifically excluded by federal statute)

Medicaid pays the bills when due and does not put the burden of collection from a third party on the Medicaid client. Individuals eligible for Medicaid assign their rights to third-party payments to the state Medicaid agency. States are required to take all reasonable measures to ensure that the legal liability of third parties to pay for care and services is met before funds are made available under the state Medicaid plan. Healthcare providers are obligated to inform Medicaid of any known third parties who might have liability. When states have determined that a potentially liable third party exists, the state is required to **cost avoid** or **pay and chase claims**. Cost avoidance is the process by which the healthcare provider bills and collects from liable third parties before sending the claim to Medicaid. Pay and chase is used when the state Medicaid agency goes ahead and pays the medical bills and then attempts to recover these paid funds from liable third parties. States generally are required to cost-avoid claims unless they have a waiver approved by CMS that allows them to use the pay-and-chase method. To learn more about third-party liability (TPL), cost avoidance, and collection, refer to Websites to Explore at the end of this chapter.

In the case of third-party liability, certain blocks of the CMS-1500 form are filled out differently (Table 8-4). This information is generic, and the health insurance professional must follow the specific Medicaid guidelines in his or her state.

As mentioned previously, in a case in which the patient has dual eligibility for Medicaid and Medicare (Medi-Medi), Medicare is primary. In this case, the claim is submitted first to Medicare, which pays its share and then "crosses it over" to Medicaid. More information on **Medicare-Medicaid crossover claims** is given in Chapter 9.

TABLE 8-4	CMS-1500 Guidelines for Medicaid Secondary Claims
Block 4	Enter the primary policyholder's complete name (last, first, middle initial) as it appears on the ID card
Block 9	Enter the primary policyholder's complete name (last, first, middle initial) as it appears on the ID card. If it is the same as the patient's, key "SAME"
Block 9a	Enter the primary insurer's policy and group numbers as indicated on the ID card
Block 9b	If the primary policyholder is other than the patient, enter his or her date of birth using the MM DD YYYY format
Block 9d	Enter the primary policy name
Block 11	Conditionally required. If the primary payer rejected the claim, enter the rejection code
Block 11d	"X" the "YES" box
Block 29	Enter the amount (if any) paid by the primary insurer. If nothing was paid by the primary policy, indicate so using zeros
Block 30	If an amount was entered in Block 29, subtract it from Block 28 and enter the balance here

What Did You Learn?

1. What is "third-party liability"?
2. List some examples of third-party entities that would be primary to Medicaid.
3. Explain the difference between "cost avoid" and "pay and chase" in reference to Medicaid claims.

COMMON MEDICAID BILLING ERRORS

The primary goal of the health insurance professional is to create and submit insurance claims so that the maximum benefits the medical record supports are received in the minimal amount of time. This is a learned process, however, and it takes an experienced individual to avoid making common errors that cause a claim to be delayed or rejected. Fig. 8-5 lists some of these common billing errors.

All claims submitted to Medicaid must pass screening criteria before they can be processed. If one or more of the following conditions are not met the claim will be returned to the provider.

Patient ID (Field 1a) There must always be an 11-digit patient number assigned by Medicaid. If this field is blank, has less than or more than 11 digits, or is invalid, the claim will be returned.

Diagnosis Code (Field 21 and 24-E) There must be a diagnosis code listed in Field 21 and/or Field 24-E. A claim with a written description without a corresponding diagnosis code is often held until staff is available to code them. If the description is not specific enough to code, the claim will be returned.

Dates of Service (Field 24-A) There must be a "From" date. If you are billing a date range, both the "From" and "To" date fields must be completed. Future service dates may not be billed.

Place of Service Code (Field 24-B) This must be a 2-digit code. If the Place of Service Code is blank, less or more than 2 digits, or an invalid code, the claim will be returned.

Procedure Code (Field 24-D) This must be a 5- or 6-digit code. If the minimum criteria are not met, the claim is returned.

Charges (Field 24-F) There must be a charge for each line billed. (**Note:** Only EPSDT claims will be accepted with a zero line submitted amount.)

Days or Units (Field 24-G) There must be a whole number in this field (no decimals).

Signature (Field 31) There must be a handwritten signature or a computer-generated name. The name may not be the provider office name; it needs to be an actual person's name who is responsible for the information submitted on the claim. Initials only are also not accepted.

Billing Date (Field 31) The date billed must be on the claim form in Field 31. If the bill date in Field 31 or the claim received date is before the latest date of service on the claim, the claim will be returned.

Total Charge (Field 28) There must be a correct total charge. Claims will be returned for no total charge or for an incorrect total charge. Each claim form must have a total.

Date Received The date received must be no earlier than the latest date of service on the claim. Do not bill for future dates. Claims received before the latest date of service on the claim will be returned to the provider.

Fig. 8-5 CMS-1500 common billing errors.

What Did You Learn?

1. What is the first goal of the health insurance professional?
2. How can the health insurance professional avoid common billing errors?

MEDICAID REMITTANCE ADVICE

Every time a claim is sent to Medicaid, a document is generated explaining how the claim was **adjudicated**, or how the payment was determined. In the past, this document was referred to as the explanation of benefits (EOB); however,

Medicaid now calls it the **remittance advice (RA)**. The RA can be in paper or electronic form (if the medical facility is set up to accept the standard electronic version) and contains information from one or several claims (Fig. 8-6). The RA typically contains several "remark codes" and "reason codes." The importance of understanding the codes and interpreting this document cannot be stressed enough. Many states generate an RA periodically (e.g., weekly), and the current status of all claims (including adjustments and voids) that have been processed during the past week is indicated. The RA format may differ from state to state; however, all states furnish basically the same information. It is the health insurance professional's responsibility to interpret this document and reconcile it with patient records. All Medicaid claims and RAs should be maintained for 6 years, or longer if mandated by state statutes of limitation.

What Did You Learn?

1. Name three Medicaid programs that serve other groups qualifying for assistance.
2. Explain the purpose of HCBS Waivers.
3. List at least 5 services provided in the HCBS waiver program.

SPECIAL BILLING NOTES

The health insurance professional must keep several things in mind when filing Medicaid claims, as described here.

Time Limit for Filing Medicaid Claims

The time limit for filing Medicaid claims varies from state to state, anywhere from 2 months to 1 year. The health insurance professional should check with the Medicaid contractor in his or her state for the "timely filing" deadline. It is good practice, however, to file all claims in a timely manner—typically right after the service has been performed, unless additional services are anticipated within the same month or eligibility period. If denial of a claim is received because of failure to meet the state's timely filing deadlines, the provider cannot bill the patient.

Copayments

Services rendered by some types of healthcare providers (e.g., podiatrists, dentists, chiropractors) often require that the Medicaid recipient make a copayment. If the health insurance professional is employed by one of these types of healthcare providers, he or she should contact the Medicaid contractor in his or her state or consult the Medicaid provider manual for information. This information usually is indicated on the Medicaid recipient's ID card. Experienced health insurance professionals suggest that if a copayment

```
PERF PROV  SERV DATE   POS NOS  PROC   MODS    BILLED    ALLOWED   DEDUCT   COINS      GRP /RC-AMT       PROV  PD
```

```
NAME  ALPHA, ALBERT         HIC 699777777A  ACNT 1111111111        ICN 1402065330030  ASG Y  MOA  MA01
W88888888  1215 121501 11   1 92547           98.00     27.22     0.00     5.44  CO-42     70.78          21.78
W88888888  1215 121501 11   1 92541           45.00     39.89     0.00     7.98  CO-42      5.11          31.91
PT RESP    13.42               CLAIM TOTALS   143.00     67.11     0.00    13.42            75.89          53.69
                                                                                                     53.69 NET
```

```
NAME  BAKER, LEEANN         HIC 699123123A  ACNT 0009              ICN 1102025001590  ASG Y  MOA  MA01  MA18
W88888888  0113 011302 11   1 J9202 GACC    600.00    446.49     0.00    89.30  CO-42    153.51         357.19
                            (J9217)
W88888888  0121 012102 11   1 J9202 CC      600.00    446.49     0.00    89.30  CO-42    153.51         357.19
                               (J9217)
PT RESP   178.60               CLAIM TOTALS 1200.00    892.98     0.00   178.60           307.02         714.38
                                                                                                    714.38 NET
```

CLAIM INFORMATION FORWARDED TO: BCBS OF MINNESOTA ❹

```
NAME  CHARLIE, CINDY        HIC 699222222A  ACNT 22222222          ICN 1402008151040  ASG Y  MOA  MA01
W88888888  0106 010602 11   1 76091  26      80.00     43.76     0.00     8.75  CO-42     36.24          35.01
W88888888  0106 010602 11   1 G0236  26      50.00      0.00     0.00     0.00  CO-B5     50.00          00.00
REM: M58
PT RESP    8.75                CLAIM TOTALS  130.00     43.76     0.00     8.75            86.24          35.01
ADJS: PREV PD    0.00  INT     0.17  LATE FILING CHARGE     0.00  ❷                                  35.18 NET
```

```
NAME  BETA, BOB             HIC 699111111A  ACNT 12345678901234567890 ICN 1402063333010  ASG Y  MOA  MA01  MA72
W88888888  0304 030402 11   1 99214          180.00     81.99    47.65     6.87  CO-42     98.01          00.00
W88888888  0304 030402 11   1 82010           30.00      0.00     0.00     0.00  CO-B7     30.00          00.00
W88888888  0304 030402 11   1 J1040           10.00      9.39     0.00     1.88  CO-42     00.61          00.00
PT RESP   56.40                CLAIM TOTALS  220.00     91.38    47.65     8.75           128.62          00.00
                                                                                                     00.00 NET
```

```
NAME  BUMAN, JAMES          HIC 699555555A  ACNT 55555555          ICN 1402065200070  ASG Y  MOA  MA01
W88888888  0304 030402 11   1 99214           75.00      0.00     0.00     0.00  PR-B7     75.00          00.00
                                                                                  OA-71    20.00
                                                                                  PR-A3   -20.00
PT RESP   55.00                CLAIM TOTALS   75.00      0.00     0.00     0.00            75.00          00.00
                                                                                                     00.00 NET
```

```
TOTALS: # OF      BILLED     ALLOWED    DEDUCT      COINS      TOTAL     PROV PD        PROV  ❸    CHECK
        CLAIMS    AMT        AMT        AMT         AMT        RC-AMT    AMT            ADJ AMT      AMT
        5         1768.00    1095.23    47.65       209.52     672.77    803.08         108.50      749.56
```

```
PROVIDER ADJ DETAILS:  PLB REASON CODE    FCN             HIC          AMOUNT  ❶
                           CS             1402063333010   699111111A    34.98
                           CS             1402065200070   699555555A    20.00
                           WO             7101347082956                 53.69
                           L6                                           -0.17
```

GLOSSARY: Group, Reason, MOA, Remark and Adjustment Codes:
CO   Contractual Obligation. Amount for which the provider is financially liable. The patient may not be billed for this amount.
PR   Patient Responsibility. Amount that may be billed to a patient or another payee.
OA   Other Adjustment.
A3   Medicare Secondary Payer liability met.
B5   Claim/Service denied/reduced because coverage guidelines were not met or were exceeded.
B7   This provider was not certified for this procedure/service on this date of service.
42   Charges exceed our fee schedule or maximum allowable amount.
71   Primary Payer amount.
M58   Please resubmit the claim with the missing/correct information so that it may be processed.
MA01   If you do not agree with what we approved for these services, you may appeal our decision. To make sure that we are fair to you, we require another individual that did not process your initial claim to conduct the review. However, in order to be eligible for a review, you must write to us within 6 months of the date of this notice, unless you have a good reason for being late.
MA119   Provider level adjustment for late claim filing applies to this claim.
MA18   The claim information is also being forwarded to the patient's supplemental insurer. Send any questions regarding supplemental benefits to them.
MA72   The beneficiary overpaid you for these assigned services. You must issue the beneficiary a refund within 30 days for the difference between his/her payment to you and the total of the amount shown as patient responsibility and as paid to the beneficiary on this notice.
CS   Adjustment
WO   Withholding
L6   Interest

3/25/02

Fig. 8-6 Standard paper remittance (SPR) advice notices, revised format.

is required, it should be collected before services are rendered. Also, the new rules under the DRA Act impose copayments and premiums to certain categories of Medicaid recipients.

Accepting Assignment

As mentioned previously, Medicaid payments are made directly to the healthcare provider. Contractors in most states point out, however, that it is still important that assignment is accepted on all Medicaid claims. If Block 27 on the CMS-1500 form is not checked "Yes," the claim may be denied. Providers participating in Medicaid must accept the Medicaid reimbursement as payment in full. **Balance billing**, billing the recipient for any amount not paid by Medicaid, is not allowed. Additionally, according to federal law, a provider who accepts Medicaid payment for services furnished to an ill or injured individual has no right to additional payment from a liable third party even if Medicaid has been reimbursed.

Services Requiring Prior Approval

Prior approval may be required for some Medicaid services, products, and procedures to verify medical necessity, with the exception of some emergency situations. If prior approval is required, the provider must request and obtain prior approval before rendering the service, product, or procedure in order to seek Medicaid payment. Obtaining prior approval *does not* guarantee payment or ensure recipient eligibility on the date of service. The recipient must be Medicaid eligible on the date that the service, product, or procedure is provided. Requests for prior approval must be submitted as specified by the local Health and Human Services office or the Medicaid contractor in the particular state in which the services are rendered.

Preauthorization

Preauthorization is required for all inpatient hospitalization, unless the hospitalization was due to an emergency. In the case of an emergency, most Medicaid contractors require 24-hour notification. Normally, a preadmission/preprocedure review is performed by the provider before the patient is admitted to the hospital and the procedure or service is performed. Costs of services that require review will not be paid unless the claim denotes that review has been performed, the admission is medically necessary, and the setting is appropriate. The Medicaid contractor provides a preauthorization number, which should be entered in Block 23 of the CMS-1500 form. The health insurance professional should review and be aware of what procedures and services require a preadmission/preprocedure review and preauthorization. This information usually can be found in the Medicaid provider manual, or the health insurance professional can contact his or her local Medicaid contractor.

> ### 📁 HIPAA Tip
>
> Paper claim and Prior Authorization Request Form (PA/RF) instructions must be consistent with the Administrative Simplification provisions of the federal Health Insurance Portability and Accountability Act of 1996.

Retention, Storage, and Disposal of Records

The question "How long should a practice keep medical records?" often generates a challenging discussion. According to HIPAA's proposed privacy regulation, medical records must be maintained for 6 years. According to federal statute, the government can take criminal or civil action up to 7 years. To make it more confusing, the Department of Health and Human Services Privacy Act of 1974 established a new system of records, called the *National Provider System*. The National Provider System states that "records are retained indefinitely, except in the instance of an individual provider's death, in which case HCFA (now CMS) would retain such records for a 10-year period following the provider's death." In addition, there may be state laws and regulations giving specific time frames for medical record retention. Some practices archive paper records permanently using a photoduplicating process such as microfilm or microfiche.

Storage of medical records is also important. The healthcare staff needs to be able to find the records they are looking for easily. If dozens of boxes must be searched to find specific medical records, it would cost the practice time and money; it is important that records are stored where they can be located quickly and easily. Computerized records can be stored on electronic media such as discs, magnetic tape, and CD-ROM. Magnetic storage media do not guarantee permanency, however. Computer experts suggest using a permanent-type CD-ROM.

When it has been determined that a medical record has met all requirements (state and federal) for disposal, this process should be performed according to state statute. Typically, the rule of thumb for paper record disposal is a shredding process. It is unacceptable merely to discard paper records in a trash bin because of security violations. Records kept on magnetic media can be erased or deleted.

> ### ❓ What Did You Learn?
>
> 1. What is the time limit for filing Medicaid claims?
> 2. Name the types of providers that might require a copayment.
> 3. Preauthorization is always required for what types of Medicaid services?

FRAUD AND ABUSE IN THE MEDICAID SYSTEM

Fraud is an intentional misrepresentation or deception that could result in an unauthorized benefit to an individual or individuals and usually comes in the form of a false statement requesting payment under the Medicaid program. **Abuse** typically involves payment for items or services in which there was no intent to deceive or misrepresent, but the outcome of poor and inefficient methods results in unnecessary costs to the Medicaid program.

What Is Medicaid Fraud?

Medicaid fraud occurs when a healthcare provider such as a physician, dentist, pharmacist, hospital, nursing home, or other healthcare service engages in one or more of the following practices:

- Billing:
  - for medical services not actually performed
  - for a more expensive service than was rendered
  - separately for several services that should be combined into one billing
  - twice for the same medical service
  - for ambulance runs when no medical service is provided
- Dispensing generic drugs and billing for brand name drugs
- Giving or accepting something in return for medical services (kickbacks)
- Bribery
- Providing unnecessary services
- False cost reports
- Transporting multiple passengers in an ambulance and billing a run for each passenger

Medicaid fraud and abuse drive up healthcare costs for everyone. The health insurance professional should contact the Attorney General's Medicaid Fraud Control Unit if he or she has evidence or suspects that a healthcare provider (or patient) is committing Medicaid fraud.

Patient Abuse and Neglect

Frequent unexplained injuries or complaints of pain without obvious injury can be indicators of patient abuse and neglect, such as the following:

- Burns or bruises suggesting the use of instruments or cigarettes
- Passive, withdrawn, and emotionless behavior
- Lack of reaction to pain
- Sexually transmitted diseases or injury to the genital area
- Difficulty in sitting or walking
- Fear of being alone with caretakers
- Obvious malnutrition
- Lack of personal cleanliness
- Habitually dressed in torn or dirty clothes
- Obvious fatigue and listlessness
- Begging for food or water
- In need of medical or dental care
- Left unattended for long periods
- Bedsores and skin lesions

> ⭐ **Imagine This!**
>
> Superior Ambulance Company transports patients from the Coast View Convalescent Home to a nearby medical center. The vehicles are equipped to carry four patients at a time. Shirley Holmes, whose father (a Medicaid recipient) resides at Coast View, received a bill for $800 for an emergency transport. She was with her father at the time of transport and noted that two other residents were occupants of the ambulance at the same time her father was taken to the medical center. Mrs. Holmes discussed the charge with Coast View's administrator, and it was discovered that the ambulance company, rather than splitting the cost of the transport among the three patients who were transported on that run, charged each patient the entire $800 fee.

> 🕐 **Stop and Think**
>
> Martin Roble received a prescription for a medication that was to be filled using a generic product. The pharmacist filled the prescription with generic drugs, according to Medicaid rules, but charged Medicaid for the more expensive brand name medication. Would this be considered fraud or abuse?

The health insurance professional should learn how to recognize fraud and abuse and do everything possible to prevent it. There is a Medicaid Fraud Control Unit in every state, which is a federally funded state law enforcement entity located in the State Attorney General's office. In addition to investigating fraud committed by healthcare providers, the Medicaid Fraud Control Unit also investigates the abuse, neglect, and exploitation of elderly, ill, and disabled residents of long-term care facilities such as nursing homes, facilities for the mentally and physically disabled, and assisted living facilities. The investigation of corruption in the administration of the Medicaid program is another important responsibility of the Medicaid Fraud Control Unit. To report fraud or abuse, health insurance professionals may use the state's hotline number or contact the Medicaid Fraud Control Unit nearest them.

Extensive information on Medicaid fraud and abuse can be found on the CMS website. At the CMS home page, click on "Medicaid." Under the heading "Medicaid Integrity Programs," select the topic "State Program Integrity and Support & Assistance." Here you will find information on fraud prevention along with related links for state contacts and how to report fraud.

MEDICAID QUALITY PRACTICES

"The right care for every person every time" is how CMS defines quality. CMS is responsible for supporting State Medicaid and CHIP programs in their efforts to achieve patient-centered, safe, effective, efficient, timely, and equitable care. CMS partners with states to share best practices, provide technical assistance to improve performance measurement, evaluate current improvement efforts to inform future activities, work together with quality partners, and coordinate activities to ensure efficiency of operations. To achieve this goal, CMS developed several key strategies, as follows:

Evidenced-based care and quality measurement: CMS supports states' efforts to improve performance measurement and the quality of care through the use of evidence-based measure sets that are widely accepted in the healthcare industry.

Payment aligned with quality: CMS supports states in their efforts to implement quality based purchasing-known as pay-for-performance (P4P). P4P is a quality improvement and reimbursement process targeting payments that generate much stronger financial support for patient-focused, high-value care. P4P promotes reimbursement for quality, access efficiency, and successful outcomes.

Health information technology (HIT): HHS has a 10-year plan to transform the delivery of healthcare by building a new health information infrastructure, including electronic health records (EHRs) and a network to link health records nationwide. CMS also encourages creative uses of HIT in states' Medicaid and CHIP programs.

Information dissemination and technical assistance: Information dissemination, knowledge transfer, and technical assistance are very important in the Medicaid and CHIP programs, given that states have wide flexibility in how they run their programs. CMS shares model practices, lessons learned, and innovative approaches to emerging issues through briefs, analysis of demonstration evaluations, participating in conferences and Webcasts, and other methods.

SUMMARY CHECKPOINTS

▶ Medicaid is a combination federal and state medical assistance program designed to provide medical care for low-income individuals and families, specifically children, pregnant women, the elderly, the disabled, and parents with dependent children.

▶ The Medicaid program was created to give low-income Americans access to healthcare. It has since evolved into a large insurance program with complex eligibility rules. Today, Medicaid is a major social welfare program administered by CMS.

▶ The following are some of the changes that have occurred in the Medicaid program in recent years:
  • AFDC has been renamed TANF.
  • SSI was established in 1972 to provide federally funded cash assistance to qualifying elderly and disabled poor.
  • Medically needy groups have been expanded.
  • The healthcare reform bill will allow nearly everyone under age 65 with income up to 133% of the FPL to be eligible for Medicaid in 2014.

▶ The federal government establishes broad national guidelines for Medicaid eligibility and contributes approximately 57% of the Medicaid cost to the individual states.

▶ To be eligible for federal funds, states must provide Medicaid coverage for certain categories of individuals. The two major groups that qualify for Medicaid are the categorically needy and the medically needy.

▶ Each state can set its own guidelines for Medicaid eligibility standards, services, benefit packages, payment rates, and program administration within the broader federal guidelines. In addition to the federally mandated programs, states can have additional "state-only" programs, but these programs do not receive federal funds.

▶ The Children's Health Insurance Program (CHIP) provides federal matching funds for states to implement health insurance programs for children in families that earn too much to qualify for Medicaid but too little to reasonably afford private health coverage.

▶ The EPSDT program was developed to fit the standards of pediatric care and to meet the special physical, emotional, and developmental needs of low-income children.

▶ The PACE program provides comprehensive alternative care for noninstitutionalized elderly who otherwise would be in a nursing home.

▶ As a general rule, Medicaid pays only for services that are determined to be medically necessary. To meet this criterion, the service must be consistent with the diagnosis and in accordance with the standards of good medical practice, performed at the proper level, and provided in the most appropriate setting.

▶ Cost sharing applies to people who do not meet the income/assets requirements (medically needy) of Medicaid but may qualify for assistance by using their medical expenses to spend down their income before Medicaid considers their eligibility.

▶ Providers participating in Medicaid must accept the Medicaid reimbursement as payment in full. Each state is free to determine (within federal restrictions) how reimbursements are calculated and the resulting rates for services, with certain exceptions.

▶ Medicaid eligibility can be verified in the following ways:
• patient's Medicaid ID card
• AVR system, which uses a touch-tone phone process
• EDI, an electronic method that involves online interactive clearinghouses
• point-of-sale device, in which eligibility information is contained on a magnetic strip similar to a credit card
• computer software programs, which involves keying patient information into a computer

▶ Most very poor elderly or disabled individuals are covered under Medicaid and Medicare, commonly referred to as dual coverage, dual eligibility, or Medi-Medi. These individuals may receive Medicare services as well as other services available under their state's Medicaid program. Medicaid pays all of the cost-sharing portions (deductibles and coinsurance) of Medicare Parts A and B for dually eligible beneficiaries.

▶ A variety of health plans serve Medicaid MCOs that provide health benefits and additional services through an arrangement between a state Medicaid agency and MCOs that accept a set payment, or capitation, for these services. Approximately two-thirds of Medicaid beneficiaries are enrolled in some form of managed care, mostly in HMOs) and primary care case management (PCCM) arrangements.

▶ Medicaid, by law, is the payer of last resort. Claims must first be sent to any third parties involved, and the third parties must meet their legal obligations to pay the claims before Medicaid is billed. Common Medicaid billing errors include the following:
• incorrect patient ID numbers
• incorrect diagnosis/procedure code(s)
• incorrect dates of service format
• omission of a charge (there must be one for each line of service)
• incorrect billing date
• incorrect signature

▶ When the patient has dual eligibility for Medicaid and Medicare (Medi-Medi), Medicare is primary. The claim is submitted first to Medicare, which pays its share and then "crosses it over" to Medicaid.

▶ Every time a claim is sent to Medicaid, a document, called a remittance advice (RA), is generated explaining how the claim was adjudicated, or how the payment was determined. The RA can be in paper or electronic form and contains information from one or several claims. The RA typically contains "remark codes" and "reason codes," which the health insurance professional must be able to understand to interpret and reconcile this document with patient records.

▶ Medicaid fraud occurs when a healthcare provider engages in illegal or deceptive practices. Abuse typically involves payment for items or services in which there was no intent to deceive or misrepresent, but the outcome of poor and inefficient methods results in unnecessary costs to the Medicaid program. The health insurance professional should learn to recognize fraud and report it to the state's hotline number or contact the Medicaid Fraud Control Unit.

⟳ CLOSING SCENARIO

When they first began the chapter, Nela and Berta felt as if they were on a ship heading into uncharted waters. Looking over the chapter objectives and terms left them feeling more than slightly apprehensive. There was so much to learn; however, the study plan they laid out before starting Chapter 8 was to "bite off one chunk at a time," which worked well for them in understanding the concepts presented. In addition to what was in the chapter, they frequently visited the CMS website for more detailed information. Additionally, they consulted the Medicaid website in their state to become knowledgeable about their individual state's regulations.

Berta, because her mother-in-law was currently in a nursing home, was particularly interested in learning about the "spend down" process, which apparently her mother-in-law went through to become eligible for Medicaid. Nela's interest was in the area of programs for women and children because of her own situation. By now, the women have had enough experience with completing the CMS-1500 claim that they had few problems filling out the blocks for typical Medicaid cases. Understanding the Medicaid remittance advice proved to be more of a challenge, however, and the women admitted that it might take additional experience before they acquired the necessary skill to become efficient. Their instructor assured them that this skill would come with time. It was becoming apparent to both women that a career as a health insurance professional was going to be interesting and rewarding, albeit challenging.

WEBSITES TO EXPLORE

- For live links to the following websites, please visit the Evolve site at
  http://evolve.elsevier.com/Beik/today/
- To learn about the Medicaid program, visit the website for the Centers of Medicare and Medicaid Services at
  http://www.cms.hhs.gov/
- For a more in-depth discussion of Medicaid visit
  http://www.cms.hhs.gov/MedicaidGenInfo/03_TechnicalSummary.asp/
- To learn about the Medicaid program in your state, log on to
  http://cms.hhs.gov/medicaid/consumer.asp/
  and select the applicable state site.
- To see a timeline of Medicaid's key developments, follow the Evolve icon to
  http://www.kff.org/medicaid/medicaid_timeline.cfm/
- Access an updated fact sheet for the Medicaid program in your state at
  http://www.statehealthfacts.org/medicaid.jsp/
- To find out what the TANF program is called in your state, log on to
  http://www.acf.hhs.gov/programs/ofa/states/st_index.html/
- For state-by-state Medicaid descriptions and plans, research the following website:
  http://64.82.65.67/medicaid/states.html/
- To learn more about the Affordable Care Act, follow the Evolve icon to
  http://www.healthcare.gov/law/introduction/index.html/

- To learn the specific guidelines for the Medicaid programs offered in a particular state, log on to
  http://www.cms.hhs.gov/medicaid/consumer.asp/
  and insert the name of the state in the "select state" box.
- For complete information on the Medicare Prescription Drug, Improvement, and Modernization Act of 2003, log on to
  http://www.cms.hhs.gov/MMAUpdate/
- The CMS website provides extensive information on third-party liability, cost avoidance, and collection at
  http://www.cms.hhs.gov/ThirdPartyLiability/
- To learn more about SSI benefits, countable income, and exclusions for the SSI program, log on to
  www.socialsecurity.gov/
- The Website for MHCCM is at
  http://www.cms.hhs.gov/medicaid/hipaa/adminsimp/
- For updates on SSI benefits, log on to
  www.socialsecurity.gov/pubs/10003.pdf/

Author's Note: Websites change frequently. If any of these URLs is unavailable, use applicable guide words in your Internet search to acquire additional information on the various subjects listed.

REFERENCES AND RESOURCES

Centers for Medicare and Medicaid Services: *Deficit Reduction Act Important Facts for State Policymakers,* February 21, 2008. http://www.cms.hhs.gov/DeficitReductionAct/Downloads/Cost sharing.pdf/.

CHAPTER 9

Conquering Medicare's Challenges

Chapter Outline

I. Medicare Program
   A. Medicare Program Structure
      1. Medicare Part A
      2. Medicare Part B
   B. Enrollment
   C. Premiums and Cost-Sharing Requirements
   D. Medicare Part C (Medicare Advantage Plans)
      1. Healthcare Reform's Impact on Medicare Advantage Plans
   E. Other Medicare Health Plans
   F. Medicare Part D (Medicare Prescription Drug Benefit Plan)
   G. Changing Medicare Health or Prescription Drug Coverage
   H. Programs of All-Inclusive Care for the Elderly (PACE)
II. Medicare Combination Coverages
   A. Medicare/Medicaid Dual Eligibility
   B. Medicare Supplement Policies
      1. Medigap Insurance
         a. Standard Medigap Policies
         b. Where the Gaps Are
         c. Eligibility
      2. Medicare Secondary Payer
III. Medicare and Managed Care
   A. Medicare HMOs
      1. HMO with Point-of-Service Option
      2. Preferred Provider Organization
      3. Provider-Sponsored Organization
      4. Private Fee-for-Service Plan
      5. Special Needs Plans
   B. Advantages and Disadvantages of Medicare HMOs
      1. Advantages
      2. Disadvantages
   C. Why This Information Is Important to the Health Insurance Professional
IV. Preparing for the Medicare patient
   A. Medicare's Lifetime Release of Information Form
   B. Determining Medical Necessity
   C. Advanced Beneficiary Notice
   D. Local Coverage Determination (LCD)
   E. Health Insurance Claim Number and Identification Card
   F. Replacing the Medicare Card
V. Medicare Billing
   A. Physician Fee Schedule
   B. Medicare Participating and Nonparticipating Providers
   C. Determining What Fee to Charge
VI. Filing Medicare claims
   A. Electronic Claims
   B. Administrative Simplification Compliance Act
   C. Transition to ASC X12 Version 5010
   D. Exceptions to Mandatory Electronic Claim Submission
   E. Small Providers and Full-Time Equivalent Employee Assessments
   F. ASCA Enforcement of Paper Claim Submission
      1. Claim Status Request and Response
   G. Deadline for Filing Medicare Claims
      1. Timely Filing Rules
VII. Using the CMS-1500 Form for Medicare Claims
   A. CMS-1500 Completion Guidelines
   B. Completing a Medigap Claim
   C. Medicare Secondary Payer
      1. Insurance Primary to Medicare
      2. Completing Medicare Secondary Policy Claims
      3. MSP Conditional Payment
   D. Medigap Crossover Program
   E. Medicare/Medicaid Crossover Claims
VIII. Medicare Summary Notice
   A. Information Contained on the MSN
   B. Medicare Remittance Advice

1. Standard Paper Remittance Advice
2. Electronic Remittance Advice
   a. Enrolling in Electronic Remittance
   C. Electronic Funds Transfer
IX. Medicare Audits and Appeals
   A. Audits
   B. Recovery Audit Contractor (RAC) Program
   C. Appeals (Fee-for-Service Claims)
   D. Appeals Process (Medicare Managed Care Claims)
X. Quality Review Studies
   A. Quality Improvement Organizations
   B. Beneficiary Notices Initiative

C. Beneficiary Complaint Response Program
D. Hospital-Issued Notice of Noncoverage (HINN) and Notice of Discharge (NODMAR) and Medicare Appeal Rights Reviews
E. The Center for Medicare and Medicaid Innovation (CMI)
F. Physician Review of Medical Records
G. Physician Quality Reporting System (PQRS)
H. Medicare Billing Fraud
I. Clinical Laboratory Improvement Amendments Program

CHAPTER OBJECTIVES

After completion of this chapter, the student should be able to:

1. Describe the Medicare program and its structure.
2. List and discuss Medicare combination coverages (i.e., Medi-Medi, Medigap, and Medicare Secondary Policy).
3. Discuss Medicare managed care plans, including their advantages and disadvantages.
4. Outline specific considerations in preparation for the Medicare patient.
5. Recap the Medicare billing process.
6. Summarize the basics for filing Medicare claims electronically.
7. Establish guidelines for using the CMS-1500 paper form.
8. Compare and contrast MSNs and ERAs and the information each contains.
9. Discuss the purpose of Medicare audits and explain the five-level appeal process.
10. Explain the purpose of quality review studies.
11. Identify methods for detecting and reporting Medicare billing fraud.
12. Discuss the function of CLIA as it pertains to claims processing.

CHAPTER TERMS

adjudicated
advanced beneficiary notice (ABN)
allowable charges
beneficiary
Beneficiary Complaint Response Program
Beneficiary Notices Initiative
benefit period
claims adjustment reason codes
Clinical Laboratory Improvement Amendments (CLIA)
coordination of benefits contractor (COBC)
credible coverage
demand bills
disproportionate share
donut hole
downcoding
dual eligibles
electronic funds transfer (EFT)
electronic remittance advice (ERA)
end-stage renal disease (ESRD)
Federal Insurance Contribution Act (FICA)
fiscal intermediary (FI)
health insurance claim number (HICN)
HMO with point-of-service (POS) option
initial claims
lifetime (one-time) release of information form
local coverage determinations (LCDs)
mandated Medigap transfer
Medicare
Medicare Administrative Contractors (MACs)
Medicare gaps
Medicare HMOs
Medicare limiting charge
Medicare managed care plan
Medicare nonparticipating provider (nonPAR)
Medicare Part A
Medicare Part B
Medicare Part C (Medicare Advantage Plans)
Medicare Part D (Prescriptions Drug Plan)
Medicare participating provider (PAR)
Medicare Physician Fee Schedule
Medicare Secondary Payer (MSP)
Medicare Summary Notice (MSN)
Medicare supplement policy
network
noncovered services
open enrollment period
peer review organization (PRO)
Physician Quality Reporting System (PQRS)
Programs of All-inclusive Care for the Elderly (PACE)
quality improvement organizations (QIOs)
quality review study
Recovery Audit Contractor (RAC)
relative value unit
remittance advice (RA)
remittance remark codes
resource-based relative value system (RBRVS)
self-referring
small provider
special needs plan (SNP)
standard paper remittance (SPR)

MEDICARE PROGRAM

Medicare, a comprehensive federal insurance program, was established by Congress in 1966 to give individuals age 65 years and older financial assistance with medical expenses. In 1972 the Medicare program was expanded to include certain categories of disabled individuals younger than age 65 and individuals of any age who have **end-stage renal disease (ESRD)**, a group of permanent kidney disorders requiring dialysis or transplant. Fig. 9-1 shows important transitions in the Medicare program from its inception to 2010 enrollment.) Medicare is administered by the Center for Medicare and Medicaid Services (CMS), formerly called the

⟳ OPENING SCENARIO

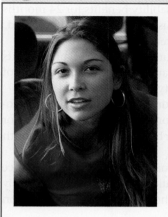

Rita Thomas, a high school dropout, attended an alternative high school to earn her general education diploma (GED). A single mother of a 3-year-old son, Rita lives with her grandmother and works as a waitress in a neighborhood bar and grill. Grandma Nan, as Rita calls her, encourages her granddaughter to enroll in night classes at the local community college. The evening schedule works well because Rita can keep her day job and Grandma Nan is available to babysit for her. Rita signs up for a health insurance course.

"Learn as much as you can about Medicare and then you can explain it all to me," Grandma Nan implores. "It's all so confusing." Encouraged by her grandmother's request, Rita enthusiastically begins her pursuit of "conquering Medicare's challenges." Until now, Medicare was just a word to Rita without much meaning. She had heard Grandma Nan and her elderly friends discussing it many times, but Rita paid little attention. She was aware, however, that these women did not understand Medicare's whole picture. Now Rita has an opportunity to do something not only for herself but also for her grandmother, who has done so much for her.

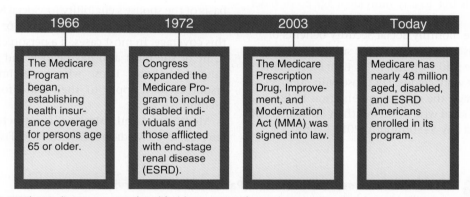

1966	1972	2003	Today
The Medicare Program began, establishing health insurance coverage for persons age 65 or older.	Congress expanded the Medicare Program to include disabled individuals and those afflicted with end-stage renal disease (ESRD).	The Medicare Prescription Drug, Improvement, and Modernization Act (MMA) was signed into law.	Medicare has nearly 48 million aged, disabled, and ESRD Americans enrolled in its program.

Fig. 9-1 The Medicare program. (Modified from Centers for Medicare and Medicaid: World of Medicare. http://cms.meridianksi.com/kc/ilc/scorm_course_launch_frm.asp?strCourseID=C00073&strUserID=FERGE002&strCredit=no-credit&strMode=normal/.)

Healthcare Financing Administration (HCFA). CMS is a federal agency within the U. S. Department of Health and Human Services (DHHS) that administers the Medicare program and works in partnership with state governments to administer Medicaid, the State Children's Health Insurance Program (SCHIP), and health insurance portability standards. To study a timeline of key developments in the Medicare Program, visit the Evolve site.

Medicare Fact: In 2010 the first "baby boomers" turned 65 and became eligible for Medicare. In the coming years, the number of patients depending on Medicare will rise from 48 million to more than 90 million Americans.

The **Federal Insurance Contributions Act (FICA)** provides for a federal system of old age, survivor, disability, and hospital insurance. The old age, survivor, and disability insurance part is financed by Social Security taxes. The hospital insurance part of Medicare is funded through taxes withheld from employees' wages and matched by employer contributions. In 2011 the FICA tax rate was lowered to 5.65% for employees. The employer rate remained unchanged, while the Social Security rate for employees was lowered to 4.20%. The Medicare contribution rate is 1.45% (amount withheld from wages). Employers must contribute a matching percentage for a total Medicare contribution of 2.9%. All wages are subject to the Medicare tax; there is no wage base limit.

Medicare is not provided free of charge; beneficiaries must meet certain conditions to qualify for benefits. Additionally, Medicare requires cost sharing in the form of premiums, deductibles, and coinsurance, all of which are discussed in this chapter.

Medicare Program Structure

Medicare is composed of four parts:

Medicare Part A—hospital insurance

Medicare Part B—medical (physicians' care) insurance (original, or traditional, Medicare); incudes healthcare provided in clinics

Medicare Part C—Medicare **Advantage** (managed care–type plans, formerly Medicare+Choice)

Medicare Part D—prescription drug program

Medicare Part A

Medicare Part A (hospital insurance) helps pay for services for the following types of healthcare (Table 9-1):

- Inpatient hospital care (including critical access hospitals)
- Inpatient care in a skilled nursing facility (SNF)
- Home healthcare
- Hospice care
- Blood

Medicare Part A does not cover custodial or long-term (nursing home) care.

Coverage requirements under Medicare state that for a service to be covered, it must be considered medically necessary—reasonable and necessary for the diagnosis or treatment of an illness or injury or to improve the functioning of a malformed body part.

Noncovered services are items or services that are not paid for by Medicare. See Table 9-2 for a list of noncovered services.

Medicare Part A is free to any individual age 65 or older who is

- eligible to receive monthly Social Security benefits or
- eligible on the basis of wages on which sufficient Medicare payroll taxes were paid. ("Sufficient" is 40 or more quarters of Social Security work credits. For those with 30 to 39 quarters of coverage, the monthly premium is $248/month. An individual who has fewer than 30 quarters of work credits must pay $450/month [2011 figures].)

Medicare Part A is also free to any disabled individual younger than age 65 who has

- received Social Security disability benefits for 24 months as a worker, surviving spouse, or adult child of a retired, disabled, or deceased worker or
- accumulated a sufficient number of Social Security credits to be insured for Medicare and meets the requirements of the Social Security disability program.

Medicare Fact: If an individual is diagnosed with amyotrophic lateral sclerosis (ALS or Lou Gehrig's disease), he or she automatically qualifies for both Parts A and B the month that disability benefits begin.

A **beneficiary** (an individual who has health insurance through the Medicare or Medicaid program) automatically qualifies for Part A if he or she was a federal employee on January 1, 1983.

Application for Medicare Part A is automatic when an individual applies for Social Security benefits. A husband or wife may also qualify for Part A coverage at age 65 on the basis of the spouse's eligibility for Social Security. If an individual is not eligible for free Part A, he or she may purchase this coverage. In most cases, if a person chooses to buy Part A, he or she must also have Part B and pay monthly premiums for both. Those who have limited income and resources may apply to their state for help in paying premiums.

Medicare Administrative Contractors (MACs), also referred to as Medicare Carriers and Fiscal Intermediaries

TABLE 9-1	2011 Medicare Hospital Insurance (Part A) Covered Services*		
SERVICES	**BENEFIT**	**MEDICARE PAYS**	**BENEFICIARY PAYS (OTHER INSURANCE MAY PAY ALL OR PART)**
Hospitalization: Semiprivate room, general nursing, miscellaneous services	First 60 days	All but $1132	$1132
	61st to 90th day	All but $283 per day	$283 per day
	91st to 150th day	All but $556 per day	$556 per day
	Beyond 150 days	Nothing	All charges
Skilled nursing	First 20 days	100% of approved	Nothing if approved
Facility care	21st to 100th day	All but $141.50 per day	$141.50 per day
	Beyond 100 days	Nothing	All costs
Home health care: Medically necessary skilled care, therapy	Part-time care	100% of approved	Nothing if approved
Hospice care for the terminally ill	As long as doctor certifies need	All but limited costs for drugs and respite care	Limited costs for drugs and respite care
Blood	Blood	All but first 3 pints	First 3 pints

*Hospital deductibles and coinsurance amounts change each year. The numbers shown in this chart are effective for 2011.
From http://www.insurance.wa.gov/publications/consumer/Medicare_Chart_A_B.pdf/.

TABLE 9-2	Medicare Part A Noncovered Services

Medical devices or **biologicals** (drugs or medicinal preparations obtained from animal tissue or other organic sources) that have not been approved by the U.S. Food and Drug Administration

Items and services that are determined to be investigational in nature: **alternative medicine**, including experimental procedures and treatments, acupuncture, and chiropractic services (except when manipulation of the spine is medically necessary to fix a subluxation of the spine—when one or more of the bones of the spine move out of position)

Most care received outside of the United States

Cosmetic surgery (unless it is needed to improve the function of a malformed part of the body)

Most dental care

Hearing aids or the examinations for prescribing or fitting hearing aids (except for implants to treat severe hearing loss in some cases)

Personal care or custodial care, such as help with bathing, toileting, and dressing (unless patient is homebound and receiving skilled care), and nursing home care (except in a skilled nursing facility if eligible)

Housekeeping services to help patient stay at home, such as shopping, meal preparation, and cleaning (unless patient is receiving hospice care)

Nonmedical services, including hospital television and telephone, a private hospital room, canceled or missed appointments, and copies of x-rays

Most non-emergency transportation, including ambulance services

Some **preventive care**, including routine foot care

Most vision (eye) care, including eyeglasses (except when following cataract surgery) and examinations for prescribing or fitting eyeglasses or contact lenses

---

(FIs), are private insurance companies that serve as the federal government's agents in the administration of the Medicare program, including the payment of claims. In the past, carriers made Medicare payments to providers including doctors and equipment suppliers, and FIs made Medicare payments to facilities such as hospitals and nursing facilities. Railroad Retirement Board Carriers (RRBC) administer Medicare benefits for railroad retirees. With the new MAC structure, there are 15 contractors by jurisdiction responsible for processing Part A and B claims. Four of the A/B MAC providers will overlap responsibility for handling Home Health and Hospice claims. The final four MAC plans will be the Durable Medical Equipment (DME) contractors. Fig. 9-2 shows a map of these MAC jurisdictions along with the name of each MAC and the states they will cover.

For updates on Medicare Parts A and B administrative contractors and MACs, visit the Evolve site.

Imagine This!

Eloise Graham went to the Argyle County Mental Health Center (ACMHC) for psychiatric counseling. Under Medicare, this is a covered service, but the adult day care services Eloise receives that are provided at ACMHC are not considered reasonable and necessary. A claim submitted to Medicare for the adult day care services was denied.

Medicare Part B

Medicare Part B is medical insurance financed by a combination of federal government funds and beneficiary premiums that help pay for the following:
- Medically necessary physicians' services
- Some preventive services
- Outpatient hospital services
- Clinical laboratory services
- Durable medical equipment (To qualify as DME, equipment must be ordered by a physician for the patient's use in the home, and items must be reusable, e.g., walkers, wheelchairs, hospital beds)
- Blood (received as an outpatient)

For a complete list of covered and noncovered Part B services, type "Medicare & You" along with the appropriate year in your Internet search engine, e.g., "Medicare & You 2013."

For a beneficiary who became eligible for Medicare on or after January 1, 2005, Medicare covers a "Welcome to Medicare" physical examination if it is performed within the first 12 months of coverage, if that individual has Part B coverage. Beginning January 2011, Part B also covers a yearly "wellness" examination for those who have had Part B for longer than 12 months in order to develop or update a personalized prevention plan based on current health and risk factors. This yearly exam is free if the healthcare provider accepts assignment. Medicare covers "wellness" exams for healthy beneficiaries every year. Part B also can help pay for many other medical services and supplies that are not covered by Medicare Part A and for home healthcare if the beneficiary is not enrolled in Part A. Medicare covers other preventive healthcare services, such as
- bone mass measurements;
- colorectal cancer screening;
- diabetes services;
- glaucoma testing;
- Pap tests, pelvic examinations, and clinical breast examinations;
- prostate cancer screening;
- screening mammograms; and
- certain vaccinations.

Table 9-3 lists additional services and supplies that Medicare Part B helps pay for and services that are not covered by Part B.

All Medicare Part B beneficiaries pay for Part B coverage. Most beneficiaries enrolled in "original" Medicare paid a

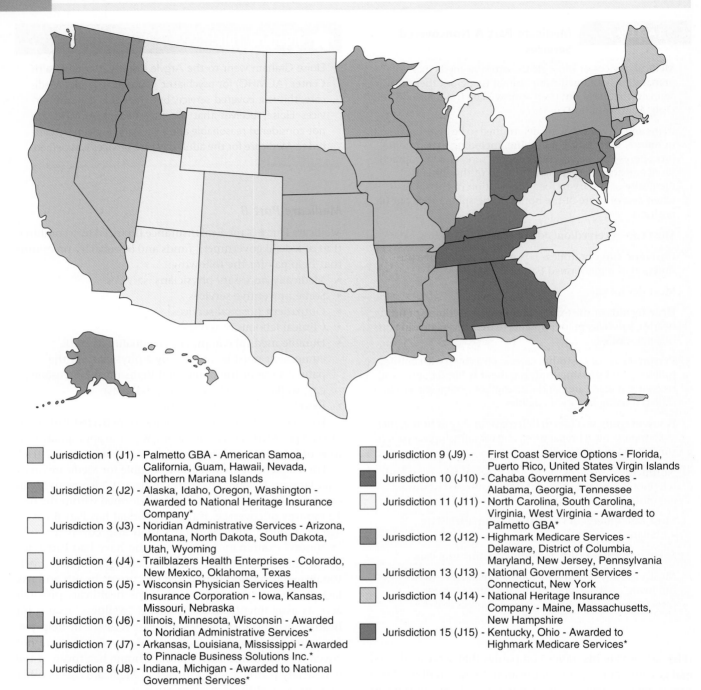

Jurisdiction 1 (J1) - Palmetto GBA - American Samoa, California, Guam, Hawaii, Nevada, Northern Mariana Islands

Jurisdiction 2 (J2) - Alaska, Idaho, Oregon, Washington - Awarded to National Heritage Insurance Company*

Jurisdiction 3 (J3) - Noridian Administrative Services - Arizona, Montana, North Dakota, South Dakota, Utah, Wyoming

Jurisdiction 4 (J4) - Trailblazers Health Enterprises - Colorado, New Mexico, Oklahoma, Texas

Jurisdiction 5 (J5) - Wisconsin Physician Services Health Insurance Corporation - Iowa, Kansas, Missouri, Nebraska

Jurisdiction 6 (J6) - Illinois, Minnesota, Wisconsin - Awarded to Noridian Administrative Services*

Jurisdiction 7 (J7) - Arkansas, Louisiana, Mississippi - Awarded to Pinnacle Business Solutions Inc.*

Jurisdiction 8 (J8) - Indiana, Michigan - Awarded to National Government Services*

Jurisdiction 9 (J9) -   First Coast Service Options - Florida, Puerto Rico, United States Virgin Islands

Jurisdiction 10 (J10) - Cahaba Government Services - Alabama, Georgia, Tennessee

Jurisdiction 11 (J11) - North Carolina, South Carolina, Virginia, West Virginia - Awarded to Palmetto GBA*

Jurisdiction 12 (J12) - Highmark Medicare Services - Delaware, District of Columbia, Maryland, New Jersey, Pennsylvania

Jurisdiction 13 (J13) - National Government Services - Connecticut, New York

Jurisdiction 14 (J14) - National Heritage Insurance Company - Maine, Massachusetts, New Hampshire

Jurisdiction 15 (J15) - Kentucky, Ohio - Awarded to Highmark Medicare Services*

Fig. 9-2 Medicare AB MAC jurisdictions.

TABLE 9-3	Services and Supplies Medicare Part B Helps Pay for and Services Not Covered by Part B
Items Medicare part B helps pay for*	Abdominal aortic aneurysm screening Ambulance services Ambulatory surgical centers Blood Bone mass measurements (bone density) (every 2 yr) Cardiovascular screenings (every 5 yr) Chiropractic services (limited) Clinical laboratory services Clinical research studies Colorectal cancer screenings Defibrillator (implantable automatic) Diabetes screenings

TABLE 9-3	Services and Supplies Medicare Part B Helps Pay for and Services Not Covered by Part B—cont'd
	Diabetes self-management training
	Diabetes supplies
	Doctor services
	Durable medical equipment
	Emergency room services
	Eye examinations for people with diabetes
	Eyeglasses (limited)
	Federally qualified health center services
	Flu shots
	Foot examinations and treatment
	Glaucoma tests
	Hearing and balance examinations
	Hepatitis B shots
	Home health services
	Kidney dialysis services and supplies
	Mammograms (screening)
	Medical nutrition therapy services
	Mental health care (outpatient)
	Occupational therapy
	Outpatient hospital services
	Outpatient medical/surgical services/supplies
	Pap tests, pelvic examinations, and clinical breast examinations
	Physical examination (one-time "Welcome to Medicare" examination)
	Physical therapy
	Pneumococcal vaccine
	Practitioner services (non-doctor)
	Prescription drugs (limited)
	Prostate cancer screenings
	Prosthetic/orthotic items
	Rural health clinical services
	Second surgical opinions
	Smoking cessation (counseling to stop smoking)
	Speech-language pathology services
	Surgical dressing services
	Telemedicine
	Tests (e.g., x-rays, MRI, CT scans, electrocardiograms)
	Transplants and immunosuppressive drugs
	Travel (emergencies when traveling outside the United States)
	Urgently needed care
Services not covered by Medicare part B[†]	Acupuncture
	Chiropractic services
	Cosmetic surgery
	Custodial care
	Deductibles, coinsurance, copayments
	Dental care and dentures
	Eye examinations (routine) and refractions
	Foot care (routine)
	Hearing aids and examinations
	Hearing tests not ordered by doctor
	Laboratory tests (screenings)
	Long-term care (custodial care in nursing homes)
	Orthopedic shoes
	Physical examinations (yearly or routine)
	Prescription drugs (refer to Medicare Part D)
	Shots to prevent illness
	Surgical procedures in ambulatory surgical centers not covered by Medicare Part B
	Syringes or insulin (some diabetic supplies)
	Travel to foreign countries

*Limitations, deductibles, and copayments may apply.
[†]With exceptions previously listed as being covered.

monthly premium of $96.40 in 2011 and $99.90 in 2012. Medicare Part B monthly premiums are subject to an increase every year.

Medicare Fact: Part B premiums are higher for those beneficiaries whose yearly income is in excess of $85,000 (single) or $170,000 (joint).

The health insurance professional should become familiar with Medicare's guidelines to determine whether a specific procedure or service is covered. If coverage is questioned, the professional should contact Medicare by phone at 1-800-MEDICARE (1-800-633-4227) or on the Internet at www.medicare.gov/.

In addition, the Websites to Explore at the end of this chapter provide several Internet links to follow for additional help and information.

The Part B MAC determines payment of Part B–covered items and services. As mentioned earlier, a MAC is a private company that contracts with CMS to provide claims processing and payment for Medicare Part B services. The local MAC also has the ability and authority to designate an item or service as noncovered for its service area or jurisdiction. For a complete list of all noncovered items or services for his or her state, the health insurance professional should contact the local MAC. (MACs and FIs are subject to periodic change.)

Enrollment

Before an individual reaches age 65, he or she must decide whether to enroll in Medicare Part A or Part B or both. If eligible beneficiaries want Medicare coverage to start the month they reach age 65, they should contact their local Social Security office 3 months before their 65th birthday. If they decide not to sign up for Medicare until after their 65th birthday, the Medicare Part B effective date is delayed.

For each 12-month period an individual delays enrollment in Medicare Part B, he or she will have to pay a 10% Part B premium penalty.

An eligible beneficiary may delay enrollment without a penalty or a waiting period, however, if the individual (or spouse) was still employed and covered by an employer's group health plan at the time of eligibility. Individuals who do not enroll within the 3-month period before becoming age 65 must wait and enroll during the general enrollment period, which is January 1 through March 31 of each year. Medicare Part B coverage becomes effective on July 1 of that year. Unless an eligible person has an employer-provided group health plan, declining Medicare may not be a good idea. If Medicare coverage is declined when the individual first becomes eligible, "late enrollment" carries two penalties. (See next section on Premiums and Cost-Sharing Requirements.)

Premiums and Cost-Sharing Requirements

Medicare Part B (medical insurance) cost-sharing requirements include a monthly premium, discussed in a previous section. This premium, which is automatically deducted from the beneficiary's monthly Social Security check, is subject to change every year. The second cost-sharing requirement in original Medicare Part B is an annual deductible of $162 (2011). After the deductible is met, Medicare pays 80% of **allowable charges**. Allowable charges are the fees Medicare permits for a particular service or supply. Table 9-4 summarizes the Medicare Part B cost-sharing amounts for various types of covered services.

A **benefit period** is the duration of time during which a Medicare beneficiary is eligible for Part A benefits for services incurred in a hospital or skilled nursing facility (SNF) or both. A benefit period begins the day an individual is

TABLE 9-4	Services Covered by Medicare Medical Insurance (Part B) for 2011		
SERVICES	**BENEFIT**	**MEDICARE PAYS**	**BENEFICIARY PAYS (OTHER INSURANCE MAY PAY ALL OR PART)**
Medical expense: physician services and medical supplies	Medical services in and out of the hospital	80% of approved (after $162 deductible)	20% of approved (after deductible) plus excess charges
Outpatient hospital treatment	Unlimited if medically necessary	Amount based on a fee schedule (after $162 deductible)	Coinsurance or copayment amount, which varies according to the service (after deductible)
Clinical laboratory	Diagnostic tests	100% of approved	Nothing if approved
Home health care: medically necessary skilled care, therapy	Part-time care	100% of approved	Nothing if approved
Durable medical equipment (DME)	Prescribed by doctor for use in home	80% of approved (after $162 deductible)	20% of approved (after deductible) plus excess charges
Blood	Blood	All but first 3 pints	First 3 pints

From http://www.insurance.wa.gov/publications/consumer/Medicare_Chart_A_B.pdf.

admitted to a hospital or SNF. The benefit period ends when the beneficiary has not received care in a hospital or SNF for 60 days in a row. If the beneficiary is readmitted to the hospital or SNF before the 60 days elapse, it is considered to be in the same benefit period. If the beneficiary is admitted to a hospital or SNF after the initial 60-day benefit period has ended, a new benefit period begins. The inpatient hospital deductible must be paid for each benefit period, but there is no limit to the number of benefit periods allowed.

As mentioned previously, Part A is free for individuals who have worked enough quarters to qualify (40 or more). Penalties may be assessed for failing to enroll at appropriate times. For Part A, the penalty applies only to those who pay for Part A coverage. If an individual does not enroll in Part A when first eligible, the monthly premium may go up 10% unless he or she is eligible for a special enrollment period. If a person is not covered by an employer-sponsored group health plan, a premium penalty is charged if he or she fails to enroll in Medicare Part B during the Initial Enrollment Period or Special Enrollment Period. The monthly premium for Part B may go up 10% for each full 12-month period that the individual was eligible for Part B but did not sign up for it. For example, a 2-year delay would be 20%; a 3-year delay would be a 30% penalty, and so on. This penalty is paid for the remainder of the individual's life.

Medicare Fact: Premiums, deductibles, and penalty amounts are subject to change every year.

Medicare Part C (Medicare Advantage Plans)

The Balanced Budget Act of 1997, which went into effect in January 1999, expanded the role of private plans under what was originally called Medicare + Choice to include managed care plans such as preferred provider organizations (PPOs), provider-sponsored organizations (PSOs), private fee-for-service (PFFS) plans, and medical savings accounts (MSAs) coupled with high-deductible insurance plans. The Medicare Prescription Drug, Improvement, and Modernization Act of 2003 renamed the program "Medicare Advantage" and created another option: regional PPOs.

Medicare Advantage is an alternative to traditional (original) Medicare that allows the government to pay insurers to manage benefits to seniors. These prepaid healthcare plans offer regular Medicare Parts A and B coverage in addition to coverage for other services. Medicare Advantage plans are run by private companies approved by Medicare. Under Medicare Part C, individuals who are eligible for Medicare Parts A and B can choose to get their Medicare benefits through a variety of plans (see previously), with the exception of individuals with ESRD, who must remain on original Medicare. The primary Medicare Part C plans include the following:

Medicare managed care plans, such as health maintenance organizations (HMOs), PSOs, PPOs, and other certified public or private coordinated care plans that meet the standards under the Medicare law.

Medicare private, unrestricted fee-for-service plans that allow beneficiaries to select certain private providers. These providers must accept the plan's payment terms and conditions.

MSA plans that allow beneficiaries to enroll in a plan with a high deductible. After the deductible is met, the MSA plan pays providers. Money remaining in the MSA can be used to pay for future medical care, including some services not usually covered by Medicare Part A and Part B, such as dentures.

Medicare Part C coverage not only includes Part A and Part B coverage but also pays for services not covered under the original Medicare plan, such as preventive care, prescription drugs, eyeglasses, dental care, and hearing aids.

For a Medicare beneficiary to qualify for one of these Medicare Advantage options, he or she must be eligible for Medicare Parts A and B and must live in the service area of the plan. As mentioned, an individual is generally not eligible to elect a Medicare Advantage plan if he or she has been diagnosed with ESRD. There are exceptions to this eligibility rule, however, such as individuals who are already members of a Medicare Advantage plan when they are diagnosed with ESRD and individuals who received a kidney transplant and no longer require a regular course of dialysis treatments.

Medicare Fact: If a beneficiary enrolls in a Medicare Part C plan, he or she does not need a supplemental plan (Medigap).

Healthcare Reform's Impact on Medicare Advantage Plans

The changes introduced in the healthcare reform bill will be phased in gradually after they began in 2011. Medicare Advantage plans were designed to save money for the government by operating like HMOs. Because Congress (in 2003) believed that subsidies would encourage providers to expand the plans into rural and less profitable markets, Medicare Advantage plans receive more federal dollars than what is paid to providers through traditional Medicare. The provisions in the healthcare reform bill are designed to bring payments to these plans more in alignment with payments to traditional Medicare. These changes will be phased in over 3 years, ideally making the transition easier for Medicare Advantage customers and insurance providers.

How will this change affect seniors? Premiums may rise, some plans may reduce the extra benefits they provide as they adjust to lower payments from the government, and some insurance companies may stop offering Medicare Advantage altogether. It is important to remember, however, that no one currently enrolled in a Medicare Advantage plan will lose his or her coverage. Under Medicare guidelines, a beneficiary can always switch to another plan if he or she prefers to stay in an Advantage plan or to have the option of enrolling in traditional Medicare.

Other Medicare Health Plans

Plans that are not Medicare Advantage Plans but are still part of Medicare are

• Medicare Cost Plans

- Demonstration/pilot programs
- Programs of All-Inclusive Care for the Elderly (PACE)

Some plans provide both Parts A and B coverage and some also provide prescription drug coverage (Part D). Details of the Medicare Cost Plans and Demonstration/Pilot Programs are explained on page 83 respectively of the *Medicare and You* handbook for 2012.

The PACE program is discussed later in this chapter.

Medicare Part D (Medicare Prescription Drug Benefit Plan)

Medicare Part D offers prescription drug coverage to all seniors eligible for Medicare. These plans are run by insurance companies or other private organizations approved by Medicare. The cost of drugs within each plan can vary.

There are two ways to get prescription drug coverage:

1. Medicare Prescription Drug Plans (sometimes called PDPs) that add drug coverage to original Medicare, some Medicare Cost Plans, some Medicare PFFS plans, and MSA plans.
2. Medicare Advantage Plans (e.g., HMOs or PPOs) or other Medicare plans that offer prescription drug coverage as a plan benefit.

When beneficiaries enroll in Medicare Part D, they pay an additional premium, which can be deducted from their monthly Social Security check or paid separately. Premiums vary depending on the plan, with a national average of $32.34 in 2011. Individual plans, such as group health insurance plans, that include prescription coverage must, however, offer no less than the standard Medicare benefit, referred to as **credible coverage**. Medicare's standard benefits under Part D are shown in Table 9-5. These figures are subject to change every year. It should be noted here that many plans offer more comprehensive coverage than Medicare's basic coverage.

Owing to the new healthcare reform law, the Standard Part D benefit now provides some coverage in the "**donut hole**"—between the point at which Medicare Part D stops paying for prescriptions and the point at which catastrophic coverage for drugs becomes effective. Although Part D does not provide a benefit for brand name drugs in the donut hole

until 2013, the manufacturers of the brand-named drugs will provide a 50% discount to most Part D enrollees. By 2020, the Part D donut hole will be completely phased out through the combination of the additional Part D benefit and brand discount.

Individuals qualifying for both Medicare and Medicaid benefits (**dual eligibles**, sometimes referred to as Medi-Medi) who receive the full Medicaid benefits package no longer have prescription drug coverage under Medicaid but can enroll in Medicare Part D. Medicare pays the Part D deductible for all dual eligibles and for their monthly premiums, if they enroll in an average or low-cost Part D plan. These subsidies eliminate the gap in coverage (donut hole) for dual eligibles that Medicare beneficiaries who do not qualify for Medicare and Medicaid face. Dual eligibles are responsible, however, for small copays ranging from $2.50 to $6.30. Dual eligibles residing in nursing homes or other institutions are exempt from copays because they already are contributing all but a small portion of their income to the cost of their nursing home care.

Changing Medicare Health or Prescription Drug Coverage

Beneficiaries can change their Medicare health or prescription drug coverage during the annual open enrollment period. Beginning in the fall of 2011, the annual enrollment period dates changed, giving enrollees more time to join or switch their Medicare health or prescription drug plan. Rather than November 15 to December 31, the new enrollment period is between October 15 and December 7. Therefore, if a change was made during this period in 2011, new coverage will began on January 1, 2012.

Programs of All-Inclusive Care for the Elderly (PACE)

Programs of All-Inclusive Care for the Elderly (PACE) is a combination Medicare/Medicaid program that provides community-based long-term care services to eligible recipients. If an individual qualifies for Medicare, all Medicare-covered services are paid for by Medicare. If he or she also qualifies for Medicaid, he or she must pay either a small monthly payment or pay nothing for the long-term care portion of the PACE benefit. Those who are not Medicaid-eligible must pay a monthly premium to cover the long-term care portion of the PACE benefit and a premium for Medicare Part D drugs. However, there is no deductible or copayment for any drug, service, or care approved by the PACE team.

PACE is available only in areas where a PACE organization is under contract to deliver services. To be eligible for the program, an individual must meet the following criteria:

- Is 55 years or older
- Meets the medical need criteria
- Lives in an area serviced by a PACE organization
- Can be safely served in the community according to the PACE organization

TABLE 9-5	Medicare Part D Standard Benefit Table	
	2010	**2011**
Deductible	$310.00	$310.00
Initial coverage limit	$2830.00	$2840.00
Out-of-pocket threshold	$4550.00	$4550.00
Minimum copays (catastrophic portion of benefit):		
Generic preferred drug	2.50	2.50
All other	6.30	6.30

To view the fact sheet "Quick Facts about Programs of All-Inclusive Care for the Elderly (PACE)," visit the Evolve site.

> ### What Did You Learn?
>
> 1. What are Medicare's two primary parts?
> 2. Name four common services Medicare B does not cover.
> 3. What are the cost-sharing requirements for traditional Medicare Part B?
> 4. What type of service does Medicare Advantage cover that fee-for-service Medicare does not?
> 5. List the eligibility requirements for PACE.

MEDICARE COMBINATION COVERAGES

Because Medicare does not cover some services and there are deductibles and copayments that patients must pay out of pocket for most services, beneficiaries often have added health insurance coverage to help with the gaps in Medicare's coverage. This extra coverage can be one of the following:

- Medicare/Medicaid dual eligibility
- Medicare supplement policies
- Medicare Secondary Payer (MSP)

The following sections explain each of these supplemental types of healthcare coverage.

Medicare/Medicaid Dual Eligibility

Dual eligibility, as stated earlier, refers to the status of individuals who qualify for benefits under both the Medicare and Medicaid programs. Most dual eligibles are low-income elderly or individuals younger than 65 years with disabilities. Medicare does not pay for all health services, just basic physician and hospital care. In addition, Medicare beneficiaries have to meet a yearly deductible and pay a monthly premium and a 20% copayment (cost sharing) for all covered services. Dual eligibles rely on Medicaid to pay Medicare premiums and cost-sharing (deductibles and copays) expenses and to pay for the needed benefits Medicare does not cover such as long-term care.

Medicare Supplement Policies

The traditional Medicare program provides valuable coverage of healthcare needs, but it leaves uninsured areas with which elderly and disabled Americans need additional help. To ensure that they are adequately protected, many seniors purchase a **Medicare supplement policy** (also referred to as a Medigap policy). A Medicare supplement policy is a health insurance plan sold by a private insurance company to help pay for healthcare expenses not covered by Medicare and Medicare's deductibles and coinsurance. An individual may qualify for supplemental insurance through an employer-sponsored retirement plan or, more commonly, through a Medigap plan.

Medigap Insurance

Medigap insurance is designed specifically to supplement Medicare benefits and is regulated by federal and state law. A Medigap policy must be clearly identified as Medicare supplemental insurance, and it must provide specific benefits that help fill the gaps in Medicare coverage. Other kinds of insurance may help with out-of-pocket healthcare costs, but they do not qualify as Medigap plans.

In June of 2010, the types of Medigap plans available changed. There are two new Medigap Plans, Plans M and N. Plans E, H, I, and J are no longer available to buy. Beneficiaries who purchased one of these discontinued plans before June 1, 2010, can keep that plan, however. Each plan has a different set of benefits. Plan A is the basic plan, and it has the least amount of benefits. Plan F, the most comprehensive, provides 100% of the gaps in Medicare; there are no deductibles, no copays, and no coinsurance with any healthcare provider who accepts Medicare.

Table 9-6 shows the 10 Medigap plans currently available and what each covers.

When an individual buys a Medicare supplement policy, he or she pays a premium to the private insurance company. This premium is above and beyond the Medicare Part B premium. If the individual has a Medicare Advantage plan, it is not necessary to have a Medicare supplement policy, because these plans typically include much of the same coverages as Medigap.

Standard Medigap Policies

The 10 standard Medigap policies were developed by the National Association of Insurance Commissioners and incorporated into state and federal law. The plans cover specific expenses not covered or not fully covered by Medicare. Insurance companies are not permitted to change the combination of benefits or the letter designations of any of the plans.

All states must allow the sale of plan A, and all Medigap insurers must make plan A available if they are going to sell any Medigap plans in their state. Although not required to offer any of the other plans, most insurers do offer several of these alternate plans to pick from; some offer all 10. Insurers can decide which of the optional plans they will sell as long as the state in which the plans are sold approves. Although insurers must offer the same coverage in each plan, they do not have to charge the same premium rates; it is strongly suggested that individuals shop around and compare prices before purchasing a Medigap policy.

Where the Gaps Are

Box 9-1 describes the **Medicare gaps** in various types of care.

Eligibility

If an individual enrolls in Medicare Part B when he or she turns 65, federal law forbids insurance companies from denying eligibility for Medigap policies for 6 months. This

TABLE 9-6   Ten Standard Medicare Supplemental Plans

BENEFITS	A	B	C	D	F*	G	K	L	M	N
Basic Benefits										
Part A: Hospital coinsurance costs up to an additional 365 days after Medicare benefits end	X	X	X	X	X	X	X	X	X	X
Part A: Hospice care coinsurance or copay	X	X	X	X	X	X	50%	75%	X	X
Part B: Coinsurance or copay	X	X	X	X	X	X	50%	75%	X	X‡
Medicare preventive care Part B coinsurance	X	X	X	X	X	X	X	X	X	X
Parts A & B: Blood (first 3 pints)	X	X	X	X	X	X	50%	75%	X	X
Additional Benefits										
Skilled nursing facility coinsurance			X	X	X	X	50%	75%	X	X
Part A deductible		X	X	X	X	X	50%	75%	50%	X
Part B deductible			X		X					
Part B excess charges					X	X				
Foreign travel emergency (up to plan limits)			X	X	X	X			X	X
Out-of-pocket yearly limit†							$4,640	$2,320		

*Plan F also offers a high-deductible plan. This means beneficiary pays for Medicare covered costs up to the deductible amount ($2,000 in 2011) before the Medicare Supplement plan pays anything.

†After beneficiary meets the out-of-pocket yearly limit and the yearly Part B deductible ($162 in 2011), the Medicare Supplement plan pays 100% of covered services for the rest of the calendar year. Out-of-pocket limit is the maximum amount beneficiary would pay for coinsurance and copays.

‡Plan N pays 100% of the Part B coinsurance except up to $20 copays for office visits and up to $50 copays for emergency room visits (if the hospital admits the patient, the plan waives the emergency room copays).

Note: Out-of-pocket annual limit for Plans K and L increases each year with inflation.

Box 9-1

Medicare Gaps by Care Type

During a hospital stay, Medicare Part A does not pay the
- yearly deductible;
- coinsurance amount for each day of hospitalization more than 60 days and up to 90 days for any one benefit period;
- coinsurance amount for each day of hospitalization more than 90 days and up to 150 days, for any one benefit period past a 150-day hospitalization;
- anything past a 150-day hospitalization;
- the cost of 3 pints of blood, unless replaced; or
- medical expenses during foreign travel.

During a stay in a skilled nursing facility, Medicare Part A does not pay the
- coinsurance amount for each day in the facility more than 20 days and up to 100 days for any one benefit period or
- anything for a stay of more than 100 days.

For home healthcare, Medicare Part A does not pay

- 20% of the approved cost of DME or approved nonskilled care or
- anything for nonmedical personal care services.

For physicians, clinics, laboratories, therapies, medical supplies, and equipment, Medicare Part B does not pay
- yearly deductible;
- 20% of the Medicare-approved amount;
- 15% above the Medicare-approved amount if provider does not accept assignment;
- preventive or routine examinations and testing, except for the "Welcome to Medicare" examination if received within the first 6 months of eligibility;
- treatment that is not considered medically necessary;
- prescription medication that can be self-administered;
- general dental work;
- routine eye or hearing examinations; or
- glasses or hearing aids.

6-month period is called the **open enrollment period**. If the individual did not enroll in Medicare Part B when turning 65, he or she can sign up for it later, during the yearly general enrollment period—January to March. The individual has a 6-month open enrollment period for Medigap policies beginning July 1 of that year. Individuals who were covered by a group health insurance plan when they turned 65 have a 6-month open enrollment period for Medigap policies beginning the date their Part B coverage begins, regardless of when they sign up for it. An insurance company must sell eligible applicants the policy of their choice without any medical screening, regardless of their medical history. The company is not permitted to place any extra limits on the coverage offered, and they must offer the policy for the same monthly premium as everyone else buying the same policy when first eligible for Medicare.

Medicare Secondary Payer

Medicare Secondary Payer is the term used when Medicare is not responsible for paying first because the beneficiary is covered under another insurance policy. The MSP program, enacted in 1980, was created to preserve Medicare funds and to ensure that funds would be available for future generations. Since the program's beginning, a series of federal laws has changed the coordination of benefits provision between Medicare and other insurance carriers. These federal laws take precedence over individual state law and private insurance contracts. For certain categories of individuals, Medicare is the secondary payer regardless of state law or plan provisions. Medicare most likely would be the secondary payer in any of the following situations:

- Workers' compensation (injury or illness that occurred at work)
- Working aged (age 65 years and older) who are covered by a group health plan through their own or their spouse's current employment
- Disabled individuals age 64 and younger who are covered by a large group health plan (more than 100 employees) through their own or a family member's current employment
- Medicare beneficiaries with permanent kidney failure covered under a group health plan
- Individuals with black lung disease covered under the Federal Black Lung Program
- Veterans Administration benefits
- Federal Research Grant Program

It is often the responsibility of the health insurance professional to determine, in cases in which the Medicare beneficiary has other insurance coverage, to which third-party payer the electronic or CMS-1500 paper claim is submitted first. Many medical practices use a structured form such as a MSP questionnaire to simplify this process. (An example MSP questionnaire is shown in Fig. 9-3).

? What Did You Learn?

1. List three kinds of Medicare combination coverage.
2. What categories of people make up the "dual eligible" classification?
3. How does Medicaid assist Medicare beneficiaries?
4. How many standard Medigap policies are currently available?
5. What do most Medigap plans cover?
6. Name four payers that typically would be primary to Medicare.

MEDICARE AND MANAGED CARE

We have learned that Medicare-eligible individuals have a choice whether to receive Medicare benefits through traditional (original) Medicare or through a managed care plan. A **Medicare managed care plan** is an HMO, a PPO, a PFFS, or a **Special Needs Plan (SNP)** (see later) that uses Medicare to pay for part of its services for eligible beneficiaries. Medicare managed care plans fill the gaps in basic Medicare much as Medigap policies do; however, Medicare managed care plans and Medigap policies function differently. Medigap policies work along with Medicare to pay for medical expenses. Medical claims are sent to Medicare and then to a Medigap insurer, and each pays a portion of the approved charges. Medicare managed care plans provide all basic Medicare benefits, plus some additional coverages (depending on the plan), to fill the gaps Medicare does not pay. The extent of coverage beyond Medicare, the size of premiums and copayments, and decisions about paying for treatment all are controlled by the managed care plan itself, not by Medicare.

When a patient enrolls in a Medicare managed plan, he or she agrees to receive care only from an approved list of physicians, hospitals, and other providers, called a network, in exchange for reduced overall healthcare costs. There are several types of Medicare managed care plans. Some have tight restrictions concerning members' visiting specialists or seeing providers outside the network. Others give members more freedom to choose when they see providers and which providers they may consult for treatment.

Medicare HMOs

Similar to the structure of the HMOs we learned about in Chapter 7, **Medicare HMOs** maintain a network of physicians and other healthcare providers. The HMO member/enrollee must receive care only from the providers in the network except in emergencies. If a member sees a provider outside the network, the HMO usually pays nothing toward the bill. Because an HMO plan member has technically withdrawn from traditional Medicare by opting to join the managed care organization, Medicare also pays nothing. The result in this case is that the plan member must pay the entire bill out of pocket.

Medicare Secondary Payer Questionnaire

Patient Name: _____ Date: _____

HICN: _____

Medicare law requires that we determine if your medical services might be covered by another insurer. In order to assist us in the correct billing of these services, please answer the following questions:

1. Is your injury/illness due to:

A. Work-related accident/condition?
☐ No
☐ Yes, name and address of workers' compensation plan:_____
_____
_____
Policy or ID#: _____
Accident date: _____

B. A condition covered under the Federal Black Lung Program?
☐ No
☐ Yes

C. An automobile accident?
☐ No
☐ Yes, name and address of auto insurance: _____
_____
_____
Name of insured: _____
Policy or ID#: _____
Accident date: _____ Accident location: _____

D. An accident other than an automobile accident?
☐ No
☐ Yes, name and address of no-fault insurer:_____
_____
_____
Name of insured: _____
Policy or ID#: _____
Accident date: _____ Accident location: _____

E. The fault of another party?
☐ No
☐ Yes, name and address of no-fault insurer:_____
_____
_____
Name of insured: _____
Policy or ID#: _____
Accident date: _____ Accident location: _____

DMERC Region D Supplier Manual *(Rev. 1/2001) Exhibit 1*

Fig. 9-3 MSP questionnaire. (From U.S. Department of Health and Human Services, Centers for Medicare and Medicaid Services.)

Continued

Medicare Secondary Payer Questionnaire (cont'd)

2. Are you eligible for coverage under the Veterans' Administration?
    ☐ No
    ☐ Yes

3. Are you employed?
    ☐ No. Date of retirement: _____
    ☐ Yes, employer name and address: _____
    _____

    Do you have employer group health plan coverage?
    ☐ No
    ☐ Yes, insurer name and address: _____
    _____

        Policy #: _____
        Group #: _____

4. Is your spouse employed?
    ☐ No. Date of retirement, if applicable: _____
    ☐ Yes, spouse's name: _____
    Employer name and address: _____

    Are you covered under your spouse's employer group health plan?
    ☐ No
    ☐ Yes, insurer name and address: _____
    _____

        Policy #: _____
        Group #: _____

5. Are you a dependent covered under a parent's/guardian's employer group health plan?
    ☐ No
    ☐ Yes, employer name and address: _____
    _____

        Insurer name and address: _____
        _____

        Name of insured: _____
        Policy #: _____
        Group #: _____

Thank you for your cooperation in ensuring that your medical services will be billed to the proper insurer(s).

Exhibit 1 (Rev. 1/2001)   *DMERC Region D Supplier Manual*

Fig. 9-3—cont'd

HMO with Point-of-Service Option

One type of HMO has a significant modification that makes it more popular, albeit more costly, than the standard HMO plan. This plan offers what is referred to as an **HMO with point-of-service (POS) option**. A member is allowed to see providers who are not in the HMO network and to receive services from specialists without first going through a primary care physician. This method is called **self-referring**. When a member does go outside the network or sees a specialist directly, however, the plan pays a smaller portion of the bill than if the member had followed regular HMO procedures. The member pays a higher premium for this plan than for a standard HMO plan and a higher copayment each time the self-referral option is used.

Preferred Provider Organization

A PPO works much the same as an HMO with POS option. If a member receives a service from a PPO's network of providers, the cost to the member is lower than if the member sees a provider outside the network; however, a member does not have to go through a primary care physician for referrals to specialists. PPO patients usually are allowed to self-refer to specialists. PPOs tend to be more expensive than standard HMOs, charging a monthly premium and a higher copayment for non-network services.

Provider-Sponsored Organization

A PSO is a group of medical providers—physicians, clinics, and hospitals—that skips the insurance company middleman and contracts directly with patients. As with an HMO, members pay a premium and a copayment each time a service is rendered. Some PSOs in urban areas are large groups of physicians and hospitals that offer a wide choice of providers. Some PSOs are small networks of providers that contract through a particular employer or other large organization or that serve a rural area where no HMO is available.

Private Fee-for-Service Plan

Under a PFFS plan, the Medicare beneficiary can go to any Medicare-approved physician or hospital that accepts the plan's payment terms and agrees to treat him or her. When joining a PFFS plan that has a network, patients can also see any of the network providers who have agreed to treat plan members.

Special Needs Plans

A Special Needs Plan (or SNP, often pronounced "snip") is a type of Medicare Advantage plan designed to attract and enroll Medicare beneficiaries who fall into a certain special needs classification. There are two types of SNPs: The exclusive SNP enrolls only those beneficiaries who fall into the special needs demographic. The other type is the **disproportionate share** SNP. (A disproportionate share is a payment adjustment to compensate hospitals for the higher operating costs they incur in treating a large share of low-income patients.)

Advantages and Disadvantages of Medicare HMOs

Medicare Advantage plans provide the same benefits as traditional Medicare; however, they can charge lower costs because of how HMO plans are structured. HMO plans typically provide a managed treatment approach to care that is designed to minimize unnecessary costs and services. This design allows HMO Advantage plan enrollees to pay lower premium rates than those charged by traditional Medicare plans. And although insurance rates and coverages vary from state to state, required copay and deductible amounts under HMO Advantage plans normally run less than those for traditional plans. (It should be noted here that even though Advantage plan enrollees typically pay lower premiums, they still have to pay the Medicare Part B monthly premium.)

As with most areas of healthcare insurance, there are advantages and disadvantages to enrolling in a Medicare HMO.

Advantages

- HMOs may cover services that traditional Medicare does not cover, such as eyeglasses, hearing aids, prescriptions, and dental coverage.
- Enrollees do not need Medigap insurance.
- Paperwork is limited or nonexistent, in contrast to traditional Medicare coverage.
- HMOs often pay additional coverage for hospital stays that exceed the limits set by traditional Medicare.

Disadvantages

- Choice of healthcare providers and medical facilities is limited.
- Members/enrollees are covered only for healthcare services received through the HMO except in emergency and urgent care situations.
- Prior approval is usually necessary from a primary care physician for a specialist's services, surgical procedures, medical equipment, and other healthcare services, which is not required under traditional Medicare.
- Enrollees who travel out of the HMO's service area do not receive coverage except in emergency and urgent care situations.

If an enrollee decides to switch from the HMO to the traditional Medicare plan, coverage does not begin until the first day of the month after the disenrollment request. When a Medicare beneficiary has traditional Medicare as well as a Medicare supplement plan (Medigap), this picture changes. Table 9-7 illustrates how traditional Medicare with a Medigap policy (Plan F) compares with Medicare Advantage.

Medicare Fact: In 2010, nearly 12 million people were enrolled in Medicare Advantage, compared with approximately 48 million enrolled in traditional Medicare.

TABLE 9-7	Traditional Medicare with Medigap Policy vs. Medicare Advantage	
ORIGINAL "FEE-FOR-SERVICE" MEDICARE WITH A MEDIGAP (EXAMPLE: PLAN F)	**COMPARISON POINT**	**MEDICARE ADVANTAGE: HMO, PPO, OR PFFS (PRIVATE MEDICARE PLANS)**
Beneficiary must have Parts A and B. Usually companies may deny, but must accept all applicants, all ages, during Medigap Open Enrollment and Guaranteed Issue periods.	Eligibility	Member must have Parts A and B and live in service area. Takes all applicants except those with end-stage renal disease (some exceptions).
Premium varies with gender and health and goes up with age. Companies may underwrite (add to premium). Generally, no copay costs at time of service. No out-of-pocket maximum.	Costs: Premium/copay/coinsurance/out-of-pocket maximum	All plan members pay same premium regardless of age, gender, or health. Cost sharing (copays) must be paid for most medical services. Many plans have an out-of-pocket annual maximum.
No network: Patient may go to any provider that accepts Medicare. No referrals required for specialist visits. It may be hard to find providers accepting Original Medicare in some areas. Plan may be used for treatments at major medical facilities, such as Mayo Clinics.	Provider choice and availability (Always ask providers what insurance they accept!)	HMOs and PPOs maintain provider network; they must have available providers in order to accept new members. PFFS plan has no provider network; it may be hard to find providers who accept it in some areas. HMO: Generally covers in-network only. Referrals may be required for specialist visits. PPO: Covers out of network, but then costs may be higher. No referrals required.
Not included. If beneficiary wants Rx coverage, may enroll in any stand-alone (PDP) available.	Prescription drug coverage (Make sure the choice covers Rx!)	If member wants Rx coverage, must enroll in the included Rx coverage if choosing an HMO or PPO. (VA-eligible excepted.) With PFFS, member may choose either the plan's Rx coverage, if offered, or a stand-alone PDP.
Yes, guaranteed renewable as long as premium is paid and the application was correct. Benefits never change. No election season for Medigaps.	Renewable?	No, benefits may change yearly. However, member usually remains in a plan unless disenrolls at election times.
Covers only same as original Medicare. No routine dental care, vision care, or physical examinations; no alternative medicine.	Extras?	Some plans include routine dental care, vision care, or physical examinations. Some offer additional alternative medicine package.
Good for travelers or "snow birds." May save money for people needing high-cost or frequent care. Beneficiary should customize elements of the Medicare picture – choose doctors and drug plan.	Whom it may be best for	Network plans may be good for people who otherwise cannot find a Medicare provider. May save money unless frequent appointments or treatments are needed. Having a packaged plan may simplify choices.
Because Medigaps are standardized, price and customer service are the only differences. Comparison shopping a few competitively priced plans is recommended.	At www.medicare.gov go to the Medicare Options Compare link. Enter ZIP code for a list of Medicare supplements and Medicare Advantage plans authorized to operate in your area.	Plans are not standardized—use comparison pages at www.medicare.gov. Plans are regulated by Medicare/CMS.

CMS, Center for Medicare and Medicaid Services; HMO, health maintenance organization; PDP, prescription drug plan; PFFS, private fee-for-service; PPO, preferred provider organization; Rx, drug.
Modified from http://www.oregon.gov/DCBS/SHIBA/docs/comparison_chart.pdf?ga=t.

Why This Information Is Important to the Health Insurance Professional

As a health insurance professional, you will be doing more than sitting at a desk entering data into a computer. In your job, you no doubt will become a liaison between many third-party payers and the entire healthcare team. Additionally, you must be able to answer patients' questions about Medicare accurately. The Medicare program and all its various parts and choices can be confusing to people, especially the elderly. Although it is important that the health insurance professional learn all the intricacies of the Medicare program from the provider standpoint, he or she also must become an expert from the beneficiaries' perspective. The fact alone that the fee-for-service (called *original* or *traditional* Medicare) plan covers 80% of *allowed charges* is enough to create confusion. When you present an elderly patient with an advanced beneficiary notice (ABN) or begin discussing Medicare's lifetime release of information form, you must be prepared to answer questions in layman's language.

⭐ Imagine This!

Arlene Sorensen had been told by her gynecologist when she was younger that it was important to receive a Pap smear every year. After she became eligible for Medicare, she told her family practice provider that she wanted to continue this practice. The first Pap smear was covered by Medicare; however, a subsequent Pap smear a year later was not. When she questioned her physician, he referred her to the health insurance professional, who informed Mrs. Sorensen that Medicare considers Pap smears "medically necessary" only every 2 years, unless the patient is considered high risk.

❓ What Did You Learn?

1. Name four kinds of Medicare managed care plans.
2. When patients enroll in a Medicare managed care plan, they typically agree to choose healthcare providers from an approved list called a _____.
3. A type of Medicare Advantage plan designed to attract and enroll Medicare beneficiaries who fall into a certain special needs classification is called a _____.
4. Which type of Medicare plan has a higher enrollment, traditional Medicare or Medicare Advantage?
5. Explain why it is important for the health insurance professional to be knowledgeable about the specifics of both original Medicare and Medicare Advantage?

PREPARING FOR THE MEDICARE PATIENT

When a Medicare beneficiary comes to the office for an appointment, the procedure for handling the encounter is basically the same as with non-Medicare patients, with a few exceptions.

Medicare's Lifetime Release of Information Form

The medical facility should maintain a current release of information for every patient. Among other things, this approach allows the health insurance professional to complete and submit the insurance form legally. Typically, a release of information is valid for only 1 year; however, with Medicare, a **lifetime (one-time) release of information form** may be signed by the beneficiary, eliminating the necessity of annual updates. Fig. 9-4 is an example of a lifetime release of information.

Determining Medical Necessity

Before Medicare pays for a service or procedure, it must be determined whether it is medically necessary. To meet Medicare's definition of medical necessity, the service or procedure must be:

- Consistent with the symptoms or diagnosis of the illness or injury being treated
- Necessary and consistent with generally accepted professional medical standards
- Not furnished primarily for the convenience of the patient or physician
- Furnished at the most appropriate level that can be provided safely to the patient

CMS has the power to determine whether the method of treating a patient in a particular case is reasonable and necessary on a case-by-case basis. Even if a service is reasonable and necessary, coverage may be limited if the service is provided more frequently than allowed under a national coverage policy, a local medical policy, or a clinically accepted standard of practice.

Claims for services that are not medically necessary are denied, but not getting paid is not the only risk. If Medicare or other payers determine that services were medically unnecessary *after* payment has already been made, the payment is treated as an *overpayment*, and the beneficiary will have to refund the money, with interest. If a pattern of such claims is evident, and the provider knows or should have known that the services were not medically necessary, the provider may face large monetary penalties, exclusion from the Medicare program, and possibly criminal prosecution.

One of the most common reasons for denial of Medicare claims is that the provider did not know the services provided were not medically necessary. Lack of knowledge is not a defense, however, because a general notice to the medical community from CMS or a MAC (including a Medicare report or special bulletin) that a certain service is not covered

LIFETIME AUTHORIZATION AND REQUEST FOR MEDICAL INFORMATION

I hereby release Charles H. Shaw, M.D., P.A. DBA Gainesville Orthopaedic Group to release my records to the physician individual I direct verbally or in writing.

RELEASE OF MEDICAL INFORMATION
I, the below named patient, hereby authorize Charles H. Shaw, M.D./D. Troy Trimble, D.O., Gainesville Orthopaedic Group to release to my referring physician and/or family physician and any third party payer (such as an insurance company or government agency, e.g., Blue Cross or Medicare) any medical information and records concerning my treatment when requested or by such third party payer or other entity for use in connection with making or determining claim payment for such treatment and/or diagnosis.

ASSIGNMENT OF BENEFITS AND GUARANTEE OF PAYMENT
I, the below named patient/subscriber, hereby absolutely assign payments directly to Charles H. Shaw, M.D./D. Troy Trimble, D.O., Gainesville Orthopaedic Group and any group and/or individual surgical and/or major medical benefits herein specified and otherwise payable to me for their services as described.

Medicare/Medicaid: I certify that the information given me in applying for payment under title XVIIIVXIX of the Social Security Administration or its intermediaries or carriers any information needed for this or a related Medicare claim. I request that payment of authorized benefits be made on my behalf. I assign the benefits payable for physician's services to Charles H. Shaw, M.D./D. Troy Trimble, D.O., Gainesville Orthopaedic Group.

I/We hereby guarantee payment of all charges incurred for the below named patient from the date of the first treatment until discharged from care by Charles H. Shaw, M.D./D. Troy Trimble, D.O., Gainesville Orthopaedic Group. I/We agree that should the amount of insurance benefit to be insufficient to cover the expenses, I/We will be responsible for the entire amount due for services rendered. I/We understand that statements are due when received unless other arrangements have been made with Charles H. Shaw, M.D./D. Troy Trimble, D.O. DBA Gainesville Orthopaedic Group. I/We understand that if there is no response or payment from the insurance company within 60 days of billing, I/we will be responsible for the balance due on account.

_____   _____
Subscriber (insured person) Signature   Date

                                                   ☐ Checking this box indicates a digital signature.
_____
Subscriber Printed Name

_____   _____
Patient Signature (if different from the subscriber) Date

_____
Patient Printed Name

Fig. 9-4 CMS lifetime (one-time) release authorization for Medicare beneficiaries.

is considered sufficient notice. This is why it is important for the health insurance professional to attend periodic educational seminars, read all Medicare/Medicaid-related publications, and make every effort to keep up with these changes. Additionally, if a provider fails to read Medicare's publications, but delegates that responsibility to others, the physician or the professional corporation may still be held liable for what the physician should have known.

🕐 Stop and Think

Gladys Larson calls the office to schedule an appointment to "have Dr. Clifford remove all these ugly spots on my chest." Looking through her health record, you notice the physician's reference to "benign keratosis." How do you determine whether an ABN is necessary?

Health insurance professionals can protect the physicians they work for by obtaining up-to-date information on services covered by Medicare from several sources. CMS publishes a periodical called *The CMS Quarterly Provider Update*, which includes all changes to Medicare instructions that affect physicians, provides a single source for national Medicare provider information, and gives physicians advance notice on upcoming instructions and regulations. (See Websites to Explore at the end of this chapter.) Additionally, to keep informed, providers can subscribe to the CMS weekly email updates at cmlists@subscriptions.cms.hhs.gov/.

Advanced Beneficiary Notice

If, after checking the coverage rules, the health insurance professional believes that it is likely that Medicare *would not* pay for a test or procedure the provider orders, the patient should be asked to sign an **advanced beneficiary notice (ABN)**. An ABN should also be offered to a Medicare patient before he or she is provided a service that Medicare ordinarily covers but is likely to be denied on this particular occasion (e.g., when the health insurance professional has good reason to expect the procedure will be denied on the basis of other Medicare denials and/or local coverage determination [LCD; see later] policies, or because the patient's diagnosis or procedure does not meet the Medicare program standards for medical necessity).

The ABN is intended to inform the patient in advance that it is likely that coverage for the procedure will be denied and allows the patient to make an informed decision whether to receive the service for which he or she may be personally responsible to pay. If the service is denied and a signed ABN is not on file, the physician may not hold the patient responsible for payment. Fig. 9-5 is an example of a typical ABN.

When patients are asked to sign an ABN, they have two options:

- They may choose to receive the test or procedure, agree to be responsible for payment, and sign the ABN.
- They may choose not to receive the test or procedure, refuse to be responsible for payment, and sign the ABN.

When a patient is given an ABN, the health insurance professional should be able to answer questions about financial responsibility and payment options so that the patient can make an informed decision about his or her healthcare.

> ### ⭐ Imagine This!
>
> Shelly Jennings, a health insurance professional employed by Medical Specialties, Inc., asked all Medicare patients receiving a "screening" colonoscopy to sign an ABN because when she first started working at the facility, Medicare did not cover this procedure unless there were symptoms indicating a problem. After several patients complained, Medicare made an inquiry. Shelly's excuse was that she did not have time to read all the publications Medicare sent or attend periodic educational seminars and did not realize that Medicare now paid for a colonoscopy screening every 10 years, unless the patient is considered high risk.

Local Coverage Determination (LCD)

A **local coverage determination (LCD)** consists only of information pertaining to when a procedure is considered medically reasonable and necessary. Most of Medicare's policies are established at the local level, giving MACs a great deal of authority over payment policy in a given state. Through development of local Medicare policy, MACs and FIs can determine whether a procedure is considered appropriate in an attempt to clarify specific coverage guidelines, particularly when a carrier has identified overutilization of

a procedure. These policies were formerly called Local Medical Review Policies (LMRPs).

Health Insurance Claim Number and Identification Card

The Medicare beneficiary's **health insurance claim number (HICN)** is in the format of nine numerical characters, usually the beneficiary's Social Security number, followed by one alpha character. It also might be a 6-digit or 9-digit number with one or two letter prefixes or suffixes. This type of coding allows the health insurance professional to look at the patient's identification (ID) card and immediately determine what the coverage is. These codes may appear on correspondence that Social Security sends out about a Medicare card, but they will never appear on a Social Security card. Once a person is eligible for Medicare, this number (along with the alpha or alphanumeric code) will be used on all Medicare claims. For example, if a wage earner applies for benefits, and his or her SS number is 123-45-6789, the claim number is then 123-45-6789A. If the status of a beneficiary changes, his or her SS number will not change, but it is possible for the prefix or suffix of his or her claim number to change. Fig. 9-6 shows an example of a Medicare ID card, and Table 9-8 lists some of the more common alpha codes for HICNs and what they stand for.

When patients present Medicare cards, the information on the front shows whether they are enrolled in Hospital (Part A), Medical (Part B) or both along with the dates of eligibility. Patients belonging to a Medicare Advantage do not have the traditional ID card, but instead use the ID card of the plan in which they are enrolled.

Patients who have both traditional Medicare and a Medigap policy will have two cards; therefore, when they visit the medical office, they should provide both cards. The official Medicare red, white, and blue card has a cardboard-type composition and only has information on the front. The health insurance professional does not need to make a copy of the back; however, the Medigap card is usually plastic (like a credit card), and it often has pertinent important information on the back (depending on the issuing insurer). If this is the case, a photocopy of both the back and the front of the Medigap card should be made, along with any other photo identification the patient provides.

Replacing the Medicare Card

If a Medicare enrollee loses his or her Medicare card or if it gets worn to such a degree so that the information is no longer legible, a replacement can be requested from the local Social Security office. A replacement card can also be requested online on the Social Security website. Once the request has been made, it takes about 30 days for the replacement card to arrive in the mail.

(A) Notifier(s):

(B) Patient Name: *(C)* Identification Number:

ADVANCE BENEFICIARY NOTICE OF NONCOVERAGE (ABN)

<u>NOTE</u>: If Medicare doesn't pay for *(D)*_____ below, you may have to pay.

Medicare does not pay for everything, even some care that you or your health care provider have good reason to think you need. We expect Medicare may not pay for the *(D)*_____ below.

*(D)*_____	*(E)* Reason Medicare May Not Pay:	*(F)* Estimated Cost:

WHAT YOU NEED TO DO NOW:

- Read this notice, so you can make an informed decision about your care.
- Ask us any questions that you may have after you finish reading.
- Choose an option below about whether to receive the *(D)*_____ listed above.
  Note: If you choose Option 1 or 2, we may help you to use any other insurance that you might have, but Medicare cannot require us to do this.

(G) OPTIONS: Check only one box. We cannot choose a box for you.

❑ **OPTION 1.** I want the *(D)*_____ listed above. You may ask to be paid now, but I also want Medicare billed for an official decision on payment, which is sent to me on a Medicare Summary Notice (MSN). I understand that if Medicare doesn't pay, I am responsible for payment, but **I can appeal to Medicare** by following the directions on the MSN. If Medicare does pay, you will refund any payments I made to you, less co-pays or deductibles.

❑ **OPTION 2.** I want the *(D)*_____ listed above, but do not bill Medicare. You may ask to be paid now as I am responsible for payment. **I cannot appeal if Medicare is not billed**.

❑ **OPTION 3.** I don't want the *(D)*_____ listed above. I understand with this choice I am **not responsible for payment**, and **I cannot appeal to see if Medicare would pay.**

(H) Additional Information:

This notice gives our opinion, not an official Medicare decision. If you have other questions on this notice or Medicare billing, call **1-800-MEDICARE** (1-800-633-4227/**TTY**: 1-877-486-2048).
Signing below means that you have received and understand this notice. You also receive a copy.

(I) Signature:	*(J)* Date:

Form CMS-R-131 (03/08)   Form Approved OMB No. 0938-0566

Fig. 9-5 Example of an advance beneficiary notice.

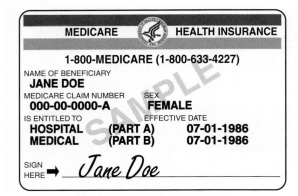

Fig. 9-6 Sample Medicare ID card.

TABLE 9-8	Traditional Medicare HICN Alpha Code Types
CODE	**IDENTIFICATION**
A	Primary claimant (wage earner)
B	Aged wife, age 62 or over
B1	Aged husband, age 62 or over
B2	Young wife, with a child in her care
C1-C9	Child—includes minor, student, or disabled child
D	Aged widow, age 60 or over
D1	Aged widower, age 60 or over
D6	Surviving divorced wife, age 60 or over
E	Widowed mother
E1	Surviving divorced mother
E4	Widowed father
E5	Surviving divorced father
F1	Parent (father)
F2	Parent (mother)
F3	Stepfather
F4	Stepmother
F6	Adopting father
F6	Adopting mother
HA	Disabled claimant (wage earner)
HB	Aged wife of disabled claimant, age 62 or over
M	Uninsured—premium health insurance benefits (Part A)
M1	Uninsured—qualified for but refused Health Insurance Benefits (Part A)
W	Disabled widow
W1	Disabled widower
W6	Disabled surviving divorced wife

What Did You Learn?

1. What are the criteria for meeting Medicare's "medically necessary" guidelines?
2. What are LCDs?
3. When should an ABN be used?
4. How is the HICN structured?

MEDICARE BILLING

Billing for services rendered to Medicare beneficiaries is slightly different from that of non-Medicare patients. The health insurance professional should use the *Medicare Physician Fee Schedule* rather than the regular fee schedule used by the practice. The fees contained in this special fee schedule for the services performed by the healthcare provider are calculated using a complex formula worked out by the federal government and printed periodically.

Physician Fee Schedule

CMS publishes an updated **Medicare Physician Fee Schedule** every year. In the past decade, the Medicare fee schedule was changed from fee-for-service to a **resource-based relative value system (RBRVS)**. This means that each of the payment values is found within a range of payments. Medicare physician fee schedules vary from one region to another. Table 9-9 shows a portion of a page from the 2011 *Medicare Physician Fee Schedule* for WPS Health Insurance (J5 MAC Part B–Iowa, Kansas, Missouri, and Nebraska).

Payment for each service in the fee schedule is based on three factors:

1. A nationally uniform relative value for the specific service calculated with use of components of work, practice overhead, and professional liability—referred to as a **relative value unit**.
2. A geographically specific modifier that considers variation in different areas of the country. Each area of

TABLE 9-9	Sample Portion of a Medicare Fee Schedule*		
PROC	**S**	**PAR**	**NONPAR**	**LIMITING CHARGE**
97001	A	69.45	65.98	75.88
97002*	A	38.29	36.38	41.84
97003*	A	76.43	72.61	83.50
97004	A	46.22	43.91	50.50

A, primary claimant; NonPAR, nonparticipating provider; PAR, participating provider;
*These amounts apply when service is performed in a facility setting.
From U.S. Department of Health and Human Services, Centers for Medicare and Medicaid Services.

the United States has its own geographic practice cost indices for each of the relative value factors of work, practice overhead, and professional liability.

3. A nationally uniform conversion factor that is updated annually.

RBRVS and the relative value unit are discussed in more detail in Chapter 17.

Medicare Participating and Nonparticipating Providers

In its simplest explanation, a **Medicare participating provider (PAR)** or supplier is one who has signed a contract with Medicare; a **Medicare nonparticipating provider (nonPAR)** or supplier has not. Medicare PARs agree to accept Medicare's allowed amount as payment in full. Medicare nonPARs and suppliers may choose whether to accept Medicare's approved amount as payment on a case-by-case basis. If they do not accept the approved amount, the beneficiary can be charged the full billed amount. The "full billed" amount cannot exceed the **Medicare limiting charge**, however, which is 115% of Medicare's allowed amount.

After the beneficiary's annual deductible has been met, Medicare pays 80% of the fee schedule amount for a physician's service, and the beneficiary is responsible for 20%. Medicare PARs benefit from the following advantages:

- Their Medicare fee schedule is 5% higher than that of nonPARs.
- They are provided with toll-free lines if they submit claims electronically.
- Their names are listed in the *Medicare Participating Physician/Supplier Directory*, which is furnished to senior citizen groups.

Medicare providers are generally required to submit claims for beneficiaries whether they are PAR or nonPAR and regardless of whether or not they accept assignment. Furthermore, the law does not allow the provider to charge for this service. Problems with claims processing occur when a service has been rendered by a provider who is not enrolled with the Medicare program. The most common service rendered by a non-enrolled provider is an influenza shot. In such cases, beneficiaries must typically submit claims to Medicare on their own behalf. Some non-enrolled providers will, however, submit claims for beneficiaries.

Determining What Fee to Charge

It is important that the health insurance professional know how to interpret the Medicare fee schedule so that he or she can determine the correct fee to charge the patient. Using the example fee schedule shown in Table 9-9 and choosing CPT code 97001 (a physical therapy evaluation), the amount Medicare allows a PAR to charge the patient is the amount shown in column 3 under the heading "PAR," or $69.45. A Medicare nonPAR accepting assignment can charge the amount in the next column under the heading "NonPAR," or $65.98. The limiting charge for providers *not accepting*

assignment is the amount in the next column under the heading "Limiting," or $75.88—15% more than the nonPAR amount.

> ### ? What Did You Learn?
>
> 1. Who uses Medicare's "limiting charge"?
> 2. List three advantages of becoming a Medicare PAR.
> 3. How does a health insurance professional determine what fee to charge for a Medicare-eligible service?

FILING MEDICARE CLAIMS

Medicare Fact: Beneficiaries who are enrolled in a Medicare Advantage Plan do not have to file claims, because Medicare pays these private insurance companies a set amount every month.

Electronic Claims

Medicare claims must be submitted electronically from a provider's office to an MAC, a DME MAC, or a **Fiscal intermediary (FI)** through the use of computer software that meets two specific electronic filing requirements. The electronic filing requirement established by the Health Insurance Portability and Accountability Act of 1996 (HIPAA) claim standard and the CMS requirements contained in the provider enrollment and certification category (as stated in the EDI Enrollment page of the CMS website) must be met before claims can be submitted electronically to Medicare. Providers that bill FIs can also submit claims electronically using direct data entry (DDE) screens. (DDE is discussed in detail in Chapter 16.)

Administrative Simplification Compliance Act (ASCA)

The Administrative Simplification Compliance Act (ASCA) requires that all **initial claims** for Medicare be submitted electronically, with limited exceptions. Initial claims are those submitted to a Medicare contractor for the first time, including resubmission of previously rejected claims, claims with paper attachments, **demand bills**, Medicare secondary claims, and nonpayment claims. A demand bill is a request form a beneficiary can send to a MAC or FI requesting a review of a noncoverage determination (see example in Fig. 9-7). Initial claims do not include adjustments submitted to contractors on previously submitted claims or appeal requests.

Medicare will not pay on claims submitted on paper that do not meet the limited exception criteria. Claims denied for this reason will contain a **claim adjustment reason code** (an explanation why the claim or service line was paid differently from how it was billed) and a **remittance remark code**

DEPARTMENT OF HEALTH AND HUMAN SERVICES
CENTERS FOR MEDICARE & MEDICAID SERVICES

MEDICARE RECONSIDERATION REQUEST FORM

1. Beneficiary's Name:_____

2. Medicare Number:_____

3. Description of Item or Service in Question: _____

4. Date the Service or Item was Received: _____

5. I do not agree with the determination of my claim. MY REASONS ARE:

_____

_____

_____

6. Date of the redetermination notice_____
   (If you received your redetermination more than 180 days ago, include your reason for not making this request earlier.)

_____

_____

_____

7. Additional Information Medicare Should Consider:_____

_____

_____

_____

8. Requester's Name:_____

9. Requester's Relationship to the Beneficiary: _____

10. Requester's Address: _____

_____

11. Requester's Telephone Number: _____

12. Requester's Signature: _____

13. Date Signed: _____

14. ❑ I have evidence to submit. (Attach such evidence to this form.)
   ❑ I do not have evidence to submit.

15. Name of the Medicare Contractor that Made the Redetermination:_____

NOTICE: Anyone who misrepresents or falsifies essential information requested by this form may upon
conviction be subject to fine or imprisonment under Federal Law.

Form CMS-20033 (05/05) EF (05/2005)

Fig. 9-7 Sample demand bill.

(a supplemental explanation for an adjustment already described by a claim adjustment reason code, indicating that the claim will not be considered unless submitted electronically). Claims required to be submitted electronically must comply with the appropriate claim standards adopted for national use under HIPAA.

Transition to ASC X12 Version 5010

The Secretary of the HHS, along with CMS, has adopted ASC X12 Version 5010 (replacing Version 4010/4010A1) as the next standard for HIPAA covered transactions. The final rule was published on January 16, 2009. Full compliance for the implementation of Version 5010 is June 30, 2012. The health information professional should check the CMS website periodically to see if this compliance date has been extended.

Exceptions to Mandatory Electronic Claim Submission

The following is a list of exceptions to ASCA's mandatory electronic claim submission:
- Small provider claims.
- Roster billing of inoculations covered by Medicare (except for those companies that agreed to submit these claims electronically as a condition for submission of flu shots administered in multiple states to a single carrier).
- Claims for payment under a Medicare demonstration project that specifies that claims be submitted on paper.
- Medicare Secondary Payer Claims when there is more than one primary payer and one or more of those payers made an "Obligated to accept as payment in Full" (OTAF) adjustment.
- Claims submitted by Medicare beneficiaries or Medicare Managed Care Plans.
- Dental claims.
- Claims for services or supplies furnished outside the United States by non-U.S. providers.
- Disruption in electricity or communication connections that are outside a provider's control and expected to last more than 2 business days.
- Claims from providers that submit fewer than 10 claims per month on average during a calendar year.

Small Providers and Full-Time Equivalent (FTE) Employee Assessments

A **small provider** is defined as
- a provider of services—as defined in section 1861(u) of the Social Security Act—with fewer than 25 full-time equivalent (FTE) employees or
- a physician, practitioner, facility, or supplier that is not otherwise a provider under the section with fewer than 10 FTEs.

ASCA Enforcement of Paper Claim Submission

MACs are required to monitor and enforce the ASCA regulations and to conduct a quarterly analysis of the number of paper claims received. Following the analysis, notices are mailed to any provider who submitted a large number of paper claims the previous quarter, asking the provider to explain which exception is applicable to the practice and to provide documentation to support that exception. If the provider does not respond with an acceptable response to prove eligibility for submitting paper claims, all paper claims will be rejected. This decision cannot be appealed.

For more details on this topic, visit the Evolve site.

Providers can purchase the software required for electronic claims submission from a vendor, contract with a billing service or a clearinghouse that offers software and programming support, or use HIPAA-compliant free billing software supplied by Medicare carriers, DME MACs, and FIs. Medicare contractors maintain a list on their providers' web page that contains the names of vendors whose software is currently being used successfully to submit HIPAA-compliant claims to Medicare.

Medicare Fact: Medicare contractors are allowed to collect a fee to recoup their costs up to $25 if a provider requests a Medicare contractor to mail an initial disk or update disks for this free software.

📁 HIPAA Tip

Covered entities may disclose protected health information about non-Medicare patients without their permission when the information involves Quality Improvement Organizations' quality-related activities under its contract. (Under HIPAA, a "covered entity" is a health plan, healthcare clearinghouse, or healthcare provider who transmits information in electronic form.)

HHS has posted the final rule for the Health Insurance Reform; Modifications to the updated version of the HIPAA Electronic Transaction Standards in the *Federal Register*, Vol. 74, No. 11 dated January 16, 2009. This document can be accessed through the Evolve site.

Medicare Fact: Although the majority of providers use electronic claims submission, a significant number of providers are considered small enough to still submit paper claims.

⏱ Stop and Think

You are employed by a two-physician practice. In addition to you, the health insurance professional, there is a medical receptionist, two medical assistants, and a registered nurse. You have just completed transferring all patient accounts over to a computerized patient accounting system. Are you now required to submit all Medicare claims electronically?

Claim Status Request and Response

Providers have several options to obtain claim status information from Medicare contractors. These options allow providers to:

- Use provider help lines to call the local MAC/FI in order to speak to a customer service representative.
- Enter data via Interactive Voice Response (IVR) telephone systems operated by Medicare contractors.
- Enter claim status queries via DDE screens maintained by Medicare contractors.
- Submit a Health Care Claim Status Request (276 transaction) electronically and receive a Health Care Claim Status Response (277 transaction) back from Medicare.

The electronic 276/277 process is recommended if the provider is able to automatically generate and submit 276 queries when necessary. This procedure eliminates the need for manual inquiry entries or phone calls to a contractor to obtain this information. This electronic process is normally less expensive for both the provider and Medicare. In addition, the 277 response enables automatic posting of the status information directly to patient accounts, eliminating the need for manual data entry. The Medicare electronic claims processing manual can be found through the Evolve site.

📁 HIPAA Tip

With the implementation of HIPAA, it is possible to submit an electronic claim and to submit a separate paper attachment for that claim. When an electronic claim is filed, an attachment control number is assigned. The paper attachment is sent with a cover page containing the attachment control number.

Deadline for Filing Medicare Claims

Medicare Fact: Medicare's fiscal year is the same as that of the federal government; it begins on October 1 and ends September 30 of the following year.

Timely Filing Rules

The Patient Protection and Affordable Care Act included a provision that limited timely filing of claims to 1 year from the date of services. This change significantly shortens the time providers previously had to file Medicare claims.

Providers should be aware of these timely filing rules, especially if they are holding claims for some reason, because they shorten the time to file claims. If providers have concerns or questions they should contact their MAC. *MLN Matters Article #MM7080* contains information about timely filing requirements and how CMS implements them. This article can be accessed on the Evolve site.

Medicare regulations allow exceptions to timely filing requirements made in case of a Medicare program's

administrative error as well as Retroactive Entitlements to Medicare coverage.

💬 What Did You Learn?

1. What does Medicare consider an "initial" claim to be?
2. The date for full compliance for the implementation of Version 5010 is _____.
3. List those entities that are considered by ASCA to be "small providers."
4. What is the revised deadline for filing Medicare claims?

USING THE CMS-1500 FORM FOR MEDICARE CLAIMS

The CMS-1500 (08-05) form is the standard paper claim form used by a non-institutional provider or supplier to bill MACs and DME MACs when a provider qualifies for a waiver from the ASCA requirement for electronic submission of claims. It is also used to bill some Medicaid state agencies.

CMS does not supply CMS-1500 forms to providers for claim submission. Claim forms can be purchased at the U.S. Government Printing Office (1-866-512-1800), local printing companies, and/or office supply stores. The National Uniform Claim Committee (NUCC) is responsible for the design and maintenance of the CMS-1500 form. NUCC also provides detailed step-by-step instructions for completing the CMS-1500.

The only acceptable claim forms are those printed in the official OCR Red ink. Although a copy of the CMS-1500 form can be downloaded from the Internet, copies of the form cannot be used for submitting claims. The majority of paper claims are scanned using Optical Character Recognition (OCR) technology. (See OCR rules outlined in Chapter 5.)

CMS-1500 Completion Guidelines

To ensure accurate and quick claim processing, the following guidelines should be followed for paper claims:

- Do not staple, clip, or tape anything to the CMS-1500 claim form.
- Place all necessary documentation in the envelope with the claim form.
- Include the patient's name and Medicare number on each piece of documentation submitted.
- Use dark ink.
- Use only uppercase (CAPITAL) letters.
- Use 10- or 12-pitch standard fonts.
- Do not mix character fonts on the same form.
- Do not use italics or script.
- Avoid using old or worn print bands.
- Do not use dollar signs, decimals, or punctuation.
- Enter all information on the same horizontal plane within the designated field.

- Do not print, handwrite, or stamp any extraneous data on the form.
- Ensure that data are in the appropriate fields and do not overlap into other fields.
- Remove pin-fed edges at side perforations, if applicable.
- Use only an original red-ink-on-white-paper CMS-1500 claim form.

Submission of paper claims that do not meet the carrier's requirements may delay payments.

The process of completing the CMS-1500 form for Medicare claims is similar to that of a commercial claim, with a few exceptions. Complete Medicare claims filing instructions, which are essentially the same as those provided on the NUCC website, can be found in Appendix B. Fig. B-3 in Appendix B shows an example of a completed Medicare "simple" claim—a claim for a patient with Medicare coverage only. The link to the CMS Manual System (Pub. 100-04) can be found on the Evolve site.

🗀 HIPAA Tip

The determining factor for the correct place of service (POS) for Medicare beneficiaries is determined by the status of the patient. When a patient is registered as an inpatient (POS 21) or outpatient (POS 22), one of these POS codes must be used to bill Medicare.

The CMS-1500 paper claim form is being revised to accommodate crosswalking to Version 5010.

Completing a Medigap Claim

Completion of Blocks 9 through 9d on the CMS-1500 form is conditional for insurance information related to Medigap. Only PARs are required to complete Block 9 and its subdivisions and only when the patient wishes to assign his or her benefits under a Medigap policy to the PAR. PARs of service and suppliers must enter information required in Block 9 and its subdivisions if requested by the beneficiary. (PARs sign an agreement with Medicare to accept assignment of Medicare benefits

for *all* Medicare patients. NonPARs can accept assignment on a case-by-case basis.)

A claim for which a beneficiary elects to assign his or her benefits under a Medigap policy to a PAR is called a **mandated Medigap transfer**. If a PAR and the patient want Medicare payment data forwarded to a Medigap insurer under a mandated Medigap transfer, all of the information in Blocks 9, 9a, 9b, and 9d must be complete and accurate. Otherwise, Medicare cannot forward the claim information to the Medigap insurer.

If the health insurance professional wishes to use the statement "Signature on File" in Block 13 in lieu of the patient's actual signature, a statement must be signed and dated by the patient and maintained in the practice's records (Fig. 9-8). Table 9-10 contains instructions for completion of blocks that are affected by Medigap policies. A completed CMS-1500 claim form for a patient with both Medicare and Medigap coverage is shown in Fig. B-5 in Appendix B. The Medigap Crossover Program is discussed in a separate section.

Medicare Secondary Payer

When Medicare is the secondary payer, the claim must be submitted first to the primary insurer. The primary insurer processes the claim in accordance with the coverage provisions in the contract. If, after processing the claim, the primary insurer does not pay in full for the services, the claim may be submitted to Medicare electronically or via a paper claim for consideration of secondary benefits. It is the provider's responsibility to obtain primary insurance information from the beneficiary and to bill Medicare appropriately. Claim filing extensions are not granted because of incorrect insurance information.

Insurance Primary to Medicare

Circumstances under which Medicare payment may be secondary to other insurance include the following:
- Group health plan coverage: working aged, disability (large group health plan), and ESRD
- No fault or other liability insurance
- Work-related illness/injury: workers' compensation, black lung, and veterans benefits

---

(Name of Beneficiary) (Health Insurance Claim Number) (Medigap Policy Number)

I request that payment of authorized Medigap benefits be made either to me or on my behalf to the provider of service and (or) supplier for any services furnished to me by the provider of service and (or) supplier. I authorize any holder of Medicare information about me to release to (Name of Medigap Insurer) any information needed to determine these benefits payable for related services.

_____
(Signature) (Date)

Fig. 9-8 Example of "signature on file" statement.

TABLE 9-10	**Modifications to the CMS-1500 Form for a Medigap Claim**
Block 9	Enter the last name, first name, and middle initial of the Medigap enrollee, if it is different from that shown in Block 2. Otherwise, enter the word "SAME."
Block 9a	Enter the policy and/or group number of the Medigap insured preceded by MEDIGAP, MG, or MGAP. *Note:* Block 9d must be completed if a policy and/or group number is in Block 9a.
Block 9b	Enter the Medigap enrollee's birth date (MMDDCCYY) and sex. Can leave blank if birth date is the same as Block 3.
Block 9c	Disregard "employer's name or school name," which is printed on the form. Enter the claims processing address for the Medigap insurer. Use an abbreviated street address, 2-letter state postal code, and Zip Code copied from the Medigap insured's Medigap ID card. For example: 1257 Anywhere Street, Baltimore, MD 21204, is shown as "1257 Anywhere St MD 21204." *Note:* If a carrier-assigned unique identifier of a Medigap insurer appears in Block 9d, Block 9c may be left blank.
Block 9d	Enter the name of the Medigap insured's insurance company or the Medigap insurer's unique identifier provided by the local Medicare carrier. If you are a participating provider of service or supplier, and the beneficiary wants Medicare payment data forwarded to a Medigap insurer under a mandated Medigap transfer, all of the information in Block 9 and its subdivisions must be complete and correct. Otherwise, the claim information cannot be forwarded to the Medigap insurer.
Block 12	Block 12 must be completed in all Medicare/Medigap claims. Failure to include an appropriate signature and 6-digit date or a "signature on file" statement results in claim rejection. A Medigap authorization signature in Block 13 does not satisfy the Block 12 signature requirement. If a valid signature is on file, no date is necessary.
Block 13	Completion of this block is conditional for Medigap. The signature in Block 13 authorizes payment of mandated Medigap benefits to the PAR of service or supplier if required Medigap information is included in Block 9 and its subdivisions. The patient or his or her authorized representative signs this block, or the signature must be on file as a separate Medigap authorization. The Medigap assignment on file in the participating physician or supplier's office must list the name of the specific Medigap insurer. It may state that the authorization applies to all occasions of service until it is revoked.

The rest of the form for a Medigap claim is completed using the Medicare guidelines provided in Table 9-10.

For a paper claim to be considered for MSP benefits, a copy of the primary payer's EOB notice must be forwarded along with the claim form.

Stop and Think

Franklin Elmore is a new patient in your office. When he filled out the patient information form, he indicated that he was born February 26, 1939, and is employed full-time at Alamo Distributing Company. Under the insurance section, Mr. Elmore lists Medicare as his primary insurer and group coverage with Amax Quality Assurance through his employer as his secondary insurance. Is Mr. Elmore's information form correct? Which insurer should receive the CMS-1500 claim first?

Completing Medicare Secondary Policy Claims

When Medicare is the secondary payer, the primary payer's EOB typically includes the following information:
- Name and address of the primary insurer
- Name of subscriber and policy number
- Name of the provider of services
- Itemized charges for all procedure codes reported
- Detailed explanation of any denials or payment codes
- Date of service

A detailed explanation of any primary insurer's denial or payment codes must be submitted with the claim to Medicare. If the denial/payment code descriptions or any of the previously listed information is not included with the claim, there may be a delay in processing or denial of the claim. If the beneficiary is covered by more than one insurer primary to Medicare (e.g., a working aged beneficiary who was in an automobile accident), the EOB statements from those plans must be submitted with the claim.

To submit MSP claims electronically, the health insurance professional should refer to the American National Standards Institute's (ANSI) *Version 005010X212 Implementation Guide* or the *National Standard Format Specifications* for reporting requirements.

For submission of a paper claim to Medicare as the secondary payer, the following instructions apply:
- The CMS-1500 form must indicate the name and policy number of the beneficiary's primary insurance in Blocks 11 through 11c.
- Providers, whether they are PAR or nonPAR, must submit a claim to Medicare if a beneficiary provides a copy of the primary EOB.
- The claim must be submitted to Medicare for secondary payment consideration with a copy of the EOB. If the beneficiary is not cooperative in supplying the EOB, the beneficiary may be billed for the amount Medicare would pay as the secondary payer.

- Providers must bill the primary insurer and Medicare the same charge for rendered services. If the primary insurer is billed $50.00 for an office visit and they pay $35.00, Medicare cannot be billed the remaining $15.00. Medicare also must be billed for the $50.00 charge, and a copy of the primary insurer's EOB must be attached to the completed claim form.

It was stated previously that when paper or electronic claims are submitted for Medicare, Block 11 must be completed. By completing this block, the physician/supplier acknowledges having made a good faith effort to determine whether Medicare is the primary or secondary payer. A claim without this information would be returned.

When there is insurance primary to Medicare, as in the MSP situation, the health insurance professional should enter the insured's policy or group number in Block 11 and proceed to Blocks 11a through 11c. (When there is no insurance primary to Medicare, enter the word "NONE" in Block 11 and proceed to Block 12.) Completion of Blocks 11b and 11c is conditional for insurance information primary to Medicare. Table 9-11 gives instructions for how Blocks 11a through 11d should be completed for MSP claims. (A completed CMS-1500 claim for a patient with group coverage primary to Medicare (MSP) is shown in Fig. B-6 in Appendix B.)

MSP Conditional Payment

Medicare may make a conditional payment if they know that another insurer is primary to Medicare but that the primary payer has not made prompt payment (within 120 days) or has denied the claim for a reason Medicare considers acceptable. (This conditional payment is applicable, however, only for black lung, workers' compensation, and accidents.) From a reimbursement standpoint, a claim paid conditionally pays the same as if there were no insurance other than Medicare. To learn more about how to apply for an MSP conditional payment, contact the local COBC by phone or mail. This information can also be found on the CMS website.

TABLE 9-11	Modifications to the CMS-1500 for Medicare Secondary Payer Claims
Block 11a	Enter the insured's birth date (MMDDCCYY) and sex, if different from Block 3.
Block 11b	Enter the employer's name, if applicable. If there is a change in the insured's insurance status, such as retired, enter the 6-digit retirement date (MMDDYY) preceded by the word "RETIRED."
Block 11c	Enter the *complete* insurance plan or program name (e.g., Blue Shield of [State]). If the primary payer's EOB does not contain the claims processing address, record the primary payer's claims processing address directly on the EOB.
Block 11d	Can be left blank. Not required by Medicare.

Medigap Crossover Program

Effective October 2007, CMS transferred the mandatory Medicare supplemental (Medigap) insurance crossover program from its Medicare contractors to the national **COBC**. The Medigap crossover process, which is mandated by the Social Security Act, is activated when (1) a PAR Medicare provider includes a specific identifier on the beneficiary's claim and (2) payment benefits are assigned to that provider. This process ensures data consistency among the many organizations that transmit Medicare data. A Medigap claim-based COBA ID is a unique identifier associated with each contract. As previously mentioned, COBA IDs are five-digit numbers in the range 55000 through 59999 that are assigned by the COBC. After a healthcare provider enrolls in this program, an ID is provided. The Medigap policy information should be shown in Blocks 9 through 9d on the CMS-1500 claim form as follows:

- The word "Medigap" (or MG or MGAP) and the individual Medigap policy number must be present in Item 9a on the CMS-1500 form.
- The Medigap COBA ID number must be present in Item 9d on the CMS-1500 Form.

A list of Medigap companies and their corresponding COBA ID numbers is available on the CMS website at http://www.cms.gov/COBAgreement/ in the PDF document entitled "Medigap Claim-based COBA IDs for Billing Purposes." For more information on COBA and unique identifiers, visit the Evolve site.

Medicare/Medicaid Crossover Claims

Modifications must be made on the CMS-1500 form for dual-eligible beneficiaries. The claim is sent to Medicare first, which determines its liability portion of the charges. Then the claim is automatically crossed over to Medicaid directly from the Medicare carrier. The following blocks are affected:

Block 1: The Medicare and Medicaid boxes should be checked.

Block 10d: The abbreviation MCD should be entered, followed by the beneficiary's Medicaid ID number.

Block 27: PARs and nonPARs should place an "X" in the "YES" box, because assignment must be accepted on Medicare/Medicaid crossover claims.

Note: It is a good idea to check with the state Medicaid FI for any special instructions for submitting claims for dual eligibles.

A completed CMS-1500 claim for a patient with both Medicare and Medicaid coverage is shown in Fig. B-4 in Appendix B.

Other than the blocks noted earlier, the Medicare/Medicaid claim is completed as directed by the Medicare claims completion guidelines listed in Appendix B.

Medicare Fact: Because Medicare Advantage claims do not automatically cross over to Medicaid, plan providers must submit claims to the State Medicaid Program in order to receive payment for any Medicaid cost-sharing obligation.

MEDICARE SUMMARY NOTICE

When a Medicare claim is filed, the beneficiary receives a document called the **Medicare Summary Notice (MSN)**, as shown in Fig. 9-9. The MSN form is an easy-to-read statement that lists Part A and B claims information, including what Medicare paid and the patient's deductible status. The health insurance professional should make it clear to the patient that the MSN is not a bill and that he or she should not send any money to the provider or supplier until a statement is received.

Medicare also has a website where beneficiaries can view an electronic MSN online and print copies from their home computers. The electronic MSN does not replace the paper MSN, which is mailed every 3 months for claims covering services provided to the beneficiary (if any) during that period, but it is a quick and convenient way for beneficiaries to track their claims. Beneficiaries can view their electronic MSNs by visiting www.MyMedicare.gov/. This website provides additional valuable information for Medicare beneficiaries. Seniors who do not own a computer can visit their local library or senior center to look up this information. Another valuable source of information for Medicare beneficiaries is the State Health Insurance Assistance Program (SHIP). SHIP's toll free phone number is printed on the back cover of the *Medicare & You* handbook.

Information Contained on the MSN

The MSN gives a breakdown of Medicare claims billed on the patient's behalf and processed by the MAC or FI. In addition to listing the services received along with the name of the provider, the MSN lists:

- the total amount billed by providers,
- Medicare's approved payment amount for services,
- amount paid to the beneficiary or his or her provider,
- costs the beneficiary is responsible for, and
- deductible information.

If there is a supplemental insurance policy or Medigap, the insurer for this coverage may also need a copy of the MSN to process its share of the bill. This is normally done electronically via the Medicare/Medigap crossover process, which is mandated by the Social Security Act and activated when a participating Medicare provider includes a specific identifier on the beneficiary's claim and the beneficiary assigns benefits to that provider.

The health insurance professional should know how to read the MSN so that he or she can answer any questions beneficiaries might have. Detailed instructions on how to read the MSN can be found on the CMS website as well as the Medicare.gov/ website.

Medicare Remittance Advice

When a claim has gone through the processing stage, Medicare notifies the provider as to how the claim was **adjudicated** (how the decision was made about the payment). This notification is referred to as a **remittance advice (RA)**. The RA is notification that Medicare sends to the provider and includes a list of all claims paid and claims rejected or denied during a particular payment period. A paper RA is generated for all providers whether they file paper or electronic claims. The only exception is when the provider has been approved to receive the RA electronically.

Each RA contains a list of claims that Medicare has cleared for payment since the last RA was generated as well as any claims that have moved to a "deny status" since the last RA was sent. RAs are generated in a weekly cycle. Each claim listed on the RA contains detailed processing information. A reimbursement amount, Claim Adjustment Reason Codes, and Remittance Remark Codes are included for each claim. Claim adjustment reason codes and remittance remark codes are used in the **electronic remittance advice (ERA)** and the **standard paper remittance advice (SPR)** to relay information relevant to the adjudication of Medicare Part B claims. Reason codes detail the reason why an adjustment was made to a healthcare claim payment by the payer, and remark codes represent nonfinancial information crucial to understanding the adjudication of the claim.

Standard Paper Remittance Advice

The SPR is the standard form CMS uses for provider payment notification. The form was created to (1) provide a document that is uniform in content and format and (2) ease the transition to the electronic remittance format. The SPR displays the same reason codes, remark codes, messages, and other data as the ERA for Medicare Part A providers.

Fig. 9-10 shows an example SPR along with a list of the various fields depicted on the SPR and their definitions. One claim is listed in each block of the remittance and is separated from other claims with a line. The claims on the remittance are organized in alphabetical order, by beneficiary name within each type of claim (i.e., Inpatient, Part A). At the end of each type of claim, there is a subtotal of the

CMS
CENTERS for MEDICARE & MEDICAID SERVICES

Medicare Summary Notice

BENEFICIARY NAME
STREET ADDRESS
CITY, STATE   ZIP CODE

BE INFORMED: Beware of telemarketers offering free or discounted Medicare items or services.

CUSTOMER SERVICE INFORMATION

Your Medicare Number: 111-11-1111A

If you have questions, write or call:
Medicare
555 Medicare Blvd., Suite 200
Medicare Building
Medicare, US XXXXX-XXXX

Local: (XXX) XXX-XXXX
Toll-free: 1-800-XXX-XXXX
TTY for Hearing Impaired: 1-800-XXX-XXXX

This is a summary of claims processed from 5/10/2011 through 6/10/2011.

PART B MEDICAL INSURANCE – ASSIGNED CLAIMS

Dates of Service	Services Provided	Amount Charged	Medicare Approved	Medicare Paid Provider	You May Be Billed	See Notes Section
Claim Number: 12435-84956-84556						
Paul Jones, M.D., 123 West Street,						a
Jacksonville, FL 33231-0024						
Referred by: Scott Wilson, M.D.						
04/19/XX	1 Influenza immunization (90724)	$5.00	$3.88	$3.88	$0.00	b
04/19/XX	1 Admin. flu vac (G0008)	5.00	3.43	3.43	0.00	b
	Claim Total	**$10.00**	**$7.31**	**$7.31**	**$0.00**	
Claim Number: 12435-84956-84557						
ABC Ambulance, P.O. Box 2149,						a
Jacksonville, FL 33231						
04/25/XX	1 Ambulance, base rate (A0020)	$289.00	$249.78	$199.82	$49.96	
04/25/XX	1 Ambulance, per mile (A0021)	21.00	16.96	13.57	3.39	
	Claim Total	**$310.00**	**$266.74**	**$213.39**	**$53.35**	

PART B MEDICAL INSURANCE – UNASSIGNED CLAIMS

Dates of Service	Services Provided	Amount Charged	Medicare Approved	Medicare Paid You	You May Be Billed	See Notes Section
Claim Number: 12435-84956-84558						
William Newman, M.D., 362 North Street						a
Jacksonville, FL 33231-0024						
03/10/XX	1 Office/Outpatient Visit, ES (99213)	$47.00	$33.93	$27.15	$39.02	c

THIS IS NOT A BILL – Keep this notice for your records.

Fig. 9-9 Example of Medicare Summary Notice Part B. (From U.S. Department of Health and Human Services, Centers for Medicare and Medicaid Services.)

EXAMPLE OF STANDARD PAPER REMITTANCE

(1)
NHIC, Corp
ADDRESS 1
ADDRESS 2
CITY, STATE ZIP
(999) 111-2222

MEDICARE
REMITTANCE
NOTICE

PROVIDER NAME
ADDRESS 1
ADDRESS 2
CITY, STATE ZIP

PROVIDER #: 1234567890
PAGE #: 1 OF 10
DATE: 06/05/XX
CHECK/EFT #: 12345678901234567890
REMITTANCE #: 12345678901234567890 (NOT A REQUIRED FIELD)

(2)

WELCOME TO THE MEDICARE PART B STANDARD PAPER REMITTANCE

(3)

PERF PROV	SERV DATE	POS	NOS	PROC	MODS	BILLED	ALLOWED	DEDUCT	COINS	GRP/ RC AMT	PROV PD

NAME: BUNYAN, PAUL   HIC 123456789   ACNT 123456789234567890   ICN 123456789012345   ASG Y   MOA

| 123456ABC | 0225 0225XX | 11 | 1 | 99213 | | 66.00 | 49.83 | 0.34 | 9.97 CO-42 | 16.17 | $39.52 |

PT RESP   10.31   CLAIM TOTALS   66.00   49.83   0.34   9.97   16.17   **$39.52 NET**

NAME: FISCHER, BENNY   HIC 999999999   ACNT FISC6123133-01   ICN 0202199306850   ASG Y   MOA MA01 MA07

| 123456ABC | 0117 0117XX | 11 | 1 | 99213 | | 66.00 | 49.83 | 0.00 | 9.97 PR-96 | 16.17 | $39.86 |

PT RESP   9.97   CLAIM TOTALS   66.00   49.83   0.00   9.97   16.17

CLAIM INFORMATION FORWARDED TO: MEDICAID   **$39.86 NET**

NAME: HURT, I.M.   HIC 999999999   ACNT HURT5-329   ICN 0202199326870   ASG Y   MOA MA01

| 123456ABC | 0117 0117XX | 11 | 1 | 90659 | | 25.00 | 3.32 | 0.00 | 0.00 CO-42 | 21.68 | $3.32 |
| 123456ABC | 0117 0117XX | 11 | 1 | G0008 | | 10.00 | 4.46 | 0.00 | 0.00 CO-42 | 5.54 | $4.46 |

27.22   **$7.78 NET**

PT RESP   0.00

NAME: FINE, R.U.   HIC 999999999   ACNT FINE7-002   ICN 0202199000150   ASG Y   N257 MA130

| 123456ABC | 0526 0526XX | 11 | 1 | 73560 | LT | 79.00 | 0.00 | 0.00 | 0.00 CO-16 | 79.00 | |

REM: N257
PT RESP   0.00   CLAIM TOTALS   79.00   0.00   0.00   0.00   79.00   0.00

(4)

TOTALS:	# OF BILLED CLAIMS	ALLOWED AMT	DEDUCT AMT	COINS AMT	TOTAL AMT	PROV PD RC-AMT	PROV AMT	CHECK ADJ AMT	AMT
	4	167.00	107.44	0.34	19.94	59.56	87.16	0.00	$87.16

(5)
PROVIDER ADJ DETAILS: PLB REASON CODE   FCN   HIC   AMOUNT

(6)
GLOSSARY: Group, Reason, MOA, Remark and Offset Codes
CO-42   Contractual Obligation. Amount for which the provider is financially liable. The patient may not be billed for this amount. Claim/service denied/reduced because this procedure/service is not paid separately. Charges exceed our fee schedule or maximum allowable amount.
M80   We cannot pay for this when performed during the same session as another approved procedure for this beneficiary
MA07   The claim information has also been forwarded to Medicaid for review.
MA28   Receipt of this notice by a physician who did not accept assignment is for information only and does not make the physician a party to the determination. No additional rights to appeal this decision, above those rights already provided for by regulation/instruction, are conferred by receipt of this notice
MA130   Your clam contains incomplete and/or invalid information, and no appeal rights are afforded
N257   Missing/incomplete/invalid billing provider/supplier primary identifier.

Fig. 9-10 Example of Standard Paper Remittance Advice (SPRA). (From U.S. Department of Health and Human Services, Centers for Medicare and Medicaid Services.)

information included on the remittance. At the end of the remittance is a total summation. Visit the Evolve site to view the 2010 CMS SPR Guide.

Electronic Remittance Advice

An ERA is one of several different types of electronic formats that are generated in place of a paper document. Information contained in an ERA furnishes basically the same information as that contained on the SPR. An ERA allows automatic posting of claims payment information directly into the facility's practice management computer system. ERAs eliminate the need for manual posting of Medicare payment information, saving the provider time and money. Automatic ERA information transfer also eliminates errors made by manual posting of information from the SPR to the patient ledger accounts.

Medicare provides free software to read the ERA and print an equivalent of an SPR. Institutional and professional providers can get this software from their MACs or FIs. These software products enable providers to view and print remittance advices when needed, thus eliminating the need to request or await mail delivery of SPRs. The *Medicare Claims Processing Manual* (Pub.100-04), Chapters 22 and 24, provides further remittance advice information. The link to this manual can be found on the Evolve site.

Medicare Fact: Any provider or supplier enrolled in the Medicare program who submits claims electronically may receive ERAs. Additionally, providers may allow a billing agent (billing service or clearinghouse) to receive ERAs on their behalf.

Enrolling in Electronic Remittance

Receiving ERAs is not automatic. The provider first must go through an enrollment process, as follows:

1. Providers must contact their software vendor to determine whether ERA capability is available for the facility's practice management system. Special programming is usually required to extract the information from the electronic remittance file and automatically post it to the patient accounts.
2. The provider must complete an ERA enrollment form (Fig. 9-11).

CMS offers free software to providers that will convert the ERA file to a readable and printable format.

Electronic Funds Transfer

Payments from Medicare may be automatically deposited to a provider's designated bank account using **electronic funds transfer (EFT)**. Each EFT transaction is assigned a unique number, which functions the same way as a Medicare check number. The EFT number appears on the RA (paper or electronic) in the same field/location as the Medicare check number. EFT is available to all providers who bill Medicare. Providers must request an EFT enrollment form from their Medicare carrier. A request for EFT authorization form is shown in Fig. 9-12.

What Did You Learn?

1. What is an MSN?
2. Explain the difference between the MSN and the Medicare RA.
3. Who is eligible to receive an ERA?
4. What is an EFT?
5. Who can receive ERAs?

MEDICARE AUDITS AND APPEALS

Audits

Medicare audits are generally designed to determine whether a provider has been reimbursed by the Medicare program for services that are properly reimbursable, that is, medically necessary. These audits are typically based on (1) random reviews, (2) prior problems or unusual billing patterns, or (3) a certain kind of billing problem that the carrier is focusing on.

Medicare audits fall into two broad categories: prepayment audits, which as the name suggests review claims before Medicare pays the provider, and postpayment audits, which analyze claims after Medicare reimbursement. Some medical facilities believe they can avoid audits if they report lower-level evaluation and management codes on claims that result in billing Medicare a lesser fee; this practice is referred to as **downcoding**. Many audits target physicians' offices that practice downcoding because this type of practice "raises a red flag" to auditors. Downcoding on a claim is discouraged when the reason for doing so is simply that documentation in the health record does not meet the carriers' guidelines. If a particular code accurately describes the service or procedure performed, a provider should not voluntarily lower the code simply because he or she fears a documentation deficiency.

Stop and Think

You are having lunch with your friend Nellie Shumway, who works for a family practice clinic across the courtyard from your building. Over lunch one day, Nellie confides, "In our office, we code all new Medicare patient visits at Level 1 (99201). It's so much easier, and we don't have to worry about Medicare auditing our records." What, if anything, might you tell your friend?

Postpayment audits are most commonly triggered by statistical irregularities. A postpayment audit can result if a provider uses a certain code much more frequently or less frequently than other providers of the same specialty in the same area. Patient complaints can also trigger audits and reviews.

CMS
CENTERS for MEDICARE & MEDICAID SERVICES

HIGHMARK®
MEDICARE SERVICES
A CMS CONTRACTOR

5010 Electronic Remittance Advice (ERA) Migration Form

Submitter Name: ______________________________

Address: ______________________________

Contact Name: ____________________ **Contact Phone Number:** ____________________

Highmark Medicare Services Electronic Data Interchange (EDI) requires a minimum of one business day advance notice to complete your migration request. Business hours are from 8:30AM to 4:30PM. This form should only be used by EXISTING ERA customers requesting to be migrated from version 4010A1 to version 5010.

Effective ____________ 20XX, please update my existing submitter number ____________ to production version 5010 835 ERA. As of this effective date, I understand that I will no longer receive version 4010A1 ERA.

Signature:

By signing below, I attest to the fact that I am authorized to sign the document on behalf of the party identified above.

Signature ______________________________ Date ____________________

Printed Name ______________________________ Title ____________________

Please fax your completed 5010 ERA Migration Form to Highmark Medicare Services EDI at (717) 302-4252.
Your request must be received one business day prior to your requested effective date.
Incomplete 5010 ERA Migration forms, or those signed incorrectly, will not be processed.

Fig. 9-11 Example of an ERA enrollment form. (From U.S. Department of Health and Human Services, Centers for Medicare and Medicaid Services.)

Recovery Audit Contractor (RAC) Program

The **Recovery Audit Contractor (RAC)** Program is a result of the Medicare Modernization Act and the Tax Relief and Healthcare act of 2006. The job of an RAC is to detect and correct past improper payments so that CMS and carriers, FIs, and MACs can implement actions that will prevent future improper payments. Providers who bill Medicare on a fee-for-service basis will be subject to review by RACs. Visit the Evolve site for the link to an overview of the RAC Program.

Appeals (Fee-for-Service Claims)

Medicare regulations allow providers and beneficiaries who are dissatisfied with Medicare's determination (of a fee-for-service claim) to request that the determination be reconsidered. Through the appeals process, Medicare attempts to ensure that the correct payment is made or that a clear and adequate explanation is given supporting nonpayment.

A physician or supplier providing items and services payable under Medicare Part B may appeal an initial determination if

- he or she accepted assignment;
- he or she did not accept assignment on a claim that was denied on the basis of not being reasonable and necessary;
- the beneficiary did not know or could not have been expected to know that the service would not be covered, requiring the provider/supplier to refund the beneficiary any payment received for the services; or
- he or she did not accept assignment, but is acting as the authorized representative of the beneficiary, and indicates this status in the appeal (attaching a copy of the beneficiary's MSN indicates that the provider/ supplier is authorized to act on the beneficiary's behalf).

AUTHORIZATION AGREEMENT FOR ELECTRONIC FUNDS TRANSFER (EFT)

Reason for Submission: ❑ New EFT Authorization
   ❑ Revision to Current Authorization *(i.e. account or bank changes)*
   ❑ EFT Termination Request

Chain Home Office: ❑ Check here if EFT payment is being made to the Home Office of Chain Organization
    (Attach letter Authorizing EFT payment to Chain Home Office)

Physician/Provider/Supplier Information

Physician's Name _____

Provider/Supplier Legal Business Name _____

_____

Chain Organization Name _____

Home Office Legal Business Name *(if different from Chain Organization Name)* _____

_____

Tax ID Number: *(Designate SSN* ❑ *or EIN* ❑*)* ___ ___ ___ ___ ___ ___ ___ ___ ___

Doing Business As Name_____

Medicare Identification Number *(OSCAR, UPIN, or NSC only)* _____

Depository Information (Financial Institution)

Depository Name _____

Account Holder's Name _____

Street Address _____

City _____ State _____ Zip Code _____

Depository Telephone Number_____

Depository Contact Person _____

Depository Routing Transit Number *(nine digit)* ___ ___ ___ ___ ___ ___ ___ ___ ___

Depositor Account Number _____

Type of Account *(check one)* ❑ Checking Account   ❑ Savings Account

Please include a voided check, preprinted deposit slip, or confirmation of account information on bank letterhead with this agreement for verification of your account number.

Authorization

I hereby authorize the Medicare contractor, _____, hereinafter called the COMPANY, to initiate credit entries, and in accordance with 31 CFR part 210.6(f) initiate adjustments for any credit entries made in error to the account indicated above. I hereby authorize the financial institution/bank named above, hereinafter called the DEPOSITORY, to credit and/or debit the same to such account.

If payment is being made to an account controlled by a Chain Home Office, the Provider of Services hereby acknowledges that payment to the Chain Office under these circumstances is still considered payment to the Provider, and the Provider authorizes the forwarding of Medicare payments to the Chain Home Office.

If the account is drawn in the Physician's or Individual Practitioner's Name, or the Legal Business Name of the Provider/Supplier, the said Physician/Provider/Supplier certifies that he/she has sole control of the account referenced above, and certifies that all arrangements between the DEPOSITORY and the said Physician/Provider/Supplier are in accordance with all applicable Medicare regulations and instructions.

FORM CMS-588 (09/03)

Fig. 9-12 Authorization agreement for electronic funds transfer (EFT). (From U.S. Department of Health and Human Services, Centers for Medicare and Medicaid Services.)

Continued

This authorization agreement is effective as of the signature date below and is to remain in full force and effect until the COMPANY has received written notification from me of its termination in such time and such manner as to afford the COMPANY and the DEPOSITORY a reasonable opportunity to act on it. The COMPANY will continue to send the direct deposit to the DEPOSITORY indicated above until notified by me that I wish to change the DEPOSITORY receiving the direct deposit. If my DEPOSITORY information changes, I agree to submit to the COMPANY an updated EFT Authorization Agreement.

Signature Line

Authorized/Delegated Official Name *(Print)* _____

Authorized/Delegated Official Title _____

Authorized/Delegated Official Signature_____Date_____

PRIVACY ACT ADVISORY STATEMENT

Sections 1842, 1862(b) and 1874 of title XVIII of the Social Security Act authorize the collection of this information. The purpose of collecting this information is to authorize electronic funds transfers.

The information collected will be entered into system No. 09-70-0501, titled "Carrier Medicare Claims Records," and No. 09-70-0503, titled "Intermediary Medicare Claims Records" published in the Federal Register Privacy Act Issuances, 1991 Comp. Vol. 1, pages 419 and 424, or as updated and republished. Disclosures of information from this system can be found in this notice.

Furnishing information is voluntary, but without it we will not be able to process your electronic funds transfer.

You should be aware that P.L. 100-503, the Computer Matching and Privacy Protection Act of 1988, permits the government, under certain circumstances, to verify the information you provide by way of computer matches.

According to the Paperwork Reduction Act of 1995, no persons are required to respond to a collection of information unless it displays a valid OMB control number. The valid OMB control number for this information collection is 0938-0626. The time required to complete this information collection is estimated to average 2 hours per response, including the time to review instructions, search existing data resources, gather the data needed, and complete and review the information collection. If you have any comments concerning the accuracy of the time estimate(s) or suggestions for improving this form, please write to: CMS, Attn: PRA Reports Clearance Officer, 7500 Security Boulevard, Baltimore, MD 21244-1850.

FORM CMS-588 (09/03)

Fig. 9-12—cont'd

Claims submitted with incomplete or invalid information are not given appeal rights and are returned as unprocessable. The provider has two options for correcting the claim:
- Submit an entirely new claim (electronic or paper) with complete, valid information
- Submit corrections in writing

Five levels of appeal action are available if the provider and/or the beneficiary disagrees with a coverage or payment decision made by Medicare. This appeal process is illustrated in the flow chart shown in Fig. 9-13.

Office addresses where to send the completed forms and appropriate accompanying completed form(s) and/or documentation can be found on the Department of Health and Human Services or the CMS website.

More detailed information regarding the Medicare appeals process can be found in the Appeals Process Brochure. To download a copy of this brochure, visit the Evolve site.

Appeals Process (Medicare Managed Care Claims)

Medicare Part C (Medicare Advantage) health plans must meet the requirements for grievance and appeals processing under Subpart M of the Medicare Advantage regulations. If a Medicare health plan denies service or payment, the plan is required to provide the enrollee with a written notice of its determination. Additionally, Medicare health plan enrollees receiving covered services from an inpatient hospital, SNF, home health agency, or comprehensive outpatient rehabilitation facility have the right to an expedited appeal if they think their Medicare-covered services are ending too soon. Plans and providers have certain responsibilities related to notifying beneficiaries of Medicare appeal rights.

Fig. 9-14 shows a flow chart for the Medicare Managed Care determination/appeals process.

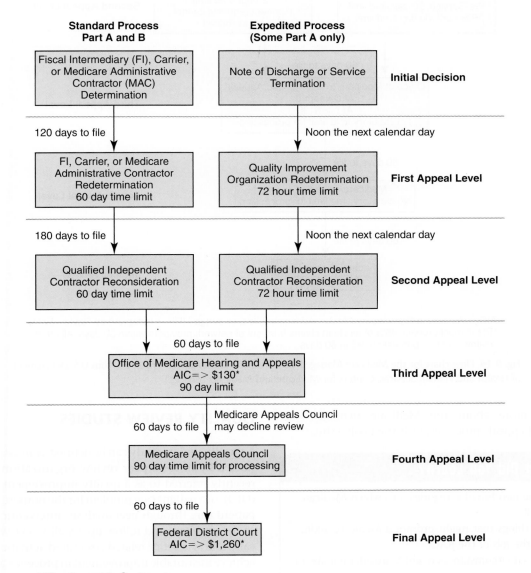

AIC = Amount in Controversy

Fig. 9-13 Original Medicare (Parts A and B Fee-for-Service) Appeals Process. (From U.S. Department of Health and Human Services, Centers for Medicare and Medicaid Services.)

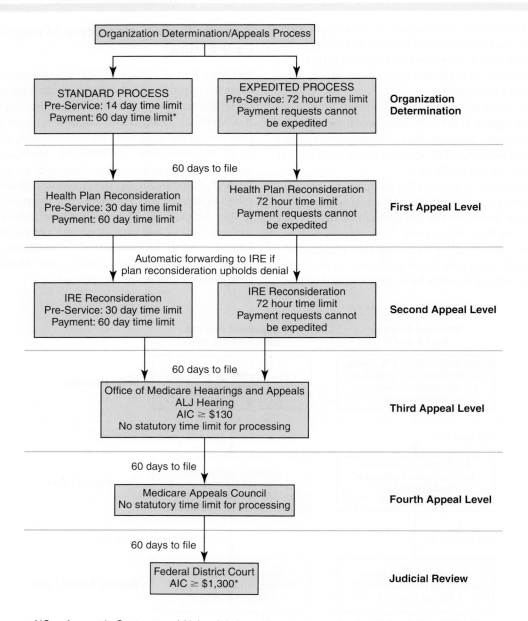

Organization Determination/Appeals Process

STANDARD PROCESS
Pre-Service: 14 day time limit
Payment: 60 day time limit*

EXPEDITED PROCESS
Pre-Service: 72 hour time limit
Payment requests cannot
be expedited

Organization Determination

60 days to file

Health Plan Reconsideration
Pre-Service: 30 day time limit
Payment: 60 day time limit

Health Plan Reconsideration
72 hour time limit
Payment requests cannot
be expedited

First Appeal Level

Automatic forwarding to IRE if
plan reconsideration upholds denial

IRE Reconsideration
Pre-Service: 30 day time limit
Payment: 60 day time limit

IRE Reconsideration
72 hour time limit
Payment requests cannot
be expedited

Second Appeal Level

60 days to file

Office of Medicare Heaarings and Appeals
ALJ Hearing
AIC ≥ $130
No statutory time limit for processing

Third Appeal Level

60 days to file

Medicare Appeals Council
No statutory time limit for processing

Fourth Appeal Level

60 days to file

Federal District Court
AIC ≥ $1,300*

Judicial Review

AIC = Amount in Controversy / ALJ = Administrative Law Judge / IRE = Independent Review Entity
*Plans must process 95% of all clean claims from out of network providers within 30 days. All other
claims must be processed within 60 days.

Fig. 9-14 Flow chart for the Medicare Managed Care Determination/Appeals Process. (From U.S. Department of Health and Human Services, Centers for Medicare and Medicaid Services.)

To learn more about the Medicare managed care grievance and appeals processes, visit the Evolve site.

What Did You Learn?

1. Name the two broad categories into which Medicare audits fall.
2. List two things that might prompt a Medicare audit.
3. What is the job of the RAC?
4. Under what circumstances might a provider initiate an appeal?
5. List the five appeal levels.

QUALITY REVIEW STUDIES

A **quality review study** can be defined as an assessment, conducted by or for a **peer review organization (PRO)** more recently referred to as a quality improvement organization (QIO), of a patient care problem for the purpose of improving patient care through peer analysis, intervention, resolution of the problem, and follow-up. Quality review studies typically follow a set of related structured activities designed to achieve measurable improvement in processes and outcomes of care. Improvements are achieved through interventions that target healthcare providers, practitioners, plans, or beneficiaries.

Quality Improvement Organizations

Quality Improvement Organizations (QIOs), are private, mainly not-for-profit organizations that are staffed by professionals, mostly doctors and other health care professionals, who are trained to review medical care, to help beneficiaries with complaints about the quality of care, and to make improvements in the entire range of care available. CMS contracts with one organization in each state, the District of Columbia, Puerto Rico, and the U.S. Virgin Islands to serve as that state/jurisdiction's QIO contractor. These contracts are 3 years in length.

The mission of the QIO Program, by law, is to improve the effectiveness, efficiency, economy, and quality of services delivered to Medicare beneficiaries. On the basis of this mission, CMS identifies the principal functions of the QIO Program as:

- improving quality of care for beneficiaries;
- protecting the integrity of the Medicare Trust Fund by ensuring that Medicare pays only for services and goods that are reasonable and necessary and that are provided in the most appropriate setting; and
- protecting beneficiaries by expeditiously addressing individual complaints, such as beneficiary complaints; provider-based notice appeals; violations of the Emergency Medical Treatment and Labor Act (EMTALA); and other related responsibilities as articulated in QIO-related law.

CMS is required to publish a report to Congress every fiscal year that outlines the administration, cost, and impact of the QIO Program.

HIPAA Tip

A covered entity can disclose information to a QIO on both Medicare beneficiaries and non-Medicare patients without patient permission when the information is needed for the QIO's quality-related activities under its contract.

Beneficiary Notices Initiative

Both Medicare beneficiaries and providers have certain rights and protections related to financial liability under the Fee-for-Service (FFS) Medicare and the Medicare Advantage (MA) Programs. These financial liability and appeal rights and protections, under the Beneficiary Notices Initiative, are communicated to beneficiaries through notices given by providers.

For example, beneficiaries have the right to:

- Be treated with dignity and respect
- Be protected against discrimination
- Get information they understand
- Get answers to Medicare questions
- Get culturally competent services
- Get emergency care when and where it is needed
- Learn about their treatment choices in clear, understandable language
- File a complaint
- Appeal denial of treatment or payment
- Have their personal information kept private
- Know their privacy rights

Beneficiary Complaint Response Program

The **Beneficiary Complaint Response Program** handles complaints by Medicare beneficiaries (or their representatives) that are made either in writing or by telephone. When the Program receives a complaint, a case manager is assigned who works with the beneficiary from start to finish, keeping him or her informed throughout the review process about the status of the complaint. The Program also uses physician peer review to assess clinical quality of care issues in a patient's record (referred to as *medical record review*). The focus of the Program is on individually based quality improvement efforts that, ideally, can lead to quality improvements in future care. Typical complaints that beneficiaries file may cite issues such as:

- Received the wrong, or erroneous dose of, medication
- Underwent inappropriate surgery
- Experienced an error in treatment
- Received inadequate care or treatment by any healthcare professional
- Was discharged too soon
- Received inadequate discharge instructions

Hospital-Issued Notice of Noncoverage (HINN) and Notice of Discharge (NODMAR) and Medicare Appeal Rights Reviews

When a hospital issues a Hospital-Issued Notice of Noncoverage (HINN) or an MCO issues a Notice of Discharge and Medicare Appeal Rights (NODMAR), the beneficiary, or his or her representative, may request an immediate review. The purpose of the review is to ensure that the HINN or NODMAR is correct and that the patient is not being discharged prematurely from care. Hospitals provide HINNs to beneficiaries of original Medicare prior to admission, at admission, or at any point during an inpatient stay if it is determined that the inpatient care the beneficiary is receiving, or is about to receive, is not covered.

For further information and to view a copy of the HINN form along with instructions for its completion, visit the Evolve site.

A NODMAR must include the following information:

- The specific reason why inpatient hospital care is no longer needed
- The effective date of the beneficiary's financial liability for continued inpatient care
- The enrollee's appeal rights

The Center for Medicare and Medicaid Innovation (CMI)

As part of the Affordable Care Act, CMS created the Center for Medicare and Medicaid Innovation (CMI). The focus of CMI is to test new models that will reduce costs while maintaining or improving the quality of care for Medicare, Medicaid, and Children's Health Insurance Program (CHIP) beneficiaries.

Currently the CMI is requesting new ideas that it can evaluate on the basis of potential improvements in quality of care and spending reductions. The best proposals are evaluated against CMI criteria and then tested to see whether they can achieve three critical goals. These three goals are (1) better care for people; (2) coordinating care to improve health outcomes for patients; and (3) exploring community care models to improve public health. Ideas that do not pass these criteria are terminated. Successful models that meet cost and quality tests may be expanded to all Medicare, Medicaid, or CHIPs.

Physician Review of Medical Records

Physician reviewers conduct medical record review to determine whether the care received was medically necessary and appropriate. Reviews may include utilization, coding, or quality of care issues. The reviewer is generally from the same specialty as the physician who provided the care. This peer review is an important component of the quality-of-care oversight provided by Medicare quality improvement organizations and external quality review organizations.

Physician Quality Reporting System (PQRS)

The Physician Quality Reporting System (PQRS) provides a financial incentive to eligible professionals (EPs) for voluntarily reporting data on specific quality measures for covered services furnished to Medicare beneficiaries. Initially, professionals who successfully reported a minimum number of quality measures on claims for services provided earned an incentive equivalent to 1.5% of the total allowed charges during the reporting period. For more information on the PQRS and to view a report summarizing the experience of EPs in the PQRS, as well as trends over time, visit the Evolve site.

Medicare Billing Fraud

You might ask yourself, "Where does Medicare billing fraud happen?" The answer is, "It can happen anywhere medicine is practiced." Medicare fraud can involve billing for tests or procedures that were never done, billing for a more complicated procedure than was actually done, or billing a multiple-procedure operation as if several separate procedures were performed. But how do you recognize Medicare Billing Fraud? First, you have to know the rules, and these rules are complex, confusing, and constantly changing.

It is possible to misinterpret a rule—this happens a lot, so you must be careful. It may initially appear as if the individual is guilty of Medicare billing fraud, when all that actually happened was failure to understand a regulation. But some people break the rules intentionally. This is what should be reported, and there are Medicare hotlines posted in most healthcare facilities for this purpose. If you work in a place as either staff or provider and you see potential Medicare billing fraud, you have an obligation to put a stop to it or report it accordingly.

When reporting fraud, follow the procedures posted in your facility or in the facility's procedure manual. Additionally, there is a wealth of information on the Internet—both on the CMS website and on the medicare.gov/ website. Additionally, you can access the CMS Fraud and Abuse fact sheet on the Evolve site.

Clinical Laboratory Improvement Amendments Program

Congress established the **Clinical Laboratory Improvement Amendments (CLIA)** program in 1988 to regulate quality standards for all laboratory tests performed on humans to ensure the safety, accuracy, reliability, and timeliness of patient test results regardless of where a test was performed. CMS assumes primary responsibility for financial management operations of the CLIA program. Although all clinical laboratories must be properly certified to receive Medicare or Medicaid payments, CLIA has no direct Medicare or Medicaid program responsibilities.

To enroll in the CLIA program, laboratories (including laboratories located in physician offices) first must register by completing an application, paying a fee, being surveyed if applicable, and becoming certified. CLIA fees are structured according to the type of certificate requested by the laboratory on the basis of the complexity of the tests it performs. After all these preliminary measures are taken, the laboratory is issued an 11-digit CLIA certificate number. This information is significant to the health insurance professional because the 11-digit CLIA certificate number must appear in Block 23 of the CMS-1500 form for Medicare claims when laboratory services have been performed in a physician office laboratory. To keep current on the latest CLIA regulations and guidance, visit the Evolve site.

❓ What Did You Learn?

1. Define a "quality review study."
2. What is the purpose of PROs?
3. Name the three goals of CMI.
4. What is the best practice for reporting Medicare fraud?
5. Where on the CMS-1500 form is the CLIA number entered?

SUMMARY CHECKPOINTS

▶ Medicare is a comprehensive federal insurance program established by Congress in 1966 to provide limited healthcare to people age 65, certain categories of disabled individuals younger than age 65, and individuals of any age who have ESRD. Medicare is administered by CMS.

▶ *Medicare Part A* (hospital insurance) helps pay for medically necessary services for the following types of healthcare:
  • Inpatient hospital care
  • Inpatient care in SNFs
  • Home healthcare
  • Hospice care

▶ *Medicare Part B* is medical insurance financed by a combination of federal government funds and beneficiary premiums, which helps pay for
  • medically necessary physicians' services (including clinic services),
  • outpatient hospital services,
  • DME, and
  • certain other services/supplies not covered by Part A.

▶ *Medicare Part C* (Medicare Advantage, formerly Medicare+Choice) is a managed healthcare structure that offers regular Part A and Part B Medicare coverage and other services. Primary Medicare Part C plans include
  • Medicare managed care plans;
  • Medicare private, unrestricted fee-for-service plans; and
  • MSA plans.

▶ Medicare Part C not only includes Part A and Part B coverage but also pays for services not covered under the original Medicare plan, such as preventive care, prescription drugs, eyeglasses, hearing aids, and dental care.

▶ As of January 2006, *Medicare Part D* (Prescription Drug Plan) will pay a portion of prescription drug expenses and cost sharing for qualifying individuals.

▶ *Medi-Medi* applies to individuals who qualify for benefits under both the Medicare and Medicaid Programs, sometimes referred to as dual eligibles. Most individuals who qualify for Medi-Medi coverage are low-income elderly and individuals younger than 65 with disabilities.

▶ *Medigap* is a Medicare supplement insurance policy sold by private insurance companies to fill "gaps" in the original (fee-for-service) Medicare plan coverage. There are 10 standardized plans. Medigap policies work only with original Medicare.

▶ *Medicare Secondary Payer (MSP)* is the term used when Medicare is not responsible for payment of healthcare charges first, because the beneficiary is covered under another insurance policy. Medicare is a secondary payer when the beneficiary is covered by group insurance, Workers' Compensation, VA, or other third-party liability applies.

▶ Advantages of Medicare HMOs include the following:
  • HMOs often do not health screen; enrollment may not be denied because of health status.
  • HMOs may cover services that traditional Medicare does not cover; enrollees do not need Medigap insurance.
  • There is limited or no paperwork to deal with; enrollees do not have to pay the Medicare deductibles and coinsurance.

▶ Disadvantages of Medicare HMOs include the following:
  • Choice of healthcare providers and medical facilities is limited.
  • Members are covered only for services received through the HMO except in emergency and urgent care situations.
  • Prior approval from a primary care physician is usually necessary for a specialist's services, surgical procedures, medical equipment, and other healthcare services.
  • Enrollees who travel out of the HMO's service area do not receive coverage except in emergency and urgent care situations.

▶ For a service or procedure to be determined *medically necessary* under Medicare guidelines, it must meet the following criteria:
  • Consistent with the symptoms or diagnosis of the illness or injury being treated
  • Necessary and consistent with generally accepted professional medical standards
  • Not furnished primarily for the convenience of the patient or physician
  • Furnished at the most appropriate level that can be provided safely to the patient

▶ The ABN is a form that Medicare requires all healthcare providers to use when Medicare does not pay for a service to ensure that beneficiaries have a choice about their healthcare in the event that Medicare does not pay.

▶ The health insurance professional must use the Medicare fee schedule to determine the amount that Medicare allows PARs and nonPARs accepting assignment to charge a patient for a particular service or procedure. Medicare PARs use the amount shown under the heading "PAR." NonPARs can charge the amount under the column heading "NonPAR." The limiting charge for providers *not accepting* assignment is the amount under the heading "Limiting," which is 15% more than the nonPAR amount.

▶ A *small provider* is defined as follows:
- A provider of services—as that term is defined in section 1861[u] of the Social Security Act—with fewer than 25 FTE employees
- A physician, practitioner, facility, or supplier that is not otherwise a provider under section 1861 [u] with fewer than 10 FTE employees

▶ An MSN is an easy-to-read statement sent to the patient that lists Part A and B claims information, including what Medicare paid and the patient's deductible status. A Medicare RA is the document Medicare sends to the provider of services that explains how claims were adjudicated. The RA contains detailed processing information including claims adjustment reason codes, which tell why an adjustment was made to the claim payment, and remittance remark codes, which represent nonfinancial information. The health insurance professional must be able to decipher these codes to understand why the payment is less than that shown on the claim.

▶ Any Medicare provider (PAR or nonPAR) who submits electronic claims can receive an ERA or allow a billing agent (billing service, clearinghouse) to receive ERAs on its behalf. The provider receives a paper Medicare check and SPR just as before. The check number appears on paper and electronic versions of the RA.

▶ Medicare payments can be automatically deposited to a provider's designated bank account using EFT. With EFT, each transaction is assigned a unique number, which functions the same way as a Medicare check number. EFT is instantaneous, allowing funds to become immediately available for practice or other expenses.

▶ Quality review studies are performed to (1) improve the processes and outcomes of patient care; (2) safeguard the integrity of the Medicare trust fund by ensuring payments are made only for medically necessary services; and (3) investigate beneficiary complaints.

▶ The health insurance professional has an obligation to report suspected Medicare billing fraud. He or she should be familiar with the rules for billing Medicare in order to identify fraud. When reporting fraud, the professional should follow the procedures posted in the facility or in the facility's procedure manual. There is also a lot of information on this topic on the Internet.

▶ The CLIA Program was established to set quality standards for all laboratory testing to ensure the safety, accuracy, reliability, and timeliness of patient test results regardless of where a test was performed.

CLOSING SCENARIO

Rita was relieved yet satisfied after completing the chapter on Medicare. As she had anticipated at the beginning, there was a lot to learn. Each evening after class, Grandma Nan had waited up for Rita, and they talked about what the lesson had been about that day. Grandma Nan's interest inspired Rita to listen closely, take detailed notes, and ask questions when she did not understand a particular concept. Soon, Rita found herself caught up in Medicare's challenges.

Rita became a big help to Grandma Nan and her elderly friends. When one of them brought over a Medicare Summary Notice, Rita went through it with them, explaining each detail line by line. She also was able to explain the concept of "medically necessary" and the fact that Medicare pays only 80% of "covered" charges—not *all* services and supplies. The light of understanding in their eyes was the only reward Rita needed, and she decided then and there that she wanted to work in a medical facility specializing in the treatment of elderly patients. Rita believed that she could establish a rapport with elderly patients similar to the one she had with Grandma Nan and her friends.

WEBSITES TO EXPLORE

- For live links to the following websites, please visit the Evolve site at
  http://evolve.elsevier.com/Beik/today/
- For extensive information on Medicare, log on to
  http://www.medicare.gov/
- National Medicare Coverage Policies are found on the following website:
  http://cms.hhs.gov/

- For more information about CMS log on to
  http://www.cms.hhs.gov/home/aboutcms.asp
- To peruse an issue of The CMS Quarterly Provider Update, log on to www.cms.hhs.gov/QuarterlyProviderUpdates/
- To view the NUCC step-by-step claims completion guidelines, visit
  http://www.justcms1500forms.com/files/claim_form_manual_v3-0_7-07.pdf
- The Medicare Coverage Issues Manual is searchable on the following:
  http://cms.hhs.gov/

- For information on how to submit MSP claims electronically, log on to the following website: http://www.ansi.org/ for the American National Standards Institute (ANSI) ASC X12N Implementation Guide
- Or for the National Standard Format (NSF) Specifications log on to http://www.hipaanet.com/hisb_nsf.htm
- For instructions on how to read the beneficiary MSN, log on to the following website: http://www.medicare.gov/Basics/SummaryNotice_HowToRead.asp
- Information on filing complaints for Medicare beneficiaries is available at www.medicare.gov/Publications/Pubs/pdf/10050.pdf
- For more information on CLIA, log on to the CMS website at http://www.cms.hhs.gov/ and click on CLIA in the left-hand column
- To view the electronic version of the "Medicare & You Handbook" log on to http://www.medicare.gov/Publications/Pubs/pdf/10050.pdf

Author's Note: If any of these URLs are unable to be found, use applicable guide words in your Internet search for acquiring additional information on the various subjects listed.

REFERENCES AND RESOURCES

Centers for Medicare and Medicaid Services: *Original Medical (Fee-for-service) Appeal/Overview.* Last modified 10/12/2011. http://www.cms.gov/OrgMedFFSAppeals/.

Mapping the Future: 2010: U.S. & Pan Russian Censuses—The first Baby Boomers turn 65. http://mappingthefuture.csis.org/10population.html/.

U.S. Department of Health and Human Services, Centers for Medicare and Medicaid Services: *Claim Status Request and Response.* Last modified December 14, 2005. http://www.cms.hhs.gov/ElectronicBillingEDITrans/10_ClaimStatus.asp#TopOfPage/.

U.S. Department of Health and Human Services, Centers for Medicare and Medicaid Services: *Electronic Health Care Claims.* Last modified September 17, 2009. http://www.cms.hhs.gov/ElectronicBillingEDITrans/08_HealthCareClaims.asp/.

U.S. Department of Health and Human Services, Centers for Medicare and Medicaid Services: *Form CMS-1500: Processing Manual.* http://www.medicarenhic.com/providers/pubs/CMS_1500_Claim_Form.pdf/.

U.S. Department of Health and Human Services, Centers for Medicare and Medicaid Services: *Medicare & You Handbook 2009,* Baltimore, March CMS Publication No. 10050.

CHAPTER 10

Military Carriers

Chapter Outline

I. Military Health Programs
II. TRICARE
   A. Military Health System
   B. TRICARE Management Activity (TMA)
   C. TRICARE Regional Contractors
   D. Who Is Eligible for TRICARE?
   E. Who Is Not Eligible for TRICARE?
   F. Losing TRICARE Eligibility
   G. TRICARE Program Options
   H. TRICARE Overseas Program (TOP)
   I. TRICARE Young Adult (TYA) Program
   J. What TRICARE Pays
III. TRICARE's Additional Programs
   A. TRICARE Dental Programs
     1. TRICARE Standard Nonavailability Statement
   B. Supplemental TRICARE Programs
     1. Exceptional Family Member Program
     2. TRICARE Plus
   C. TRICARE and Other Health Insurance (OHI)
   D. TRICARE Standard Supplemental Insurance
   E. TRICARE For Life
     1. TRICARE for Life Eligibility
IV. Verifying TRICARE Eligibility
V. TRICARE-Authorized Providers
   A. TRICARE PARs and NonPARs
VI. Cost Sharing
   A. TRICARE Coding and Payment System
VII. TRICARE Claims Processing
   A. Who Submits Claims

   B. Submitting Paper Claims
     1. Electronic Claims Submission
   C. Deadline for Submitting Claims
   D. TRICARE Explanation of Benefits
VIII. CHAMPVA
   A. Extending Eligibility
   B. Identifying CHAMPVA-Eligible Beneficiaries
   C. CHAMPVA Benefits
   D. CHAMPVA Cost Sharing
   E. Prescription Drug Benefit
   F. CHAMPVA In-house Treatment Initiative (CIT)
   G. CHAMPVA-TRICARE Connection
     1. Types of Health Insurance Plans Primary to CHAMPVA
   H. CHAMPVA-Medicare Connection
   I. CHAMPVA and HMO Coverage
   J. CHAMPVA Providers
   K. CHAMPVA For Life (CFL)
     1. CFL Eligibility
IX. Filing CHAMPVA Claims
   A. CHAMPVA Preauthorization Requirements
   B. CHAMPVA Claims Filing Deadlines
X. Instructions for Completing TRICARE/CHAMPVA Paper Claim Forms
   A. Claims Filing Summary
   B. CHAMPVA Explanation of Benefits
   C. Claims Appeals and Reconsiderations
XI. HIPAA and Military Insurers

↻ OPENING SCENARIO

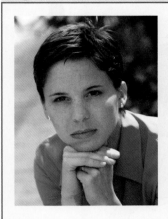

Sally Curtis is looking forward to the chapter on military insurers. She comes from a long line of military people. Both her parents are in the Army Reserves, her uncle is currently a Marine stationed in Iraq, her maternal grandfather was a Green Beret, and her great-grandfather was stationed in England during World War II. Until now, Sally was not even aware that the military had their own insurance. During a family discussion, a lot of questions about TRICARE and CHAMPVA that Sally could not answer were raised.

Sally's Aunt Betty said she was aware that there were three plans available to spouses and dependents of active service members, but she did not know which was the best plan for her. The health insurance professional working where Aunt Betty received her healthcare was of little help because she did not know much about military insurance either, and Aunt Betty wonders whether her claims were handled properly. "She calls it CHAMPUS," Aunt Betty said, "not TRICARE. What's the difference?" Sally promised her family members that she would be able to give them the answers they were looking for after she had completed Chapter 10.

CHAPTER OBJECTIVES

After completion of this chapter, the student should be able to:

1. Discuss the role of the Military Health Program.
2. Outline the TRICARE program, including eligibility and enrollment options.
3. Describe TRICARE's supplemental programs.
4. Explain the process of verifying TRICARE eligibility.
5. Distinguish between TRICARE PARs and nonPARs.
6. Recap TRICARE's cost-sharing requirements.
7. Describe the TRICARE claims process.
8. Explain the CHAMPVA program, including eligibility.
9. Discuss what the Department of Defense has done to implement HIPAA's privacy rules.

CHAPTER TERMS

accepting assignment
balance bill
catastrophic cap (cat cap)
certificate of credible coverage
CHAMPUS Maximum
    Allowable Charge
CHAMPVA for Life (CFL)
Civilian Health and Medical
    Program of the Department
    of Veterans Affairs
    (CHAMPVA)
Civilian Health and Medical
    Program of the Uniformed
    Services (CHAMPUS)
claims processor
custodial care
covered charges
Defense Enrollment Eligibility
    Reporting System (DEERS)
eZ TRICARE

Military Health System
military treatment facility
    (MTF)
nonavailability statement
    (NAS)
other health insurance
    (OHI)
regional contractor
sponsor
TRICARE
TRICARE for Life (TFL)
TRICARE Management
    Activity
TRICARE Supplemental
    Insurance
TRICARE allowable
    charge
XPressClaim

MILITARY HEALTH PROGRAMS

The federal government has provided healthcare for the military from the earliest years of U.S. history. In 1884 Congress requested that Army medical officers and surgeons attend to the families of the officers and soldiers free of charge whenever possible. During World War II, Congress authorized the creation of the Emergency Maternal and Infant Care Program, which provided maternity care and care of infants up to 1 year of age for wives and children of service members. During the Korean War, in 1956, the Dependents Medical Care Act became law. The 1966 amendments to this law initiated what later became the **Civilian Health and Medical Program of the Uniformed Services (CHAMPUS)**, a military healthcare program that existed for more than 30 years, until it was replaced with TRICARE in 1998.

TRICARE

TRICARE (TRI because it offers three different plans) is a worldwide healthcare system for the military. This wide-ranging program combines resources of the uniformed services and supplements them with networks of civilian healthcare professionals, institutions, pharmacies, and suppliers to give enrollees access to cost-efficient, high-quality healthcare. TRICARE serves nearly 10 million beneficiaries worldwide, including National Guard and Reserve members, retirees, their families, survivors, and certain former spouses. The TRICARE program is managed by **TRICARE Management Activity (TMA)** under the authority of the U.S. Assistant Secretary of Defense (Health Affairs). TRICARE is organized into six geographic parts: West, North, and South regions, and three overseas "areas": Eurasia-Africa, Latin America and Canada, and the Pacific Areas (Fig. 10-1). Each region/area has its own regional office and regional contractor. Each region/area:

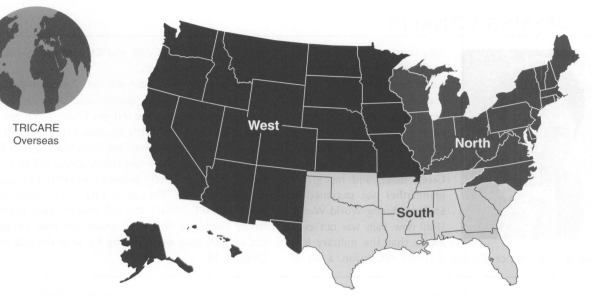

Fig. 10-1 TRICARE healthcare service regional map. (From U.S. Department of Defense, TRICARE Management Activity.)

- provides oversight of operations and health plan administration at the regional level;
- manages the contracts with regional contractors;
- supports Military Treatment Facility (MTF) Commanders;
- develops business plans for non-MTF areas (e.g., remote areas); and
- funds regional initiatives to enhance and improve delivery of healthcare.

Military Health System

Military Health System (MHS) is the name for the total healthcare infrastructure of the U.S. uniformed services under which TRICARE operates. Its mission is "to enhance the Department of Defense (DOD) and our Nation's security by providing health support for the full range of military operations and sustaining the health of all those entrusted to our care." The MHS includes **military treatment facilities (MTFs)** and various programs, such as TRICARE, within the civilian population. MTFs are clinics or hospitals operated by the DoD, located on military bases that provide care to military personnel, retirees, and dependents. The MHS provides cost-effective, quality medical care through a network of providers, MTFs, medical clinics, and dental clinics worldwide.

TRICARE Management Activity (TMA)

Since February 1998, TMA has administered the TRICARE healthcare program through the MHS. The mission of TMA is to manage TRICARE—the medical and dental programs under which members of the uniformed services, their dependents, and other beneficiaries are entitled to DoD healthcare. TMA also supports the military departments in

Source: http://www.fhpr.osd.mil/pdfs/MHS%20QDR%20Medical%20Transformation%20Roadmap.pdf

implementing its medical mission to provide, and to maintain readiness to provide, medical and dental services to members of the Armed Forces during military operations.

Like the activities of all government agencies, TMA is updated frequently, and the health insurance professional should be aware of these updates. To keep abreast of changes, visit the Evolve site.

TRICARE Regional Contractors

As mentioned, TRICARE is administered on a regional basis. Each region is headed by a **regional contractor** whose responsibility it is to provide beneficiaries with healthcare services and support in addition to what services are available at MTFs. These responsibilities include:

- Establishing provider networks
- Operating TRICARE Service Centers
- Providing customer service call centers
- Providing administrative support, e.g., enrollment, care authorization, claims processing
- Distributing educational information to beneficiaries and providers

Who is Eligible for TRICARE?

Like recipients of Medicaid and Medicare, TRICARE-eligible individuals are referred to as "beneficiaries." The service member, whether in active duty, retired, or deceased, is called the **sponsor**. The sponsor's relationship to the beneficiary (spouse, child, parent) creates eligibility under TRICARE. In addition, to be eligible for TRICARE, an individual must be registered in the **Defense Enrollment Eligibility Reporting System (DEERS)**. DEERS is a global computerized database of uniformed services members, their family members, and others who are eligible for military benefits. Enrollment in DEERS is the key to using TRICARE benefits. All sponsors are automatically registered in DEERS when they enter the military; however, it is the sponsor's responsibility to register eligible family members. Family members can update personal information such as addresses and phone numbers once they are registered.

TRICARE-eligible individuals can be classified into the following main categories:

- Active duty service members (ADSMs), who are automatically enrolled in TRICARE Prime;
- Spouses and unmarried children of ADSMs (active duty family members [ADFMs])
- Uniformed service retirees, their spouses, and unmarried children
- Medal of Honor recipients
- Unremarried former spouses and unmarried children of active duty or retired service members who have died

For more details regarding TRICARE-eligible individuals, visit the Evolve site.

Who Is Not Eligible for TRICARE?

Categories of individuals *not* eligible for TRICARE include the following:

- Most individuals who are 65 years or older and eligible for Medicare (except active duty family members). Individuals younger than 65 who are eligible for Medicare because of a disability or end-stage renal disease (ESRD) may retain eligibility until age 65 but must be enrolled in Medicare Part B.
- Parents and parents-in-law of ADSMs or uniformed services retirees or of deceased ADSMs or retirees. They may, however, be able to receive treatment in military medical facilities if space permits.
- Individuals who are eligible for benefits under the Civilian Health and Medical Program of the Department of Veterans Affairs (CHAMPVA) are not eligible for TRICARE.
- Any other person not enrolled in DEERS.

⭐ Imagine This!

Alan Workman is a Marine serving on active duty in Iraq. He has a wife and two children (2 and 7 years old) at home in the United States. In this scenario, TRICARE considers Alan the sponsor, and his wife and two children are the beneficiaries.

Losing TRICARE Eligibility

Eligibility for TRICARE may end for the following reasons:

- Sponsor separates from active duty; that is, he or she "gets out" of the military before retiring.
- Beneficiary becomes entitled to Medicare Part A but does not purchase Medicare Part B.
- Dependent child reaches age limit: Children remain eligible for TRICARE coverage up to age 21 years, or age

23 years if enrolled in college full time and the sponsor continues to provide 50% of the child's financial support. Children ages 23-26 years who are not married and not eligible for their own employer-sponsored health insurance may qualify for TRICARE Young Adult, on the basis of the sponsor's eligibility for TRICARE

- Divorce: A former spouse loses eligibility unless he or she meets specific requirements to maintain eligibility as a former spouse.
- Surviving spouse, widow, or former spouse remarries.
- DEERS information is not kept up to date: If eligibility is lost due to inaccurate or outdated information, simply updating the information restores coverage.

Note: The preceding list is not intended to be all-inclusive.

Upon loss of TRICARE eligibility, each member automatically receives a **certificate of credible coverage**, which serves as evidence of prior healthcare coverage under TRICARE, so that the individual cannot be excluded from a new health plan because of preexisting conditions.

TRICARE Program Options

Depending on the category and location of the beneficiary, he or she may be eligible for different program options. These options may change when the enrollee travels or moves, or when he or she becomes entitled to Medicare Part A, discussed later in this chapter. See Table 10-1 for details on TRICARE program options. Table 10-2 provides program information on the TRICARE programs—the type of program, enrollment and fees, and provider choice.

TRICARE Overseas Program (TOP)

TRICARE Overseas Program (TOP) has one overseas region consisting of three areas: TRICARE Eurasia-Africa, TRICARE Pacific, and TRICARE Latin America/Canada (TLAC) including the Caribbean basin. TOP provides health benefits to beneficiaries living and traveling overseas while they are eligible for TRICARE. TOP allows for significant cultural differences unique to foreign countries and their healthcare practices. The TRICARE Area Office (TAO) Director is responsible for the overall management of TOP. For more detailed information on this program, along with coverage options, visit the Evolve site.

TRICARE Young Adult (TYA) Program

Beginning May of 2011, adult children of military members and retirees younger than 26 years who are unmarried and are not eligible for their own employer-sponsored health care coverage may become eligible to purchase TRICARE Young Adult (TYA) Program coverage as long as their sponsor is still eligible for TRICARE. Initially, TRICARE Standard was the only TYA option; however, TRICARE Prime became another option for TYA enrollees effective October 1, 2011—the beginning of the federal government's new fiscal year. To use Prime, however, qualifying young adults must live in areas where a TRICARE managed-care network is available.

TABLE 10-1	TRICARE Program Options
BENEFICIARY TYPE	**PROGRAM OPTIONS**
Active duty service members (ADSMs) (Includes National Guard and Reserve members activated for more than 30 consecutive days)	TRICARE Prime TRICARE Prime Remote TRICARE Active Duty Dental Program
Active duty family members (ADFMs) (Includes family members of National Guard and Reserve members activated for more than 30 consecutive days and certain survivors)	TRICARE Prime TRICARE Prime Remote for Active Duty Family Members (TPRADFM) TRICARE Standard TRICARE Extra TRICARE For Life (TFL) (ADFMs must have Medicare Part B to participate in TFL) US Family Health Plan TRICARE Dental Program
Retired service members and eligible family members, survivors, Medal of Honor recipients, qualified former spouses, and others	TRICARE Prime TRICARE Standard TRICARE Extra TFL (if entitled to premium-free Medicare Part A on basis of age, disability, or end-stage renal disease, the beneficiary must have Medicare Part B to keep TRICARE eligibility) US Family Health Plan TRICARE Retiree Dental Program
National Guard and Reserve members and their family members (Qualified non–active duty members of the Selected Reserve, Retired Reserve, and certain members of the Individual Ready Reserve)	TRICARE Reserve Select (members of the Selected Reserve) TRICARE Retired Reserve (members of the Retired Reserve younger than 60 years) TRICARE Dental Program TRICARE Retiree Dental Program

"TRICARE" is a registered trademark of the TRICARE Management Activity. All rights reserved.

Monthly premiums for both Standard and Prime are considerably higher than what a military family typically pays to enroll in TRICARE. Cost shares, deductibles, and catastrophic cap protection are based on the sponsor's status and the type of coverage selected.

What TRICARE Pays

Like most insurers, TRICARE pays for only *allowed* services, supplies, and procedures, which are referred to as **covered charges**. TRICARE's covered charges include medical and psychological services and supplies that are considered appropriate care and are generally accepted by qualified professionals to be reasonable and adequate for the diagnosis and treatment of illness, injury, pregnancy, or mental disorders or for well-child care.

TRICARE's allowable charge, also known as the **CHAMPUS Maximum Allowable Charge (CMAC)**, is the amount on which TRICARE figures a beneficiary's cost share (coinsurance) for covered charges. TRICARE calculates this allowable charge by looking at all professional (noninstitutional) providers' fees for the same or similar services nationwide over the past year, with adjustments for specific localities. If the health insurance professional does not know what the allowable charge is for a particular service or supply, he or she can telephone the regional claims processor for this information or consult the TRICARE provider handbook. It is advisable to keep a current copy of the handbook on file for information regarding TRICARE billing and claims submission guidelines.

> ### 🗂 HIPAA Tip
>
> TRICARE/CHAMPVA beneficiaries and providers of care benefit from HIPAA in the following ways:
> - Improves uniformity and efficiency of communication among providers
> - Increases protection of patients' private, personal health information
> - Makes transferring enrollment between plans easier

> ### 💬 What Did You Learn?
>
> 1. List the 3 TRICARE regions and 3 overseas areas.
> 2. What is the Military Health System's mission?
> 3. What are the regional contractor's responsibilities?
> 4. What categories of people are eligible for TRICARE?
> 5. Name the 3 main TRICARE coverage options.
> 6. What does TRICARE pay?

TRICARE'S ADDITIONAL PROGRAMS

The three basic program options under TRICARE are TRICARE Standard, TRICARE Extra, and TRICARE Prime (Fig. 10-2). To use TRICARE Extra or TRICARE Prime, the individual receiving care must live in an area where these options are available and a civilian provider network has been established to support these plans. It is important to keep in mind that active duty, guard, and reserve members are automatically enrolled in TRICARE Prime. Military retirees and their dependents must choose the option that best suits their needs.

TRICARE Dental Programs

TRICARE also offers dental programs for both active duty and retirees. The TRICARE Active Duty Dental Program (ADDP) is available to eligible active duty service members who are either referred for care by a dental treatment facility

TABLE 10-2   **TRICARE Program Descriptions**

PROGRAM	TYPE OF PROGRAM	ENROLLMENT AND FEES	MEDICAL PROVIDER CHOICE
TRICARE Prime	Similar to a managed care or health maintenance organization option available in specific geographic areas	Enrollment required Retirees, their families, survivors, and qualifying former spouses pay annual enrollment fees Offers lowest out-of-pocket costs	Most care provided by primary care manager (PCM) at a military treatment facility (MTF) or within the TRICARE network PCM referrals required for most specialty care
TRICARE Prime Remote (includes TPRADFM)	Benefit similar to those of TRICARE Prime for active duty service members living and working in remote locations and the eligible family members residing with them	Enrollment required No annual enrollment fee Offers same low out-of-pocket costs as TRICARE Prime	Care provided by TRICARE network providers (or a TRICARE-authorized provider if a network provider is unavailable)
TRICARE Standard	Fee-for-service option available worldwide	No enrollment required No annual enrollment fee or enrollment applications Annual deductibles and cost shares apply	Care provided by TRICARE-authorized non-network providers No referrals required Some services require prior authorization May enroll in TRICARE Plus where available
TRICARE Extra	Preferred provider option in areas with established TRICARE networks Not available overseas	No enrollment required No annual enrollment fee or enrollment applications Annual deductibles and discounted cost shares apply	Care provided by TRICARE network providers No referrals required Some services require prior authorization
TRICARE Reserve Select (TRS)	Premium-based health care plan that qualified National Guard and Reserve members may purchase Available worldwide Offers member-only and member-and-family coverage	Member must qualify for and purchase TRS to participate Monthly premiums, annual deductibles, and cost shares apply	Care provided by any TRICARE-authorized provider (network or non-network) No referrals required Some services require prior authorization
TRICARE Retired Reserve (TRR)	Premium-based health care plan that qualified Retired Reserve members may purchase Available worldwide Offers member-only and member-and-family coverage	Member must qualify for and purchase TRR to participate Monthly premiums, annual deductibles, and cost shares apply	Care provided by any TRICARE-authorized provider (network or non-network) No referrals required Some services require prior authorization
TRICARE For Life	TRICARE's Medicare-wraparound coverage available to all Medicare-eligible TRICARE beneficiaries, regardless of age, provided they have Medicare Part A and Medicare Part B	No enrollment fees Must be entitled to premium-free Medicare Part A and have purchased Medicare Part B	Care provided by Medicare providers TRICARE Pharmacy Home Delivery option may be used to meet prescription needs Beneficiary may enroll in TRICARE Plus where available
US Family Health Plan (USFHP)	TRICARE Prime managed care option available through networks of community-based, not-for-profit health care systems in six areas of the United States	Enrollment required Depending on the health care system, enrollment fees may apply	Care provided by primary care providers in the health care system in which members are enrolled Primary care providers will refer for specialty care

Topic	TRICARE Prime	TRICARE Extra	TRICARE Standard
Definition	TRICARE Prime is a managed care option similar to a health maintenance organization (HMO).	TRICARE Extra is similar to a preferred provider organization (PPO) where the beneficiary selects from a network of providers.	TRICARE Standard has the same benefits and cost shares as the former CHAMPUS.
Cost vs. Choice	Least out-of-pocket costs with some restrictions on freedom of choice.	Copayment 5% less than TRICARE Standard and no deductible when using the retail network pharmacy.	Highest out-of-pocket costs with the greatest degree of freedom to choose healthcare providers.

Fig. 10-2 TRICARE's three options. (From U.S. Department of Defense, TRICARE Management Activity.)

(DTF) to a civilian dentist or have a duty location and live more than 50 miles from a DTF. ADSMs enrolled in Prime Remote are automatically eligible to use the Remote ADDP. National Guard and Reserve members are eligible only if they have active duty orders issued for a period of more than 30 consecutive days.

The TRICARE Retiree Dental Program (TRDP) is available to retired service members and their eligible family members, including retired National Guard and Reserve members. Enrollees must satisfy an initial 12-month enrollment period in order to become eligible for the full scope of benefits. New retirees who elect to enroll within 4 months after retirement are eligible for a waiver of this 12-month waiting period.

For detailed information on TRICARE health plan options, visit the Evolve site.

TRICARE Standard Nonavailability Statement

As discussed previously, military personnel and their TRI-CARE-eligible dependents typically receive healthcare at an MTF. If the needed treatment is unavailable at an MTF and it becomes necessary for the individual to seek treatment in a civilian hospital, he or she sometimes must obtain a **nonavailability statement (NAS)**. An NAS is certification from a military hospital stating that it cannot provide the care that a TRICARE beneficiary needs. If the beneficiary does not get an NAS before receiving inpatient care from a civilian source, TRICARE may not share the costs. The NAS system is now automated. This means that instead of sending a paper copy of the NAS in with the TRICARE claim, the MTF enters the NAS electronically into the DEERS computer files.

Even though an outpatient NAS is no longer required for outpatient procedures (except in specific situations, e.g., maternity), the beneficiary must obtain advance authorization

to undergo any procedures. Healthcare providers—whether or not they participate in TRICARE Standard—are required to obtain these advance authorizations. To learn more about this topic, visit the Evolve site.

📁 HIPAA Tip

HIPAA privacy applies to individually identifiable health information, including paper, electronic, and oral communications. This also applies to information that identifies the patient and relates to his or her past, present, or future health condition.

⭐ Imagine This!

In February 2003 Kim Sun Hwa, a TRICARE Standard enrollee, sought care for a serious cardiac condition at the MTF near the town where she lived. The MTF did not have the facilities to perform the needed quadruple-bypass surgery and referred her to Genesis Cardiac and Rehabilitation Center 150 miles away. The MTF filed a nonavailability statement with DEERS; however, the health insurance professional at Genesis advised Kim that an NAS was no longer necessary for beneficiaries enrolled in TRICARE Standard. After the procedure, Kim experienced postsurgical depression and returned to Genesis for outpatient psychotherapy. Because she did not need an NAS from the MTF for her surgery, Kim assumed she would not need an NAS for the treatment of her mental health condition; however, without the NAS, TRICARE refused the second claim.

Supplemental TRICARE Programs

TRICARE offers supplemental programs tailored specifically to beneficiary health concerns or conditions. Many of these programs have specific eligibility requirements based on beneficiary category, plan, or status. They include health promotion programs such as alcohol education, smoking cessation, and weight loss. Some are for specific populations, such as the Foreign Force Member Health Care Option and the Pre-activation Benefit for National Guard and Reserve. Other programs are for certain health conditions, such as the Cancer Clinical Trials. Many programs are limited to a certain number of participants or a particular geographic location. The following sections discuss two of these special programs. For detailed information on all of these special TRICARE programs, visit the Evolve site.

Exceptional Family Member Program

The Exceptional Family Member Program (EFMP) is a mandatory enrollment program based on specifically defined rules. EFMP works with other military and civilian agencies to provide comprehensive and coordinated medical, educational, housing, community support, and personnel services to families with special needs. An *exceptional family member* is a dependent, regardless of age, who requires medical services for a chronic condition; receives ongoing services from a specialist; has mental health concerns/social problems/psychological needs; receives education services provided by means of an Individual Education Program (IEP); or a family member receiving services provided through an Individual Family Services Plan (IFSP). To learn more about EFMP, visit the Evolve site.

TRICARE Plus

TRICARE Plus is a military treatment facility primary care enrollment program that is offered at selected local MTFs. This program allows beneficiaries who normally are only able to get care at MTFs on a space-available basis, and who are not enrolled in a TRICARE Prime option, to enroll and receive primary care appointments at the MTF within the same primary care access standards as beneficiaries enrolled in a TRICARE Prime option. Non-enrollment in TRICARE Plus does not affect TRICARE For Life benefits or other existing programs. (TRICARE For Life is discussed later in this chapter.)

TRICARE and Other Health Insurance (OHI)

If a TRICARE-eligible beneficiary has other healthcare coverage besides TRICARE Standard, Extra, or Prime through an employer, an association, or a private insurer, or if a student in the family has a healthcare plan through his or her school, TRICARE considers this coverage to be **other health insurance (OHI)**. It also may be called *double coverage* or *coordination of benefits*. Any OHI a TRICARE enrollee has in addition to TRICARE coverage is considered primary health insurance. If a TRICARE beneficiary has OHI, he or she should tell the healthcare provider and regional contractor. Keeping the regional contractor informed about OHI will allow TRICARE to better coordinate benefits and will help ensure that there is no delay in payment of claims.

TRICARE Fact: OHI does not include TRICARE supplemental insurance or Medicaid. These programs are not primary to TRICARE.

TRICARE Standard Supplemental Insurance

TRICARE Supplemental Insurance policies, similar to Medicare supplemental insurance policies, are health benefit plans designed specifically to supplement TRICARE benefits. These plans are frequently available from military associations or other private organizations. Although TRICARE supplement plans have their own rules, they generally pay most or all of whatever is left after TRICARE has paid its share of the cost of covered services and supplies. Such policies are not specifically for retirees and may be advantageous for other TRICARE-eligible families as well.

TRICARE For Life

TRICARE For Life (TFL) is TRICARE's Medicare-wraparound coverage available to all Medicare-eligible TRICARE beneficiaries regardless of age or place of residence provided that they have both Medicare Part A and Part B. Medicare is the primary insurer, but TRICARE acts as secondary payer, minimizing out-of-pocket expenses. TFL benefits include covering Medicare's coinsurance and deductible. Whether the beneficiary uses either a provider who does participate in Medicare (PAR) or one who does not (nonPAR), the provider files claims with Medicare. Medicare pays its portion first and electronically forwards the claim to the TFL claims processor. TFL pays the provider directly for TRICARE-covered services. TFL has no enrollment fees and no monthly premium cost, and is a permanent healthcare benefit for all uniformed service branches.

TRICARE For Life Eligibility

TFL is available for *all* dual TRICARE-Medicare–eligible uniformed services retirees, including:

- retired members of the Reserve Component who are in receipt of retirement pay,
- Medicare-eligible family members, and
- Medicare-eligible widows/widowers, certain former spouses, and beneficiaries younger than 65 years who are also entitled to Medicare Part A because of a disability or chronic renal disease.

Dependent parents and parents-in-law are not eligible for TRICARE Prime, Standard, or Extra or TRICARE For Life. They are eligible, however, to receive care under the sponsor's TRICARE benefits at an MTF on a space-available basis. Care received outside the MTF must be covered by another form of insurance. They may also be eligible for TRICARE Senior Pharmacy benefits if they are entitled to Medicare Part A, if they turned 65 on or after April 1, 2001, and if they are enrolled in Medicare Part B.

TRICARE Fact: ADFMs are not required to have Medicare Part B to remain eligible for TRICARE. Once the sponsor reaches age 65, Medicare Part B must be in effect no later than the sponsor's retirement date to avoid a break in TRICARE coverage.

For a more comprehensive look at TFL, visit the Evolve site.

⭐ Imagine This!

Benjamin Hudson, a dual-eligible enrollee under TRICARE and Medicare, visited Dr. Alton Simmons, an ophthalmologist, for vision problems. Benjamin subsequently opted to receive laser surgery to correct his myopia. When he received a statement for the entire fee, he telephoned the health insurance professional in Dr. Simmons' office stating that because he had Medicare and TRICARE coverage, one or the other should pay. Under the impression that an error had been made, Benjamin insisted that the claim be resubmitted; however, the health insurance professional informed him that because laser surgery was a noncovered expense under Medicare, TRICARE would not pay it either. Mr. Hudson refused to pay the bill on the grounds that the health insurance professional should have informed him that this was a noncovered service before the procedure. Dr. Simmons ultimately adjusted the charge off Benjamin's account.

❓ What Did You Learn?

1. List TRICARE's three options for healthcare.
2. Into which option are active service members automatically enrolled?
3. When is it necessary for a TRICARE beneficiary to obtain an NAS?
4. List two supplemental TRICARE program options.
5. True or false: OHI is secondary to TRICARE.
6. Who is eligible for TFL?

VERIFYING TRICARE ELIGIBILITY

Patient eligibility for TRICARE must be confirmed at the time of service; therefore, when a patient comes to the office for an appointment and informs the health insurance professional that he or she is eligible for benefits under one of the military's healthcare programs, it should be verified immediately. Ensure that the patient has a valid Common Access Card (CAC), uniformed service ID Card, or eligibility authorization letter. Dependent eligibility can be authenticated with a valid photo ID of the dependent accompanied by a copy of the sponsor's activation orders (when he/she has been activated for more than 30 consecutive days). Beneficiaries younger than 10 years are not routinely issued ID cards. The parent's proof of eligibility may serve as proof of the child's eligibility. Following are suggestions for verifying eligibility:

- Check the expiration dates on CACs and ID cards, and copy both sides of the cards.
- Because the ID card alone is not sufficient to prove eligibility, access the appropriate carrier website, e.g., www.humana-military.com/ or www.triwest.com/provider/.
- Retain a printout of the eligibility verification screen for the provider's files.
- Use the sponsor's Social Security number when verifying eligibility.

Box 10-1 describes military ID cards and how to interpret the information on them. Fig. 10-3 shows examples of military ID cards. Samples of military ID cards can also be found on the Evolve site. Box 10-2 lists some suggestions for verification of TRICARE/CHAMPUS eligibility.

❓ What Did You Learn?

1. How can TRICARE eligibility be verified?
2. What color is an ADSM's card? A military retiree's card?
3. True or false: It is illegal to copy a TRICARE ID card.

TRICARE-AUTHORIZED PROVIDERS

A *TRICARE-authorized provider* is a hospital or institutional provider, physician, or other provider of services or supplies specifically authorized to provide benefits under TRICARE. An authorized provider must have a valid state license and a national organization accreditation (if needed). Medicare-certified providers are considered TRICARE-authorized providers. TRICARE regional contractors are responsible for verifying a provider's authorized status. Beneficiaries who visit a provider who is not TRICARE-authorized are responsible for the full cost of care. Non-institutional TRICARE-authorized providers may charge more than the TRICARE maximum allowable charge for TRICARE-covered services. However, by law, they cannot charge more than 15% above the TRICARE maximum allowable charge.

Beneficiaries can contact their regional contractor to find a TRICARE-authorized provider.

There are two types of authorized providers: network and non-network. Network providers are TRICARE-authorized providers who have signed an agreement with the regional contractors to provide care at a prenegotiated rate. Additionally, network providers will file claims on the beneficiary's behalf.

Non-network providers must be certified, but they do not sign a contractual agreement with the TRICARE regional contractors. There are two types of non-network providers:

- Participating providers agree to file claims for beneficiaries, to accept payment directly from TRICARE, and to accept the TRICARE maximum allowable charge as payment in full for their services.
- Nonparticipating providers do not agree to accept the TRICARE maximum allowable charge or file beneficiary claims.

Box 10-1

Interpreting the Uniformed Services ID Card

The Uniformed Services ID card incorporates a digital photographic image of the bearer, barcodes containing pertinent machine-readable data, and printed ID and entitlement information.

ID Card Color

- Active duty family members (ADFMs): tan
- TAMP-eligible members: tan
- Retiree family members: tan
- Retirees: blue
- National Guard and Reserve family members: red

ID Card Key Fields

- SSN or Sponsor SSN (or last 4 digits of SSN)
  - Providers should use the SSN when verifying the card bearer's eligibility
- Expiration Date:

- Check the expiration date. It should read "INDEF" (i.e., indefinite) for retirees. If the card is expired, the beneficiary must immediately update his or her information in the Defense Eligibility Enrollment Recording System (DEERS) and get a new card. Eligibility for TRICARE benefits will be determined by the eligibility response received from DEERS and not from the information on the ID card.
- Civilian:
  - Check the back of the ID card to verify eligibility for TRICARE civilian care. The center section of the card should read "YES" under the box titled "CIVILIAN."
  - *Note:* If a beneficiary using TRICARE For Life (TFL) has an ID card that reads "NO" in this block, the beneficiary is still eligible for TFL if he or she has both Medicare Part A and Medicare Part B coverage.

Box 10-2

Suggestions for Verifying TRICARE/CHAMPUS Eligibility

- Ask to see a Uniformed Services ID card or a family member's Uniformed Services ID card. Anyone 10 years old or older should have a personal ID card.
- Check the back of the card for TRICARE/CHAMPUS eligibility and the expiration date.
- A Prime enrollee must show his or her Uniformed Services ID card and TRICARE Prime ID card. The Prime ID card does not specify the beneficiary's period of eligibility, so the health insurance professional needs to verify the current eligibility status by calling the beneficiary services hotline. Failure to verify eligibility may result in claim denial.
- The Prime sponsor's Social Security number is included in the 11-digit number on the Prime ID card. Verify the Prime sponsor's Social Security number with the patient. It should match the final 9 digits of the number given on the TRICARE Prime ID card.
- If you are the patient's PCM, you also should verify that you are the PCM listed on the Prime card and note the effective date of the coverage.
- In most cases, active duty personnel must seek nonemergency healthcare from their host MTF. Under certain circumstances, such as nonavailability of needed services at the MTF, active duty personnel may obtain Prime benefits from civilian providers under the Supplemental Healthcare Program. Because active duty personnel are not issued Prime ID cards, they must show their green (active duty) ID cards to verify eligibility.
- Make a copy of the front and back of all ID cards for your records.

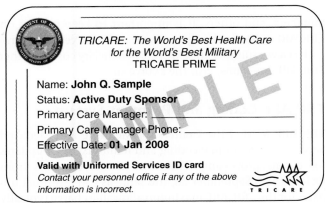

Fig. 10-3 Samples of Military ID cards. (From U.S. Department of Defense, TRICARE and Humana Military Healthcare Services.)

Non-network providers can choose to participate on a claim-by-claim basis.

TRICARE PARs and nonPARs

Healthcare providers who participate in TRICARE, also referred to as **accepting assignment**, agree to accept the **TRICARE allowable charge (TAC)** (including the cost share and deductible, if any) as payment in full for the healthcare services provided and cannot balance bill—bill for the difference between the provider's usual fee and the TRICARE allowable amount. Individual providers who do not accept assignment on all claims can participate in TRICARE on a case-by-case basis. As mentioned, nonPARs may charge up to 15% above the TAC for their services, and TRICARE beneficiaries are financially responsible for these additional charges.

PARs and nonPARs who accept assignment must file the claim for the patient, and TRICARE sends the payment (if any) directly to the provider. Hospitals that participate in Medicare, by law, also must participate in TRICARE Standard for inpatient care. For outpatient care, hospitals may choose whether or not to participate. TRICARE-authorized providers are not required to participate in the TRICARE network; however, they must be certified as authorized providers in the region where care is given.

? What Did You Learn?

1. What are the criteria for a TRICARE-authorized provider?
2. By law, a non-institutional TRICARE-authorized provider cannot charge more than _____% above the TRICARE maximum allowable charge.
3. True or false: A TRICAR PAR must accept the TAC as payment in full and cannot balance bill.

COST SHARING

Beneficiaries are responsible for cost shares and deductibles for care that is covered under TRICARE Standard. A **catastrophic cap** (cat cap) is the annual upper limit a family will have to pay for TRICARE Standard–covered services in any fiscal year. The cat cap for families of active duty service members is $1000; for all others it is $3000. The cat cap applies only to allowable charges for covered services and does not apply to services that are not covered or to the total amount of what nonPAR providers may charge above the TAC. Table 10-3 provides examples of cost shares for families who use civilian providers and facilities under each of the three TRICARE options. It should be noted that these listed fees are subject to change. Table 10-4 provides examples of cost shares for retirees (younger than 65 years), their family

TABLE 10-3	Cost Shares for Families using Civilian Providers/Facilities		
	TRICARE PRIME	**TRICARE EXTRA**	**TRICARE STANDARD**
Annual deductible	None	$150/individual or $300/family for E-5 and above $50/$100 for E-4 and below	$150/individual or $300/family for E-5 and above $50/$100 for E-4 and below
Annual enrollment fee	None	None	None
Civilian outpatient visit	No cost	15% of negotiated fee	20% of allowed charges for covered service
Civilian inpatient admission	No cost	Greater of $25/charge per admission or $15.65/day	Greater of $25/charge per admission or $15.65/day
Civilian inpatient mental health	No cost	Greater of $25/charge per admission or $20/day	Greater of $25/charge per admission or $20/day
Civilian inpatient skilled nursing facility care	$0 per diem charge per admission No separate copayment/cost share for separate billed professional charges	Greater of $25/charge per admission or $15.65/day	Greater of $25/charge per admission or $15.65/day

members, and others. It is important to keep current on TRICARE because changes may occur from year to year.

To view a summary of TRICARE beneficiary costs for other TRICARE programs, visit the Evolve site.

TRICARE Coding and Payment System

TRICARE follows the Centers for Medicare and Medicaid Services (CMS) annual coding and reimbursement updates for claims processing. TRICARE's fiscal year runs from October 1 to September 30, the same as CMS. Annual updates for the TRICARE maximum allowable charge typically occur between February 1 and April 1. New codes are usually

TABLE 10-4	Cost Shares for Retirees (< 65 Years), Family Members, and Others		
	TRICARE PRIME	**TRICARE EXTRA**	**TRICARE STANDARD**
Annual deductible	None	$150/individual or $300/family	$150/individual or $300/family
Annual enrollment fee	$230/individual $460/family	None	None
Civilian copays		20% of negotiated fee	25% of allowed charges for covered service
Outpatient emergency care mental health visit	$12 $30 $25 $17 (group visit)	20% of negotiated fee	25% of allowed charges for covered service
Civilian inpatient cost share	$11/day ($25 minimum) charge per admission	Lesser of $250/day or 25% of negotiated charges plus 20% of negotiated professional fees	Lesser of $535/day or 25% of billed charges plus 25% of allowed professional fees
Civilian inpatient skilled nursing facility care	$11/day ($25 minimum) charge per admission	$250 per diem co-payment or 20% cost-share of total charges, whichever is less, institutional services, plus 20% of cost-share of separately billed professional charges	25% cost share of allowed charges for institutional services, plus 25% cost share of allowable separately billed professional charges
Civilian inpatient mental health	$11/day ($25 minimum)	20% of institutional and negotiated professional fees	Lesser of $193/day or 25% of allowable fees

"TRICARE" is a registered trademark of the TRICARE Management Activity. All rights reserved.

implemented on January 1 to align with the Medicare implementation of new Current Procedural Terminology (CPT) codes. Other code structures, such as Healthcare Common Procedure Coding System (HCPCS) codes, are subject to a quarterly update and can undergo code and pricing changes every 3 months during the fiscal year. To view the TRICARE fee schedule/reimbursement file, which posts information on CMAC along with all other reimbursement methodologies defined for TRICARE, visit the Evolve site.

TRICARE Fact: *TRICARE Provider News* (published by the TRICARE Management Activity) is a periodical that helps keep providers up to date on TRICARE.

What Did You Learn?

1. True/false: Beneficiaries are responsible for cost shares and deductibles for care that is covered under TRICARE Standard.
2. The cat cap for families of ADSMs is _____ per year.
3. TRICARE's fiscal year runs from _____ to _____, the same as CMS's fiscal year.

TRICARE CLAIMS PROCESSING

The designated contractor who processes medical claims for care received within a particular state or region is called a **claims processor**. In some regions, such contractors are called TRICARE contractors or fiscal intermediaries (FIs). All claims processors have toll-free phone numbers to handle questions that a health insurance professional might have regarding TRICARE claims. It cannot be stressed enough that the health insurance professional should have the latest TRICARE handbook on file or should log on to the TRICARE website and download an electronic version of the handbook. In addition to the handbook, a file should be kept that has an up-to-date list of telephone numbers and addresses to assist claims processing. A copy of the *TRICARE Provider Handbook* can be downloaded from the link on the Evolve site, or a hard copy can be requested from the TRICARE contractor in the region. Changes to TRICARE programs are continually made as public law and/or federal regulations are amended, so it is important to keep up to date.

Who Submits Claims

If the patient is enrolled in TRICARE Prime and goes to a Prime provider, the provider submits the claim. After the claim is submitted, the beneficiary and provider receive an explanation of benefits (EOB) from the claims processor showing the services performed and the adjudication.

Patients using TRICARE Standard may be responsible for submitting their own claims to the appropriate claims processor, depending upon the status of the provider. If the patient has access to the Internet, the appropriate form (CHAMPUS Claim Patient Request for Medical

Payment Form 2642) can be downloaded from the TRI-CARE website. It may be necessary first to download the Adobe Reader software. Instructions for downloading and installing the software are available at the site. If they receive care from nonPARs, TRICARE Standard patients must file their own claims. In this case, the reimbursement check is sent to the patient, and it is his or her responsibility to ensure that the provider's bill is paid.

To view Form 2642, visit the Evolve site.

TRICARE requires that claims be filed electronically with the appropriate Health Insurance Portability and Accountability Act of 1996 (HIPAA)–compliant standard electronic claims format, but if a non-network provider must submit claims on paper, TRICARE requires that they be submitted on either a CMS-1500 (for professional charges) or a UB-04 (institutional charges) claim form.

Palmetto Government Business Administrators (PGBA), based in South Carolina, processes claims and provides customer service for about 65% of the nation's TRICARE claims for medical services. PGBA serves as a claims-processing subcontractor, administering the TRICARE North Region for Health Net Federal Services and the South Region for Humana Military Healthcare Services. In addition to TRICARE, PGBA processes Medicare Advantage claims.

Stop and Think

Ruth Carson is a 36-year-old teacher and a TRICARE Standard beneficiary. On March 30, she visits her family physician, Dr. Bennett, for a routine yearly examination. As Dr. Bennett's health insurance professional, you must advise Ruth that Dr. Bennett does not accept assignment on TRICARE claims and that Ruth will have to file her own claim. Ruth asks you how to file the claim. What are your instructions?

Submitting Paper Claims

TRICARE network providers are required to submit claims electronically. Non-network providers still have the option to submit paper claims; however, they are encouraged to consider the benefits of electronic filing options. Providers submitting paper claims should use the standard CMS-1500 claim form. As mentioned, patients who file their own claims must use Form 2642, which can be downloaded from the TRICARE website. If the patient files his or her own claim, the provider's detailed itemized statement and an NAS (if necessary) must be attached. Completed claims are sent to the TRICARE claims processor in the region in which the enrollee resides. Fig. 10-4

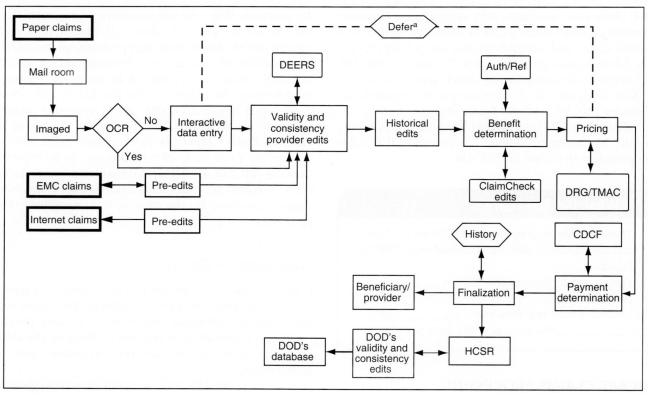

Source: GAO.

Fig. 10-4 Process that TRICARE paper claims undergo. (Source: U.S. Department of Defense, TRICARE Management Activity.)

illustrates the process that TRICARE paper claims undergo. For information on where to file paper claims, visit the Evolve site for a link to the TRICARE claims website.

Electronic Claims Submission

Like other third-party payers, TRICARE prefers claims to be filed electronically. The advantages to electronic claims filing include the following:

- Saves time by sending claims directly into the TRICARE processing system
- Saves money with no-cost or low-cost claims filing options
- Improves cash flow with faster payment turnaround
- Expedites claim confirmation—usually the next day with batch processing
- Reduces postage costs and mailing time
- Reduces paper handling
- Provides a better audit trail (the electronic media claims response reports show which claims were accepted for processing and which were denied)

XPressClaim is a secure, streamlined World Wide Web–based system that allows providers to submit single TRICARE claims electronically and, in most cases, receive immediate results. XPressClaim is a fast and efficient way to have TRICARE claims processed, and it is free. Filing a TRICARE claim with XPressClaim is relatively easy if the provider is already a member of *myTRICARE claims for Providers*.

eZ TRICARE: For uploading of batches of TRICARE claims directly from a practice management system to the TRICARE claims contractor, eZ TRICARE is available. With eZ TRICARE, there is no software to install, no data entry, and no cost to the provider. eZ TRICARE can accept a variety of claims formats, including the latest HIPAA National Standard Format as well as a CMS-1500 print file.

Claims clearinghouses: TRICARE contractors receive claims from a large number of electronic media claims (EMC) clearinghouses. If this is the preferred method of claims submission, the provider can contact the clearinghouse of choice to find out what is needed to send TRICARE claims to the appropriate contractor.

Electronic Data Interchange (EDI) Gateway: If the provider's system can create HIPAA-compliant claims formats, and it is preferable to send claims directly to the payer, then PGBA's EDI Gateway may be the preferred choice. EDI Gateway can handle all inbound and outbound HIPAA-compliant EDI transactions.

Deadline for Submitting Claims

It is a good practice to submit TRICARE claims within 30 days from the date of services or as soon as possible after the care is rendered. No payment is made for incomplete claims or claims submitted *more than 1 year* after services are rendered by PARs and nonPARs. In addition, PARs are required to participate in Medicare (accept assignment) and

submit claims on behalf of TRICARE and Medicare beneficiaries. It is important for TRICARE providers to adhere to specific guidelines in claims preparation to ensure smooth and timely processing and payment of claims.

The sooner the TRICARE contractor receives the claim forms and other papers, the sooner the claim is paid. As mentioned, the contractor must receive claims within 1 year of the date the service was rendered or, in the case of inpatient care, within 1 year of the date of an inpatient's discharge. If the claim covers several different medical services or supplies that were provided at different times, the above-mentioned 1-year deadline applies to each item on the claim. When a claim is submitted on time, but the claims contractor returns it for more information, the claim must be resubmitted, along with the requested information, so that it is received by the contractor no later than 1 year after the medical services or supplies were provided, or 90 days from the date the claim was returned, whichever is later.

TRICARE Explanation of Benefits

If there are no problems with the claim, the contractor usually sends a written notice, known as an EOB, in about 1 month. The EOB shows the following (Fig. 10-5):

- What the provider billed
- The TRICARE allowable charge at the time of care
- How much of the patient's annual deductible has been met
- How much the patient has paid toward the annual cost cap
- The patient's cost share for the care
- How much TRICARE paid
- Any reasons for denying services on a claim

Note: TRICARE beneficiaries can now view paperless EOBs online. For more information on viewing EOBs on the Internet, visit the Evolve site.

What Did You Learn?

1. The designated contractor who processes medical claims for care received within a particular state or region is commonly called a _____.
2. True or false: Patients using TRICARE Standard may be responsible for submitting their own claims.
3. List advantages of filing claims electronically.
4. Name two systems commonly used for submitting electronic claims.
5. What is the deadline for filing TRICARE claims?
6. List 6 items of information contained on a TRICARE EOB.

CHAMPVA

The **Civilian Health and Medical Program of the Department of Veterans Affairs (CHAMPVA)** is a federal health-care benefits program administered by the Department of Veterans Affairs (VA). Established in 1973, it now provides

T R I C A R E

TRICARE EXPLANATION OF BENEFITS

This is a statement of the action taken on your TRICARE Claim.
Keep this notice for your records.

PGBA or WPS
TRICARE Claims Administrator for Your Region

1*

2*

Date of Notice:	August 02, 2012
Sponsor SSN:	000-00-0000
Sponsor Name:	NAME OF SPONSOR
Beneficiary Name:	NAME OF BENEFICIARY

3*

4*

5*

7*   Benefits were payable to:

6*

PATIENT, PARENT/GUARDIAN
ADDRESS
CITY STATE ZIP CODE

PROVIDER OF MEDICAL CARE
ADDRESS
CITY STATE ZIP CODE

8*

Claim Number: 919533693-00-00

Services Provided By Date of Services		Services Provided		Amount Billed	TRICARE Approved	See Remarks
9*		10*		11*	12*	13*
PROVIDER OF MEDICAL CARE						
07/08/2012	1	Office/outpatient visit, est	(99213)	$ 45.00	$ 38.92	1
07/08/2012	1	Comprehen metabolic panel	(88054)	20.00	19.33	1
07/08/2012	1	Automated hemogram	(85025)	12.00	12.00	1
Totals:				**$ 77.00**	**$ 70.25**	

Claim Summary	Beneficiary Liability Summary	Benefit Period Summary
	15*	16*

				Fiscal Year Beginning:		
Amount billed:	77.00	Deductible	0.00	October 01, 2011		
TRICARE Approved:	70.25	Copayment:	0.00		Individual	Family
Non-Covered: 14*	6.75	Cost Share	17.56	Deductible:	150.00	150.00
Paid by Beneficiary:	0.00			Catastrophic Cap:		
Other Insurance:	0.00			**Enrollment Year Beginning:**		
Paid to Provider:	52.69			December 01, 2011		
Paid to Beneficiary:	0.00				Individual	Family
Check Number:		POS Deductible:			300.00	600.00
		Prime Cap:				856.32

Remarks 17*

1 – CHARGES ARE MORE THAN ALLOWABLE AMOUNT

1-888-XXX-XXXX 18*

THIS IS NOT A BILL
If you have questions regarding this notice, please call or write us at the telephone number/address listed above.

1.   PGBA or WPS processes all TRICARE claims depending on the region where you live.

2.   Prime Contractor: The name and logo of the company that provides managed care support for the region where you live will appear here.

3.   Date of Notice: PGBA or WPS prepared your TRICARE Explanation of Benefits (TEOB) on this date.

4.   Sponsor SSN/Sponsor Name: Your claim is processed using the Social Security Number of the military service member (active duty, retired or deceased) who is your TRICARE sponsor.

5.   Beneficiary Name: The patient who received medical care and for whom this claim was filed.

Fig. 10-5 TRICARE example of benefits. (Source: U.S. Department of Defense, TRICARE Management Activity.)

Continued

TRICARE Explanation of Benefits

6. Mail To Name and Address: We mail the TRICARE Explanation of Benefits (TEOB) directly to the patient (or patient's parent or guardian) at the address given on the claim. (HINT: Be sure your doctor has updated your records with your current address.)

7. Benefits Were Payable To: This field will appear only if your doctor accepts assignment. This means the doctor accepts the TRICARE Maximum Allowable Charge (TMAC) as payment in full for the services you received.

8. Claim Number: Each claim is assigned a unique number. This helps PGBA or WPS keep track of the claim as it is processed. It also helps them find the claim quickly whenever you call or write us with questions or concerns.

9. Service Provided By/Date of Services: This section lists who provided your medical care, the number of services and the procedure codes, as well as the date you received the care.

10. Services Provided: This section describes the medical services you received and how many services are itemized on your claim. It also lists the specific procedure codes that doctors, hospitals and labs use to identify the specific medical services you received.

11. Amount Billed: Your doctor, hospital or lab charged this fee for the medical services you received.

12. TRICARE Approved: This is the amount TRICARE approves for the services you received.

13. See Remarks: If you see a code or a number here, look at the Remarks section (17) for more information about your claim.

14. Claim Summary: A detailed explanation of the action taken by PGBA or WPS taken on your claim is given here. You will find the following totals: amount billed, amount approved by TRICARE, non-covered amount, amount (if any) that you have already paid to the provider, amount your primary health insurance paid (if TRICARE is your secondary insurance), benefits we have paid to the provider, and benefits paid to the beneficiary by PGBA or WPS. A Check Number will appear here only if a check accompanies your TEOB.

15. Beneficiary Liability Summary: You may be responsible for a portion of the fee your doctor has charged. If so, you'll see that amount itemized here. It will include any charges that we have applied to your annual deductible and any cost-share or copayment you must pay.

16. Benefit Period Summary: This section shows how much of the individual and family annual deductible and maximum out-of-pocket expense you have met to date. If you are a TRICARE Standard or Extra beneficiary, PGBA or WPS calculates your annual deductible and maximum out-of-pocket expense by fiscal year. See the Fiscal Year Beginning date in this section for the first date of the fiscal year. If you are a TRICARE Prime beneficiary, we calculate your maximum out-of-pocket expense by enrollment and fiscal year. See Enrollment Year Beginning date in this section for the first date of your enrollment year. (Note: the Enrollment Year Beginning will appear on your TEOB only if you are enrolled in TRICARE Prime.)

17. Remarks Explanations of the codes or numbers listed in See Remarks will appear here.

18. Toll-Free Telephone Number: Questions about your TRICARE Explanation of Benefits? Please call PGBA or WPS at this toll-free number. Their customer service representatives will assist you.

Fig. 10-5—cont'd

---

services for more than 336,000 qualifying dependents. The CHAMPVA Program provides reimbursement for most medical expenses—inpatient, outpatient, mental health, prescription drugs, skilled nursing care, and durable medical equipment (DME)—as well as a limited dental benefit (requires preauthorization) for spouse or widow/ers and the dependent children of veterans who are not TRICARE eligible and fall into one of the following categories:

- the spouse or child of a veteran who has been rated permanently and totally disabled for a service-connected disability by a VA regional office;
- the surviving spouse or child of a veteran who died from a VA-rated service-connected disability;
- the surviving spouse or child of a veteran who was at the time of death rated permanently and totally disabled; or
- the surviving spouse or child of a military member who died in the line of duty, not as a result of misconduct (in most of these cases, these family members are eligible for TRICARE, not CHAMPVA).

CHAMPVA eligibility can be lost if certain demographic changes occur, such as when a widow (younger than 55 years) remarries, the spouse divorces the sponsor, or a sponsor or family member becomes eligible for Medicare or TRICARE. Dependent children lose their eligibility on reaching age 18 years. This age is extended to 23 years if they are attending an accredited college full time (a minimum of 12 credit hours). The Patient Protection and Affordability Care Act (PPACA) included a request to extend the time of coverage until the dependent's 26th birthday, so that CHAMPVA dependents are eligible for the same benefits as dependents whose parents carry private insurance.

Under CHAMPVA, the VA shares the cost of covered healthcare services and supplies with eligible beneficiaries. An eligible CHAMPVA sponsor may be entitled to receive medical care through the VA healthcare system on the basis of his or her own veteran status. Additionally, as the result of a recent policy change, if the eligible CHAMPVA sponsor is the spouse of another eligible CHAMPVA sponsor, both are

Department of Veterans Affairs Health Administration Center **VA** CHAMPVA	**Open Access** **No Referral Required**
Beneficiary Name	
Include this Member Number on all claims and letters **"Patient SSN"**	
This is your CHAMPVA Identification Card	
Effective Date	Expiration Date	1-800-733-8387 www.va.gov/hac

CHAMPVA is secondary to most other health plans. Include an explanation of benefits from other insurers. CHAMPVA is primary to Medicaid.

For Electronic Claims Filing please follow the instructions at: www.va.gov/hac/forproviders under "How to File a Claim."

For Mental Health/Substance Abuse Preauthorization
Call 1-800-424-4018—Preauthorization is required:
• After 23 outpatient mental health visits in a calendar year
• For all other mental health/substance abuse services

For Durable Medical Equipment (DME) Preauthorization
Call 1-800-733-8387—Preauthorization is required:
• For DME purchase or rental over $2,000

Fig. 10-6 Sample CHAMPVA Member ID card. (From U.S. Department of Veterans Affairs, Health Administration Center, CHAMPVA: Fact Sheet 01-16: For Health Care Providers and Office Managers. http://www.va.gov/hac/factsheets/champva/FactSheet01-16.pdf/.)

now eligible for CHAMPVA benefits. Because, as previously mentioned, CHAMPVA eligibility can be affected by changes such as marriage, divorce from the sponsor, and eligibility for Medicare or TRICARE, CHAMPVA recipients should report any changes in status to CHAMPVA immediately.

CHAMPVA Fact: CHAMPVA is managed by the VA's Health Administration Center in Denver, Colorado.

CHAMPVA Fact: There is no cost to CHAMPVA beneficiaries when they receive healthcare treatment at a VA facility.

📁 HIPAA Tip

TRICARE and MTFs are required to give health information about any individual to the U.S. Department of Health and Human Services for use in an investigation of a complaint.

🕐 Stop and Think

Harold and Patsy Yates were divorced 12 years ago. Harold, a double-amputee Vietnam veteran, was rated by the regional VA office as having a permanent and total service-connected disability. Harold and Patsy are eligible for CHAMPVA; however, Patsy plans to remarry. How, if at all, would marriage affect her eligibility?

🕐 Stop and Think

Suppose that Harold Yates had been killed in Vietnam, rather than disabled, and he and Patsy were married at the time of his death, which makes her eligible for CHAMPVA benefits. In this scenario, if Patsy remarries, how would the marriage affect her eligibility?

Extending Eligibility

In addition to the eligibility criteria outlined in the previous subsection, individuals must meet the following conditions in order for benefits to be extended past age 65 years:

• If the individual turned 65 before June 5, 2001, and has only Medicare Part A coverage, he/she will be eligible for CHAMPVA without needing Medicare Part B coverage.
• If the individual turned 65 before June 5, 2001, and has Medicare Part A and B coverage, he/she must keep both Medicare Parts to be eligible for CHAMPVA.

To see a fact sheet on CHAMPVA eligibility requirements, visit the Evolve site.

Identifying CHAMPVA-Eligible Beneficiaries

Every CHAMPVA beneficiary has a member ID card that looks like the one shown in Fig. 10-6. Eligibility can also be confirmed with the use of the CHAMPVA Interactive Voice Response (IVR) system. CHAMPVA also accepts electronic data interchange (EDI) requests to validate eligibility through its clearinghouse, Emdeon.

📁 HIPAA Tip

After the date for full compliance with HIPAA's final rule is issued by HHS, the Health Administration Center will accept only HIPAA-compliant ASC X12 5010 claims and transactions. The Health Administration Center will still maintain its EDI payer IDs with Emdeon as 84146 for Medical claims and 84147 for Dental claims, and will support all of the transactions listed above in the same manner.

CHAMPVA Benefits

In general, CHAMPVA covers 75% of most healthcare services and supplies that are medically and psychologically necessary. Prescription medications by mail (Meds by Mail) are free to 100% disabled veterans and their dependent family members who do not have prescription drug insurance; however, over-the-counter medications are not covered. CHAMPVA benefits normally do not include dental or most eye care. Exceptions are limited to services directly related to treatment of certain medical conditions of the eyes or mouth. CHAMPVA-eligible patients may see any provider of their choice as long as the provider is properly licensed.

CHAMPVA Cost Sharing

Although many veterans qualify for cost-free healthcare services on the basis of a service-connected condition or other qualifying factor, most are required to complete an annual financial assessment or "Means Test" to determine whether they qualify for cost-free services. Veterans whose gross household income and net worth exceed the established thresholds as well as those who choose not to complete the financial assessment must agree to pay the required copays to become eligible for VA services. Along with their enrollment confirmation and priority group assignment, enrollees will receive information regarding their copay requirements, if applicable.

To view CHAMPVA's 2011 "Copay Requirements at a Glance" chart, visit the Evolve site.

For the most part, CHAMPVA has two cost-sharing responsibilities for outpatient services: an annual deductible and a copayment. If the provider does not accept assignment (nonPAR), the beneficiary is responsible for paying the annual deductible, a copayment, and any provider-billed amount that exceeds CHAMPVA's total allowable amount. For professional services that are not covered by CHAMPVA, the beneficiary pays the full allowable amount. If the provider agrees to accept CHAMPVA's allowable amount as payment in full, he or she cannot balance bill.

The annual outpatient deductible is $50 per beneficiary, or a maximum of $100 per family per year. The annual deductible must be paid before CHAMPVA begins paying its 75% of the allowable amount. As claims are processed for covered services, charges are automatically credited to individual and family deductible requirements for each calendar year. Under the CHAMPVA In-house Treatment Initiative (CITI), there is no deductible for inpatient services, ambulatory surgery, partial psychiatric day programs, hospice services, or services provided by VA medical facilities.

To provide financial protection against a potential financial crisis of a long-term illness or serious injury, CHAMPVA has established an annual cat cap of $3000 per calendar year. This is the maximum out-of-pocket expense that a beneficiary or a family can incur in 1 year for CHAMPVA-covered services. After the $3000 limit is reached, copays for covered services are waived for the remainder of the calendar year, and CHAMPVA pays 100% of the allowable amount. Table 10-5 is a cost summary showing what beneficiaries have to pay when they have no other health insurance (OHI). Table 10-6 is a cost summary of cost sharing with OHI.

The following is a recap of CHAMPVA's basic benefits and cost sharing:
- major medical plan, inpatient, outpatient, mental health, substance abuse, prescription medication (includes those on Medicare) and hospice;
- annual deductible: $50 individual, $100 family;
- cost share (copay): beneficiary pays 25% of allowable charges, unless care is provided by the Veterans Affairs, such as
  - CITI
  - Meds by Mail
  - Durable medical equipment
- $3000 annual catastrophic cap; and
- freedom to choose any provider.

Beneficiaries do *not* need to see a VA doctor—CHAMPVA covers visits to private providers as long as they are appropriately licensed. No prior approval is necessary for referrals to specialists or for diagnostic tests as long as they are considered medically necessary. (See CHAMPVA Payment Summary in Table 10-7).

CHAMPVA does not cover:
- routine dental care;
- routine vision care, unless disease is present;
- chiropractic care;
- routine physical examinations except school physicals; or
- custodial/domiciliary care (nursing homes, long term care).

Preauthorization is required for certain types of services, such as:
- Dental care (other than the exceptions mentioned previously)
- Durable medical equipment with a total purchase price or total rental price of more than $2000, e.g., wheelchairs, hospital bed, and specialized lifts
- Hospice services
- Mental health/substance abuse services
- Organ and bone marrow transplants

TABLE 10-5	Beneficiary Cost Sharing with No Other Health Insurance

BENEFITS	DEDUCTIBLE	PATIENT/MEMBER PAYS
Ambulatory surgery	No	25% of CHAMPVA allowable amount
Durable medical equipment (DME)	Yes	25% of CHAMPVA allowable amount
Emergency room charges	Depends (on whether the emergency care becomes part of inpatient charges or remains an outpatient charge)	The charges will be included in the inpatient charge if, once stabilized, the patient is admitted to the hospital. The payment will then be based on "inpatient services." If the patient is not admitted, the payment is based on "outpatient services."
Inpatient mental health:		
High-volume residential treatment centers	No	25% of CHAMPVA allowable amount
Low-volume treatment center	No	Lesser of: (1) per-day amount times the number of inpatient days and (2) 25% of billed amount
Inpatient services:		
Diagnosis-related group (DRG)–based	No	Lesser of: 1) per-day amount times the number of inpatient days; 2) 25% of billed amount; or 3) DRG rate
Non–DRG-based	No	25% of CHAMPVA allowable amount
Outpatient services (e.g., doctor visits, laboratory/radiology, home health, mental health services, skilled nursing visits, ambulance)	Yes	25% of CHAMPVA allowable amount after deductible
Pharmacy services (retail)	Yes	25% of CHAMPVA allowable amount
Professional services	Yes	25% of CHAMPVA allowable amount

TABLE 10-6	Beneficiary Cost Sharing with Other Health Insurance (OHI)

SERVICE	OHI PAYS	CHAMPVA PAYS	PATIENT/ MEMBER PAYS
All medical services and supplies that are covered by both the OHI and CHAMPVA	Their plan allowable	What is owed up to the CHAMPVA allowable amount	In most cases, $0
Medical services covered by the OHI, and *not* covered by CHAMPVA	Their plan allowable	$0	The OHI plan copayment
Medical services *not* covered by the OHI but covered by CHAMPVA (*Note:* Does *not* pay for services that were determined to be noncovered by the OHI because there was a failure to follow the OHI plan requirements.)	$0	The CHAMPVA allowable amount	The cost share for the type of service

TABLE 10-7	CHAMPVA Payment Summary			
BENEFITS	**DEDUCTIBLE?**	**MEMBER/PATIENT PAYS**	**CHAMPVA PAYS**	
Ambulatory surgery facility services	No	25% of CHAMPVA allowable	75% of CHAMPVA allowable	
Professional services	Yes	25% of CHAMPVA allowable after deductible	75% of CHAMPVA allowable	
Durable medical equipment (DME), non-VA source	Yes	25% of CHAMPVA allowable after deductible	75% of CHAMPVA allowable	
Inpatient services:				
Diagnosis-related group (DRG)– based	No	Lesser of: 1) per day amount × number of inpatient days; 2) 25% of billed amount; or 3) DRG rate	CHAMPVA allowable less beneficiary cost share	
Inpatient services: non–DRG-based	No	25% of CHAMPVA allowable	75% of CHAMPVA allowable	
Mental health:				
High-volume/RTC	No	25% of CHAMPVA allowable	75% of CHAMPVA allowable	
Low-volume	No	Lesser of: (1) per day amount × number of inpatient days or (2) 25% of billed amount	CHAMPVA allowable less beneficiary cost share	
Outpatient services (e.g., doctor visits, laboratory/radiology, home health, skilled nursing visits, ambulance)	Yes	25% of CHAMPVA allowable after deductible	75% of CHAMPVA allowable	
Pharmacy services	Yes	25% of CHAMPVA allowable after deductible	75% of CHAMPVA allowable	
VA source (DME, MBM, CITI)	No	Nothing	100% of VA cost	

Failure to acquire preauthorization for these services and items results in denial of the claim. On confirmation of eligibility, applicants receive program materials that specifically address covered and noncovered services and supplies. For more detailed information on CHAMPVA benefits, download the CHAMPVA handbook through the link on the Evolve site.

Prescription Drug Benefit

CHAMPVA offers a more cost-effective prescription drug benefit than Medicare Part D, and there is no monthly premium. Under CHAMPVA, the prescription plan is considered "credible coverage," and beneficiaries typically do not have to sign up for a Medicare Part D prescription drug plan. If CHAMPVA beneficiaries receive their maintenance medications through the CHAMPVA Meds by Mail program and do not routinely use a local pharmacy, their prescriptions will continue to be provided free of charge and delivered directly to their homes.

To view a comparison chart of prescription drug coverages under Medicare, CHAMPVA, and TRICARE, visit the Evolve site.

If there is any question about whether a particular service is payable under CHAMPVA guidelines, the health insurance professional should consult the most recent CHAMPVA handbook or contact the VA Health Administration Center using the toll-free phone line or go to www.va.gov/hac/contact/ and follow the directions for submitting an e-mail via the VA's Inquiry and Routing Information System (IRIS). Fact Sheet 01-16: "For Outpatient Providers and Office Managers," can be viewed and downloaded by logging on to the Evolve site.

Stop and Think

Elaine Porter is employed by Harper Products, Inc. She has single coverage under her employer's group healthcare plan. Elaine's husband, a helicopter pilot, was killed when his Chinook helicopter was shot down by an air-to-ground missile during Desert Storm. Because Elaine also is covered under CHAMPVA, which payer in this case would be primary?

CHAMPVA In-house Treatment Initiative (CIT)

CITI is a voluntary program that allows the CHAMPVA beneficiary to be treated at participating VA Medical Centers with no out-of-pocket cost. Each VA medical center that participates in the CITI program offers different services on the basis of unused capacity. Once the beneficiary locates a CITI facility he or she wants to use, the CITI Coordinator can be contacted to find out what services are offered at that specific medical center. CHAMPVA beneficiaries who are also covered by Medicare cannot participate in the CITI program, because Medicare does not pay for services provided by a VA Medical Center.

CHAMPVA-TRICARE Connection

Even though CHAMPVA and TRICARE are similar and are both federal healthcare programs, an individual who is eligible for TRICARE is not eligible for CHAMPVA. TRICARE provides coverage to the families of active duty service members, families of service members who died while on active duty, and retirees and their families, whether or not the veterans are disabled. CHAMPVA provides benefits to eligible family members of veterans who officially have been declared 100% permanently disabled from service-connected conditions, survivors of veterans who died from service-connected conditions, and survivors of service members who died in the line of duty who are not otherwise entitled to TRICARE benefits.

Types of Health Insurance Plans Primary to CHAMPVA

Unless the beneficiary is covered under one of the following plans, CHAMPVA is the primary payer:

- State Victims of Crime Compensation Program
- Indian Health Services
- Workers' compensation claim
- Injury due to automobile accident

Another exception to third-party payer priority is when a CHAMPVA-eligible beneficiary resides or travels overseas. When this is the case, if all eligibility criteria are met, CHAMPVA is the primary payer (unless there is OHI) until the individual returns to the United States. In all other cases, CHAMPVA is the secondary payer. In the case of OHI, either the provider or the beneficiary must file a claim first with the OHI. After receiving an EOB from the primary insurer, a claim may be filed with CHAMPVA for any balance remaining. The EOB from the primary insurer as well as the provider's itemized statement must accompany the CHAMPVA claim.

CHAMPVA-Medicare Connection

When a beneficiary is eligible for healthcare benefits under both Medicare and CHAMPVA, Medicare is the primary payer. In most cases, Medicare/CHAMPVA dual coverage results in no out-of-pocket expenses for the individual, and a supplement plan is unnecessary. CHAMPVA does not pay Medicare Part B premiums, however. It is important for the beneficiary to be aware that if he or she has Medicare and CHAMPVA, Medicare's rules and procedures must be followed for covered services. Failure to follow them means that the service would not be covered under CHAMPVA. If Medicare determines that the service is not medically necessary or appropriate, CHAMPVA also will deny coverage. If the beneficiary or the provider disagrees with the Medicare decision, an appeal should be made with Medicare rather than with CHAMPVA. In most cases, beneficiaries who are eligible for Medicare Part A must enroll in Part B also in order to have CHAMPVA eligibility.

CHAMPVA and HMO Coverage

If a CHAMPVA-eligible beneficiary has a health maintenance organization (HMO) or preferred provider organization (PPO) plan, CHAMPVA pays any copayments required under the HMO/PPO plan for CHAMPVA-covered services up to the CHAMPVA allowable amount. When medical services are available through the HMO/PPO, and the patient chooses to seek care outside the HMO (e.g., the patient visits a physician who is not associated with the HMO/PPO or does not follow the rules and procedures of the HMO/PPO plan), CHAMPVA will not pay for that care. Likewise, if the beneficiary has Medicare and chooses to receive care from a provider who does not accept Medicare patients, CHAMPVA will not pay. It is very important that the beneficiary follow the primary payer's guidelines when visiting HMO/PPO network or participating providers.

Changes in OHI coverage must be reported to the CHAMPVA office in Denver, Colorado, on VA Form 10-7959c. When submitting this form, the patient or health insurance professional should include a copy of the OHI copayment information or schedule of benefits. A copy of VA Form 10-7959c can be downloaded through the Evolve site.

CHAMPVA Providers

Healthcare providers may elect to participate in CHAMPVA simply by agreeing to see the beneficiary and submitting a claim to CHAMPVA on the beneficiary's behalf. Providers who accept CHAMPVA patients also must accept the CHAMPVA allowable rate as payment in full and cannot balance bill. If the provider chooses not to participate in CHAMPVA, patients typically must pay the entire bill and submit their own claims to CHAMPVA for personal reimbursement of the allowable amount. Even nonPARs must accept the allowable rate and cannot balance bill. Under the CHAMPVA program, however, the patient is responsible for paying the CHAMPVA cost share and any charges for non-covered services.

CHAMPVA For Life (CFL)

The **CHAMPVA For Life (CFL)** program became effective October 1, 2001. It is an extension of CHAMPVA benefits to those 65 years and older. CFL serves as the secondary payer to minimize out-of-pocket expenses by covering Medicare's coinsurance and deductibles. Like most health insurance, CFL is not long-term care insurance, but it will cover some of the costs. Additionally, it does not pay for **custodial care**—assistance with activities of daily living (ADL), such as bathing, dressing, and feeding, or supervision of those who are cognitively impaired. Much like Medigap insurance, CFL picks up where Medicare leaves off. CFL pays the coinsurance and deductibles but does not pay for the monthly Medicare Part B premium. TFL enrollees do not receive cash or checks from CFL. Benefits cover only medical services and are paid directly to the providers.

CFL does pay for skilled nursing care up to a limit. As with Medicare, there must be a medical condition that was treated in a hospital for 3 consecutive days, and the beneficiary must be admitted to a skilled nursing facility (SNF) within 30 days after hospitalization in order for CFL to be activated. Medicare has a 100-day limit on skilled nursing, after which CFL is the primary payer; however, it does not cover the full amount. The beneficiary should expect to pay a copayment (Table 10-8).

CFL Eligibility

The spouses of veterans must be at least 65 years old to be eligible for CFL. Seniors who turned 65 before June 5, 2001, need only Medicare Part A to be eligible. Those turning 65 after that date need both Medicare A and B. The spouse of a veteran qualifies if the veteran meets one of the following conditions:
- Has a service-connected disability rating of 100%, meaning he or she is permanently and totally disabled or died with that rating
- Has died from a VA-rated service-connected disability
- Has died in the line of duty (does not qualify if eligible for TRICARE)
- Cannot have been dishonorably discharged

A spouse loses eligibility for CFL if he or she divorces the veteran. A widow or widower who remarries also loses

eligibility; however, if the remarriage terminates, his or her eligibility is reinstated.

What Did You Learn?

1. What federal department administers CHAMPVA?
2. List the eligible categories for CHAMPVA coverage.
3. In general, CHAMPVA covers __% of most healthcare services and supplies that are medically/psychologically necessary.
4. Name CHAMPVA'S two cost-sharing responsibilities for outpatient services.
5. What is CHAMPVA's annual cat cap?
6. True or false: An individual can have both TRICARE and CHAMPVA coverage.
7. List 5 plan types that are primary to CHAMPVA.
8. When a beneficiary is eligible for both Medicare and CHAMPVA, _____ is the primary payer.

FILING CHAMPVA CLAIMS

As with TRICARE, providers accepting assignment for CHAMPVA claims must submit the claim for the beneficiary. Beneficiaries who receive treatment from nonPARs usually are required to submit their own claims. All CHAMPVA paper claims should be sent to the following address: VA Health Administration Center, CHAMPVA, PO Box 65024, Denver, CO 80206-9024.

As stated earlier, if the beneficiary has OHI, claims should be sent to the OHI first. The EOB from the OHI should then be attached to the claim and submitted to CHAMPVA.

CHAMPVA Fact: By law, CHAMPVA is always secondary payer except to Medicaid and CHAMPVA supplemental policies.

CHAMPVA claims should preferably be filed electronically using the most current HIPAA-mandated claim transaction standards. As with TRICARE claims, the status of claims can be checked electronically via the VA Health Administration Center's 24-hour IVR system, at 1-800-733-8387. Step-by-step instructions for using IVR can be found at http://www.ehow.com/how_6115284_check-status-champva-claim.html/. CHAMPVA also accepts paper claims; however, the turnaround time for payment is longer. Details on payment methodology and covered benefits for CHAMPVA health plans are covered in the policy manuals on the CHAMPVA website.

CHAMPVA Preauthorization Requirements

Preauthorization is required for certain procedures/services, such as
- Organ and bone marrow transplants
- Hospice care
- Dental care
- DME worth more than $2000
- Most mental health or substance abuse services

The CHAMPVA handbook contains a complete listing of preauthorization services and supplies.

TABLE 10-8	Beneficiary Cost Shares with Medicare and CHAMPVA For Life (CFL)		
COVERAGE DAYS	MEDICARE	CFL	INDIVIDUAL
Day 1-20	100%	0%	0%
Day 20-100	80%	20%	0%
Day 100+	0%	75%	25%

Box 10-3

Exceptions to CHAMPVA's Timely Filing Requirements

Exceptions to CHAMPVA's timely filing requirements may be granted when:

1. There is medical documentation of beneficiary incompetence and the beneficiary did not have a legal guardian.
2. There is evidence of an administrative error, e.g., the beneficiary has been prevented from timely filing owing to misrepresentation, mistake, or other accountable action of a Health Administration Center (HAC) employee acting within the scope of that individual's authority. Necessary evidence must include:
   a. A written statement describing how the error caused failure to file within the usual time limit.
   b. Copy of an agency letter or written notice reflecting the error.
3. The claimant submitted the claim to a primary health insurer, and the primary insurer delayed adjudication past the CHAMPVA deadline. In such cases, the following must be established:
   a. The claim was originally sent to the primary health insurer prior to the CHAMPVA claim filing deadline or must have been filed with CHAMPVA prior to the deadline but was returned or denied pending processing by the other health insurer.
   b. The claimant must submit a statement with the claim indicating the original date of submission to the other health insurer, the date of adjudication, and any relevant correspondence, and an EOB.

For CHAMPVA-Medicare dual-eligible individuals, specific procedures performed at free-standing ambulatory surgery centers must have Medicare prior approval. For a listing by procedure of those services, refer to the *CHAMPVA Policy Manual*, Chapter 3, Section 7.1, on the CHAMPVA website.

CHAMPVA Claims Filing Deadlines

CHAMPVA claims follow the same filing deadline specifications as TRICARE, with the exception that all CHAMPVA claims are sent to the VA Health Administration Center in Denver, Colorado. A TRICARE contractor can grant exemptions from the filing deadlines under certain circumstances. Box 10-3 lists circumstances that qualify for a timely filing exemption.

When a claim has been denied, and the denial was overturned for whatever reason, a retroactive authorization will be made. In such cases, the beneficiary has 180 days after notification of an approved retroactive authorization to file a claim.

🕐 Stop and Think

Maria Delgado received care from her family physician, Imari Deili, on July 1, 2003. Anne Jenkins, Dr. Deili's health insurance professional, neglected to file a claim until Ms. Delgado telephoned inquiring about a series of statements she received. Anne completed the claim and mailed it to the TRICARE contractor on June 30, 2004. She then told Ms. Delgado that the claim would be paid by TRICARE because it would be postmarked within the 1-year time limit. Is Anne correct?

💬 What Did You Learn?

1. True or false: Providers accepting assignment for CHAMPVA must submit the claim for the beneficiary.
2. Where does the health insurance professional send CHAMPVA claims?
3. List 4 procedures/services that require preauthorization.
4. What is the deadline for filing CHAMPVA claims?

INSTRUCTIONS FOR COMPLETING TRICARE/CHAMPVA PAPER CLAIM FORMS

CHAMPVA allows professional charges to be submitted on paper using a CMS-1500 (08/05) claim form and following TRICARE/CHAMPVA guidelines. These guidelines are provided in an Appendix B table along with a completed TRICARE simple claim (Fig. B-7) as well as a completed CHAMPVA claim (Fig. B-8). When completing the claim, the health insurance professional should remember that the "sponsor" is the member or was active-duty military. The sponsor's dependent (spouse or child) is the "patient" or "beneficiary" (these terms are often used interchangeably). These instructions are generic and may not be exactly the same as required by the claims processor in each area. The health insurance professional should obtain complete, detailed, and up-to-date claims completion guidelines from the TRICARE claims processor in his or her area or CHAMPVA to ensure that CMS-1500 forms are completed correctly to expedite reimbursement.

Claims Filing Summary

The following are important points to consider when filing claims:

- Claims should be submitted as soon as services are rendered to expedite the claims process.
- The claims filing deadline is 1 year from the date of service or 1 year from the date of discharge for inpatient hospitalization.
- Copies should be kept of all information submitted to the TRICARE claims processor or CHAMPVA.

It is not beneficial to hold multiple claims over a period of time and submit them all at once. If numerous claims are submitted and there is a problem with one, it could delay the processing of all claims.

CHAMPVA Explanation of Benefits

On completion of the processing of a CHAMPVA claim, an EOB form is sent to both the beneficiary and the provider if the claim was filed by the provider. When beneficiaries file their own claims, EOBs are sent only to them. As with a TRICARE EOB, the CHAMPVA EOB is a summary of the action taken on the claim and contains basically the same information. (See example in Fig. 10-7).

Claims Appeals and Reconsiderations

In the event that a provider or beneficiary disagrees with the manner in which a claim was processed and considers it necessary to file a claims appeal or have the processing of a claim reconsidered, such an appeal must be in writing and filed within 1 year of the date of the EOB in the case of a denial of the service or benefit, or 1 year from the date of the letter notifying denial of eligibility or service. (The EOB contains pertinent information on the procedures for filing an appeal.) The appeal request should be in writing and include the following:

- the reason why the claim is being appealed,
- a copy of the EOB or determination letter, and
- any new and relevant information not previously considered.

On receipt of the written appeal, all claims for the entire course of treatment are reviewed. After review of the appeal and supporting documentation, a written decision is sent advising of the decision. If the provider or beneficiary still disagrees with the decision, a second review can be requested. Again, the reason(s) it is believed that the decision was made in error should be identified, and any additional information that supports the request included. A second request for review must be sent within 90 days of the date of the initial decision. Second-level decisions are final. Health insurance professionals should contact the CHAMPVA office in Denver, to the attention of Appeals, for information on appeals and reconsiderations. To review a fact sheet on CHAMPVA reconsideration and appeal rights for beneficiaries, visit the Evolve site.

⭐ Imagine This!

Dr. Serjio Manya, a psychiatrist, provided psychiatric treatment to Samuel Fortune, a Gulf War veteran, for clinical depression. Samuel, who was determined to be eligible for CHAMPVA after his diagnosis, subsequently was admitted to the Trenton Mental Healthcare Facility because of a suicide attempt, where he remained for 15 months. Because Dr. Manya was a nonparticipating provider (nonPAR) and Samuel's mental condition rendered him incompetent, the claim was not filed within the time limit. Because Samuel's illness was documented by Dr. Manya, however, Samuel was able to get a filing extension and ultimately received CHAMPVA benefits.

❓ What Did You Learn?

1. All CHAMPVA paper claims must be submitted on the _____ form.
2. True or false: On the claim form, the "sponsor" is the member or was active duty military.
3. List at least 6 items of information shown on an EOB.
4. An appeal request to CHAMPVA must contain what items?

HIPAA AND MILITARY INSURERS

All MTFs have implemented the privacy rules of the Health Insurance Portability and Accountability Act of 1996 (HIPAA). Although the MHS has always had privacy standards in place to limit unauthorized access to and disclosure of personal health information, HIPAA's rules heighten awareness, raise the level of oversight, and provide a standard set of guidelines to protect the privacy of all patients.

Each MTF has an assigned, trained privacy officer available to respond to any questions or concerns that beneficiaries may have regarding HIPAA's privacy rules. The privacy officers also serve as patient advocates, ensuring that personal health information maintained by the MTF remains protected yet accessible to beneficiaries and their providers. A copy of the notice to privacy practice is available on the TRICARE website for sponsors and family members to download; copies are also available for distribution at each DoD MTF.

All MTFs now meet HIPAA transaction set standards for all programs.

📁 HIPAA Tip

HIPAA requires all employees, contractors, and volunteers of healthcare provider organizations, healthcare insurers, and healthcare clearinghouses, including those associated with TRICARE and CHAMPVA who come in contact with Protected Health Information, to be trained annually in the areas of privacy and security.

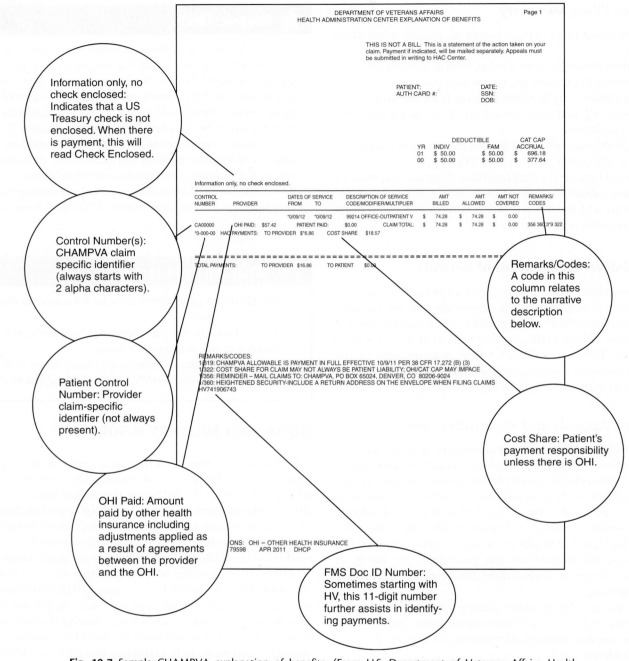

Fig. 10-7 Sample CHAMPVA explanation of benefits. (From U.S. Department of Veterans Affairs, Health Administration Center.)

SUMMARY CHECKPOINTS

▶ TRICARE is a worldwide healthcare system for the uniformed services, serving nearly 10 million beneficiaries including National Guard and Reserve members, retirees, their families, survivors, and certain former spouses. The program is managed by TRICARE Management Activity (TMA) under the authority of the U.S. Assistant Secretary of Defense (Health Affairs). TRICARE is organized into 6 geographic regions: the West, North, and South regions and 3 overseas "areas."

▶ Categories of eligibility under TRICARE's three plans (Standard, Extra, and Prime) are:
- Active duty service members (ADSMs); automatic enrollment
- Spouses and unmarried children of ADSMs
- Uniformed service retirees, their spouses, and unmarried children
- Medal of Honor recipients
- Un-remarried former spouse and unmarried children of active duty or retired service members who have died

▶ TRICARE pays for only *allowed* services, supplies, and procedures, which are referred to as covered charges. Covered charges include medical and psychological services and supplies that are considered appropriate and are generally accepted by qualified professionals to be reasonable and adequate for the diagnosis and treatment of illness, injury, pregnancy, and mental disorders or for well-child care.

▶ An NAS is a document of certification from the MTF that says it cannot provide the specific healthcare the beneficiary needs. The statements must be entered electronically in the Defense Department's DEERS computer files by the MTF. An NAS is no longer necessary for TRICARE Standard beneficiaries except for maternity cases.

▶ If a TRICARE-eligible beneficiary has other healthcare coverage through an employer, an association, or a private insurer, or if a student in the family obtained a healthcare plan through his or her school, TRICARE considers this other health insurance (OHI). In such cases, OHI is primary to TRICARE.

▶ Patient eligibility must be verified at the time of service. The patient must have a valid Common Access Card (CAC), uniformed service ID card, or eligibility authorization letter. Check the expiration date on the card.

▶ TRICARE PARs agree to accept the TRICARE allowable charge on all claims as payment in full for the healthcare services provided and not balance bill. NonPARs can participate in TRICARE on a case-by-case basis. PARs and nonPARs who accept assignment must file the claim for the patient, and TRICARE sends the payment (if any) directly to the provider.

▶ Beneficiaries are responsible for cost shares and deductibles for care that is covered under TRICARE Standard.

▶ The designated contractor who processes medical claims for care received within a particular state or region is called a claims processor, TRICARE contractor, or fiscal intermediary (FI).

▶ TRICARE network providers are required to submit claims electronically. Non-network providers still have the option to submit paper claims.

▶ The deadline for filing TRICARE claims is 1 year after services are rendered for both PARs and nonPARs.

▶ CHAMPVA is a healthcare benefits program for qualifying dependents and survivors of veterans. Under CHAMPVA, the VA shares the cost of covered healthcare services and supplies with eligible beneficiaries. CHAMPVA is managed by the VA's Health Administration Center in Denver, Colorado.

▶ Individuals who are entitled to CHAMPVA benefits include

• *the spouse or dependent child* of a veteran who has been rated by a VA regional office as having a permanent and total service-connected condition/disability;
• *the surviving spouse or dependent child* of a veteran who died as a result of a VA-rated service-connected condition or who, at the time of death, was rated permanently and totally disabled from a VA-rated service-connected condition; and
• *the surviving spouse or dependent child* of an individual who died in the line of duty and the death was not due to misconduct.

▶ There is no cost to CHAMPVA beneficiaries when they receive healthcare treatment at a VA facility.

▶ In general, CHAMPVA covers 75% of most healthcare services and supplies that are medically necessary. Prescription medications by mail are free to 100%-disabled veterans and their dependent family members who do not have prescription drug insurance; however, over-the-counter medications are not covered.

▶ CHAMPVA benefits do not normally include dental or most eye care.

▶ For the most part, CHAMPVA beneficiaries have two cost-sharing responsibilities for outpatient services: an annual deductible and a copayment.

▶ CHAMPVA and TRICARE are federal programs; however, an individual who is eligible for TRICARE is not eligible for CHAMPVA.

▶ A qualifying beneficiary can be eligible for healthcare benefits under Medicare and CHAMPVA. For healthcare services covered under both plans, there are often no out-of-pocket expenses for covered services. Also, if Medicare finds the service is not medically necessary or appropriate, CHAMPVA does not provide coverage either.

▶ Medicare is primary to CHAMPVA.

▶ Healthcare providers may elect to participate in CHAMPVA by agreeing to see the beneficiary and submitting a claim on the beneficiary's behalf. Providers who accept CHAMPVA patients also must accept the CHAMPVA allowable rate as payment in full and cannot balance bill.

▶ Providers filing paper claims should use the standard CMS-1500 claim form and follow the TRICARE/CHAMPVA guidelines for completing the form

▶ All CHAMPVA paper claims should be sent to VA Health Administration Center, CHAMPVA, PO Box 65024, Denver, CO 80206-9024.

▶ The deadline for submitting CHAMPVA claims is 1 year from the date of service. For inpatient hospital claims, the deadline is 1 year from the date of discharge.

CLOSING SCENARIO

After completing the chapter on military carriers, Sally thought she was ready to answer her Aunt Betty's questions. She agreed with her aunt that the various plans available under TRICARE can be confusing and that it may be difficult to decide which plan best suits a military spouse's or dependent's needs. First, Sally explained that CHAMPUS was the former name, and the plan was now called TRICARE (TRI because it offers three plans). Next, Sally outlined the three plans along with the advantages and disadvantages of each. She gave her aunt several Internet websites from which to get further details regarding TRICARE and suggested that she sit down with the health insurance professional at the medical clinic to resolve some of the confusion over claims.

Sally also discovered that her grandfather was eligible to receive his prescription medicine by mail through the VA. This would be a tremendous cost savings for him because he was taking seven different medications. It gave Sally a good feeling to know that she was able to help her family. Now, she looked forward to helping others through her career as a health insurance professional.

WEBSITES TO EXPLORE

- For live links to the following websites, please visit the Evolve site at
  http://evolve.elsevier.com/Beik/today/
- To find the nearest uniformed services personnel office, log on to
  http://www.dmdc.osd.mil/rsl/
- For detailed information on TRICARE, log on to
  http://www.tricare.osd.mil/hipaa/
- To view the TRICARE handbook, log on to
  http://www.tricare.osd.mil/tricarehandbook/
- For details regarding the cat cap in a particular area, log on to
  http://tricare.mil/contactus/
- To view the CHAMPVA handbook, log on to
  http://www.va.gov/hac/forbeneficiaries/champva/handbook.asp/
- Additional information on HIPAA, TRICARE, and the new privacy standards is available on the TRICARE website at
  http://www.tricare.osd.mil/hipaa/
- To report fraud, waste, or abuse in federal programs, log on to
  http://www.gao.gov/fraudnet/fraudnet.htm/

Author's Note: If any of these URLs are unable to be found, use applicable guide words in your Internet search for acquiring additional information on the various subjects listed.

REFERENCES AND RESOURCES

Humana Military Healthcare Services, TRICARE South: *TRICARE Extended Care Health Option,* August 3, 2009: http://www.humanamilitary.com/south/bene/TRICAREPrograms/echo.asp/.

Quarles, B: *PGBA Joins Group of U.S. Defense Contractors Committed to Compliance,* Columbia, SC, Jan 13, 2009, PGBA, LLC http://www.reuters.com/article/pressRelease/idUS158280+13-Jan-2009+PRN20090113./.

TRICARE Eligibility. Copyright 2009 Military Advantage. http://www.military.com/benefits/tricare/tricare-eligibility/.

TRICARE Standard Overview. Copyright 2009 Military Advantage. http://www.military.com/benefits/tricare/tricare-standard/tricare-standard-overview/.

U.S. Department of Defense, Military Health System, TRICARE Management Activity: Monthly Premiums Decrease for TRICARE Reserve Select, No. 08-114. Falls Church, VA, November 19, 2008. http://www.tricare.mil/pressroom/news.aspx?fid=480/.

U.S. Department of Defense, Military Health System, TRICARE Management Activity: *TRICARE Plus,* Falls Church, VA, July 1, 2009. http://www.tricare.mil/mybenefit/home/overview/SpecialPrograms/Plus?Other/.

U.S. Department of Defense, Military Health System, TRICARE Management Activity: *TRICARE Provider News Issue I,* Louisville, KY, 2009. http://www.humana-military.com/library/pdf/PS_Bull_09_i1_Lo.pdf/.

U.S. Department of Defense, Military Health System, TRICARE North: *Exceptional Family Member Program (EFMP) Enrollment.* https://www.hnfs.net/common/caremanagement/efmp_enrollment.htm/.

United States Department of Veterans Affairs, Health Administration Center, Chief Business Office, Veterans Health Administration: *Provider News,* February 3, 2009. http://www.va.gov/hac/forproviders/provider_news.asp/.

CHAPTER 11

Miscellaneous Carriers: Workers' Compensation and Disability Insurance

Chapter Outline

I. Workers' Compensation
  A. History
  B. Federal Legislation and Workers' Compensation
  C. Eligibility
    1. Exemptions
    2. Benefits
    3. Denial of Benefits and Appeals
    4. Time Limits
  D. Workers' Compensation Claims Process
    1. First Report of Injury
    2. Physician's Role
    3. Determining Disability
    4. Vocational Rehabilitation
    5. Waiting Periods
    6. Claim Forms
    7. Progress Reports
  E. Special Billing Notes
  F. Workers' Compensation and Managed Care
  G. Health Insurance Portability and Accountability Act and Workers' Compensation
  H. Workers' Compensation Fraud
  I. Online Workers' Compensation Service Center
II. Private and Employer-Sponsored Disability Income Insurance
  A. Defining Disability
    1. Short-Term Disability
    2. Long-Term Disability
  B. Disability Claims Process
    1. Employee's Responsibilities
    2. Employer's Responsibilities
    3. Attending Physician's Statement
    4. Health Insurance Professional's Role
III. Federal Disability Programs
  A. Americans with Disabilities Act
  B. Social Security Disability Insurance
    1. History of the Social Security Disability Insurance Program
    2. Administration and Funding
    3. Eligibility
  C. Supplemental Security Income
    1. Administration and Funding
    2. Eligibility
  D. State Disability Programs
  E. Centers for Disease Control and Prevention Disability and Health Team
  F. Ticket to Work Program
    1. Purpose
    2. How the Program Works
  G. Filing Supplemental Security Income and Social Security Disability Insurance Claims
    1. Patient's Role
    2. Role of the Healthcare Provider
    3. Role of the Health Insurance Professional

CHAPTER OBJECTIVES

After completion of this chapter, the student should be able to:

1. Explain the history and purpose of workers' compensation.
2. Identify legislation that provided benefits for various categories of federal workers.
3. Discuss workers' compensation eligibility requirements and exemptions.
4. Explain workers' compensation benefits, denial of benefits, and appeals.
5. Discuss time limits for filing workers' compensation claims.
6. Summarize the workers' compensation claim process, including special billing notes.

OPENING SCENARIO

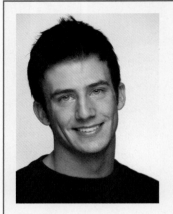

The terms "workers' compensation" and "disability insurance" were familiar to Jim Lightfoot. His father had been a construction worker on a high-rise apartment building and had fallen to his death 6 years earlier. Even though Jim was young at the time, he remembers the monthly benefit checks his mother received, which were so vital in helping pay living expenses for the family. Jim was anxious to learn as much as he could about the various types of disability listed in the chapter outline.

Tammy Hansen, a classmate, did not share Jim's enthusiasm for the subject at first, but her uncle was an insurance salesman. The day before Jim and Tammy were to begin the chapter on workers' compensation and disability insurance, Uncle Niles stopped by her house and Tammy overhead her father and uncle discussing disability income insurance. "I can't afford to have disability insurance," her father stated, to which her uncle replied, "With your growing family, you can't afford not to!" The tone of her uncle's voice made Tammy sit up and listen. Why, she wondered, did her uncle believe that disability income insurance was important? Perhaps this chapter might be more informative and interesting than she first thought.

7. Discuss workers' compensation and managed care.
8. Explain HIPAA's connection to workers' compensation.
9. State methods for preventing workers' compensation fraud.
10. Discuss how disability is determined and the various responsibilities of the employer, employee, and physician.
11. Differentiate between Social Security Disability Insurance and Supplemental Security Income.
12. Discuss miscellaneous programs, including State Disability, and Disability and Health Team.
13. Describe the Ticket to Work Program, its purpose, and how it works.
14. Outline the process for filing Social Security Disability Insurance and Supplemental Security Income claims.

CHAPTER TERMS

activities of daily living (ADLs)
Americans with Disabilities Act (ADA)
benefit cap
Black Lung Benefits Act
casual employee
coming and going rule
Disability and Health Team
disability income insurance
earned income
egregious
employment network
exemptions
Federal Employment Compensation Act (FECA)
Federal Employment Liability Act (FELA)
financial means test
instrumental activities of daily living (IADLs)

interstate commerce
job deconditioning
Longshore and Harbor Workers' Compensation Act
long-term disability
Merchant Marine Act (Jones Act)
modified own-occupation policy
no-fault insurance
occupational therapy
ombudsman
own-occupation policy
permanent and stationary
permanent disability
permanent partial disability
permanent total disability
progress or supplemental report

protected health information (PHI)
short-term disability
Social Security Disability Insurance (SSDI)
Supplemental Security Income (SSI)
temporarily disabled

temporary disability
temporary partial disability
temporary total disability
Ticket to Work Program
treating source
vocational rehabilitation
workers' compensation

WORKERS' COMPENSATION

Workers' compensation is a type of insurance regulated by state laws that pays medical expenses and partial loss of wages for workers who are injured on the job or become ill as a result of job-related circumstances. If death results, benefits are payable to the surviving spouse and dependents as defined by law. Most U.S. workers are covered by the Workers' Compensation Law. In many states, the employer, not the employee, pays the premiums. Each state sets up its own workers' compensation laws and regulations; however, they are basically the same from state to state.

History

Workers' compensation began in Germany in the 1800s when it was determined that something needed to be done to take care of injured workers to limit their physical and financial suffering from injuries or illnesses resulting from their jobs. Workers' compensation became common in the United States in the 1930s and 1940s, and it exists today in all 50 states and territories.

When workers' compensation was first proposed, U.S. companies were hesitant to accept full responsibility for paying the premiums. Their argument was that on top of the premium expense, they still could be financially liable in a worker-initiated lawsuit. A compromise was reached between businesses and workers: Companies would pay the premiums for the insurance that protected workers, and the workers would give up the right to sue the employer for damages resulting from a job-related illness or injury. This principle continues essentially intact today. Workers' compensation is not considered a "benefit"; rather, it is a legally mandated right of the worker.

Companies that meet specific state requirements must provide workers' compensation for all employees. Businesses that do not provide coverage as required by law can incur fines and other penalties. Workers' compensation can be purchased from several sources—private insurance companies, state funds, insurance pools, and self-insurance programs. Most states require employers to purchase workers' compensation insurance in the state in which their business operates. State statutes establish the framework and set up the laws for most workers' compensation insurance. As mentioned earlier, these laws provide benefits not only for workers but also for dependents of workers who are killed or die as a result of job-related accidents or illnesses. Many state laws also protect employers and their fellow workers by limiting the amount an injured employee can recover from an employer and by eliminating the liability of coworkers in most accidents.

For more detailed information on the history of workers' compensation, visit the Evolve site.

⭐ Imagine This!

Pirates, contrary to popular myth, proved to be highly organized and entrepreneurial. Before their assignment to the ranks of outlaws, they were considered highly prized allies of the government, plundering and sharing the spoils with governors of the pre-Revolutionary colonies, giving them a safe port.

Privateering (the gentleman's term for piracy) was a dangerous occupation; taking booty away from those who did not want to give it up leads to sea battles, hand-to-hand combat, and injury. Because of the ever-present chance of impairment, a system was developed to compensate injured "employees." There was one catch: He or she (there were female pirates as well) had to survive the wounds to collect because there was no recorded compensation for death.

Piratesinfo.com provides some information regarding the amount of payment made to the injured: loss of an eye—100 pieces of eight (Spanish dollar); loss of a finger—100 pieces of eight; loss of left arm—500 pieces of eight; loss of right arm—600 pieces of eight; loss of left leg—400 pieces of eight; and loss of right leg—500 pieces of eight.

Average weekly wage for colonial Americans of this period equated to approximately 2 pieces of eight per week. Loss of an eye or finger would merit payment approximating 50 weeks of wages. The right arm was worth 300 weeks (a little less than 6 years). These compare closely with modern compensation schedules.

In addition to being compensated, injured crew members were allowed to remain on board and offered less strenuous duty. The first return-to-work program was created.

Federal Legislation and Workers' Compensation

Workers' compensation programs are offered at the state level. In addition, there are several categories of federal programs for workers who do not fall under the umbrella of covered employees under state laws.

The **Federal Employment Compensation Act (FECA)** provides workers' compensation for nonmilitary federal employees. Many of the provisions are similar to state workers' compensation laws; however, awards are limited to disability or death incurred while in the performance of the employee's duties but not caused willfully by the employee, by intoxication, or other illegal acts. FECA covers medical expenses resulting from the disability and can require the employee to undergo job retraining. Under this act, a disabled employee receives two thirds of his or her normal monthly salary during the disability period and may receive more for permanent physical injuries or if he or she has dependents. FECA provides compensation for survivors of employees who are killed while on the job or die from a job-related illness or condition. FECA is administered by the Office of Workers' Compensation Programs.

Although not a workers' compensation statute, the **Federal Employment Liability Act (FELA)**, states that companies in which railroads are engaged in **interstate commerce** (trade that involves more than one state) are liable for injuries to their employees if they have been negligent. The **Merchant Marine Act (Jones Act)** provides seamen (individuals involved in transporting goods by water between U.S. ports) with the same protection from employer negligence that FELA provides railroad workers. Congress enacted the **Longshore and Harbor Workers' Compensation Act** to provide workers' compensation to specified employees of private maritime employers. The Office of Workers' Compensation Programs administers the act.

The **Black Lung Benefits Act** provides compensation for miners with black lung (pneumoconiosis, also called *anthracosis*). The Black Lung Benefits Act requires liable mine operators to award disability payments and establishes a fund administered by the Secretary of Labor providing disability payments to miners in cases in which the mine operator is unknown or unable to pay. The Office of Workers' Compensation Programs regulates the administration of the act.

Eligibility

In the United States, any employee who is injured on the job or develops an employment-related illness that prevents the employee from working is likely to be eligible to collect workers' compensation benefits. The benefits also apply to the spouse and dependents of a family member who dies because of a job-related accident or illness. If the disability is permanent or the employee has dependents, benefits include a specific percentage (often two-thirds) of regular wages or salary.

As with many rules and regulations, there are exceptions. Benefits are awarded only for disability or death occurring while the employee was in the process of performing lawful duties. If any horseplay, drunken stumbling, or illegal drugs are involved, workers' compensation usually does not pay. Workers' compensation does not pay for self-inflicted injuries and for injuries incurred while a worker is off the job, committing a crime, or violating company policy.

Exemptions

Not all business organizations are required to purchase workers' compensation insurance for their employees. Criteria for **exemptions** vary from state to state. The following list presents various exemption classifications (these classifications are not nationwide but vary from state to state):

- Employers with a minimum number of full-time employees (fewer than three and up to five, depending on the state)
- Executive officers
- Individuals who are business partners (coverage is optional)
- Sole proprietors (most states allow optional coverage)
- Casual employees

A **casual employee** is one who is not entitled to paid holiday or sick leave, has no expectation of ongoing employment, and for whom each engagement with the employer constitutes a separate contract of employment. Casual employees often receive a higher rate of pay to compensate for a lack of job security and benefits.

- Volunteers
- Part-time domestic employees, agricultural workers, and emergency relief workers

These categories of employees are typically excluded, but employees can obtain workers' compensation and employers' liability insurance coverage by agreement between their employer and an insurance carrier.

The previous list is not all inclusive. For additional information on workers' compensation exemptions, visit the Evolve site.

Benefits

Workers' compensation insurance is **no-fault insurance**. Benefits are paid to the injured (or ill) worker regardless of who is to blame for the accident or injury, barring the exceptions mentioned previously. There are four major benefit components to workers' compensation:

1. Medical expense—pays the expenses involved for hospitalization, physicians' visits, and any necessary medical treatment
2. Disability pay—can be temporary or permanent if it is determined that the worker will never fully recover
3. Vocational rehabilitation—if the injury or illness results in the worker being unable to perform the usual duties of his or her occupation, retraining may be necessary for the worker to enter into a new trade or business; also, physical therapy may be necessary
4. Death benefits—paid to surviving dependents

Because workers' compensation imposes strict liability without inquiry into fault, an employer could be penalized if the cause of injury or illness was **egregious**, meaning the employer was conspicuously negligent, such as violating federal or state safety standards, failing to correct known defects, or exhibiting other careless conduct.

Most state workers' compensation laws exclude coverage for injuries sustained while an employee is commuting to and from work. This exclusion is referred to as the **coming and going rule**. There are exceptions to this rule, however, such as when the scope of the employee's duties includes travel or when the employee is running an errand for the employer during the commute. Inquiry as to whether the coming and going rule applies to a particular situation should be made before simply ruling out the possibility of coverage for an accident that occurred during a worker's commute to or from work. If an employee is injured during a lunch period, it is usually considered outside the scope of the employment relationship. In the case of an automobile accident, workers' compensation might deny the claim, indicating that the automobile insurance carrier of the at-fault party is the primary payer.

🕐 Stop and Think

Carol Brown, bookkeeper at the Memorial Health Clinic, drops off the bank deposit each evening on her way home from work. One evening, as she is in the process of making the deposit, she slams her hand in the depository door, sustaining a laceration to her middle and index fingers. Several weeks later, as Carol is on her way to the bank to make the daily deposit, she stops at a convenience store for a cup of coffee and a donut. In her haste, she spills the coffee, sustaining second-degree burns to her torso. Does either of these scenarios represent a legitimate workers' compensation claim?

📁 HIPAA Tip

HIPAA requirements do not apply to certain types of benefit plans known as excepted benefits, which include coverage only for accidents (including accidental death or dismemberment) or certain categories of disability income insurance.

Denial of Benefits and Appeals

Employees who believe they have been wrongly denied workers' compensation benefits can appeal or resort to litigation. Some states have an **ombudsman**, who is an individual responsible for investigating and resolving workers' complaints against the employer or insurance company that is denying the benefits.

Most work injuries result in granted benefits' because it is usually obvious when an injury is work related. In these cases, if the claim is filed in a timely manner and according to a company's work rules, benefits are awarded. However, various situations may justify an employer or the insurer contesting a claim for workers' compensation benefits. It may be believed that an injury or resulting disability does not meet one or more of the legal requirements for entitlement to benefits. In these cases, a notice that the claim has been denied, containing reasons for the denial, must be issued promptly to the worker by the employer or by the employer's workers' compensation insurance company.

The appeal process differs from state to state. In many states, if the employee disagrees with the decision to deny the claim, he or she may appeal, but it must be done within a specified time, depending on state statutes. The appeal process can be started by contacting the appropriate state agency or by hiring an attorney. If all attempts at appeal do not reverse the decision and the denial becomes final, the worker is responsible for payment of all medical bills. If the individual has other health insurance, a claim can be submitted to that insurer. Most health insurance companies ask that a copy of the workers' compensation claim denial be included with the claim.

For more detailed information on workers' compensation by state, visit the Evolve site.

⭐ Imagine This!

Louise Carson has been a teacher at Harrison Junior High School for 10 years. At her yearly physical examination, her healthcare provider informs her that she is dangerously hypertensive. Louise attributes her hypertension to stress from her teaching responsibilities plus increasing pressure from her supervisor to maintain better discipline in the classroom. Louise's blood pressure does not respond to conventional antihypertensive medication, so her physician suggests a 6-week leave of absence from her job. Louise files a workers' compensation claim with the Harrison City School District; however, the claim is denied. The reason for denial, TEL-Abbot, Harrison's insurer, informs her, is that high stress is a normal part of the teaching profession.

🕐 Stop and Think

Benjamin Abbott, owner of Abbott Manufacturing, holds an annual Christmas party every year in the company cafeteria. Attendance to the party is optional, but Mr. Abbott uses this occasion to hand out the employee Christmas bonuses. Night shift foreman Ken Carter sustains a back injury while doing the limbo at the party. Abbott's insurer denies the claim stating that even though, technically, the injury occurred at work, it was not during regular work hours, and the employee was not engaged in his usual work duties. Can Ken appeal this decision?

Time Limits

Each state has rules established under which an employee is required to file a claim within a certain time limit. Usually traumatic claims must be brought within a time frame that runs from the date of the accident, date of last medical treatment, or date of the last payment of benefits. In cases where a job-related disease does not manifest immediately (i.e., lung cancer, toxic disease, or mesothelioma [a type of lung disease caused by asbestos exposure]), the time limit may extend from the date of the last exposure, date of the first symptoms of the disease, or date the diagnosis was determined. The time limits for filing claims and issuing appeals are established by individual state statutes and vary from state to state; the health insurance professional needs to become familiar with the workers' compensation regulations in the state in which he or she is employed.

Workers' Compensation Claims Process

The workers' compensation claims process can be long and arduous. Various steps must be followed, and report forms must be completed. This process can be facilitated if the individual steps are adhered to carefully and the forms are completed correctly and in a timely manner. The following sections discuss the steps for successful workers' compensation claim processing.

First Report of Injury

Employees who are injured, suspect they have been injured, or have contracted a disease they believe is related to their job should take immediate steps to protect their rights and to ensure that their claim is processed properly. Failure to seek timely medical treatment within the workers' compensation network may cause a delay in claim processing and perhaps denial of benefits. Injured workers should be transported to a medical treatment facility without delay in the case of an emergency. For nonemergency situations, the employee should take the following steps:

- The injured or ill worker should notify a supervisor of the incident immediately and provide the names of witnesses, if any.
- The injured or ill worker should complete the initial accident report or necessary paperwork. It does not matter whether the injury is severe or minor; it must be documented. The employer should supply the necessary forms (Fig. 11-1).
- The employer should report the incident to his or her workers' compensation carrier.
- The injured or ill worker should be sent to a medical facility for treatment or diagnosis, if not already done.

The procedure for reporting injuries and filing claims may vary from state to state. Contact the workers' compensation department in the state in which you reside and request specific guidelines for your state.

Physician's Role

Physicians have two distinct roles in the workers' compensation process:

1. To diagnose and treat work-related injuries and illnesses
2. To provide claims administrators opinions in response to specific medical and legal questions about work-related injuries or illnesses

WORKERS COMPENSATION - FIRST REPORT OF INJURY OR ILLNESS

Employer (Name & Address with Zip Code)	Carrier/Administrator Claim Number	Report Purpose Code
	Jurisdiction	Jurisdiction Claim Number

	Insured Report Number	

SIC Code	Employer Fein	Employer's Location Address (If different)	Location #:
			Phone #

CARRIER/CLAIMS ADMINISTRATOR

Carrier (Name, Address & Phone No)	Policy Period To Check if Appropriate ☐ Self-Insurance	Claims Administrator (Name, Address & Phone Number)

Carrier Fein	Policy/Self-Insured Number	Administration Fein

Agent Name & Code Number

EMPLOYEE / WAGE

Name (Last, First, Middle)	Birth Date	Social Security Number	Hire Date	State of Hire

Address (include Zip Code)	Sex	Marital Status	Occupation/Job Title
			Employment Status
			NCCI Class Code
Phone	# Dependents		

Rate Per ☐ Day ☐ Month ☐ Week ☐ Other:	# Days Worked/Week	Full Pay for Day of Injury? ☐ Yes ☐ No Did Salary Continue? ☐ Yes ☐ No

OCCURANCE/TREATMENT

Time Employee Began Work	Date of Injury/Illness	Time of Occurrence AM PM	Late Work Date	Date Employer Notified	Date Disability Began

Contact Number/Phone Number	Type of Injury/Illness	Part of Body Affected
Did Injury/Illness Exposure Occur on Employer's Premises? Yes ☐ No ☐	Type of Injury/Illness Code	Part of Body Affected Code

Department or Location Where Accident or Illness Exposure Occurred	All Equipment, Materials, or Chemicals Employee Was Using When Accident or Illness Exposure Occurred
Specific Activity the Employee was Engaged in When the Accident or Illness Exposure Occurred	Work Process the Employee Was Engaged in When Accident or Illness Exposure Occurred

How Injury or Illness/Abnormal Health Condition Occurred. Describe the Sequence of Events and Include Any Objects or substances that Directly Injured the Employee or Made the Employee ILL	Cause of Injury Code

Date Return(ed) To Work	If Fatal, Give Date of Death	Were Safeguards or Safety Equipment Provided? ☐ Yes ☐ No Were They Used ☐ Yes ☐ No
Physician/Health Care Provider (Name & Address)	Hospital (Name & Address)	Initial Treatment

Witness (Name & Phone #)

Date Administrator Notified	Date Prepared	Preparer's Name & Title	Phone Number

Fig. 11-1 Sample workers' compensation first report of injury form.

Employer's Instructions
DO NOT ENTER DATA IN SHADED FIELDS

Preferred Formats for Date and Time: Dates should be entered as MM/DD/YYYY, and times as HH:MM a (am) / p (pm)

SIC Code: This is the code which represents the nature of the employer's business which is contained in the Standard Industrial Classification Manual published by the Federal Office of Management and Budget.

Carrier: The licensed business entity issuing a contract of insurance and assuming financial responsibility on behalf of the employer of the claimant.

Claims Administrator: Enter the name of the carrier, third party administrator, state fund, or self-insured responsible for administering the claim.

Agent Name & Code Number: Enter the name of your insurance agent and his/her code number if known. This information can be found on your insurance policy.

Employee/Wage Section: When filling in Social Security Number, do **NOT** include dashes.

Occupation/Job Title: This is the primary occupation of the claimant at the time of the accident or exposure.

Employment Status: Indicate the employee's work status. The valid choices are:

Apprenticeship Full-Time	Apprenticeship Part-Time	Disabled	Full-Time
Not Employed	On Strike	Part-Time	Piece Worker
Retired	Seasonal	Unknown	Volunteer

Date Disability Began: The first day on which the claimant originally lost time from work due to the occupation injury or disease or otherwise deigned by statute.

Contact Name/Phone Number: Enter the name of the individual at the employer's premises to be contacted for additional information.

Type of Injury/Illness: Briefly describe the nature of the injury or illness (e.g. Lacerations to the forearm).

Part of Body Affected: Indicate the part of body affected by the injury/illness (e.g. Right forearm, lower back). Part of Body Affected Code does not allow multiple body parts to be selected. Please choose the most dominant body part affected from the list.

Department or Location Where Accident or Illness Exposure Occurred: (e.g. Maintenance Dept or Client's Office at (address). If the accident or illness exposure did not occur on the employer's premises, enter address or location. Be specific.

All Equipment, Material or Chemicals Employee Was Using When Accident or Illness Exposure Occurred: (e.g. Acetylene cutting torch, metal plate). List of all the equipment, materials, and/or chemicals the employee was using, applying, handlings or operating when the injury or illness occurred. Be specific, for example: decorator's scaffolding, electric sander, paintbrush, and paint. Enter "NA" for not applicable if no equipment, materials, or chemicals were being used. NOTE: The items listed do not have to be directly involved in the employee's injury or illness.

Specific Activity the Employee Was Engaged in When the Accident or Illness Exposure Occurred: (e.g. Cutting metal plate for flooring). Describe the specific activity the employee was engaged in when the accident or illness exposure occurred, such as sanding ceiling woodwork in preparation for painting.

Work Process the Employee Was Engaged in When Accident or Illness Exposure Occurred:
Describe the work process the employee was engaged in when the accident or illness exposure occurred, such as building maintenance. Enter "NA" for not applicable if employee was not engaged in a work process (e.g. walking along a hallway).

How Injury or Illness/Abnormal Health Condition Occurred. Describe the Sequence of Events and Include Any Objects or Substances That Directly Injured the Employee or Made the Employee Ill:
(Worker stepped back to inspect work and slipped on some scrap metal. As worker fell, worker brushed against the hot metal.) Describe how the injury or illness/abnormal health condition occurred. Include the sequence of events and name any objects of substance that directly injured the employee or made the employee ill. For example: Worker stepped to the edge of the scaffolding to inspect work, lost balance and fell six feet to the floor. The worker's right wrist was broken in the fall.

Date Return(ed) To Work: Enter the date following the most recent disability period on which the employee returned to work.

Fig. 11-1—cont'd

The physician may be asked the following questions:

- Was the injury or illness caused by the employee's work?
- Is the condition **permanent and stationary**, meaning has the employee reached a state of maximal medical improvement?
- If a condition is permanent and stationary, has the injury caused permanent disability that limits the ability to compete in the open labor market?
- Can the employee return to his or her usual and customary work assignment? If not, does he or she need some type of accommodations because of work restrictions, or does the employee need to be retrained for a new job?
- Will the employee who has a permanent and stationary condition require access to future medical treatment for the condition?

Usually a single physician fills both of the above-listed roles in workers' compensation cases; however, an independent medical evaluator may address the specific medical and legal questions. When an injured or ill employee visits the medical facility, the attending physician should

- obtain a complete history of the condition, including preexisting conditions or disability;
- obtain a thorough work history, including any exposures as they pertain to the chief complaint;
- perform a physical examination, focusing on the system or systems involved;
- consider restrictions (e.g., no typing for more than 1 hour) before taking the patient off work to prevent **job deconditioning** (i.e., the patient psychologically or physically loses his or her ability to perform normal job duties at the previous level of expertise as a result of being absent from work);
- make a diagnostic evaluation; and
- complete all paperwork promptly because the patient may have no source of income if the paperwork is delayed (Fig. 11-2).

Determining Disability

When an injured or ill worker visits the healthcare facility for treatment, the provider completes an attending physician statement (as discussed in the previous section), which should indicate any physical or mental impairments resulting from the incident. The classification of workers' compensation disability cases, mandated by federal law, is as follows:

- Medical treatment only—this category comprises minor injuries or illnesses that are resolved quickly, resulting in a minimal loss of work time with no residual limitations. Compensation is made for medical expenses rendered that are necessary to cure and relieve the effects of the injury or illness.
- **Temporary disability**—benefits in this category are paid so long as the physician's opinion concurs with that claim

of status. Temporary disability includes two subcategories:

- **Temporary total disability**—the worker's ability to perform his or her job responsibilities is totally lost, but on a temporary basis.
- **Temporary partial disability**—an injury or illness impairs an employee's ability to work for a limited time. The impairment is such that the individual is able to perform limited employment duties and is expected to recover fully.
- **Permanent disability**—the ill or injured employee's condition is such that it is impossible to return to work. Compensation is awarded to the worker for the loss of value of his or her skills in the open labor market. As with temporary disability, permanent disability has two subcategories:
  - **Permanent partial disability**—prevents the individual from performing one or more occupational functions but does not impair his or her capability of performing less demanding employment.
  - **Permanent total disability**—the employee's ability to work at any occupation is totally and permanently lost.

🕐 Stop and Think

George Meade makes his living as a concert pianist. To relax between concerts, George takes up woodworking and inadvertently severs his right index finger, preventing him from performing. Into what classification would George's disability fall?

Vocational Rehabilitation

When employees cannot return to their previous job because of a workers' compensation injury or illness, they often are entitled to **vocational rehabilitation** services if it is reasonable to assume that these individuals can be trained for some alternative type of employment. The goal of vocational rehabilitation is to return the injured worker to some sort of suitable, gainful employment that he or she can reasonably achieve and that offers an opportunity to restore the injured worker to maximum self-support as soon as practical and as near as possible to what it was before the incident.

Waiting Periods

Workers' compensation benefits normally do not begin immediately. Most states have a waiting period that applies before benefits to the injured (or ill) employee begin. Of the 54 jurisdictions (50 states, District of Columbia, Puerto Rico, Virgin Islands, and Guam), only 1 jurisdiction, the Virgin Islands, does not have a waiting period. In 24 jurisdictions, there is a 3-day waiting period, and

Health Care Provider Report
See Instructions on Reverse Side
(WHEN COMPLETED RETURN TO REQUESTER)

H C 0 1

DO NOT USE THIS SPACE

Please PRINT or TYPE your responses.
Enter dates in MM/DD/YYYY format.

SOCIAL SECURITY NUMBER	DATE OF INJURY
EMPLOYEE	EMPLOYER
INSURER/SELF-INSURER/TPA	INSURER CLAIM NUMBER

INSURER ADDRESS

CITY	STATE	ZIP CODE

REQUESTER must specify all items to be completed by health care provider. ☐ Items: _____ ☐ MMI (#9) ☐ PPD (#10)

HEALTH CARE PROVIDER TO COMPLETE ITEMS REQUESTED ABOVE

1.   Date of first examination for this injury by this office: _____ (date)

2.   Diagnosis (include all ICD-10-CM codes):

3.   History of injury or disease given by employee:

4.   In your opinion (as substantiated by the history and physical examination) was the injury or disease caused, aggravated or accelerated by the employee's alleged employment activity or environment?   ☐ No   ☐ Yes

5.   Is there evidence of pre-existing or other conditions that affect this disability?   ☐ No   ☐ Yes   If yes, describe:

6.   Is further treatment of this injury or referral to another doctor planned?   ☐ No   ☐ Yes   If yes, describe:

7.   Has surgery been performed?   ☐ No   ☐ Yes   If yes, date and describe: _____ (date)

8.   Attach the most recent Report of Work Ability. Date of report: _____ (date)

9.   **Has the employee reached maximum medical improvement?**   ☐ No   ☐ Yes   Date reached: _____
     (If yes, complete item #10) (See definition on back)

10. **Has the employee sustained any permanent partial disability from the injury?**   ☐ No   ☐ Yes   ☐ Too early to determine
     The permanent partial disability is _____ % of the whole body. This rating is based on Minn. Rules:

5223.	%	5223.	%
5223.	%	5223.	%

NAME (Type or Print)	SIGNATURE		DEGREE
ADDRESS	STATE	LICENSE #/REGISTRATION #	
CITY STATE ZIP CODE	AREA CODE TELEPHONE #	DATE SIGNED	

MN HC01 (7/01)

Fig. 11-2 Sample healthcare provider report.

the waiting period is 7 days in 23 jurisdictions. Idaho, Massachusetts, Mississippi, and Nevada have a 5-day waiting period. North Dakota and Montana have a 4-day waiting period. Most states allow for retroactive compensation when disability continues for a certain period from the date of injury or illness.

Occupational therapy is different from vocational rehabilitation. Occupational therapy is a treatment that focuses on helping individuals achieve independence in all areas of their lives. An occupational therapist works with individuals with varying disabilities and provides treatment for individuals to relearn physical skills lost as a result of an illness or accident—ideally so that they can return to some form of gainful employment or an independent, productive life.

Claim Forms

In contrast to most major third-party payer claims, there is no universal form to use when filing a workers' compensation claim. Some states allow workers' compensation claims to be submitted on the CMS-1500 form. Private insurance carriers typically have their own forms. The health insurance professional should determine if it is acceptable to submit a workers' compensation claim on the CMS-1500 form; if not, the health insurance professional should ask the patient to request the required form from his or her employer or insurer.

⭐ Imagine This!

Frank Turner sustains a serious cut to his right hand while operating a band saw at work. Frank's injury qualifies him for workers' compensation benefits, which start 1 week after the incident occurred. Larry Boggs, a coworker in the millroom with Frank, becomes ill the same week. Thinking he was just suffering from a minor cold, Larry does not file for workers' compensation; however, 2 weeks later, his cold is no better. Larry returns to his physician, who determines he has pneumonia. Larry subsequently is hospitalized for 1 week, during which time further tests reveal that Larry's condition is caused by breathing minute particles of sawdust. When Larry is discharged from the hospital, he files a workers' compensation claim. The claim is approved, but Larry's benefits do not begin until 4 weeks after his illness began.

Normally, multiple copies of all workers' compensation reports are essential for proper distribution as follows:
1. Original form to the insurance carrier
2. One copy to the appropriate state agency
3. One copy to the patient's employer
4. One copy to be retained in the healthcare provider's files
   When special claim forms should be used, instructions usually are provided—often on the back side of the form. If instructions do not come with the form, the health

insurance professional should ask the patient to obtain detailed guidelines from the employer or insurer.

Because thousands of different forms are used for workers' compensation claims in the United States, to avoid confusion, instructions for completing the standard CMS-1500 claim form are used in this chapter. These instructions can be found in Appendix B along with an example of a completed claim for a workers' compensation case. These instructions are generic, and the health insurance professional should obtain exact guidelines from the employer, the insurer, or the particular state in which the claim occurs to prevent delays or rejections.

Before completing the blocks, the health insurance professional should determine the name and address of the insurer to whom the claim will be sent. This information should appear in the upper-right-hand corner of the claim form.

Progress Reports

Keeping the employer and insurance carrier apprised of the patient's treatment plan, progress, and status is a priority in workers' compensation cases. The health insurance professional should be well versed in the particulars of workers' compensation reporting so that written communications meet all accepted legal standards. After the initial visit to the physician has occurred and the attending physician report has been filed, unless the employee has returned to work full-time, periodic reports have to be filed. These are referred to as **progress or supplemental reports** (Fig. 11-3). Often, there are no special printed forms for progress reports; copies of clinical notes from the patient's health record or a letter from the attending physician giving a detailed account of the patient's progress are acceptable. When the patient's disability ends, and he or she is able to return to work, the physician submits a final report.

Special Billing Notes

Most states have a fee schedule that providers must use when billing a workers' compensation claim, and as long as a workers' compensation claim is pending, the provider cannot bill the patient. Additionally, balance billing is not allowed on workers' compensation claims. If the claim has been denied, and all efforts for appeal have been exhausted, the health insurance professional should issue a letter of reply immediately, after which direct billing to the patient or the patient's private insurance company for the services rendered is allowed. The workers' compensation fee schedule does not apply to denied claims; instead, the provider's usual and customary fees apply. Workers' compensation claims are handled differently in each state, and the health insurance professional must follow the guidelines set forth by the law in his or her state. Also, rules and regulations and appropriate forms may change from year to year, which makes it vitally important for the health insurance professional to keep up-to-date with the most current laws in the state in which he or she is employed.

**Workers' Compensation
Medical Progress Report**

Claim Number	Health Care Provider

Employee Last Name	First Name	
Mailing Address (include zip code)		Telephone (include area code)
Occupation	Date of Birth	Sex
Description of injury/illness	Date of Exam	Social Security Number
Employer	Employer Contact Person	
Employer Address		Phone #
Insurer Name	Claim Representative	
Insurer Address		Phone #

Current Work Ability: ☐ Fit for regular work duties   ☐ Unfit for regular work duties

Start date for return to regular work duties (dd/mm/yy)

Duration of modified duties: ☐ 1-7 days   ☐ 8-14 days   ☐ 15-21 days   ☐ More

Start date for modified duties (dd/mm/yy)

Subjective Information
Objective Information
Past diseases/injuries

Diagnostics (Lab/x-rays, CT, etc.)	ICD Code:

Prescribed treatment/advice/referrals

Please give details for the following questions when the answer is Yes

Has worker been hospitalized?   ☐ Yes   ☐ No   Dates:_____ to _____

Has an operation been performed?   ☐ Yes   ☐ No   Date(s):

Any factors delaying recovery?   ☐ Yes   ☐ No   Explain:

Is permanent disability probable?   ☐ Yes   ☐ No

Would you suggest an examination by a WC doctor?   ☐ Yes   ☐ No

Will worker be seen again?   ☐ Yes   ☐ No   Date:

I hereby certify that the above is a correct statement of services personally rendered by me.

Health Care Professional Signature _____ Date _____

Name of Physician	EIN #
Address	NPI #

Fig. 11-3 Sample workers' compensation medical progress report.

Sandra Cotter was injured at work when a filing cabinet fell on her foot. The human relations officer advised Sandra to see her own physician because the company did not have a specific workers' compensation physician. Sandra was treated at the Heartland Medical Clinic, which billed her health insurer, Blue Cross and Blue Shield. Blue Cross and Blue Shield refused payment, so Heartland billed Sandra. Sandra refused to pay the bill, stating that it was a workers' compensation case. Heartland argued that they had not received a call from Sandra's employer authorizing treatment. Still, Sandra refused to pay. After sending Sandra statements for 6 months, Heartland sent her a certified letter stating they were refusing all future medical treatment at the clinic. Sandra filed a complaint with the State Workers' Compensation Board, and the case eventually was resolved; however, Heartland still refused to see Sandra for subsequent visits.

Workers' Compensation and Managed Care

As an alternative to the traditional approach to workers' compensation insurance coverage, some employers choose a managed care system (e.g., health maintenance organization or preferred provider organization) to provide medical care to injured employees, which can be a cost savings to the employer. Some states, such as New Jersey, have a Workers' Compensation Managed Care Organization that manages the use of care and costs associated with claims covered by workers' compensation insurance. Employers can typically realize a savings in premium costs by selecting the managed care option if offered in the state and approved by the state workers' compensation board.

Health Insurance Portability and Accountability Act and Workers' Compensation

The Health Insurance Portability and Accountability Act (HIPAA) Privacy Rule does not apply to workers' compensation insurers, workers' compensation administrative agencies, or employers. The Privacy Rule recognizes the legitimate need for insurers and other entities involved in the workers' compensation system to have access to injured workers' **protected health information (PHI)** as authorized by state or other law. Workers' compensation patients may or may not be required to sign a release of information form for a claim form to be filed. Additionally, employers and claims adjusters retain the right of access to workers' compensation files. If the health insurance professional encounters a workers' compensation case for an established patient who already has a health record in that office, a new record should be created and kept separate from that individual's regular health record. Some medical offices color code or flag workers' compensation records or file them in a separate area to avoid confusion. The health insurance professional should check the regulations in his or her state regarding PHI regulations.

Workers' Compensation Fraud

As with any type of insurance, fraud occurs in workers' compensation cases. Most states require workers' compensation insurers, self-insured employers, and third-party administrators to report fraud to the State Insurance Commissioner's office or to the local District Attorney's office or both. Anyone can report workers' compensation fraud, however. When fraud is suspected, a report should be made within a reasonable time frame, usually within 30 days from the time the individual reporting knows or reasonably believes he or she knows the identity of a person or entity that has committed workers' compensation fraud or has knowledge that such fraud has been committed. This report often can be accomplished by a telephone call to either of the previously named offices.

Online Workers' Compensation Service Center

The Online Workers' Compensation Service Center is a national website that provides workers' compensation news and information for employees, employers, insurers, and medical providers. Anyone can use this research center to locate an insurance provider, get information on a program in a particular state, and find professional help relating to workplace injuries and disabilities in the United States. To learn about workers' compensation laws in your state, go to the Evolve site.

❓ What Did You Learn?

1. How did workers' compensation originate?
2. Who is eligible for workers' compensation benefits?
3. List four exemption classifications.
4. What is no-fault insurance?
5. What does an ombudsman do?

PRIVATE AND EMPLOYER-SPONSORED DISABILITY INCOME INSURANCE

Most people think about insurance coverage as it relates to health, life, home, or automobile, but the most crucial aspect of personal and family finances is **earned income**—income from employment. If an illness or injury occurred, and this income stopped, most people would quickly find it difficult or impossible to maintain a home and provide for their family. **Disability income insurance** replaces a portion of earned income when an individual is unable to perform the requirements of his or her job because of injury or illness (that is not work related).

⭐ Imagine This!

Paul Graham, a self-employed auto mechanic, purchased private disability income insurance from Excel Coverage Experts. When he became disabled because of a shoulder injury, his monthly disability benefits paid his house and car payments. Stanley Morgan, Paul's neighbor, fell from a ladder while fixing his roof, resulting in multiple fractures in both legs. Stanley did not have disability income insurance. Stanley was disabled for 6 months, during which time the bank foreclosed on his house because he could not pay the mortgage.

Disability insurance can be purchased privately through a commercial insurance company, or it is sometimes furnished by the employer. There are two major types of disability coverage:

1. **Short-term disability**, which provides an income for the early part of a disability—typically 2 weeks to 2 years
2. **Long-term disability**, which helps replace income for a longer time—5 years or until the disabled individual turns 65

Defining Disability

Disability is commonly defined one of two ways:

1. An individual is unable to perform in the occupation or job that he or she was doing before the disability occurred. This definition of disability is covered in what is referred to as **own-occupation policies**. A variation is the **modified own-occupation policy**, which covers workers for their own occupation as long as they are not gainfully employed elsewhere.
2. An individual is unable to perform any occupation for which he or she is suited by education and experience.

The distinction between these two definitions can be crucial. If a surgeon loses a hand, he or she may be unable to perform surgery. In the case of an own-occupation policy, the surgeon would be able to recover because he or she was able to work as a physician in a nonsurgical field. With the inability to perform any occupation, there would be no recovery, even if the surgeon could work as a tour guide.

Short-Term Disability

Short-term disability pays a percentage of an individual's wages or salary if he or she becomes **temporarily disabled**, meaning that the individual is unable to work for a short time because of sickness or injury (excluding job-related illnesses or injuries). A typical short-term disability policy pays one-half to two-thirds salary or wages for a specific number of weeks, depending on the policy. Most short-term disability policies have a **benefit cap**, meaning there is a maximum benefit amount paid per month.

A worker generally begins receiving money from a short-term disability policy within 1 to 14 days after becoming sick or disabled. The actual time elapsed before payments begin depends on the stipulations in the policy. Often, if the individual sustains an injury, benefits begin immediately. It usually takes longer with an illness because there needs to be enough time to show that the illness is severe enough to be disabling. If the disability insurance is furnished by the employer, there may be additional restrictions as to when the short-term disability benefits begin. The employer may require all sick days to be used up before the employee begins receiving disability payments. Typically, if the condition worsens over time, the individual would receive disability pay retroactive to the first sick day.

Long-Term Disability

As with short-term disability, a long-term disability insurance policy protects an individual from the loss of ability to earn an income because of an illness or injury that is not work related. It pays a monthly amount to help cover expenses when an individual is unable to perform his or her job or function in a chosen occupation or profession.

There are two major types of individual long-term disability insurance: no cancelable and guaranteed renewable. With both no cancelable and guaranteed renewable policies, the insurer cannot cancel or refuse to renew the policy as long as the required premiums are paid on time. The key difference between the two major types of policies is that under a no cancelable contract, the individual has the extra security that premiums can never be increased above those shown in the policy as long as the required premiums are paid. With a guaranteed renewable policy, the premiums can be increased, but only if the change affects an entire class of policyholders. For this reason, initial premiums for guaranteed renewable policies can be less expensive than no cancelable policies.

Disability Claims Process

As with workers' compensation, there are several steps to the disability claims process. To allow this process to work efficiently and effectively, the employee and the employer must attend to certain responsibilities.

Employee's Responsibilities

First, the worker must notify the proper party that he or she intends to file a disability claim. To do this, the individual first needs to submit a claim request. If disability insurance is provided through the employer, a claim form may be obtained from the company's human resources department. Some insurers allow telephone or electronic submission of claims. In this case, the human resources department should provide a toll-free number or website and specific instructions for submitting the claim. In the case of an individual or private disability policy, a claim form may be obtained from the insurance company where the policy was purchased. The claim request should include everything needed to process the claim, including

1. information the employee provides (Fig. 11-4),
2. information the employer provides (Fig. 11-5),
3. the attending physician statement (Fig. 11-6), and
4. Claimant's Authorization to Disclose Health Information (Figure 11-7).

EMPLOYEE'S CLAIM FOR COMPENSATION

ANSWER ALL QUESTIONS FULLY - PRINT OR TYPE CLEARLY

IMPORTANT: Your Social Security Number Must Be Entered:

IMPORTANTE: El Numero de su Seguro Social Debe Ser Indicado:

WCB Case No. (If known)_____ Carrier Case No. (if known)_____

A. **Injured person**	1. Name.. First Name Middle Name Last Name 2. Mailing Address... Number and Street (includeApartment No.) City State Zip Code. 3. Sex ☐Male ☐Female Date of Birth...Telephone No. ( )............... 4. Do you speak English? ☐Yes ☐No If no, what language do you speak?............................... 5. Name of union and local number, if member.. 6. State what your regular work/occupation was... 7. Wages or average earnings per day, including overtime, board, rent and other allowances............ 8. Were you paid full wages for the day of injury? ☐Yes ☐No 9. Your work week at time of injury was: ☐Five day ☐Six day ☐Seven day ☐Other...............
B. **Employer(s)**	1. Employer..Telephone No. ( )............... 2. Employer's Address... 3. Were you employed by any other employer or employers at the time of your injury/illness? ☐Yes ☐No 4. If yes, did you lose time from work at this other employment as a result of your injury/illness? ☐Yes ☐No
C. **Place/Time**	1. Address where injury occurred...County................... 2. Date of Injury.......................................at.............o'clock, ☐ AM ☐ PM
D. **The Injury**	1. How did injury/illness occur?... ....
E. **Nature and Extent of Injury/ Illness**	1. State fully the nature of your injury/illness, including all parts of body injured............................... .... 2. Date you stopped work because of this injury/illness?... 3. Have you returned to work? ☐ Yes ☐ No If yes, on what date?.. 4. Does injury/illness keep you from work? ☐Yes ☐No 5. Have you done any work during period of disability? ☐ Yes ☐ No 6. Have you received any wages since your injury/illness? ☐Yes ☐ No

F. **Medical Benefits**	1. Did you receive or are you now receiving medical care? ☐ Yes ☐No
	2. Are you now in need of medical care? ☐Yes ☐No
	3. Name of attending doctor..
	   Doctor's address...
	4. If you were in a hospital, give the dates hospitalized..
	   Name of hospital..
	   Hospital's address...

G. **Comp. Payments**	1. Have you received or are you now receiving workers' compensation payments for the injury reported above? ☐Yes ☐No 2. Do you claim further workers' compensation payments? ☐Yes ☐No
H. **Notice**	1. Have you given your employer (or supervisor) notice of injury? ☐Yes ☐No 2. If yes, notice was given ☐orally ☐in writing, on.. to ....

ANY PERSON WHO KNOWINGLY AND WITH INTENT TO DEFRAUD PRESENTS, CAUSES TO BE PRESENTED, OR PREPARES WITH KNOWLEDGE OR BELIEF THAT IT WILL BE PRESENTED TO, OR BY AN INSURER, OR SELF INSURER, ANY INFORMATION CONTAINING ANY FALSE MATERIAL STATEMENT OR CONCEALS ANY MATERIAL FACT SHALL BE GUILTY OF A CRIME AND SUBJECT TO SUBSTANTIAL FINES AND IMPRISONMENT.

Signed by...Dated...

(Claimant)

C-3 (2-04)

Fig. 11-4 Employee's statement form.

EMPLOYER'S REPORT OF NON-WORK-RELATED ACCIDENT/OCCUPATIONAL DISEASE

Send this notice directly to the Chair, Workers' Compensation Board at the address shown on the reverse side within ten (10) days after an accident occurs. ANSWER ALL QUESTIONS FULLY. A copy should also be provided to or retained by your workers' compensation insurance carrier.

Any employer who fails to timely file Form C-2, as required by Section 110 of the Workers' Compensation Law, is subject to a fine of not more than $1,000. In addition, the Board or Chair may impose a penalty of up to $2,500.

TYPEWRITER PREPARATION IS STRONGLY RECOMMENDED - INCLUDE ZIP CODE IN ALL ADDRESSES-EMPLOYEE'S S.S.NO. MUST BE ENTERED BELOW ↓

WCB CASE NO.(If Known)	CARRIER CASE NO.	CARRIER CODE NO.	WC POLICY NO.	DATE OF ACCIDENT	EMPLOYEE'S S.S. NO.
		W		m m d d y y	

1.(a) EMPLOYER'S NAME | (b) EMPLOYER'S MAILING ADDRESS | (c) OSHA CASE/FILE NO.

(d) LOCATION (If Different From Mailing Address) | (e) NATURE OF BUSINESS (Principal Products, Services, etc.) | (f) NY UI EMPLOYER REG. NO. | (g) FEIN - if UI Emp. Reg. No. Unknown

2.(a) INSURANCE CARRIER | (b) CARRIER'S ADDRESS

3.(a) INJURED EMPLOYEE (First, M.I., Last) | (b) ADDRESS (Includes No. & Street, City, State, Zip & Apt. No.)

ACCIDENT

4. (a) ADDRESS WHERE ACCIDENT OCCURRED | (b) COUNTY | (c) WAS ACCIDENT ON EMPLOYER'S PREMISES? ☐ Yes ☐ No

5. HOUR EMP. BEGAN WORK h h : m m ☐ AM ☐ PM | 6. TIME OF ACCIDENT h h : m m ☐ AM ☐ PM | 7. DEPT. WHERE REGULARLY EMPLOYED | 8.(a) DATE STOPPED WORK BECAUSE OF THIS INJURY/ILLNESS m m d d y y | (b) WAS EMPLOYEE PAID IN FULL FOR DAY? ☐ Yes ☐ No

INJURED PERSON

9. SEX ☐ Male ☐ Female | 10. DATE OF BIRTH m m d d y y | 11.OCCUPATION (Specific job title at which employed) | 12. DATE HIRED m m d d y y

13.(a) AVERAGE EARNINGS PER WEEK? $, .0 0 | (b) TOTAL EARNINGS PAID DURING 52 WEEKS PRIOR TO DATE OF ACCIDENT (Include bonuses, overtime, value of lodging, etc.) $, .0 0 | 14. (a) EMPLOYEE IS: ☐ Full Time ☐ Part Time | (b) INJURED EMPLOYEE'S WORK WEEK (Check days usually worked.) Mon ☐ Tue ☐ Wed ☐ Thu ☐ Fri ☐ Sat ☐ Sun ☐

NATURE OF INJURY

15. NATURE OF INJURY AND PART(S) OF BODY AFFECTED | 16. (a) DID YOU PROVIDE MEDICAL CARE? ☐ Yes ☐ No | (b) IF YES, WHEN?

17. WAS EMPLOYEE TREATED IN AN EMERGENCY ROOM? ☐ Yes ☐ No | 18. WAS EMPLOYEE HOSPITALIZED OVERNIGHT AS AN IN-PATIENT? ☐ Yes ☐ No

19. (a) NAME AND ADDRESS OF DOCTOR | (b) NAME AND ADDRESS OF HOSPITAL

20. (a) HAS EMPLOYEE RETURNED TO WORK? ☐ Yes ☐ No | (b) IF YES, GIVE DATE: m m d d y y | (c) AT WHAT WEEKLY WAGE? $, .0 0

NOTE: FORM C-11 MUST BE FILED EACH TIME THERE IS A CHANGE IN EMPLOYMENT STATUS

CAUSE OF ACCIDENT

21. WHAT WAS EMPLOYEE DOING WHEN INJURED? (Please be specific. Identify tools, equipment or material the employee was using.)

22. HOW DID THE ACCIDENT OR EXPOSURE OCCUR? (Please describe fully the events that resulted in injury or occupational disease. Tell what happened and how it happened. Please use separate sheet if necessary.)

23. OBJECT OR SUBSTANCE THAT DIRECTLY INJURED EMPLOYEE. e.g., the machine employee struck against or which struck him/her, the vapor or poison inhaled or swallowed, the chemical that irritated his/her skin. In cases of strains, the thing (s)he was lifting, pulling, etc.

FATAL CASES

24. (a) DATE OF DEATH m m d d y y | (b) NAME AND ADDRESS OF NEAREST RELATIVE | (c) RELATIONSHIP

PREPARATION

DATE EMPLOYER/SUPERVISOR FIRST KNEW OF INJURY m m d d y y | DATE OF THIS REPORT m m d d y y | IF FORM IS SUBMITTED BY EMPLOYER, COMPLETE A & B BELOW. IF FORM IS SUBMITTED BY THIRD PARTY, COMPLETE A,B,C & D BELOW.

A. EMPLOYEE PREPARING FORM OR SUPPLYING INFORMATION TO THIRD PARTY | B. TITLE | TELEPHONE NUMBER & EXTENSION

C. IF REPORT PREPARED BY THIRD PARTY, COMPANY NAME AND ADDRESS

D. THIRD PARTY CONTACT NAME | TELEPHONE NUMBER & EXTENSION

Fig. 11-5 Sample employer's statement form.

Health Care Provider Report
See Instructions on Reverse Side
(WHEN COMPLETED RETURN TO REQUESTER)

Please PRINT or TYPE your responses.
Enter dates in MM/DD/YYYY format.

SOCIAL SECURITY NUMBER	DATE OF INJURY
EMPLOYEE	EMPLOYER
INSURER/SELF-INSURER/TPA	INSURER CLAIM NUMBER
INSURER ADDRESS	
CITY STATE ZIP CODE	

REQUESTER must specify all items to be completed by health care provider. ☐ Items: _____ ☐ MMI (#9) ☐ PPD (#10)

HEALTH CARE PROVIDER TO COMPLETE ITEMS REQUESTED ABOVE

1. Date of first examination for this injury by this office: _____ (date)

2. Diagnosis (include all ICD-10-CM codes):

3. History of injury or disease given by employee:

4. In your opinion (as substantiated by the history and physical examination) was the injury or disease caused, aggravated or accelerated by the employee's alleged employment activity or environment? ☐ No ☐ Yes

5. Is there evidence of pre-existing or other conditions that affect this disability? ☐ No ☐ Yes   If yes, describe:

6. Is further treatment of this injury or referral to another doctor planned? ☐ No ☐ Yes   If yes, describe:

7. Has surgery been performed? ☐ No ☐ Yes   If yes, date and describe: _____ (date)

8. Attach the most recent Report of Work Ability. Date of report: _____ (date)

9. **Has the employee reached maximum medical improvement?** ☐ No ☐ Yes   Date reached: _____
   (If yes, complete item #10) (See definition on back)

10. **Has the employee sustained any permanent partial disability from the injury?** ☐ No ☐ Yes ☐ Too early to determine
    The permanent partial disability is _____ % of the whole body. This rating is based on Minn. Rules:

5223.	%	5223.	%
5223.	%	5223.	%

NAME (Type or Print)	SIGNATURE		DEGREE
ADDRESS	STATE	LICENSE #/REGISTRATION #	
CITY STATE ZIP CODE	AREA CODE	TELEPHONE #	DATE SIGNED

MN HC01 (7/01)

Fig. 11-6 Attending physician's statement form.

CLAIMANT'S AUTHORIZATION TO DISCLOSE HEALTH INFORMATION
(Pursuant to HIPAA)

INSTRUCTIONS

To the Claimant: The Health Insurance Portability and Accountability Act of 1996 (HIPAA) set standards for guaranteeing the privacy of individually identifiabl ehealth information and the confidentiality of patient medical records. By completing and signing this form, you authorize your health care provider to file medical reports with the parties that you choose (such as the Workers' Compensation Board, your employer's insurance carrier, your attorney or representative, etc.) by checking the appropriate boxes below.

You have the right to refuse to sign this Authorization. If you sign, you have the right to revoke this Authorization at any time by mailing a request to revoke to the health care provider. You have the right to receive a copy of this Authorization.

IMPORTANT: Failure to execute this authorization may interfere with your ability to obtain workers' compensation benefits.

CLAIMANT'S NAME	CLAIMANT'S SOCIAL SECURITY NUMBER	CLAIMANT'S DATE OF BIRTH

LIST ALL WCB CASE NUMBER(S) AND CORRESPONDING DATE(S) OF ACCIDENT FOR WHICH YOU ARE GRANTING AUTHORIZATION

I, _____, hereby authorize my treating health provider,
       Claimant's Name

_____, to disclose the following described health information:
       Health Provider's Name

_____

_____

_____

This information can be disclosed to the following parties: *(check all that apply; give names and addresses, if known)*

☐ New York State Workers' Compensation Board

☐ My current/former employer _____

☐ Workers' compensation insurance carrier(s) _____

☐ Third-party administrator _____

☐ My attorney/licensed representative _____

☐ The Uninsured Employer's Fund (this fund is responsible for paying the medical bills and lost wage benefits when an employer is uninsured.)

☐ Special Funds Conservation Committee (for cases under Section 25-a or 15-8 of the Workers' Compensation Law)

   Section 25-a: If your claim is being reopened after being previously closed, the Special Fund for Reopened Cases may be responsible for paying your medical bills and lost wage benefits.

   Section 15-8: If you had a medical condition that existed prior to this injury, the Special Fund for Second Injuries may be responsible for reimbursing your employer's insurance carrier after a period of time has elapsed.

Redisclosure: I understand that once the above-referenced health care provider discloses health information based on this Authorization, that health information is no longer protected by HIPAA and the Privacy Rule.

Expiration Date: This Authorization expires upon the final closing of the workers' compensation claim(s) for which it is executed.

I have had the opportunity to review and understand the content of this Authorization. By signing this Authorization, I confirm that it accurately reflects my wishes.

| _____ | _____ | _____ |
| Printed Name of Claimant or Legal Representative | Signature of Claimant or Legal Representative | Date |

If Authorization signed by a legal representative on behalf of claimant, state relationship to claimant_____and
basis for authority (e.g. claimant is a minor; patient is deceased and representative is the claimant in a workers' compensation proceeding or represents the estate) _____

TO THE HEALTH PROVIDER: Keep the original of this Authorization on file. A copy must be given to the patient/claimant upon request.

Fig. 11-7 Sample disclosure form.

Employer's Responsibilities

If the disability insurance is provided by the employer, a statement that helps identify the benefits available should accompany the claim. The employer also must provide detailed information regarding the type of coverage, policy number, division/class number, and division/class description.

Attending Physician's Statement

It is important that the injured or ill worker be examined by a physician as soon as possible after the disability has occurred and within the time limit allowed by the insurer. The physician must determine that the individual is disabled as defined by the policy. An attending physician's statement must be completed, which typically includes information such as

- the diagnosis,
- the first day the individual was unable to work,
- whether or not the illness or injury was work related,
- the nature of the treatment or suggested treatment, and
- restrictions and limitations.

Health Insurance Professional's Role

Frequently, disability claim handling gets tied up in time-consuming tasks such as document processing, record keeping, written correspondence, telephone inquiries, photocopying, and sending faxes. The process involves a lot of human interaction, which complicates the process, especially if all phases are not properly documented and monitored. Everyone involved can become quickly frustrated and impatient. It is the health insurance professional's responsibility to see that everything possible is done to facilitate the claims process for the benefit of the medical practice and the disabled patient. The health insurance professional attends to this responsibility by seeing to it that claim forms and statements are completed correctly and submitted promptly and all necessary documentation is included.

The health insurance professional's role also might be to educate the patient regarding disability benefits. With disability insurance, the insurer does not reimburse the patient

strictly according to the fees charged for medical services rendered by the attending physician. Disability insurance benefits are paid to compensate for loss of income from wages. Periodic payments (typically monthly) are made directly to the patient to use for expenses as he or she sees fit. Ideally, the patient has a separate health insurance policy to pay the cost of needed healthcare.

What Did You Learn?

1. What do disability income insurance benefits pay?
2. What items should a typical claim request include?
3. List five things the attending physician's statement should address.
4. What is the health insurance professional's role in the disability claims process?

FEDERAL DISABILITY PROGRAMS

Federal disability programs provide services such as cash support, healthcare coverage, and direct supportive services to eligible individuals with disabilities. These programs typically are limited to individuals younger than age 65. There are nine major federal disability programs that include sizable proportions of individuals age 50 to 64, as follows:

1. Social Security Disability Insurance (SSDI)
2. Supplemental Security Income (SSI)
3. Medicare
4. Medicaid
5. Workers' compensation
6. Black Lung
7. Department of Veterans Affairs (VA) Disability Compensation Program
8. VA Pension Programs
9. VA Health Services Program

An individual may receive benefits from more than one program if he or she meets all the eligibility requirements. Specific eligibility requirements typically vary, depending on the purpose of the program, and eligibility requirements may change over time, as the result of amendments to the law, new regulations, or court decisions that affect eligibility criteria.

Disability under the federal programs generally is defined as significant difficulty with performing or the inability to perform certain day-to-day functions as a result of a health condition or impairment. For adults age 18 through 64, these functions often involve working or keeping house. For individuals age 65 and older, the functions may involve the inability to carry out routine daily tasks. Some commonly used factors federal programs look at in assessing disability are the following:

- Sensory impairments—difficulty with or the inability to see, hear, or speak
- Cognitive or mental impairments—the presence of or resulting disabilities from cognitive or mental

impairments (e.g., Alzheimer's disease, mental illness, mental retardation)

- Functioning of specific body systems—capacity of specific body systems (e.g., climbing stairs, walking 3 blocks, lifting more than 10 lb)
- **Activities of daily living (ADLs) and instrumental activities of daily living (IADLs)**—difficulty with or the inability to perform without the help of another person or a device ADLs (e.g., bathing, dressing, eating, toileting, and walking); or IADLs (e.g., using the telephone, shopping, preparing meals, keeping house, and managing medications)
- Working—inability to work; limitations in the amount or kind of work; or ability to work only occasionally, irregularly, or part-time

Americans with Disabilities Act

The intent of the **Americans with Disabilities Act (ADA)** of 1990 is to protect the civil rights of individuals with disabilities. Equal opportunity provisions pertain to employment, public accommodation, transportation, state and local government services, and telecommunications. Disability is present for purposes of the ADA if an individual meets one of the following three criteria:

1. The individual has a physical or mental impairment that substantially limits one or more major life activities.
2. A record exists of such an impairment.
3. The individual is regarded as having an impairment.

Social Security Disability Insurance

Social Security Disability Insurance (SSDI) is the primary federal insurance program that protects workers from loss of income as a result of disability. SSDI provides monthly cash benefits to disabled workers younger than age 65 and to certain of their dependents. SSDI is intended for workers who retire before age 65 because of a disability.

History of the Social Security Disability Insurance Program

The 1935 Social Security Act established the federal Social Security system to provide old-age benefits for retired workers. The SSDI program was enacted in 1956 to provide benefits to workers age 50 through 64 who retired early because of a disability. Subsequent amendments broadened SSDI coverage to include certain dependents and workers younger than age 50.

Administration and Funding

SSDI is federally administered by the Social Security Administration. Funding is provided through the disability insurance (SSDI) portion of the Social Security payroll tax on wages. Generally, the Federal Insurance Contribution Act (FICA) taxes are collected at a rate of 7.65% on gross earnings (i.e., earnings before any deductions). The breakdown of FICA is 6.2% for Social Security (Old-Age, Survivors, and Disability Insurance [OASDI]) and 1.45% for Medicare. In 2011, the FICA tax rate for employees was reduced to 5.65%. The employer tax rate remained unchanged, and the Social Security rate for employees was reduced to 4.20%. The wage base limit for Social Security (OASDI parts) was $106,800. There is no wage base limit for the Medicare Part A (hospital insurance) payroll tax.

Note: This lower FICA tax rate is temporary.

Eligibility

To become eligible for SSDI, individuals must meet two criteria:

1. They must have worked enough Social Security–covered work quarters.
2. They must have a severe impairment that makes them unable to do their previous work or any other kind of substantial financially gainful activity.

Social Security–covered work quarters are credited annually for the years during which an individual works, is covered by Social Security, and earns a specified amount, which is adjusted upward each year. No more than four quarters can be credited per year. Workers must be fully insured (based on Social Security contributions) and (except for individuals who are blind or who are over 31 years old) must have at least 20 quarters of coverage during the 40-quarter period up to the time of disability to receive SSDI. Individuals who are fully insured under Social Security have at least one quarter of coverage for every four quarters up to the time of disability. Individuals who have 40 quarters are fully insured for life. Workers younger than age 31 and individuals who are blind need fewer quarters, but a minimum of six quarters is required. Disability for SSDI is defined as the inability to do any substantial gainful activity by reason of any medically determinable physical or mental impairment that can be expected to result in death or that has lasted or can be expected to last for a continuous period of not less than 12 months.

After it has been established that the applicant has enough quarters and is not earning more than the "substantial gainful activity amount," a State Disability Determination unit examines medical evidence to determine if the applicant's mental or physical impairment is severe enough to have more than a minimal effect on the applicant's ability to work. If so, the applicant's medical condition is compared with a Social Security Administration listing of more than 100 impairments (e.g., loss of two limbs; fracture of vertebra with spinal cord involvement, substantiated by appropriate sensory and motor loss; vision of 20/200 or less after correction).

Applicants whose medical conditions are at least as severe as the conditions in the Social Security Administration listing are considered disabled. Applicants who are not found disabled at this point are evaluated two additional steps. First, a determination is made regarding whether or not the applicant can do his or her past work. This decision is based on assessments of factors such as physical abilities (e.g., strength, walking, standing) or mental abilities (e.g., the ability to carry out and remember instructions or to respond appropriately in work settings).

For applicants who cannot perform past work, an assessment is done to determine their ability to perform other jobs that exist in the national economy. This assessment is based on the individual's functional capacity, age, education, and work experience. Generally, individuals younger than age 50 are considered to be able to adapt to new work situations.

Dependent coverage and survivor benefits are offered through SSDI to certain qualifying individuals. Disabled individuals can receive SSDI in three ways:

1. On their own as disabled workers (described previously)
2. As widows or widowers (who are age 50 to 59) of insured individuals
3. As adults age 18 through 64 who became disabled in childhood whose parents receive SSDI, are Social Security retirees, or who are deceased (but had been insured under Social Security)

⭐ Imagine This!

After teacher Louise Carson had her workers' compensation claim denied, she quit her job and filed for SSDI. SSDI found Louise to be disabled at her teaching position; however, they determined that she could perform at a "new work" situation that was less stressful and suggested that Louise use her education and training to work in a library or become a private tutor.

Supplemental Security Income

The **Supplemental Security Income (SSI)** program provides monthly cash payments to low-income aged, blind, and disabled individuals. The SSI program was established by the 1972 amendments to the Social Security Act, which replaced earlier federal grants to the states for old-age assistance, aid to the blind, and aid to the permanently disabled.

Administration and Funding

The SSI program is administered by the Social Security Administration. Funding comes from general federal revenues. Many states have chosen the option to supplement federal SSI payments with their own funds.

Eligibility

In contrast to SSDI, individuals receiving SSI because of blindness or disability have no work requirements, but they must meet a **financial means test**, a detailed and comprehensive questionnaire that establishes financial need. The SSI financial means test depends on income and resources. Individuals younger than age 65 must meet disability and financial means criteria, whereas individuals age 65 or older need to meet only the financial means criteria. Individuals may receive SSI payments either as individuals or as couples. Both members of a couple must be aged, blind, or disabled and must meet the financial means criteria to collect

payments. Other than these provisions for couples, there are no dependent or survivor benefits in SSI.

The determination of disability under SSI for adults is identical to the one used in the SSDI program. For children younger than age 18, the determination of disability is based on a standard of comparable severity. The methods of counting various types of income and resources are complex, but generally the maximum unearned monthly income in 2011 for individuals applying for SSI was $694 and $1011 for couples if they received only Social Security and $1433 for individuals and $2107 for couples if their income was only from wages. Countable resources are limited to $2000 for individuals and $3000 for couples.

The SSDI and SSI programs share various concepts and terms; however, there are many important differences in the rules affecting eligibility and benefit payments. These differences are important because many persons may apply or be eligible for benefits under both programs. To view a table summarizing the differences between the SSDI and SSI programs, visit the Evolve site.

📁 HIPAA Tip

As a "covered entity" under HIPAA, the Social Security Administration, which oversees the federal disability programs such as SSDI and SDI, must comply with HIPAA's medical information standards.

State Disability Programs

A few states (California, Hawaii, New Jersey, New York, and Rhode Island) and Puerto Rico have disability programs at the present time that provide short-term benefits for employees. These state programs are set up to supplement Social Security disability benefits. Because Social Security disability benefits do not cover the first 6 months of the disability, these state plans provide benefits to qualifying disabled individuals until Social Security payments begin. The funds are financed by a combination of the employees' payroll deductions and employer contributions. An employee's contributions are based on his or her earnings and are withheld from wages by the employer and transferred to the state fund. There are severe penalties for failing to withhold the contributions. With the exception of Rhode Island, an employer can opt out of the state plan and put the employee's contributions into a private plan. Private plans must meet state requirements regarding coverage, eligibility, contribution amounts, and employee approval.

Centers for Disease Control and Prevention Disability and Health Team

The **Disability and Health Team** is part of the National Center on Birth Defects and Developmental Disabilities at the Centers for Disease Control and Prevention (CDC) in Atlanta. The focus of the team is promoting the health of individuals who are living with disabilities. The CDC Disability and Health Team activities include the following:

- Assessing and monitoring disability prevalence
- Assessing the health status and quality of life for individuals with disabilities
- Describing risk factors and costs associated with secondary conditions and poor health
- Developing health promotion interventions to reduce secondary conditions and evaluate intervention effectiveness and costs
- Offering training to healthcare professionals interested in the field of disability and public health
- Supporting conferences to facilitate and encourage discussion, circulate and exchange information, establish research and policy priorities, and outline and undertake further action

To learn more about the Disability and Health Team, visit the Evolve site.

Ticket to Work Program

The **Ticket to Work Program** was created with passage of the federal Ticket to Work and Work Incentives Improvement Act of 1999. Ticket to Work is a voluntary program that gives certain individuals with disabilities greater choice in selecting the service providers and rehabilitation services they need to help them keep working or get back to work.

Purpose

Ticket to Work was created to help individuals who receive SSDI or SSI benefits find and keep employment by offering them more options for services and supports. Many individuals receiving SSDI or SSI choose not to work because they are concerned about losing their benefits. Ticket to Work gives these individuals an opportunity to choose services to meet their unique needs and obtain benefits-planning assistance so that they can make informed choices about employment. Individuals receiving SSDI or SSI disability benefits may participate in Ticket to Work.

How the Program Works

Ticket to Work participants receive a paper document or "ticket" that explains the program and includes some personal information about them. They can take their ticket to an approved employment network to receive the services they want. An **employment network** can be a public agency or private organization that has agreed to provide services under the Ticket to Work program guidelines. For more detailed information on this program, visit the Evolve site.

Filing Supplemental Security Income and Social Security Disability Insurance Claims

Patient's Role

The patient initiates the SSI or SSDI claim. The best way to begin the process is to file a Social Security disability claim at the nearest Social Security office in person. An alternative method is to contact Social Security by telephone and arrange for a telephone interview to file the claim.

A claim for Social Security disability benefits may be filed on the same day that an individual becomes disabled. There is no reason to file a Social Security disability claim for a minor illness or one that is unlikely to last 1 year or more. An individual who has a serious illness or injury and expects to be out of work for 1 year or more should not delay in filing a claim for Social Security disability benefits.

Unless the disability is catastrophic (e.g., terminal cancer, a serious heart condition requiring transplant, total paralysis of both legs), there is no easy way to tell whether an individual would be found disabled by Social Security. Individuals should make the decision about whether or not to file for Social Security disability on the basis of their own belief regarding their condition. If an individual believes that he or she is truly disabled and is not going to be able to return to work in the near future, the individual should file for Social Security disability benefits.

After a Social Security disability claim is filed, the case is sent to a disability examiner at the Disability Determination Agency in that state, who works with a physician to make the initial decision on the claim based on a thorough clinical examination and interviews. If the claim is denied and the individual requests reconsideration, the case is sent to a second disability examiner at the Disability Determination Agency, where it goes through a similar process. If a claim is denied at reconsideration, the individual may request a hearing. At this point, the case is sent to an administrative law judge who works for Social Security. The administrative law judge makes an independent decision on the claim, which is usually final.

An individual can hire an attorney to represent him or her on Social Security disability claim denials. The National Organization of Social Security Claimants' Representatives offers a referral service at 1-800-431-2804 during regular Eastern Standard Time business hours.

Applicants for SSI or SSDI benefits should obtain the free booklet Social Security Disability Benefits (Social Security Administration Publication No. 05-10029). This booklet suggests ways to help shorten the process by knowing what documents to include when applying for benefits.

Role of the Healthcare Provider

The disability determination process relies on the participation of healthcare providers in many ways. One of the most important ways is as a **treating source** that provides the long-term medical information (called medical evidence of record), which is normally required in every claim for disability benefits. In addition to providing evidence as a treating source, the healthcare provider can assist the disability programs in the following ways:

- As a member of the state Disability Determination Services disability evaluation team that makes the initial or continuing disability determination
- As a reviewer of the state decision

- As a consultative examiner for the Disability Determination Services
- As a medical expert for an administrative law judge

Healthcare providers who serve as medical experts may be asked to give verbal testimony or provide answers to questions on claim reviews. Frequently, the final decision to allow or deny a Social Security disability claim rests on the advice and medical opinions provided by these medical experts.

📁 HIPAA Tip

HIPAA protects against gaps in insurance coverage, allowing the freedom to move from one job to another or the freedom to move from SSI or SSDI status to employment.

Role of the Health Insurance Professional

The health insurance professional needs to know the Social Security regulations so that he or she is able to provide the exact information needed for evaluation of an individual's disability. There are many steps in the application process, which can be time-consuming and confusing, and knowledgeable healthcare team members should do all they can to facilitate this process.

Similar to workers' compensation claims, there is no standard form for billing disability claims. When a patient comes to the medical facility for the purpose of getting the physician's medical opinion regarding disability, the health insurance professional should advise the patient to bring the necessary forms provided by the Social Security office. Additional responsibilities of the health insurance professional include

- procuring the patient's authorization to release information,
- acquiring the necessary information for claims processing,
- ensuring that the attending physician forms are complete and signed,
- photocopying all forms for the patient's health record,
- maintaining a well-documented health record, and
- answering the patient's questions.

⏱ Stop and Think

Amy Turner, a health insurance professional for Dr. Laura Nelson, wants to be able to help patients through the often complicated process of filing for SSI or SSDI benefits. What would you suggest Amy do to become knowledgeable in this area?

💬 What Did You Learn?

1. List six federal disability programs.
2. How do federal programs define disability?
3. ADA considers disability present if an individual meets what three criteria?
4. What is the difference between SSI and SSDI?
5. List the five states that provide short-term disability benefits.

SUMMARY CHECKPOINTS

▶ Workers' compensation is a type of insurance regulated by state laws that pays medical expenses and partial loss of wages for workers who are injured on the job or become ill as a result of job-related circumstances.

▶ Any employee who is injured on the job or develops an employment-related illness that prevents the individual from working is usually eligible to receive workers' compensation benefits. A spouse and dependents of an employee who dies because of a job-related accident or illness are also eligible for benefits.

▶ Most employers must purchase workers' compensation insurance coverage for their workers; however, there are certain classifications of exemptions, depending on state statutes. Common types of exemptions include the following:
  - Employers with a minimum number of full-time employees (individual states determine this number)
  - Executive officers
  - Individuals who are business partners
  - Sole proprietors
  - Casual employees

▶ The four major benefit components to workers' compensation are as follows:
  - Medical expense—pays expenses related to hospitalization, physicians' visits, and any necessary medical treatment
  - Disability pay—can be temporary or permanent if it is determined that the worker will never fully recover
  - Vocational rehabilitation—if the injury or illness results in the worker being unable to perform the usual duties of his or her occupation, retraining may be necessary for the worker to enter into a new trade or business; also, physical therapy may be necessary
  - Death benefits—paid to surviving dependents

▶ The reporting requirements for filing a workers' compensation claim include the following steps:
- Employee notifies a supervisor of the incident immediately and provides the names of any witnesses.
- Employee completes a detailed accident report on a form furnished by the employer.
- Employer reports the incident to the company's workers' compensation carrier.
- Employee is sent to a medical facility for treatment or diagnosis. (In emergencies, this should be the first step.)
- Attending physician completes statement and distributes copies.
- Follow-up progress reports are submitted until the employee returns to work, after which a final report is filed.

▶ When the injured or ill worker visits the healthcare facility for treatment, the attending physician takes a history, performs an examination, makes a diagnosis, and completes a statement indicating any physical or mental impairments resulting from the incident. Disability is determined on the basis of these reports.

▶ The purpose of disability income insurance is to replace a portion of salary or wages earned income when an individual is unable to perform the requirements of his or her job because of injury or illness that is not work related.

▶ SSDI is a federal insurance program that pays monthly cash benefits to disabled workers younger than age 65 and to certain dependents who have lost their income because of disability. Individuals applying for SSDI must meet two criteria:
- They must have worked a specific number of Social Security–covered work quarters.
- They must have a severe impairment that makes them unable to perform their previous work or any other kind of financially gainful activity.

▶ SSI provides monthly cash payments to low-income aged, blind, and disabled individuals. There are no work requirements for SSI, but individuals must answer a detailed and comprehensive questionnaire that establishes financial need, called a financial means test. Disability determination for adults is the same under SSDI and SSI.

▶ Ticket to Work was created to help recipients of SSDI or SSI find and keep employment by offering them more options. The program gives individuals an opportunity to choose services to meet their unique needs and obtain benefits-planning assistance so that they can make informed choices about employment. Participants receive a paper document (ticket) that explains the program and includes some personal information about them. They can take their ticket to an approved employment network to receive the desired services.

▶ The patient initiates an SSI or SSDI claim by going to the nearest Social Security office in person or by telephoning and arranging for a telephone interview to file the claim. After the claim is filed, the case is sent to a disability examiner who works with a physician to make the initial decision on the claim based on a thorough clinical examination and interviews.

▶ The health insurance professional's responsibilities for facilitating disability claims processing include the following:
- Obtaining the patient's authorization to release information
- Acquiring the necessary information and forms for claims processing
- Ensuring that the attending physician reports are complete and signed
- Photocopying all forms and correspondence for the patient's health record
- Maintaining a well-documented health record
- Answering the patient's questions

CLOSING SCENARIO

Jim and Tammy had discussed their individual areas of interest before beginning the chapter. Tammy visited with her Uncle Niles several times to learn all she could about disability income insurance, and she shared what she learned with Jim. Meanwhile, Jim researched the workers' compensation websites available on the Internet. By the end of the chapter, the two students thought that they had acquired a good knowledge base for workers' compensation and private and federal disability income insurance. Jim now has a better understanding of the payment system that kept his family going after his father's death.

Jim and Tammy realize that acquiring a solid foundation in all areas of insurance is a benefit not only to health insurance professionals but also to the entire healthcare team. By becoming well informed, health insurance professionals can help educate patients to alleviate the cumbersome task of filing and maintaining all of the documents necessary for workers' compensation and disability insurance.

WEBSITES TO EXPLORE

- For live links to the following websites, please visit the Evolve site at http://evolve.elsevier.com/Beik/today
- To find out about the workers' compensations laws in your state, log on to
  http://www.workerscompensation.com
- The U.S. Department of Labor provides an overview of State Workers' Compensation Laws in a Portable Document Format (PDF) file at
  http://www.dol.gov (*Note:* You must download and install a free Adobe Acrobat Reader to view and print PDF files.)
- Wikipedia provides information on workers' compensation including statutory law and its history at

http://en.wikipedia.org/wiki/Workers'_compensation
- To learn about SSI and SSDI similarities and differences, log on to
  http://www.ssa.gov/pubs/10003.html
- To keep aware of changes in the SSDI and SSI programs, log on to
  http://www.ssa.gov
- For more information on the CDC Disability and Health Team Program, log on to the CDC website at
  http://www.cdc.gov

Author's Note: Websites change frequently. If any of these URLs is unavailable, use applicable guide words in your Internet search to acquire additional information on the various subjects listed.

Diagnostic Coding

Chapter Outline

I. Introduction to International Classification of Diseases Coding System
   A. Three Major Coding Structures
II. History of International Classification of Diseases Coding
   A. Uses of Coded Data
III. Two Diagnostic Coding Systems
   A. Comparing the Two Systems
   B. Guidelines
IV. ICD-9-CM Coding Manual
   A. Volume 2, Alphabetic List (Index)
      1. Code Structure
   B. Three Sections of Volume 2
      1. Section I, Index to Diseases and Injuries
         a. Eponyms
         b. Essential Modifiers
         c. Nonessential Modifiers
         d. Conventions for Volume 2, Alphabetic Index
         e. Hypertension and Neoplasm Tables
      2. Section II, Table of Drugs and Chemicals
      3. Section III, Index to External Causes of Injury and Poisoning (E Codes)
   C. National Coverage Determinations and Local Coverage Determinations
V. Process of Classifying Diseases
   A. Volume 1, Tabular List
      1. Organization of Volume 1 Codes
      2. Color Coding
   B. Supplementary Sections of Volume 1
      1. V Codes
      2. E Codes
   C. Locating a Code in the Tabular List (Volume 1)
VI. Symbols and Conventions Used in Volume 1
   A. Typefaces
   B. Instructional Notes
VII. Essential Steps to Diagnostic Coding
VIII. Special Coding Situations

A. Coding Signs and Symptoms
B. Etiology and Manifestation Coding
C. Combination Codes
D. Coding Late Effects
E. Coding Neoplasms
F. Coding Hypertension
IX. Overview of ICD-10 Coding System
   A. ICD-10-CM Code Structure
   B. Format of ICD-10-CM Manual
      1. Alphabetic Index
         a. Main Terms
         b. Essential and Nonessential Modifiers
      2. Conventions Used in Alphabetic Index
         a. Parentheses
         b. Cross-References (*see* and *see also*)
X. Coding steps for Alphabetic Index
XI. Tabular List
   A. Format and Structure of Codes
      1. Placeholder Character
      2. 7th Character
   B. Tabular List Conventions
      1. Abbreviations
         a. NEC ("Not Elsewhere Classifiable")
         b. NOS ("Not Otherwise Specified")
      2. Punctuation
         a. Brackets
         b. Parentheses
         c. Colons
         d. Dashes
         e. Point Dash
      3. Instructional Notes
   C. Manifestation Codes
      1. Etiology/Manifestation Convention ("Code First," "Use Additional Code," and "In Diseases Classified Elsewhere" Notes)
      2. "Code Also" Note

D. Morphology Codes

E. Default Codes

XII. ICD-10-CM General Coding Guidelines and Chapter-Specific Guidelines

  A. Codes from A00.0 through T88.9, Z00-Z99.89

    1. Signs and Symptoms

    2. Conditions That Are an Integral Part of a Disease Process

    3. Conditions That Are Not an Integral Part of a Disease Process

      a. Acute and Chronic Conditions

      b. Combination Codes

    4. Late Effects (Sequelae)

    5. Impending or Threatened Condition

      a. Laterality

XIII. Diagnostic Coding and Reporting Guidelines for Outpatient Services

  A. Selection of First-Listed Condition

  B. Outpatient Surgery

  C. Observation Stay

  D. Codes That Describe Symptoms and Signs

  E. Encounters for Circumstances Other than a Disease or Injury

  F. Level of Detail in Coding

    1. Codes with 3, 4, or 5 Digits

    2. Use of Full Number of Digits

  G. Code for Diagnosis, Condition, Problem, or Other Reason for Encounter/Visit

    1. Uncertain Diagnosis

    2. Chronic Diseases

  H. Code All Documented Conditions That Coexist

    1. Patients Receiving Diagnostic Services Only

    2. Patients Receiving Therapeutic Services Only

    3. Patients Receiving Preoperative Evaluations Only

    4. Ambulatory Surgery

    5. Routine Outpatient Prenatal Visits

    6. Encounters for General Medical Examinations with Abnormal Findings

    7. Encounters for Routine Health Screenings

XIV. Health Insurance Portability and Accountability Act and Coding

  A. Code Sets Adopted as Health Insurance Portability and Accountability Act Standards

  B. Implementation of ICD-10

XV. Importance of Learning Both Diagnostic Coding Systems

CHAPTER OBJECTIVES

After completion of this chapter, the student should be able to:

1. Discuss the meaning of a diagnosis and where it can be found in a patient record.
2. Name the three major coding structures and state the purpose of each.
3. Discuss the history and development of diagnostic coding.
4. Provide a brief comparison of the two diagnostic coding systems.
5. Outline the format of the *International Classification of Diseases, 9th Revision, Clinical Modification* (ICD-9-CM) manual and the organization of Volumes 1 and 2.
6. Describe the process of classifying diseases.
7. Explain the format and structure of ICD-9-CM codes in the Tabular List.
8. Define and provide examples for symbols and conventions used in ICD-9-CM Volume 1.
9. List the essential steps to diagnostic coding.
10. Identify and explain special coding situations.
11. Summarize the structure and format of the *International Classification of Diseases, 10th Revision, Clinical Modification* (ICD-10-CM) coding manual.
12. Outline the coding steps for the Alphabetic Index in ICD-10-CM.
13. Explain the format and structure of codes and conventions in ICD-10-CM Tabular List.
14. Discuss ICD-10-CM general coding guidelines and chapter-specific guidelines.
15. State important diagnostic coding and reporting guidelines for outpatient services in ICD-10-CM.
16. Explain the connection between the Health Insurance Portability and Accountability Act (HIPAA) and diagnostic coding.
17. Display an understanding of the importance of learning both diagnostic coding systems.

CHAPTER TERMS

category

code set

combination code

contraindication

conventions

default code

diagnosis

E codes

eponyms

essential modifiers

etiology

first-listed diagnosis

laterality

Local Coverage Determinations (LCDs)

main term

manifestation

morphology

National Coverage Determinations (NCDs)

neoplasm

NEC ("not elsewhere classifiable")

nonessential modifiers

NOS ("not otherwise specified")

notes

placeholder character

principal diagnosis

sequela (*pl.* sequelae)

7th character

subcategory

subclassification

V codes

OPENING SCENARIO

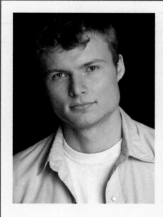

When Park Chalmers was a little boy, he had wanted to be a doctor; however, when he fainted after witnessing a bicycle accident that severely injured his best friend's arm, Park realized that the clinical side of medicine was not for him. Still, the field of medicine intrigued him. After high school, Park moved from one dead-end job to another. He soon faced the fact that without specialized career training, his prospects for living comfortably in an apartment of his own were dim.

In his search for more meaningful employment, Park noticed an advertisement in the classified section of the newspaper for a coder at a local medical clinic. The position required course work or on-the-job experience in ICD and CPT coding. The pay range noted in the ad was enticing to Park; however, he had no idea what ICD or CPT coding was. The terms themselves were "codes" to Park.

Curious about the meaning of ICD and CPT coding, Park made inquiries when he attended a job fair at the community college. He was directed to the health careers booth where current health insurance students, with the aid of an instructor, answered all his questions and gave a brief demonstration on diagnostic coding.

"I think I can learn this coding stuff," Park decided, and he headed for the Student Services Department to enroll in the upcoming health insurance program.

INTRODUCTION TO INTERNATIONAL CLASSIFICATION OF DISEASES CODING SYSTEM

In the healthcare profession, there is a recognized process of transforming descriptions of a patient's disease process, disorder, or injury into universal numerical or alphanumerical formats—codes—that are understood by all healthcare entities, including providers, government health programs, private health insurance companies, and workers' compensation carriers. In very basic language, a **diagnosis** is the reason that brought the patient to the healthcare facility, such as a rash, sore throat, or chest pains. A final diagnosis after examination can be a much more precise statement.

The diagnosis can be taken from a variety of sources within the medical record, such as the clinical notes, laboratory tests, radiological results, and other sources. The diagnosis must be determined by the healthcare professional providing the medical care. Table 12-1 lists examples of medical diagnoses.

When the healthcare insurance professional generates an insurance claim for payment of the provider's services, the diagnosis itself does not appear on the claim—only the code appears. It is very important that the code describes the diagnosis accurately and to the greatest specificity to receive maximum reimbursement for the provider and patient and that the diagnosis justifies the medical necessity of the procedure codes documented on the insurance claim.

Three Major Coding Structures

The U.S. healthcare system currently uses three major coding structures. The *International Classification of Diseases, 9th Revision, Clinical Modification* (ICD-9-CM) diagnosis codes (Volumes 1 and 2) and ICD-9-CM procedure codes (Volume 3). ICD-9-CM Volumes 1 and 2 are used to code diagnoses in physicians' offices and outpatient settings along with *Current Procedural Terminology, 4th revision* (CPT-4) codes to determine third-party payment for related services and procedures for reimbursement purposes. These codes also help establish the ambulatory payment classifications (APCs) used by most providers for related services and procedures in the outpatient setting. The procedure codes in Volume 3 establish diagnosis-related groups (DRGs) that most third-party payers use to determine payment for related services and procedures in an inpatient hospital setting. (DRGs and APCs are discussed in detail in Chapter 17.)

This chapter provides the basics of diagnostic coding. After completing the assigned readings and exercises, students should have a working knowledge of both the ICD-9-CM and the ICD-10-CM systems with the ability to generate valid codes for simple diagnoses. Students who wish to pursue a career in coding and become certified should explore the opportunities available in local coding programs or online. Visit the Evolve site for more information on becoming certified in coding.

TABLE 12-1	Examples of Medical Diagnoses
Diaper dermatitis	
Streptococcal sore throat	
Intercostal chest pain	
Fracture of neck of scapula	
Systemic lupus erythematosus	
Acute thyroiditis	

📁 HIPAA Tip

HIPAA requires that diagnosis codes be included on all Medicare claims billed to Part B carriers with the exception of ambulance claims. Providers and suppliers rely on physicians to provide a diagnosis code or narrative diagnostic statement on orders or referrals.

❓ What Did You Learn?

1. On the most basic level, what is a diagnosis?
2. Where might a patient's diagnosis be located?
3. Both the written diagnosis and the code must appear on the insurance claim. True or false?
4. Name the three major coding structures currently used in healthcare.

HISTORY OF INTERNATIONAL CLASSIFICATION OF DISEASES CODING

The history of the International Classification of Diseases (ICD) system dates back to the late 19th century in Europe when it was determined that there was a need for the standardization of medical concepts and terminology. The ICD system resulted from a group effort between the World Health Organization and 10 international centers so that medical terms reported on death certificates by physicians, medical examiners, and coroners could be grouped together for statistical purposes. The purpose of this system was to promote a way of comparing the collection, classification, processing, and presentation of mortality (death) statistics.

The first ICD system (ICD-1) was put into use in 1900. Since then, the ICD has been modified approximately once every 10 years with the exception of the 20-year period between the last two revisions—ICD-9 and ICD-10 (Table 12-2). The rationale for these periodic revisions has been to reflect advances in medical science and changes in diagnostic terminology. In 1999, the United States replaced ICD-9 with ICD-10 for coding on death certificates; however, the U.S. Department of Health and Human Services (HHS) did not publish the final rule for full adoption of the ICD-10 in the United States until January 2009. Until that time, the United States was one of the few countries that was not using ICD-10. Visit the Evolve site to read the HHS Final Rule for ICD-10 and to find more information on the history and development of the ICD coding system.

The compliance date for implementation of the ICD-10 coding system is (as of this writing) October 1, 2014, for all covered entities. Students should visit http://cms.gov/icd10/ periodically to keep abreast of further changes to this compliance date.

TABLE 12-2	International Classification of Diseases Implementation in the United States
DESIGNATION	**YEARS IN EFFECT**
ICD-1	1900-1909
ICD-2	1910-1920
ICD-3	1921-1929
ICD-4	1930-1938
ICD-5	1939-1948
ICD-6	1949-1957
ICD-7	1958-1967
ICD-8*	1968-1978
ICD-9	1979-2013
ICD-10	1999 (death certificates only); 2013

*The United States generally accepted the World Health Organization revisions except for the 8th Revision; the United States disagreed with some parts of the classification system, specifically some categories in the diseases of the circulatory system. As a result, the United States produced its own version of the ICD, referred to as ICDA-8.

Key Note:

The National Center for Health Statistics is responsible for maintaining the diagnostic codes (Volumes 1 and 2) of the ICD-10-CM; the Centers for Medicare and Medicaid Services (CMS) is responsible for maintaining the procedures codes (Volume 3).

Uses of Coded Data

Coding of healthcare data allows access to health records according to diagnoses and procedures for use in clinical care, research, and education. Following is a list of other common uses of codes in healthcare:

- Measuring the quality, safety, and effectiveness of care
- Designing payment systems and processing claims for reimbursement
- Conducting research, epidemiological studies, and clinical trials
- Setting healthcare policies
- Operational and strategic planning and designing healthcare delivery systems
- Monitoring resource use
- Improving clinical, financial, and administrative performance
- Preventing and detecting healthcare fraud and abuse
- Tracking public concerns and assessing risks of adverse public health events

? What Did You Learn?

1. When was the first ICD coding system put into use?
2. List five uses of coded data.

TWO DIAGNOSTIC CODING SYSTEMS

In this chapter, we look at two different diagnostic coding systems: ICD-9-CM and ICD-10-CM. After a comparison of the two systems and a brief discussion of the history of diagnostic coding, the ICD-9 system is presented followed by ICD-10. The reason both systems are discussed is because ICD-9 is still being used, and the health insurance professional needs to know how to use it until the transition to ICD-10.

Comparing the Two Systems

Primary concern with the current ICD-9 system is the lack of specificity of the information expressed in the codes. For example, if a patient is seen for treatment of an injury to the left leg, the ICD-9 diagnosis code does not distinguish left or right leg. If the patient is seen a few weeks later for another injury, this time on the right leg, the same ICD-9 diagnosis code would be reported. Additional documentation would likely be required when a claim is submitted to explain that the injury treated the second time is different from the one that was treated previously. In the ICD-10 diagnosis code set, characters within the code identify right versus left, initial encounter versus subsequent encounter, and other clinical information.

Another issue with ICD-9 is that it is running out of available code numbers in some chapters. ICD-10 codes have increased character length, which greatly expands the number of codes that are available for use. With more available codes, it is less likely that chapters will run out of codes in the future. Other issues that are addressed in ICD-10 include the use of full code titles, reflecting advances in medical knowledge and technology. Additionally, diagnosis coding under ICD-10-CM uses 3 to 7 digits instead of the 3 to 5 digits used with ICD-9-CM, but the format of the code sets is similar. Table 12-3 provides a comparison of the features of the ICD-9 and ICD-10 code sets.

Examples in Table 12-4 provide a comparison of the formats of the ICD-9 and ICD-10 diagnosis codes. Note the use of alpha characters and longer codes in ICD-10. In contrast to ICD-9, the alpha characters in ICD-10 are not case sensitive.

Guidelines

The Centers for Medicare and Medicaid Services (CMS) and the National Center for Health Statistics (NCHS), two departments within HHS, provide guidelines for coding and reporting using the ICD-9-CM and ICD-10-CM coding systems. Guidelines for both diagnostic coding systems can be found

TABLE 12-3	Comparisons of the Diagnosis Code Sets
ICD-9	**ICD-10**
3-5 characters in length	3-7 characters in length
Approximately 13,000 codes	Approximately 68,000 available codes
First digit may be alpha (E or V) or numeric; digits 2-5 are numeric	Digit 1 is alpha; digits 2 and 3 are numeric; digits 4-7 are alpha or numeric
Limited space for adding new codes	Flexible for adding new codes
Lacks detail	Very specific
Lacks laterality	Has laterality (codes identifying right and left)

TABLE 12-4	Comparison of Formats of ICD-9 and ICD-10 Code Sets
ICD-9 DIAGNOSIS CODE	**ICD-10 DIAGNOSIS CODE**
382.9 Acute otitis media	B01.2 Varicella pneumonia
540.9 Acute appendicitis	K21.0 Gastro-esophageal reflux disease with esophagitis
780.01 Coma	O30.003 Twin pregnancy, unspecified, third trimester

From American Medical Association, 2010. http://www.ama-assn.org/ama1/pub/upload/mm/399/icd10-icd9-differences-fact-sheet.pdf

on the websites of these two government entities. These guidelines should be used as a companion document to the official version as published by the U.S. Government Printing Office. To view these guidelines, enter "ICD-9 Guidelines" in the search box on CDC website (www.cdc.gov/). The CMS website (http://www.cms.gov/) has extensive information and guidelines for the new ICD-10 system. To access relevant information on ICD-10, type "ICD-10" in the CMS home page search box.

? What Did You Learn?

1. Name the two diagnostic coding systems.
2. Diagnosis coding under ICD-10-CM uses _____ digits instead of the _____ digits used with ICD-9-CM.
3. Name the two government entities that provide guidelines for using the ICD-9 and ICD-10 coding systems.

ICD-9-CM CODING MANUAL

The ICD-9-CM currently consists of three volumes:
- Volume 1 is the Tabular List, which lists all diagnostic codes in numerical order: first codes for diseases (001 to 999.9), followed by V codes (Supplementary Classification of Factors Influencing Health Status and Contact with Health Services—V01 to V91.99), and lastly E codes (Supplementary Classification of External Causes of Injury and Poisoning—E800 to E999).
- Volume 2 is the Alphabetic Index listing all diagnoses alphabetically by their basic description.
- Volume 3 contains Procedure Codes used for hospital inpatient procedure coding.

Although all three volumes are available in a single book, most publishers combine Volumes 1 and 2 in a separate manual. Typically, insurance companies do not require the use of Volume 3 for physician and outpatient billing; however, Volume 3 is still used for hospital inpatient coding. Medicare Part B (physician services) does not accept codes from Volume 3; if they are used, the claim is denied. It is important that the health insurance professional obtain and use the most recent version of the ICD-9-CM for effective and accurate coding. Any questions regarding which volume to use on an insurance claim should be addressed to the appropriate carrier, fiscal intermediary, or billing consultant.

Before any attempt is made to code a diagnosis, the health insurance professional must become familiar with the contents and structure of the ICD-9 manual. The format of the ICD-9 differs among publishers regarding how the material is arranged; however, the basic information is the same. The prefacing instructions given here are from the *2012 ICD-9-CM, Volumes 1, 2, & 3, Professional Edition* by Carol J. Buck, published by Saunders, which was current at the time of this writing.

Although the ICD-9-CM manual used as reference in this chapter contains all three volumes, we discuss only Volumes 1 and 2, which deal with diagnostic coding in all healthcare settings, in this chapter. Volume 3, used for inpatient hospital procedural coding, is addressed briefly in Chapter 18.

The contents of the Buck 2012 ICD-9-CM manual discussed in this chapter are as follows:

- Guide to Using the 2012 ICD-9-CM
- Symbols and Conventions
- Guide to the 2012 ICD-9-CM Updates
- Part I, Introduction
- Part II, Alphabetic Index Volume 2
  - Section I, Index to Diseases and Injuries
  - Section II, Table of Drugs and Chemicals
  - Section III, Index to External Causes of Injury (E-Codes)
- Part III, Diseases: Tabular List Volume 1
  - Infectious and Parasitic Diseases
  - Neoplasms
  - Endocrine, Nutritional, and Metabolic Diseases and Immunity Disorders
  - Diseases of the Blood and Blood-Forming Organs

- Mental, Behavioral, and Neurodevelopmental Disorders
- Diseases of the Nervous System and Sense Organs
- Diseases of the Circulatory System
- Diseases of the Respiratory System
- Diseases of the Digestive System
- Diseases of the Genitourinary System
- Complications of Pregnancy, Childbirth, and the Puerperium
- Diseases of the Skin and Subcutaneous Tissue
- Diseases of the Musculoskeletal System and Connective Tissue
- Congenital Anomalies
- Certain Conditions Originating in the Perinatal Period
- Symptoms, Signs, and Ill-Defined Conditions
- Injury and Poisonings
- Supplementary Classification of External Causes of Injury and Poisoning (E-Codes)
- Appendices
  - Appendix A, Morphology of Neoplasms
  - Appendix B, Glossary of Mental Disorders (deleted as of October 2004)
  - Appendix C, Classification of Drugs by American Hospital Formulary Service List Number and their ICD-9-CM Equivalents
  - Appendix D, Classification of Industrial Accidents According to Agency
  - Appendix E, List of Three-Digit Categories
  - Table A, Table of Bacterial Food Poisoning

It is important that the health insurance professional thoroughly study the prefacing information contained in the introductory pages because it serves as a basic foundation for diagnostic coding and aids in assigning diagnosis codes correctly.

Volume 2, Alphabetic List (Index)

Because Volume 2, the Alphabetic List, is presented before Volume 1, Tabular List, we discuss it first. Volume 2 contains an alphabetic listing that provides instructions to assist the coder in determining if a diagnosis requires the use of additional or alternative codes. Although it is the starting point for the coding process, a diagnosis should *never* be coded strictly from the Alphabetic List. After the diagnosis has been abstracted from the patient's health record, the Alphabetic List is used to guide the coder to the appropriate page in Volume 1 where codes are arranged in numerical order. The exact code can be determined from this numerical list (Volume 1).

Code Structure

A diagnosis code in the ICD-9 structure consists of three to five characters, depending on whether a 3-digit, 4-digit, or 5-digit code best represents the patient's diagnosis. ICD-9-CM codes range from 001 to V91.99 (2012) and identify symptoms, conditions, problems, complaints, or other reasons for the procedure, service, or supply provided. It is crucial that a diagnosis is coded to the "highest level of specificity." By consulting the Alphabetic List first, the health insurance professional can determine more accurately whether a 3-digit code sufficiently describes the diagnosis or whether additional numbers are required for specificity. Diagnoses that are coded inadequately or inappropriately can result in a claim being underpaid, overpaid, delayed, or denied.

Three Sections of Volume 2

As discussed previously, Volume 2 (Alphabetic List) is organized alphabetically by medical terms and contains three separate sections or indexes.

Section I, Index to Diseases and Injuries

The largest section, the Index to Diseases and Injuries, is organized alphabetically by main terms, which are always printed in boldface type (in the Buck 2012 manual, they are in red font) for easy reference. Main terms include the following:

- Diseases such as influenza or bronchitis
- Conditions such as fatigue, fracture, or injury
- Nouns such as disease, disturbance, syndrome, or eponyms
- Adjectives such as double, large, or kinked

Anatomic sites are not listed as main terms. If a patient has a diagnosis of deviated nasal septum, it would be found in the Alphabetical Index under the main term "deviation," rather than "nasal." Ankle sprain would be located under "sprain," rather than "ankle." Fig. 12-1 shows a sample page from Volume 2.

> ### ⏱ Stop and Think
>
> Marlee Davis is employed as a health insurance professional for cardiologist Ferris Barnes. Marlee is in charge of all the billing, coding, and insurance. While preparing to submit an insurance claim for patient Eloise Hardy, Marlee notes that the patient's healthcare record documents a diagnosis of "congestive heart failure." Identify the "main term" in this diagnosis.

Many conditions can be found in more than one place in the Alphabetic Index, which can be confusing. Obstetric conditions can be found under the name of the condition and under the entries for "delivery," "pregnancy," and "puerperal" (after delivery). Fig. 12-2 provides examples of how each of these three terms is shown in Volume 2. Complications of medical and surgical care are indexed under the *name of condition* and under *complications*.

Eponyms

Eponyms are diseases, procedures, or syndromes named for individuals who discovered or first used them. They typically are located alphabetically by the individual's name and by the common name. Vincent disease (trench mouth) can be found under "Vincent," "disease," and "trench" (Fig. 12-3).

nails 703.8
urinary stream 788.61
Spoiled child reaction (*see also*
   Disturbance, conduct) 312.1
Spondylarthritis (*see also* Spondylosis)
   721.90
Spondylarthrosis (*see also* Spondylosis)
   721.90
Spondylitis 720.9
   ankylopoietica 720.0
   ankylosing (chronic) 720.0
   atrophic 720.9
      ligamentous 720.9
   chronic (traumatic) (*see also* Spondy-
      losis) 721.90
   deformans (chronic) (*see also* Spondy-
      losis) 721.90
   gonococcal 098.53
   gouty 274.00
   hypertrophic (*see also* Spondylosis)
      721.90
   infectious NEC 720.9
   juvenile (adolescent) 720.0
   Kummell's 721.7
   Marie Strümpell (ankylosing) 720.0
   muscularis 720.9
Spondylopathy
   inflammatory 720.9
      specified type NEC 720.89
   traumatic 721.7
	Spondylose rhizomelique 720.0
	Spondylosis 721.90
	   with
	      disproportion 653.3
	         affecting fetus or newborn
	            763.1
	      causing obstructed labor 660.1
	         affecting fetus or newborn
	            763.1
	   myelopathy NEC 721.91
	   cervical, cervicodorsal 721.0
	      with myelopathy 721.1
	
	Main Term
	
	(in bold-faced type)
	
	   inflammatory 720.9
	   lumbar, lumbrosacral 721.3
	      with myelopathy 721.42
	   sacral 721.3
	      with myelopathy 721.42
	   thoracic 721.2
	      with myelopathy 721.41
	   traumatic 721.7
		Sponge
		   divers' disease 989.5
		   inadvertently left in operation wound
		      998.4
		      regular 626.5
		   interpalpebral 372.53
		   Koplik's 055.9
		   liver 709.09
		   Mongolian (pigmented) 757.33
		   of pregnancy 649.5
		   purpuric 782.7
		   ruby 448.1
		Spotted fever - *see* Fever, spotted
		Sprain, strain (joint) (ligament) (muscle)
		   (tendon) 848.9
		   abdominal wall (muscle) 848.8
		   Achilles tendon 845.09
		   acromioclavicular 840.0
		   ankle 845.00
		      and foot 845.00
		   anterior longitudinal, cervical 847.0
		   arm 840.9
		      upper 840.9
		         and shoulder 840.9
		   astragalus 845.00
		   atlanto-axial 847.00
		   atlanto-occipital 847.0
		   atlas 847.0
		   axis 847.0
		   back (*see also* Sprain, spine) 847.9
		   breast bone 848.40

Fig. 12-1 Sample page of section of the ICD-9 Volume 2. (Data from International Classification of Diseases, 9th Revision. U.S. Department of Health and Human Services, Public Health Service, Centers for Medicare and Medicaid Services.)

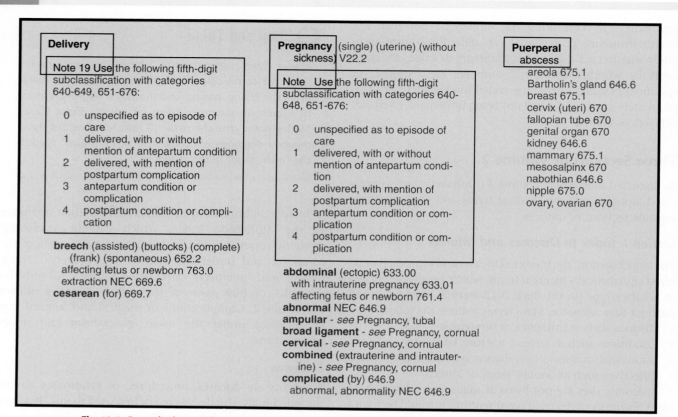

Delivery

Note 19 Use the following fifth-digit subclassification with categories 640-649, 651-676:

0   unspecified as to episode of care
1   delivered, with or without mention of antepartum condition
2   delivered, with mention of postpartum complication
3   antepartum condition or complication
4   postpartum condition or complication

breech (assisted) (buttocks) (complete) (frank) (spontaneous) 652.2
   affecting fetus or newborn 763.0
   extraction NEC 669.6
cesarean (for) 669.7

Pregnancy (single) (uterine) (without sickness) V22.2

Note   Use the following fifth-digit subclassification with categories 640-648, 651-676:

0   unspecified as to episode of care
1   delivered, with or without mention of antepartum condition
2   delivered, with mention of postpartum complication
3   antepartum condition or complication
4   postpartum condition or complication

abdominal (ectopic) 633.00
   with intrauterine pregnancy 633.01
   affecting fetus or newborn 761.4
abnormal NEC 646.9
ampullar - *see* Pregnancy, tubal
broad ligament - *see* Pregnancy, cornual
cervical - *see* Pregnancy, cornual
combined (extrauterine and intrauterine) - *see* Pregnancy, cornual
complicated (by) 646.9
   abnormal, abnormality NEC 646.9

Puerperal
   abscess
      areola 675.1
      Bartholin's gland 646.6
      breast 675.1
      cervix (uteri) 670
      fallopian tube 670
      genital organ 670
      kidney 646.6
      mammary 675.1
      mesosalpinx 670
      nabothian 646.6
      nipple 675.0
      ovary, ovarian 670

Fig. 12-2 Example showing how each of the above three terms is shown in Volume 2. (Data from International Classification of Diseases, 9th Revision. U.S. Department of Health and Human Services, Public Health Service, Centers for Medicare and Medicaid Services.)

Vincent's
   angina 101
   bronchitis 101
   disease 101
   gingivitis 101
   infection (any site) 101
   laryngitis 101
   stomatitis 101
   tonsillitis 101
Vinson-Plummer syndrome (sideropenic dysphagia) 280.8
Viosterol deficiency (*see also* Deficiency, calciferol) 268.9
Virchow's disease 733.99

Fig. 12-3 Example of an eponym listing. (Data from International Classification of Diseases, 9th Revision. U.S. Department of Health and Human Services, Public Health Service, Centers for Medicare and Medicaid Services.)

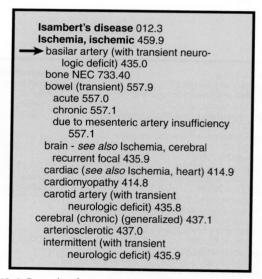

Isambert's disease 012.3
Ischemia, ischemic 459.9
   → basilar artery (with transient neurologic deficit) 435.0
   bone NEC 733.40
   bowel (transient) 557.9
      acute 557.0
      chronic 557.1
      due to mesenteric artery insufficiency 557.1
   brain - *see also* Ischemia, cerebral
      recurrent focal 435.9
   cardiac (*see also* Ischemia, heart) 414.9
   cardiomyopathy 414.8
   carotid artery (with transient neurologic deficit) 435.8
   cerebral (chronic) (generalized) 437.1
      arteriosclerotic 437.0
      intermittent (with transient neurologic deficit) 435.9

Fig. 12-4 Example of an essential modifier. (Data from International Classification of Diseases, 9th Revision. U.S. Department of Health and Human Services, Public Health Service, Centers for Medicare and Medicaid Services.)

Essential Modifiers

Essential modifiers are indented under the main term as shown in the example in Fig. 12-4. They modify the main term describing different sites, **etiology** (the cause or origin of a disease or condition), and clinical types. Essential modifiers must be a part of the documented diagnosis.

Nonessential Modifiers

Nonessential modifiers are terms in parentheses after the main terms. They typically give alternative terminology

for the main term and are provided to assist the coder in locating the applicable main term. Fig. 12-5 shows an example of how nonessential modifiers are depicted in Volume 2. Nonessential modifiers are usually not a part of the diagnostic statement; however, nonessential modifiers can provide an example of wording that might be in the provider's notes

Porocephaliasis 134.1
Porokeratosis 757.39
  disseminated superficial actinic (DSAP)
    692.75
Poroma, eccrine (M8402/0) - *see* Neoplasm, skin, benign
Porphyria (acute) (congenital) (constitutional) (erythropoietic) (familial) (he-
  patica) (idiopathic) (idiosyncratic)
  (intermittent) (latent) (mixed hepatic) (photosensitive) (South Afri-
  can genetic) (Swedish) 277.1
  acquired 277.1
  cutaneatarda
    hereditaria 277.1
    symptomatica 277.1
  due to drugs
    correct substance properly adminis-
      tered 277.1
    overdose or wrong substance given
      or taken 977.9
    specified drug - *see* Table of Drugs
      and Chemicals
  secondary 277.1
  toxic NEC 277.1
  variegata 277.1
Porphyrinuria (acquired) (congenital)
  (secondary) 277.1
Porphyruria (acquired) (congenital) 277.1

Fig. 12-5 Section of page from Volume 2 showing nonessential modifiers using porphyria. (Data from International Classification of Diseases, 9th Revision. U.S. Department of Health and Human Services, Public Health Service, Centers for Medicare and Medicaid Services.)

or diagnostic statement and can reassure the coder that the correct main term has been chosen in the index that directs him or her to the appropriate diagnostic code.

Conventions for Volume 2, Alphabetic Index

Parentheses. Nonessential modifiers are enclosed in parentheses.

Example:

Drip, postnasal (chronic).

Essential modifiers are not enclosed in parentheses and are subterms that do affect the selection of the appropriate code.

Example:

Functioning, borderline intellectual.

See. "See" is a cross-reference directing the coder to look elsewhere for the appropriate code.

Example:

Connective tissue—*see* condition.

See Also. "See also" is a cross-reference directing the coder to locate another main term in the event adequate information cannot be located under the first main term entry. Fig. 12-6 shows examples of how *see* and *see also* are used in Volume 2.

See Category. "See category" is a cross-reference directing the coder to the Tabular List (Vol. 1) for important information applicable to the use of the specific code.

Example:

Delivery—completely normal case—*see* category 650.

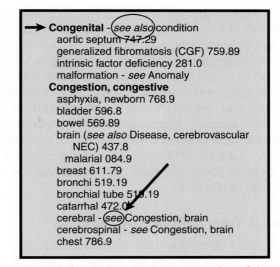

Fig. 12-6 Example from Volume 2 using congestive heart failure. (Data from International Classification of Diseases, 9th Revision. U.S. Department of Health and Human Services, Public Health Service, Centers for Medicare and Medicaid Services.)

Cross-Reference Notes. Cross-reference **notes** such as *see, see also, see condition,* and *see category* refer the coder to continue the search under another main term. Referring to the patient described in the Stop and Think box with a diagnosis of *congestive heart failure,* the main term "congestive" and the essential modifier "heart" are located in the Alphabetic Index, and there is a parenthetical notation (*see also* Failure, heart 428.0). This notation guides the coder to an alternate page in the Index, where the main term "failure, failed" is located. After the essential modifiers ("heart" and "congestive") code 428.0 is located, the coder must cross-reference this code to the Tabular List to determine if 428.0 describes this diagnosis to its "greatest specificity" or if a fifth digit is necessary.

Other Conventions. Other conventions used in the Alphabetic Index include "*Note,*" which defines terms and provides coding instructions; "*omit code,*" which directs the coder not to assign a code for that particular condition; and **NEC** ("**not elsewhere classifiable**"), which means that ICD-9-CM does not have a code that describes the condition.

Hypertension and Neoplasm Tables

The Alphabetic Index to Diseases also contains two tables: (1) Hypertension Table and (2) Neoplasm Table. If a patient is diagnosed with essential hypertension (high blood pressure from no apparent cause), the health insurance professional must locate the specific type in the hypertension table and make the determination if it is "malignant," "benign," or "unspecified" as indicated in the columnar codes (401.0, 401.1, or 401.9). If the patient's diagnosis is essential benign hypertension complicating pregnancy, childbirth, or the puerperium, the ICD-9 code would be 642.0. As with other code searches, hypertension and **neoplasm** (new growth) coding does not stop with the indexed tables in Volume 2. In the Buck 2012 manual, a red bullet behind the code indicates additional digits may be necessary to code to the greatest specificity.

Section II, Table of Drugs and Chemicals

Section II of Volume 2 consists of the Table of Drugs and Chemicals, which contains the Alphabetic Index to Poisoning and External Causes of Adverse Effects of Drugs and Other Chemical Substances. Codes in this table are used when documentation in the health record indicates a poisoning, overdose, wrong substance given or taken, or intoxication. The table also lists external causes of adverse effects resulting from ingestion or exposure to drugs or other chemical substances.

Section III, Index to External Causes of Injury and Poisoning (E Codes)

Section III is the Alphabetic Index to External Causes of Injury and Poisoning, which contains **E codes**. Codes in this section are used to classify environmental events, circumstances, and other conditions that are the cause of injury and other adverse effects. E codes are organized by main terms that describe the accident, circumstance, event, or specific agent causing the injury or adverse effect and should be used in addition to a code from the main body of the classification (Chapters 1 to 17).

🕐 Stop and Think

Bob Timmerman, 20 years old, was driving his 1978 Trans-Am on a two-lane country road at dusk when he accidentally struck a slow-moving Amish carriage, injuring a 4-year-old child. The child sustained a fractured ulna and multiple lacerations and contusions. In what section of ICD-9 would the health insurance professional look to begin the search for the appropriate diagnostic code?

National Coverage Determinations and Local Coverage Determinations

In addition to assigning the correct diagnostic code, it is also important to be knowledgeable of Medicare's **National Coverage Determinations (NCDs)** and **Local Coverage Determinations (LCDs)**, formerly known as Local Medical

Review Policies (LMRPs). NCDs are Medicare's standard national rules; LCDs are local carriers' versions of NCDs. These rules specify the services that are allowed for certain diagnoses. Databases of Medicare carriers screen ICD-9/CPT coding pairs to ensure they correspond to LCDs and automatically deny coding pairs that do not correspond. Because LCDs do not exist for all services and focus primarily on diagnostic tests, some claims are not affected by this screening method.

LCDs can change frequently; it is important to keep up-to-date by frequently checking the Medicare website by following the link available on the Evolve site. Select both the NCDs and LCDs boxes in the first section of the search page. Private payer rules can differ from Medicare rules in allowing certain services with a particular diagnosis. Most payers post their determinations on their websites.

❓ What Did You Learn?

1. List the three volumes contained in ICD-9.
2. *True or false:* Most insurance companies do not require the use of Volume 3 for physician and outpatient billing; however, Volume 3 is still used for hospital inpatient coding.
3. The Tabular List (Vol. 2) contains _____ sections including E-Codes and appendices.
4. *True or false:* A diagnosis should *never* be coded strictly from the Alphabetic List.
5. Codes used to classify environmental events, circumstances, and other conditions that are the cause of injury and other adverse effects are called _____.

PROCESS OF CLASSIFYING DISEASES

The first thing that the coder must do in the coding process is to locate the diagnosis in the health record. This task can be straightforward sometimes because many encounter forms list the more frequently used diagnoses within a certain medical specialty along with their corresponding ICD-9 codes (Fig. 12-7). Other times, the coder may have to refer to the clinical notes to locate the diagnosis. If the notes are handwritten, deciphering the healthcare professional's handwriting sometimes can be challenging (Fig. 12-8). With practice and experience, locating the diagnosis within the clinical notes and translating a physician's handwriting become easier.

After the diagnosis has been determined, the main term within the diagnosis should be identified. For example, if the diagnosis is "breast mass," the main term would be "mass." (The anatomic site "breast" is not used in the Alphabetic Index to Diseases.) Fig. 12-9 illustrates how the main term "mass" appears in Volume 2.

DIAGNOSIS: Chk or 1 = Primary		2 = Secondary					
						Chlamydia / GC Screen	86631
						Digoxin	80162
						Dilantin	80185
Abdominal Pain	789.00	COPD	496	Hypothyroidism	244.9	MSAFP	82105
Allergies	995.3	CVA, Old	438.9	Long term med use	V58.69	Pap Smear	88150
Anemia	285.9	Depression	311	Nasophyaryngitis	460	RA	86430
Anticoagulation Therapy	V58.61	Dermatitis	692.9	Otitis Media	382.00	T-4, Free-RIA	84439
Anxiety	300.00	Diabetes (Non-Insulin)	250.00	Pharyngitis	462	Sensitivity	87186
Arthritis	716.90	Diabetes (Insulin-Depend.)	250.01	Physical Exam	V70.0	Theophylline	80198
Arthritis, degen.	715.90	Dizziness	780.4	Physical, Athletic	V70.3	Urine Culture	87086

Arthritis, Rheumatoid	714.0	Elevated BP	796.2	Physical, Preemployment	V70.5	☐ Cash ☐ Credit Card	INITIALS
Asthma	493.90	Fatigue	780.79	Pneumonia	486	Check # 3204	GSM
Atrial Fibrillation	427.31	Gastroenteritis, viral	008.8	Pregnancy	V22.2		
Backache, unspec.	724.5	Gastroesophageal Reflux	530.81	Routine Child Exam	V20.0	PREVIOUS BALANCE	.00
Bronchitis	490	GYN Exam w/Pap	V72.3	Sinusitis, Acute	461.9		.00
CAD	414.00	Headaches	784.0	Sinusitis, Chronic	473.9	CREDIT BALANCE	
Chest Pain	786.50	Hypercholesterolemia	272.0	Tonsillitis	463	TODAY'S	
CHF	428.0	Hyperlipidemia	272.4	URI	465.9	CHARGES	47.00
Conjunctivitis	372.30	Hypertension, Benign	401.1	UTI	599.0		

OTHER DIAGNOSIS (NOT LISTED)			CODE			
					PAYMENT ON TODAY'S CHARGES	47.00
					PAYMENT ON PREVIOUS BALANCE	

OFFICE RETURN		LAB RETURN	NEW BALANCE
10 15 20 30 40 OTH_____			
_____ _____ _____ FU _____		DAYS WEEKS MONTHS	
DAYS WEEKS MONTHS PE WITH:		TESTS:	

Fig. 12-7 Portion of an encounter form showing list of diagnoses.

1. Right inguinal hernia, incarcerated

2. Anginal Syndrome

3. hip and tuberculosis right cellulcutitis right

Fig. 12-8 Examples of handwritten diagnoses.

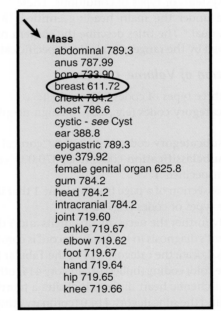

Mass
  abdominal 789.3
  anus 787.99
  bone 733.90
  breast 611.72
  cheek 784.2
  chest 786.6
  cystic - *see* Cyst
  ear 388.8
  epigastric 789.3
  eye 379.92
  female genital organ 625.8
  gum 784.2
  head 784.2
  intracranial 784.2
  joint 719.60
    ankle 719.67
    elbow 719.62
    foot 719.67
    hand 719.64
    hip 719.65
    knee 719.66

Fig. 12-9 Section of Volume 2 showing "Mass, breast." (Data from International Classification of Diseases, 9th Revision. U.S. Department of Health and Human Services, Public Health Service, Centers for Medicare and Medicaid Services.)

⭐ Imagine This!

Marlee Davis, the health insurance professional in Dr. Barnes' office, deciphered one of the physician's handwritten diagnoses as "atrophic arthritis," rather than "aortic arteritis." The error was not caught before the submission of the claim, and the insurance company rejected the claim because the procedures listed on the claim form did not coincide with the diagnosis. When the patient received an explanation of benefits from his insurance carrier that the claim was denied, he phoned the office with a complaint. Marlee had to apologize to the patient and resubmit the CMS-1500 claim form.

Note the numbers 611.72 following "breast" shown in the portion of Volume 2 in Fig. 12-10. This is the 5-digit diagnosis code for breast mass. The number one cardinal rule in coding is *never* to code from the Alphabetic Index (Volume 2) alone. Before assigning this code, it is important to read any special notes or instructions, after which the health insurance professional turns to Volume 1, the Tabular Index, and locates the code 611.72.

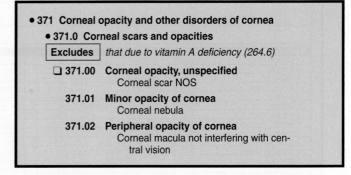

Fig. 12-10 Portion of tabular listing in Volume 2 showing the above code. (Data from International Classification of Diseases, 9th Revision. U.S. Department of Health and Human Services, Public Health Service, Centers for Medicare and Medicaid Services.)

Volume 1, Tabular List

Volume 1, the Tabular List, contains 17 sections representing anatomic systems or types of conditions. These 17 sections were listed under the main heading entitled "ICD-9-CM Coding Manual." The titles describe the content of the section followed by the range of codes in a specific category.

Organization of Volume 1 Codes

There are three types of codes in Volume 1:
- 3-digit **category** codes (e.g., 220, "benign neoplasm of ovary")
- 4-digit **subcategory** codes (e.g., 370.0, "corneal ulcer")
- 5-digit **subclassification** codes (e.g., 370.00, "corneal ulcer, unspecified")

Study the section of a page from Volume 1 that illustrates these three types of codes (Fig. 12-11).

To clarify further the necessity of 4 digits and 5 digits, say that a patient's diagnosis in the health record is coronary atherosclerosis. Locate the category 414 in the Tabular List (Volume 1). The color coding (bullet) of category 414 (other forms of chronic ischemic heart disease) indicates a fourth digit is necessary, and the subcategory 414.0 (coronary atherosclerosis) needs a fifth digit to describe the patient's diagnosis to the greatest specificity. It must be determined which of the subclassifications (414.00 through 414.07) best describes the patient's heart condition. If the 4-digit code (414.0) is submitted to the insurer, the claim no doubt would be rejected and returned unpaid because a fifth digit is necessary.

Color Coding

Most ICD-9 manuals use color coding in Volume 1 to alert the coder to special edits and other important issues. In the 2012 Buck manual, a red bullet preceding a 3-digit or 4-digit code indicates that an additional digit is required. Other publications may use a different indicator, such as circle with either a 4 or a 5 inside to indicate additional digits

Fig. 12-11 Section of a page from Volume 1 showing 3-digit, 4-digit, and 5-digit codes. (Data from International Classification of Diseases, 9th Revision. U.S. Department of Health and Human Services, Public Health Service, Centers for Medicare and Medicaid Services.)

are necessary. Refer to the bottom of the page in the Tabular list for other types of color coding and various symbols used for reference. "Unspecified Code," "Other Specified Code," and "Manifestation Code" also have special color coding in the ICD-9 manual.

Remember: A 3-digit code must not be used if a 4-digit code is available, and a 4-digit code must not be used if a 5-digit code is available.

Supplementary Sections of Volume 1

V Codes

The **V codes**, Supplementary Classification of Factors Influencing Health Status and Contact with Health Services (V01-V91.99 in Buck 2012), follow the aforementioned 17 sections. Codes in this section are used when circumstances other than a disease or injury classifiable to categories 001 through 999 are recorded as a diagnosis or problem; this can appear in the health record in one of three ways:
1. When an individual who is not currently sick visits the medical facility for a specific purpose, such as donating a tissue sample or to receive a vaccination.
2. When an individual with a known disease or injury comes in for specific treatment for that problem, such as dialysis for kidney disease, chemotherapy for cancer, or a cast change.
3. When there is a problem that influences the individual's health status but is not in itself a current illness or injury. An example is an individual with a history of a certain disease or an individual who has an artificial heart valve, which may affect his or her present condition.

When terms such as "examination," "problem with," "vaccination," and "observation" are seen as the diagnosis in a health record, it is usually a clue that a V code is necessary. Some V codes can be used alone, and some require a medical diagnosis from the main ICD-9 sections. Examples of common V code diagnoses include the following:
- Family history of malignant neoplasm
- Health supervision of infant or child
- Normal pregnancy
- Supervision of high-risk pregnancy

E Codes

The Supplementary Classification of External Causes of Injury and Poisoning, referred to as E codes (codes E800 through E999.1 in Buck 2012), follows the section on V codes. Codes in this section classify external causes of environmental events, circumstances, or conditions that resulted in the injury, condition, poisoning, or adverse effect being described, such as how an accident occurred or whether a drug overdose was accidental or intentional. Additionally, E codes can indicate the place of occurrence.

E codes are never used alone or as the primary diagnosis on a claim. They typically are combined with a code from one of the main chapters of the ICD-9 that indicates the nature of the condition. Healthcare providers usually are not required to assign E codes, unless there is an adverse reaction to a medication that has been taken according to directions. A typical example of this might be as follows:

780.4 Dizziness due to

E939.4 Benzodiazepine-based tranquilizers

Note the blue bullet preceding the E code in the Buck 2012 manual. Referring to the reference symbols and conventions at the bottom of the page, a blue bullet indicates "unacceptable principal diagnosis," meaning it cannot be used alone—it must be used in conjunction with a code from one of the main chapters (001 through 999.9). Also, some third-party payers prefer that E codes not be used at all on claims. The health insurance professional should contact the third-party carrier to determine if E codes are allowed.

The steps for selecting the correct E code for the adverse effects in the previous example are as follows:

1. Locate the drug (benzodiazepine) in the Table of Drugs and Chemicals.
2. Search for the code in the column titled "Therapeutic Use."
3. Verify the code.
4. Do not use an E code as the first diagnosis; rather, use the code for the diagnosis "dizziness."

> ### 📁 HIPAA Tip
>
> Always protect the confidentiality of all ICD-9 codes because these codes are part of the patient's record. HIPAA addresses coding issues and sets standards for their use, along with other issues regarding confidentiality in dealing with patient health records.

Locating a Code in the Tabular List (Volume 1)

Codes in Volume 1 are arranged numerically, so they are relatively easy to find. Use the numeric range descriptors at the top corners of each page to narrow down your search (Fig. 12-12). First, locate the 3-digit code that defines the category. Using the breast mass example, this would be 611, "other disorders of breast." The color coding indicates that a fourth digit is required for each subcategory. Read down through the subcategory entries until 611.7 is found, "signs and symptoms in breast." Note that a fifth digit is required. Locate the subclassification entry 611.72, "lump or mass in breast." If no other notes, symbols, or special editing codes are shown, it can be reasonable to assume that this diagnosis has been coded to its greatest specificity.

> ### 💬 What Did You Learn?
>
> 1. What is the first thing that the coder must do in the coding process?
> 2. In the diagnosis "breast mass," what is the main term?
> 3. Name the three types of codes in the Tabular List.
> 4. Most ICD-9 manuals use _____ in Volume 1 to alert the coder to special edits and other important issues.
> 5. _____ are Supplementary Classification of Factors Influencing Health Status and Contact with Health Services.

SYMBOLS AND CONVENTIONS USED IN VOLUME 1

The symbols and conventions used in Volume 1 of the ICD-9 manual include abbreviations, punctuation, symbols, footnotes, and other instructional notes. Many of these conventions are used in all three volumes; however, some are used only in Volume 2; others are used only in Volume 1. A list of symbols and conventions used in the Buck 2012 manual can be found in the first several pages of the book (xii through xviii); however, they may differ from other ICD-9-CM publications. To code accurately, the health insurance professional must understand what each of these symbols and conventions means.

Top right
Top left

610	ICD-9-CM	612.1
614	**PART III /** Diseases: Tabular List Volume 1	614.9

Fig. 12-12 Top portion of page showing range descriptors. (From Buck C: Saunders 2010 ICD-9-CM, Volumes 1, 2, and 3, Professional Edition, St Louis, 2010, Saunders.)

Typefaces

The Buck ICD-9-CM manual (and other publications) varies the format of the type to indicate other conventions, as follows:

- **Boldface:** Boldface type is used for main terms in the Alphabetic Index (Volume 2) and all codes and titles in the tabular list.
- *Italics:* Italicized type is used for all exclusion notes and to identify codes that should not be used for describing the primary diagnosis.

  Examples of these two typeface formats are shown in Fig. 12-13.

Instructional Notes

In addition to abbreviations, punctuation, and symbols, the ICD-9 manual uses instructional notes to help the health insurance professional choose the correct code (Fig. 12-14).

Bold face type ⟨

Italicized type ⟩

```
Intrathoracic - see also condition
   kidney 753.3
   stomach - see Hernia, diaphragm
Intrauterine contraceptive device
   checking V25.42
   insertion V25.1
   in situ V45.51
   management V25.42
   prescription V25.02
      repeat V25.42
   reinsertion V25.42
   removal V25.42
Intraventricular - see condition
Intrinsic deformity - see Deformity
Intruded tooth 524.34
Intrusion, repetitive, of sleep (due to
      environmenal disturbances) (with
      atypical polysomnographic features)
      307.48
Intumescent, lens (eye) NEC 366.9
   senile 366.12
Intussusception (colon) (enteric) (intes-
      tine) (rectum) 560.0
   appendix 543.9
   congenital 751.5
   fallopian tube 620.8
   ileocecal 560.0
   ileocolic 560.0
   ureter (obstruction) 593.4
```

Fig. 12-13 Example of boldface and italicized type. (Data from International Classification of Diseases, 9th Revision. U.S. Department of Health and Human Services, Public Health Service, Centers for Medicare and Medicaid Services.)

ESSENTIAL STEPS TO DIAGNOSTIC CODING

Now that the basic background for ICD-9 coding has been presented, let's look at the essential steps of diagnostic coding.

1. Locate the diagnosis in the patient's health record (or on the encounter form).
2. Determine the "main term" of the stated diagnosis.
3. Find the main term in the Alphabetic Index (Volume 2) of the most recent version of the ICD-9-CM manual.
4. Read and apply any notes or instructions contained in the Alphabetic Index. *Reminder: Never code directly from the Alphabetic Index.*
5. Cross-reference the code found in the Alphabetic Index (Volume 2) to the Tabular List (Volume 1).
6. Read and be guided by the conventions and symbols, paying close attention to any footnotes or cross-references.
7. Read through the entire category, and code to the *highest level of specificity,* taking special care to assign a fourth or fifth digit to the code if the color coding indicates it is necessary.

SPECIAL CODING SITUATIONS

Coding Signs and Symptoms

If a patient's condition has not been specifically diagnosed, the signs or symptoms must be coded. Documentation in the assessment segment of the patient record may use such terms as "probable," "questionable," "rule out," or "suspected"; however, the coder should not use any one of these terms as if it were the final diagnosis. It may take two or more visits before a specific diagnosis is confirmed.

Section 16 of the ICD-9 (codes 780 through 799) contains a list of codes classifying symptoms, signs, and ill-defined conditions for which no diagnosis classifiable elsewhere is recorded. These codes are used when no definitive diagnosis can be arrived at the conclusion of the initial encounter. Common examples of signs and symptoms include dizziness, fever, nausea, shortness of breath, and headache.

Includes	The instructional note **Includes** further defines or clarifies the content of the category, subcategory, or subclassification.
Excludes	Terms following the instructional note **Excludes** are not classified to the category, subcategory, or specific subclassification code under which it is found. The note may also provide the location of the excluded diagnosis.
Use additional code	When this note appears, an additional code(s) must be used to provide a more complete description of the diagnosis.
Code first underlying *disease*	This italicized note indicates that the description given should not be used for coding the primary diagnosis. The italicized notation is followed by the code(s) for the most common underlying disease. These codes, referred to as manifestation codes, should not be used alone or indicated as the primary diagnosis (i.e., sequenced first). They must always be preceded by another code. Record the code for the primary disease first, and then record the italicized manifestation code.
■ Nonspecified Code	Use these codes only when neither the diagnostic statement nor the documentation provides enough information to assign a more specific code. (Note: Check with the carrier or FI to see if unspecified codes are acceptable on the claim form.)
OGCR	Follow Official Guidelines for Coding and Reporting.
Code, if applicable, any causal condition first	A code with this notation may be principal if no causal condition is applicable or known.
"And" and "with"	"and" means and/or; "with" indicates another condition is included in the code.

Fig. 12-14 Examples of how boldface and italicized type and other special notations are identified. (From Buck C: Saunders 2010 ICD-9-CM, Volumes 1, 2, and 3, Professional Edition, St Louis, 2010, Saunders.)

If a patient visits the medical facility with the chief complaint of nausea, but the healthcare provider has not yet determined what is causing the nausea, the code for nausea must be used. Looking in the Alphabetic Index (Volume 1) under "nausea," we find 787.02 for nausea without vomiting and 787.01 for nausea with vomiting. Cross-referencing to the Tabular Index, we first locate the 3-digit category: "787, symptoms involving digestive system." Reading down through the subcategory and subclassification sections, note by the symbols that 5 digits are necessary. For accurate coding, it must be determined if the patient has nausea with vomiting, nausea alone, or vomiting alone; this should be documented in the clinical notes. If the clinical notes are nonspecific as to whether or not there is vomiting, it should be assumed there is not vomiting unless it is documented.

Note: Coding guidelines for inconclusive diagnoses (e.g., probable, questionable, suspected, rule out) were developed for inpatient reporting and do not apply to outpatients.

Etiology and Manifestation Coding

When the notation "code first any underlying condition" (blue highlight in Buck 2012) is seen, this indicates that the etiology (cause or origin of the disease) is coded before the **manifestation** (sign or symptom of the disease). If the

patient's diagnosis is diabetic ulcer of the heel, the underlying condition or disease process (diabetes) is coded first before the heel ulcer. Some ICD-9 manuals use the plus sign (+) to indicate a manifestation code. Slanted brackets [ ] may also be used to enclose the manifestation of an underlying condition.

Stop and Think

Lonny Chadwick noticed a suspicious-looking mole on his lower right leg and went to his dermatologist. Lonny's father died of malignant melanoma, and Lonny was concerned that his mole was also malignant. The dermatologist examined the mole and removed a section of tissue for a biopsy. When the biopsy results were returned, the laboratory report stated that the tissue sample was "abnormal, but inconclusive." Documentation in Mr. Chadwick's health record noted the fact that his father had died of malignant melanoma. The diagnosis stated "suspicious lesion, lower right leg, rule out melanoma." Subsequently, the health insurance professional submitted the claim with the diagnosis of "melanoma." What problems might arise from this incorrect coding process?

⭐ Imagine This!

Referring to Lonny Chadwick (the patient with the suspicious lesion on his lower leg), when the health insurance professional resubmitted the claim, she used the V code V10.82. Mr. Chadwick's insurance carrier returned it stating they do not pay on the basis of V codes. Subsequently, the claim had to be corrected and resubmitted a second time with the appropriate ICD-9 code. As a result of the two incorrectly coded claims, reimbursement for Mr. Chadwick's procedure took nearly 3 months.

⭐ Imagine This!

Jane Thiele went to an ophthalmologist for a routine eye examination. After the examination, she went to the reception area to pay the $150 charge. "I know my insurance won't pay for routine exams, so I'll just write you a check today," Jane told the medical receptionist. "Oh, don't worry," the receptionist replied, "Dr. Packston often finds a way to help people out, so why don't you just wait to pay." Jane was surprised and pleased when a few weeks later she received a check from her insurance company for 80% of the charge. A few years later, Jane took early retirement from her job. Because of the high cost of converting her group insurance to a COBRA policy, she applied for less costly private insurance coverage. While Jane was in the process of applying for a private policy, she was told that any problems with her eyes would not be covered. When she asked why, she was told that her medical records from Dr. Packston had indicated a diagnosis of "early cataract," which was not the case at all. Because the new insurance policy excludes all procedures involving eyes, owing to Dr. Packston's diagnosis, Jane will either have to pay for any medical services involving her eyes if problems develop or pay a much higher premium for total coverage.

Combination Codes

A **combination code** is used when more than one otherwise individually classified disease is combined with another disease and one code is assigned for both or when a single code is used to describe conditions that frequently occur together. A single (combination) code is used to classify two diagnoses or
- a diagnosis with an associated secondary process (manifestation), or
- a diagnosis with an associated complication.

An example of this is the code 034.0, "streptococcal sore throat," because a sore throat is often caused by the streptococci bacteria; however, "streptococcal" must be indicated

on the laboratory report to use 034.0. If a laboratory report does not indicate "strep," the code 462 sore throat (pharyngitis) is used. The coder should assign only the combination code when that code fully identifies the diagnostic condition involved or when the Alphabetic Index so directs. When the combination code lacks necessary specificity in describing the manifestation or complication, an additional code should be used as a secondary code. For example, if a patient has both scarlet fever and strep throat, both codes (034.0 and 034.1) must be used.

Coding Late Effects

A late effect (**sequela**) is the residual effect (condition produced) after the acute phase of an illness or injury has ended. There is no time limit on when a late effect code can be used. The residual may be apparent early, such as in cases of cerebrovascular accident, or it may occur months or years later, such herpes zoster (shingles) long after a case of childhood chickenpox. Coding of late effects generally requires two codes sequenced in the following order: The condition or nature of the late effect is sequenced first. The late effect code is sequenced second.

> *Example:*
> Gait abnormality as a late effect of hip fracture
> 781.2 Abnormality of gait
> 905.4 Late effect of fracture of lower extremity (hip)

Coding Neoplasms

A neoplasm results when abnormal cells grow uncontrollably, usually resulting in a tumor. To code neoplasms appropriately, the coder must first determine from the medical record whether the specimen in question is malignant, in situ (the cancer is confined to the immediate area where it began), benign, or of uncertain behavior. Whenever a biopsy or excisional procedure is performed for the expressed purpose of determining whether a particular tissue is malignant or not, the diagnosis should not be coded until the pathology information is present in the record. In most cases, the pathology report is clear, and the tumor is identified as either malignant or benign. However, ICD-9-CM has included two sections in the Neoplasms chapter for "Neoplasms of Uncertain Behavior" and "Neoplasms of Unspecified Nature."

When the behavior of the tissue in question has been determined, the coder should first turn to the Neoplasm Table in ICD-9-CM unless the actual histological term is documented. If so, the term (e.g., "adenoma") should be located in the Alphabetic Index, and the entries and instructional notes should be reviewed. For example, in the Alphabetic Index, the instructional note under "adenoma" tells the coder to "*see also,* neoplasm, by site, benign." The coder then refers to the Neoplasm Table by anatomical site, benign behavior, for the appropriate code. The Neoplasm Table is arranged by anatomical site for each row, and the type of histological behavior (primary, secondary, carcinoma in situ, benign, uncertain behavior, and unspecified) is described across the columns. After a code is located in the Neoplasm Table, it should always be verified in the Tabular portion of ICD-9-CM.

Example:

"Benign adenoma of the colon":

1. Locate the main term ("adenoma") in the Alphabetic Index. Note the convention *see also* "neoplasm, by site, benign."
2. Cross-reference to the Neoplasm Table.
3. Locate "colon" (listed alphabetically).
4. Cross-reference "colon" to "*see also* Neoplasm intestine, intestinal, large."
5. Assign the correct code under the "benign" column heading (211.3).

Note: V codes are sometimes used if there is a family or personal history of malignant neoplasms.

Coding Hypertension

One of the most common conditions coded is hypertension (high blood pressure). If a patient has a documented diagnosis of "hypertension, essential, benign," the steps to follow for coding this condition are as follows:

1. Locate the main term "hypertension" in the Alphabetic Index. It tells the coder to *see* Table.
2. Note the three column headings in the Table: "malignant," "benign," and "unspecified."
3. The various terms in parentheses (nonessential modifiers) listed behind the main terms in the first entry (hypertension, hypertensive) include the word "essential."
4. Because "essential" is a nonessential modifier included under the main term category, cross-reference it to the "benign" column.
5. Assign the code 401.1.

❓ What Did You Learn?

1. List four common examples of signs and symptoms.
2. Which should be coded first, the etiology or the manifestation?
3. What is a combination code?
4. Coding of sequela generally requires _____ codes with the _____ sequenced first.
5. *True or false:* In most cases, the pathology report is clear, and neoplasm (tumor) is identified as either malignant or benign.

OVERVIEW OF ICD-10 CODING SYSTEM

The ICD-10 coding system consists of two parts:
1. ICD-10-CM for diagnosis coding (used in all healthcare settings)

2. ICD-10-PCS for inpatient procedure coding (used in inpatient hospital settings only)

Diagnosis coding under ICD-10-CM uses 3 to 7 digits instead of the 3 to 5 digits used with ICD-9-CM, but the format of the code sets is similar.

Key Note:

CPT-4 codes are still used by Medicare Part B providers to describe procedures.

ICD-10-CM Code Structure

As mentioned, an ICD-10-CM code has 3 to 7 characters (Table 12-5). The first character of an ICD-10-CM code is always an alphabetic letter, and all letters of the alphabet are used except the letter "U." Alphabetic characters are not case sensitive.

Key Note:

The letter "U" has been reserved to assign codes to new diseases whose etiology (the cause of the disease) is unknown (U00 through U49) and for bacterial agents that are resistant to antibiotics (U80 through U89).

Codes longer than 3 digits always have a decimal point after the first 3 characters. Each additional character adds more specificity to the disease or condition. The additional characters add to the clinical detail and address information about previously classified diseases or conditions discovered since the last edition.

For more information on how ICD-10-CM codes are structured, visit the Evolve site. ⓔ

Format of ICD-10-CM Manual

As with ICD-9-CM, before any attempt is made to code a diagnosis, the health insurance professional must become familiar with the contents and structure of the coding manual. The format of the ICD-10-CM manual may differ among publishers regarding how the material is arranged in the introduction or preface; however, the basic information is the same. The prefacing instructions used in this chapter follow *2010 ICD-10-CM (Draft)* by Carol J. Buck, published by Saunders (2010). The information, coding instructions, and codes were current at the time of this writing. To keep up-to-date on ICD-10-CM coding practices, the health insurance professional should always consult the most recently published ICD-10-CM coding manual.

The first several pages of the ICD-10-CM manual contain the following:

- Table of Contents
- Symbols and Conventions

TABLE 12-5 Code Structure of ICD-10-CM

ICD-10-CM codes may consist of up to 7 digits, with the 7th digit extensions representing visit/encounter or sequelae for injuries and external causes

ICD-10-CM Code Format

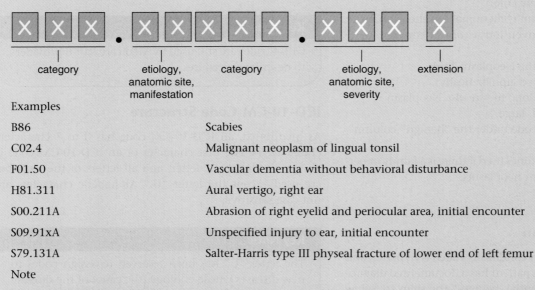

Examples

B86	Scabies
C02.4	Malignant neoplasm of lingual tonsil
F01.50	Vascular dementia without behavioral disturbance
H81.311	Aural vertigo, right ear
S00.211A	Abrasion of right eyelid and periocular area, initial encounter
S09.91xA	Unspecified injury to ear, initial encounter
S79.131A	Salter-Harris type III physeal fracture of lower end of left femur

Note

When coding fractures, the 7th character classification can indicate type, status, and encounter (initial, subsequent, and sequela). The 7th character can also represent the type of fracture and the present status of the fracture

- Part I—Introduction (containing ICD-10-CM Official Guidelines for Coding and Reporting)
- Netter Anatomy Plates
- Part II—Alphabetic Index (Index to Diseases and Injuries)
  - Table of Neoplasms
  - Table of Drugs and Chemicals
  - External Cause Index
- Part III—Tabular List of Diseases and Injuries (21 Chapters)

Note: The link for the complete ICD-10-CM Official Guidelines for Coding and Reporting can found on the Evolve site.

Alphabetic Index

The Alphabetic Index (hereafter referred to as the *Index*) contains a list of terms arranged alphabetically along with their corresponding codes. Each page of the Index is divided into three columns. At the extreme top right (or left) corner of each page is a guide word, similar to a dictionary, to assist the coder in locating the appropriate page (Fig. 12-15). For example, Fig 12-16 shows the location of the term "Paraplegia" in *2010 ICD-10-CM (Draft)* by Buck. The guide word on the left-hand page is "Paranoid," and the guide words on the right-hand page are "Perforation,

perforated." Paraplegia is located alphabetically within these two pages.

Main Terms

The first step in diagnostic coding is to identify the **main term** (sometimes referred to as the "lead term") of the diagnostic statement. This term can typically be found in the patient's medical record. The coder must locate the main term from the medical record in the Index. Main terms are generally not organized by anatomical site. When locating an anatomical term such as shoulder, the Index says "*see* condition." Main terms typically include:

- a disease (bronchitis or influenza);
- a condition (fracture, fatigue, or injury);
- an adjective (double, large, or kinked);
- a noun (a disease, disturbance, or syndrome); or
- an eponym (Larsen's syndrome).

If a patient has a diagnosis of deviated nasal septum, the main term would be "deviated" and would be found in the Index under "deviation." Main terms in the Index are printed in bold type to assist the coder in locating the desired disease or condition (Fig. 12-17).

For clarification, let's walk through this process with a patient whose diagnosis has been identified as "heart failure." "Heart" is an anatomical site. If you locate it in the Index, it will say "*see* condition." The first step is to locate "failure" in the Index.

Fig. 12-15 Sample partial page from ICD-10 Index showing guide terms at top of page. (From Buck CJ: 2010 ICD-10-CM Draft, Standard Edition, St Louis, 2010, Saunders.)

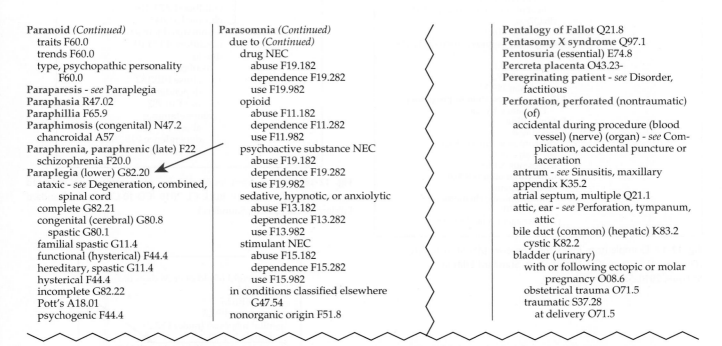

INDEX TO DISEASES AND INJURIES DRAFT / Paranoid   INDEX TO DISEASES AND INJURIES DRAFT / Perforation, perforated

Paranoid *(Continued)*
    traits F60.0
    trends F60.0
    type, psychopathic personality
        F60.0
Paraparesis - *see* Paraplegia
Paraphasia R47.02
Paraphillia F65.9
Paraphimosis (congenital) N47.2
    chancroidal A57
Paraphrenia, paraphrenic (late) F22
    schizophrenia F20.0
Paraplegia (lower) G82.20
    ataxic - *see* Degeneration, combined,
        spinal cord
    complete G82.21
    congenital (cerebral) G80.8
        spastic G80.1
    familial spastic G11.4
    functional (hysterical) F44.4
    hereditary, spastic G11.4
    hysterical F44.4
    incomplete G82.22
    Pott's A18.01
    psychogenic F44.4

Parasomnia *(Continued)*
    due to *(Continued)*
        drug NEC
            abuse F19.182
            dependence F19.282
            use F19.982
        opioid
            abuse F11.182
            dependence F11.282
            use F11.982
        psychoactive substance NEC
            abuse F19.182
            dependence F19.282
            use F19.982
        sedative, hypnotic, or anxiolytic
            abuse F13.182
            dependence F13.282
            use F13.982
        stimulant NEC
            abuse F15.182
            dependence F15.282
            use F15.982
    in conditions classified elsewhere
        G47.54
    nonorganic origin F51.8

Pentalogy of Fallot Q21.8
Pentasomy X syndrome Q97.1
Pentosuria (essential) E74.8
Percreta placenta O43.23-
Peregrinating patient - *see* Disorder,
    factitious
Perforation, perforated (nontraumatic)
    (of)
    accidental during procedure (blood
        vessel) (nerve) (organ) - *see* Com-
        plication, accidental puncture or
        laceration
    antrum - *see* Sinusitis, maxillary
    appendix K35.2
    atrial septum, multiple Q21.1
    attic, ear - *see* Perforation, tympanum,
        attic
    bile duct (common) (hepatic) K83.2
        cystic K82.2
    bladder (urinary)
        with or following ectopic or molar
            pregnancy O08.6
        obstetrical trauma O71.5
        traumatic S37.28
            at delivery O71.5

Fig. 12-16 Sample partial Index page showing guide words wherein the term "Paresis" can be located. (From Buck CJ: 2010 ICD-10-CM Draft, Standard Edition, St Louis, 2010, Saunders.)

> **Key Note:**
>
> Categories of injuries are arranged alphabetically under the main term "Injury," rather than by type of injury as in ICD-9-CM.

Essential and Nonessential Modifiers

Any relevant subterms or essential modifiers are indented under the main terms. Indented subterms are always used in combination with the main term. They describe different sites, etiology, and clinical types. Essential modifiers must be a part of the documented diagnosis (Fig. 12-18).

Frequently, a main term is immediately followed by an additional word or words in parentheses, or nonessential modifiers. Nonessential modifiers that appear in parentheses do not affect the code number assigned but are provided to assist the coder in locating the correct code (Fig. 12-19).

In our example diagnosis of heart failure, note the nonessential modifiers in parentheses immediately following "heart." These subterms do not affect the diagnostic code assigned and are given to assist the coder in locating the correct code. They may or may not be a part of the documented

diagnosis. Also note that the 4-character code I50.9 follows the parenthetical nonessential modifiers. If no other words appear in the stated diagnosis in the patient record, the next step would be to cross-reference the code to the Tabular List—the section containing diagnosis codes arranged alphanumerically and divided into chapters based on body system (anatomical site) or condition (etiology)—to finalize the process of assigning the correct code. Further steps in locating the correct code in the Tabular List are discussed later in this chapter.

> **Key Note:**
>
> If a code has only three characters (e.g., B03 Smallpox), the coder can generally assume that the category has not been subdivided further.

There are additional indented statements under the subterm "heart." To use any one of these terms, it must be identified in the stated diagnosis. For example, if the diagnostic statement in the patient's record was "arteriosclerotic heart failure," without any further description, the code would be I70.90—unspecified atherosclerosis.

Main Term (in bold-faced type)

Exstrophy *(Continued)*
  bladder *(Continued)*
    specified type NEC Q64.19
    supravesical fissure Q64.11
Extensive - *see* condition
Extra - *see also* Accessory
  marker chromosomes (normal individual) Q92.61
    in abnormal individual Q92.62
  rib Q76.6
    cervical Q76.5
Extrasystoles (supraventricular) I49.49
  atrial I49.1
  auricular I49.1
  junctional I49.2
  ventricular I49.3
Extrauterine gestation or pregnancy - *see* Pregnancy, by site
Extravasation
  blood R58
  chyle into mesentery I89.8
  pelvicalyceal N13.8
  pyelosinus N13.8
  urine (from ureter) R39.0
  vesicant agent
    antineoplastic chemotherapy T80.810
    other agent NEC T80.818

Fig. 12-17 Example from Index showing examples of main terms. (From Buck CJ: 2010 ICD-10-CM Draft, Standard Edition, St Louis, 2010, Saunders.)

Insolation (sunstroke) T67.0
Insomnia (organic) G47.00
  adjustment F51.02
  adjustment disorder F51.02
  behavioral, of childhood Z73.819
    combined type Z73.812
    limit setting type Z73.811
    sleep-onset association type Z73.810
  childhood Z73.819
  chronic F51.04
    somatized tension F51.04
  conditioned F51.04
  due to
    alcohol
      abuse F10.182
      dependence F10.282
      use F10.982
    amphetamines
      abuse F15.182
      dependence F15.282
      use f15.982

Fig. 12-18 Example from Index showing main terms with indented essential modifiers. (From Buck CJ: 2010 ICD-10-CM Draft, Standard Edition, St Louis, 2010, Saunders.)

Key Note:

The coder should *never* code directly from the Index but should locate the code found in the Index in the Tabular List to ensure the diagnosis has been coded to the optimal specificity.

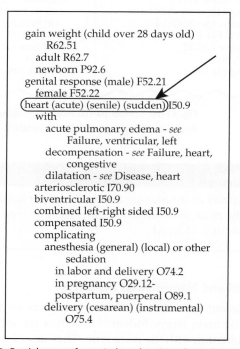

  gain weight (child over 28 days old) R62.51
    adult R62.7
    newborn P92.6
  genital response (male) F52.21
    female F52.22
  heart (acute) (senile) (sudden) I50.9
    with
      acute pulmonary edema - *see* Failure, ventricular, left
      decompensation - *see* Failure, heart, congestive
      dilatation - *see* Disease, heart
    arteriosclerotic I70.90
    biventricular I50.9
    combined left-right sided I50.9
    compensated I50.9
    complicating
      anesthesia (general) (local) or other sedation
      in labor and delivery O74.2
      in pregnancy O29.12-
      postpartum, puerperal O89.1
    delivery (cesarean) (instrumental) O75.4

Fig. 12-19 Partial page from Index showing the subterm "heart" followed by nonessential modifiers (acute, senile, sudden). (From Buck CJ: 2010 ICD-10-CM Draft, Standard Edition, St Louis, 2010, Saunders.)

Conventions Used in Alphabetic Index
Parentheses

Parentheses in the Index have a special meaning. A term that is followed by other terms in parentheses is classified to the given code number whether any of the terms in parentheses are reported in the diagnostic statement or not. For example, Fig. 12-20 shows a partial page where the term "brain abscess" is located in the Index. (Remember, the main term would be "abscess" because "brain" is an anatomical site.) Brain abscess is classified to G06.0 regardless of the part of the organ affected and whether or not the abscess is described as any of the terms in parentheses (e.g., embolic, infective, metastatic, multiple, pyogenic, or septic).

Cross-References (*see* and *see also*)

Some categories, mainly categories subject to notes linking them with other categories, require multiple indexing steps. To avoid repeating multiple steps for each of the additional

terms involved, a cross-reference is used. This cross-reference may take several forms, as in the following examples.

   Example:
  Inflammation
  bone—*see* Osteomyelitis

The term "Inflammation, bone" is to be coded in the same way as the term "Osteomyelitis." Looking up the second term ("bone"), the coder finds various forms of

Abscess (Continued)
abdomen, abdominal
   cavity K65.1
      wall L02.211
abdominopelvic K65.1
accessory sinus - *see* Sinusitis
adrenal (capsule) (gland) E27.8
alveolar K04.7
   with sinus K04.6
ambic A06.4
   brain (and liver or lung abscess)
      A06.6
   genitourinary tract A06.82
   liver (without mention of brain or
      lung abscess) A06.5
   lung (and liver) (without mention of
      brain abscess) A06.5
   specified site NEC A06.89
   spleen A06.89
anerobic A48.0
ankle - *see* Abscess, lower limb
anorectal K61.2
antecubital space - *see* Abscess, upper
      limb
antrum (chronic) (Highmore) - *see*
      Sinusitis, maxillary
anus K61.0
apical (tooth) K04.7
   with sinus (alveolar) K04.6
appendix K35.1
areola (acute) (chronic) (nonpuerperal)
      N61
   puerperal, postpartum or gestational
      - *see* Infection, nipple
arm (any part) - *see* Abscess, upper limb
artery (wall) I77.8
atheromatous I77.2
auricle, ear - *see* Abscess, ear, external
axilla (region) L02.41-
   lymph gland or node L04.2
back (any part, except buttock) L02.212
Bartholin's gland N75.1
   with
      abortion - *see* Abortion, by type
         complicated by, sepsis
      ectopic or molar pregnancy O08.0
      following ectopic or molar pregnancy
         O08.0
Bezold's - *see* Mastoiditis, acute
bilharziasis B65.1
bladder (wall) - *see* Cystitis, specified
      type NEC
bone (subperiosteal) - *see also* Osteomy-
      elitis, specified type NEC
   accessory sinus (chronic) - *see*
      Sinusitis
   chronic or old - *see* Osteomyelitis,
      chronic
   jaw (lower) (upper) M27.2
   mastoid - *see* Mastoiditis, acute,
      subperiosteal
   petrous - *see* Petrositis
   spinal (tuberculous) A18.01
      nontuberculous - *see* Osteomyelitis,
         vertebra
bowel K63.0
brain (any part) (cystic) (otogenic)
      G06.0
   amebic (with abscess of any other
      site) A06.6
   gonococcal A54.82
   pheomycotic (chromomycotic) B43.1
   tuberculous A17.81

Fig. 12-20 Sample partial page from the Index where "abscess, brain" is located. (From Buck CJ: 2010 ICD-10-CM Draft, Standard Edition, St Louis, 2010, Saunders.)

osteomyelitis listed (e.g., acute, acute hematogenous, chronic). When a term has many modifiers that might be listed beneath more than one term, the cross-reference (*see also . . .*) is used.

Example:
Paralysis
shaking (*see also* Parkinsonism)

If the term "shaking paralysis" is the only term noted in the diagnostic statement in the medical record, the code number is G20. If any other information is present that is not found indented below the term, reference should be made to "Parkinsonism," where alternative codes are found for the condition if further or otherwise qualified, such as "due to drugs or syphilitic."

As stated previously, anatomical sites and broad adjective modifiers are typically not used as main terms in the Index. Instead, the coder is instructed to look up the disease or injury reported on the medical record and to find the site or adjectival modifier under that term.

Example:
Abdomen, abdominal—*see also* condition
acute R10.0
angina K55.1
muscle deficiency syndrome Q79.4

The term "acute abdomen" is coded to R10.0, "abdominal angina" is coded to K55.1, and "abdominal muscle deficiency syndrome" is coded to Q79.4. For other abdominal conditions, the coder should look up the disease or injury reported.

What Did You Learn?

1. Name the two parts of the ICD-10-CM coding system.
2. The first character in an ICD-10 code is always a (an) _____.
3. List the five ways main terms are listed in the ICD-10-CM Alphabetic Index.
4. What do parentheses indicate in the Index?
5. Explain the difference between "see" and "see also."

CODING STEPS FOR ALPHABETIC INDEX

Following are coding steps for the Alphabetic Index:
- Locate the diagnostic statement in the patient's medical record.
   Examples:
   Fatigue fracture of vertebra, thoracic region
   Superficial foreign body in the shin
- Identify the main term in the diagnostic statement.
   Examples:
   Fatigue *fracture* of vertebra, thoracic region
   Superficial *foreign* body in the shin
- Locate the main term in the Index. Remember, main terms are listed alphabetically and can be diseases, conditions, adjectives, nouns, or eponyms. Anatomical sites are not considered main terms.

- After locating the main term, note any essential or nonessential modifiers. Remember, nonessential modifiers are terms that immediately follow the main term and are enclosed in parentheses: "Fracture, traumatic (abduction) (adduction) (separation)." Nonessential modifiers do not have to be a part of the listed diagnosis. Essential modifiers are indented under the main term and are also listed alphabetically; they must be included in the diagnostic statement.

  Examples:

  In "Fatigue *fracture* of vertebra, thoracic region," the essential modifiers are the condition and the anatomical site (fatigue, vertebra, and thoracic region).

  In "Superficial *foreign* body in the shin," the essential modifiers are superficial (without open wound) and shin. (*Note:* The coder can assume that unless it is specifically stated in the diagnostic statement that there is an open wound, the diagnosis would be without open wound.)

- Scan the main term entry (or applicable essential modifiers) for any instructional or cross-referencing notes (e.g., *see, see also*).

  Examples:

  In "Fatigue fracture of vertebra, thoracic region," there is an instructional note: "*see also* Fracture, stress vertebra M48.44."

  In "Superficial foreign body in the shin," there is an instructional note: "*see* Foreign body, superficial, leg." When cross-referencing to "foreign body, superficial, leg," we find "leg (lower) S80.85-"

- Select the most appropriate code, and verify the selected code by cross-reference to the Tabular List.

Key Note:

It is essential to use both the Index and the Tabular List when locating and assigning a code. The Index does not always provide the full code. The full code, including laterality and any applicable 7th character, can be selected only from the Tabular list.

❓ What Did You Learn?

Find the main term(s) in the following diagnoses, locate them in the Index, and provide the provisional codes found there.

1. Pressure ulcer of right elbow
2. Diffuse interstitial keratitis
3. Eustachian tube obstruction
4. Gestational diabetes mellitus

TABULAR LIST

The second section of the ICD-10-CM manual is the Tabular List (hereafter referred to as *Tabular*). This section contains a list of codes arranged alphanumerically and divided into chapters based on body system (anatomical site) or condition (etiology). Table 12-6 shows the 21 chapters of the ICD-10-CM Tabular List.

🕐 Stop and Think

1. Patient A has an anxiety disorder. In which chapter would the coder find the appropriate code?
2. Patient B has congenital malformation of the bladder. This applicable code for this diagnosis would be located in Chapter ___.
3. Patient C has been diagnosed with acute nephritic syndrome. Search Chapter ___ for the appropriate code for this condition.

Format and Structure of Codes

The Tabular List in the ICD-10-CM contains categories, subcategories, and codes comprising 3 to 7 characters. The first character is always a letter. Codes with 3 characters are included in ICD-10-CM as the heading of a **category** of codes that may be subdivided further by the use of 4th and 5th digits, which provide greater detail. A 3-character category that has no further subdivision is equivalent to a code (see "P09 Abnormal findings on neonatal screening"). A code is invalid if it has not been coded to the full number of characters required for that code, including the 7th character, if applicable. (See later subsection for more information on the use of the 7th character.) Each level of subdivision after a category is a **subcategory**, which can have 4 or 5 characters. The final level of subdivision is a **code** and can have up to 7 characters. All codes in the Tabular of the official version of the ICD-10-CM are in bold type. Codes that have applicable 7th characters are still referred to as codes, not subcategories. The ICD-10-CM uses an indented format for easy reference (Fig. 12-21).

Key Note:

For reporting purposes, only codes are permissible, not categories or subcategories, and any applicable 7th character is required.

TABLE 12-6	ICD-10 Tabular List
Chapter 1 (A00-B99)	Certain Infectious and Parasitic Diseases
Chapter 2 (C00-D48)	Neoplasms
Chapter 3 (D50-D89)	Diseases of the Blood and Blood-forming Organs and Certain Disorders Involving the Immune Mechanism
Chapter 4 (E00-E90)	Endocrine, Nutritional, and Metabolic Diseases
Chapter 5 (F01-F99)	Mental and Behavioral Disorders
Chapter 6 (G00-G99)	Diseases of the Nervous System
Chapter 7 (H00-H59)	Diseases of the Eye and Adnexa
Chapter 8 (H60-H95)	Diseases of the Ear and Mastoid Process
Chapter 9 (I00-I97)	Diseases of the Circulatory System
Chapter 10 (J00-J99)	Diseases of the Respiratory System
Chapter 11 (K00-K93)	Diseases of the Digestive System
Chapter 12 (L00-L99)	Diseases of the Skin and Subcutaneous Tissue
Chapter 13 (M00-M99)	Diseases of the Musculoskeletal System and Connective Tissue
Chapter 14 (N00-N99)	Diseases of the Genitourinary System
Chapter 15 (O00-O9A.53)	Pregnancy, Childbirth, and the Puerperium
Chapter 16 (P04-P94)	Certain Conditions Originating in the Perinatal Period
Chapter 17 (Q00-Q94)	Congenital Malformations, Deformations, and Chromosomal Abnormalities
Chapter 18 (R00-R99)	Symptoms, Signs, and Abnormal Clinical and Laboratory Findings, Not Elsewhere Classified
Chapter 19 (S00-T98)	Injury, Poisoning, and Certain Other Consequences of External Causes
Chapter 20 (V01-Y97)	External Causes of Morbidity
Chapter 21 (Z00-Z99-)	Factors Influencing Health Status and Contact with Health Services

Placeholder Character

The ICD-10-CM uses the letter "X" as a **placeholder character**. The letter "X" has two uses:

1. As the 5th character for certain 6-character codes. The "X" provides for future expansion without disturbing the 6th character structure.
   Examples:
   • T37.0x1A Poisoning by sulfonamides, accidental (unintentional), initial encounter
   • T56.0x2S Toxic effect of lead and its compounds, intentional self-harm, sequela
   • S03.4xxA Sprain of jaw, initial encounter
2. When a code has fewer than 6 characters and a 7th character extension is required. The "X" is assigned for all characters fewer than 6 to meet the requirement of coding to the highest level of specificity.
   Examples:
   • W85.xxxA Exposure to electric transmission lines, initial encounter
   • S17.0xxA Crushing injury of larynx and trachea, initial encounter
   • S01.02xA Laceration with foreign body of scalp, initial encounter

7th Character

Certain ICD-10-CM categories require an extension to provide further specificity about the condition being coded. The applicable **7th character** is required for all codes within the category or as the notes indicate in the Tabular instructions. This extension may be a number or letter and must always be the 7th character. If a code that requires a 7th character is not 6 characters long, a placeholder "X" must be used to fill in the empty characters (Fig. 12-22).

Examples:
• O65.0XX1 Obstructed labor due to deformed pelvis, fetus 1
• S02.110B Type I occipital condyle fracture, initial encounter for open fracture
• T17.220D Food in pharynx causing asphyxiation, subsequent encounter

Codes that require the use of a 7th character are used only in specific chapters (i.e., Chapters 13, 15, 18, 19, and 20).

Tabular List Conventions

The ICD-10-CM coding manual contains general guidelines and chapter-specific guidelines, which are applicable to all healthcare settings unless otherwise indicated. The **conventions** (rules and guidelines used in coding) and instructions of the classification take precedence over guidelines. ICD-10-CM uses four types of conventions that provide additional assistance to the coder. Before attempting to assign a code to a given diagnosis, the coder should be familiar with the following conventions and what they mean.

• Abbreviations
• Punctuation marks
• Instructional notes
• Symbols

Instructional notes can appear in both the Index and the Tabular and are similar among publishers. However, symbols

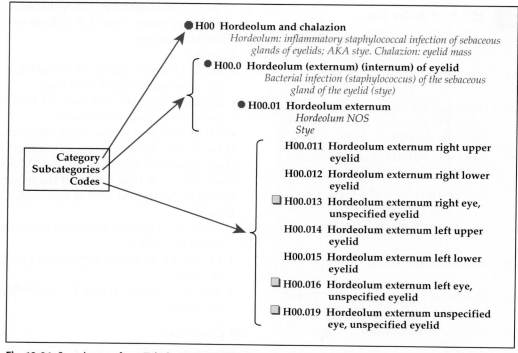

Fig. 12-21 Sample page from Tabular List identifying categories, subcategories, and codes. (From Buck CJ: 2010 ICD-10-CM Draft, Standard Edition, St Louis, 2010, Saunders.)

can differ from one publisher to the next. In *2010 ICD-10-CM Draft* by Buck, the list of symbols and their meanings are illustrated on page ix. Symbols and their meanings are also shown at the bottom of each page in the Tabular (Fig. 12-23).

Abbreviations

NEC ("Not Elsewhere Classifiable")

The abbreviation NEC ("not elsewhere classifiable") in the Index represents "other specified." When a specific code is unavailable for a condition in the Index, the coder is directed to the "other specified" code in the Tabular where an NEC entry under a code identifies it as the "other specified" code.

Example:
G93.49 Other encephalopathy
Encephalopathy NEC

Because all major components of a diagnosis are specified in ICD-10-CM, there is limited need for an NEC code option.

NOS ("Not Otherwise Specified")

The abbreviation **NOS ("not otherwise specified")** is the equivalent of unspecified, meaning that a more specific diagnosis is unavailable. Let's say that the diagnosis written in the patient's health record is simply "meningitis." Before assigning an NOS code, the coder should examine the medical record more closely or question the physician or provider for more complete documentation.

Example:
G03.9 Meningitis
Arachnoiditis (spinal) NOS

Use of NOS is restricted in ICD-10-CM because of the level of specificity that is required.

Punctuation

Brackets

Brackets, [ ], are used in the Tabular to enclose synonyms, alternative wording, or explanatory phrases. Brackets are used in the Index to identify manifestation codes.

Examples:
B06 Rubella [German measles]
J00 Acute nasopharyngitis [common cold]

Parentheses

Parentheses, ( ), are used in both the Index and the Tabular to enclose supplementary words that may be present or absent in the statement of a disease or procedure without affecting the code number to which it is assigned. The terms within the parentheses are nonessential modifiers.

Examples:
H44.611 Retained (old) magnetic foreign body in anterior chamber, right eye
I10 Essential (primary) hypertension
K51.011 Ulcerative (chronic) pancolitis with rectal bleeding

Colons

Colons, :, are used in the Tabular after an incomplete term that needs one or more of the modifiers following the colon to make it assignable to a given category.

Example:
G73.7 Myopathy in diseases classified elsewhere

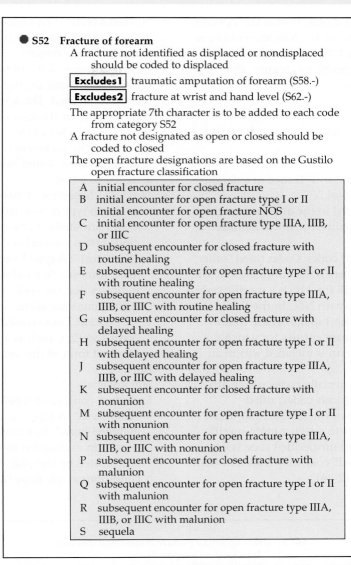

● S52   **Fracture of forearm**

A fracture not identified as displaced or nondisplaced should be coded to displaced

Excludes1 traumatic amputation of forearm (S58.-)

Excludes2 fracture at wrist and hand level (S62.-)

The appropriate 7th character is to be added to each code from category S52

A fracture not designated as open or closed should be coded to closed

The open fracture designations are based on the Gustilo open fracture classification

A   initial encounter for closed fracture
B   initial encounter for open fracture type I or II
     initial encounter for open fracture NOS
C   initial encounter for open fracture type IIIA, IIIB, or IIIC
D   subsequent encounter for closed fracture with routine healing
E   subsequent encounter for open fracture type I or II with routine healing
F   subsequent encounter for open fracture type IIIA, IIIB, or IIIC with routine healing
G   subsequent encounter for closed fracture with delayed healing
H   subsequent encounter for open fracture type I or II with delayed healing
J   subsequent encounter for open fracture type IIIA, IIIB, or IIIC with delayed healing
K   subsequent encounter for closed fracture with nonunion
M   subsequent encounter for open fracture type I or II with nonunion
N   subsequent encounter for open fracture type IIIA, IIIB, or IIIC with nonunion
P   subsequent encounter for closed fracture with malunion
Q   subsequent encounter for open fracture type I or II with malunion
R   subsequent encounter for open fracture type IIIA, IIIB, or IIIC with malunion
S   sequela

Fig. 12-22 Partial page from Tabular List showing S52 under which are listed the 7th characters and their meanings. (From Buck CJ: 2010 ICD-10-CM Draft, Standard Edition, St Louis, 2010, Saunders.)

● Unacceptable first-listed diagnosois   ● Use additional character(s)   ☐ Unspecified   **OGCR** Official Guidelines for Coding and Reporting

🔗 Complication/comorbidity   🔗 Major C/C   Excludes1   Excludes2   Includes   Use additional   Code first   Code also

Fig. 12-23 Bottom of Tabular List page showing symbols used in ICD-10. (From Buck CJ: 2010 ICD-10-CM Draft, Standard Edition, St Louis, 2010, Saunders.)

Excludes1: myopathy in:
rheumatoid arthritis (M05.32)
sarcoidosis (D86.87)
scleroderma (M34.82)
sicca syndrome [Sjögren] (M35.03)
systemic lupus erythematosus (M32.19)

Dashes

Dashes, -, are used in both the Index and the Tabular. A dash is used at the end of a code number to indicate the code is incomplete. To determine the additional character or characters, locate the code in the Tabular, review the options, and assign the appropriate code.

Example:
Fracture, pathologic
ankle M84.47-
carpus M84.44-

Point Dash

In the Tabular, the dash preceded by a decimal point, .-, indicates an incomplete code. To determine the additional character or characters, locate the referenced category or subcategory elsewhere in the Tabular, review the options, and assign the appropriate code. In the following example, the ".-" and the ".0-" after code C84 indicate that the codes are defined to a level of specificity higher than the 3-character and 4-character levels.

Example:

J43 Emphysema

Excludes1: emphysematous (obstructive) bronchitis (J44.-)

Instructional Notes

- Use of "and": When the term "and" is used in a narrative statement, it represents "and/or."
- Use of "with": The word "with" in the Index is sequenced immediately following the main term, not in alphabetical order.
- "Other" and "other specified" codes: Codes titled "other" or "other specified" are used when the information in the medical record provides detail for which a specific code does not exist. Index entries with NEC in the line designate "other" codes in the Tabular. These Index entries represent specific disease entities for which no specific code exists, so the term is included within an "other" code.
- "Unspecified" codes: Codes (usually codes with a 4th digit 9 or 5th digit 0 for diagnosis codes) titled "unspecified" are for use when the information in the medical record is insufficient to assign a more specific code. For categories where an unspecified code is not provided, the "other specified" code may represent both other and unspecified (Fig. 12-24).

- "Includes Notes": This note appears immediately under a 3-digit code title to define further, or give examples of, the content of the category.
- Inclusion terms: A list of terms is included under some codes. These terms are the conditions for which that code is to be used. The terms may be synonyms of the code title, or, in the case of "other specified" codes, the terms are a list of the various conditions assigned to that code. The inclusion terms are not exhaustive. Additional terms found only in the Index may also be assigned to a code.
- "Excludes Notes": ICD-10-CM has two types of excludes notes. Each type of note has a different definition for use, but they are similar in that they indicate that codes excluded from each other are independent of each other.
  - "Excludes1": A type 1 excludes note is a pure excludes note. It means *"not coded here!"* An Excludes1 note indicates that the code excluded should never be used at the same time as the code above the Excludes1 note. An Excludes1 note is used when two conditions cannot occur together, such as a congenital form versus an acquired form of the same condition.

Example:

B06 Rubella

Excludes1 congenital rubella (P35.0)

  - "Excludes2": A type 2 excludes note means "not included here." An Excludes2 note indicates that the condition excluded is not part of the condition represented by the code, but a patient may have both conditions at the same time. When an Excludes2 note

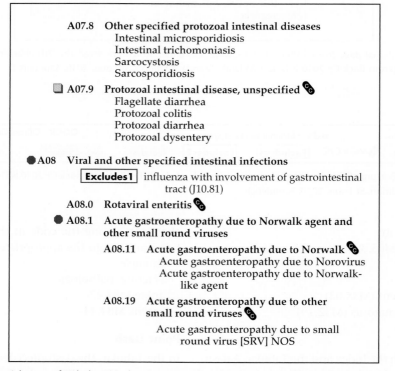

Fig. 12-24 Partial page of Tabular List showing examples of "other specified" and "unspecified" conventions use. (From Buck CJ: 2010 ICD-10-CM Draft, Standard Edition, St Louis, 2010, Saunders.)

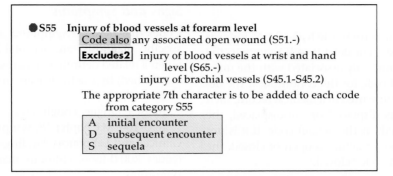

Fig. 12-25 Partial page from Tabular List showing use of "Excludes2" note. (From Buck CJ: 2010 ICD-10-CM Draft, Standard Edition, St Louis, 2010, Saunders.)

appears under a code, it is acceptable to use both the code and the excluded code together, when appropriate (Fig. 12-25).

Example:
J03 Acute tonsillitis
Excludes2 *chronic tonsillitis* (J35.0)

Manifestation Codes

In medicine, a manifestation is a sign or symptom of a disease. The Index in ICD-10-CM includes the suggestion of some manifestation codes by including the code as a second code, shown in brackets, directly after the underlying or etiology code (which should always be reported first).

Example:
Chorioretinitis—*see also* Inflammation, chorioretinal
—Egyptian B76.9 [D63.8]
—histoplasmic B39.9 [H32]

In addition, many common manifestations are included in the etiological condition by the use of combination codes in ICD-10-CM. This element helps the coder in sequencing the cause of a disease versus the signs and symptoms of a disease.

Example:
E10.21 Type 1 diabetes mellitus with diabetic nephropathy

Key Note:

Combination codes are used for both symptom and diagnosis and etiology and manifestations. An example is K50.03 Crohn's disease of small intestine with fistula. Etiology (the cause of a disease or condition) is always coded first with the manifestation code (sign or symptom of a disease) coded second.

Etiology/Manifestation Convention ("Code First," "Use Additional Code," and "In Diseases Classified Elsewhere" Notes)

Certain conditions have both an underlying etiology and multiple body system manifestations secondary to the underlying etiology. For such conditions, ICD-10-CM requires that the underlying condition be sequenced first followed by

the manifestation. Wherever such a combination exists, there is a "use additional code" note at the etiology code and a "code first" note at the manifestation code. These instructional notes indicate the proper sequencing order of the codes—etiology followed by manifestation.

In most cases, the manifestation codes have the words "in diseases classified elsewhere" in the code title. Codes with this title are a component of the etiology/manifestation convention. The code title indicates that it is a manifestation code. "In diseases classified elsewhere" codes are never permitted to be used as first-listed or principal diagnosis codes. They must be used in conjunction with an underlying condition code, and they must be listed following the underlying condition.

An example of the etiology/manifestation convention is *dementia in Parkinson's disease.* In the index, code G20 is listed first, followed by code F02.80 or F02.81 in brackets. Code G20 (Parkinson's disease) represents the underlying etiology and must be sequenced first. Codes F02.80 and F02.81 represent the manifestation of dementia in diseases classified elsewhere, with or without behavioral disturbance.

"Code Also" Note

A "code also" note tells the coder that two codes may be required to describe a condition fully, but this note does not provide sequencing direction.

Morphology Codes

In ICD-10-CM, **morphology** codes are no longer listed in the Alphabetic Index alongside the descriptors and standard codes, and they do not have a separate appendix as in ICD-9-CM. There is a note in the Tabular at the beginning of Chapter 2, Neoplasms, which discusses how morphology codes are dealt with in ICD-10-CM.

Key Note:

In medicine, morphology refers to the size, shape, and structure rather than the function of a given organ. For example, as a diagnostic imaging technique, ultrasound assists in the recognition of abnormal morphologies as symptoms of underlying conditions.

Default Codes

A code listed next to a main term in the ICD-10-CM Index is referred to as a **default code**. The default code represents the condition that is most commonly associated with the main term or is the unspecified code for the condition. If the details of a condition are documented in a medical record, such as whether a condition is displaced or nondisplaced, the coder would use "displaced" as the default code. If it is not documented as to whether a fracture is open or closed, the code would be the default code "closed."

> ### ❓ What Did You Learn?
>
> Previously, you identified the main terms and located them in the Index, providing a provisional code. Now, cross-reference to the Tabular, and assign the correct code for the following diagnoses to the greatest level of specificity:
> 1. Pressure ulcer of right elbow
> 2. Diffuse interstitial keratitis
> 3. Eustachian tube obstruction
> 4. Gestational diabetes mellitus

ICD-10-CM GENERAL CODING GUIDELINES AND CHAPTER-SPECIFIC GUIDELINES

ICD-10-CM guidelines are organized into sections. Section I includes the structure and conventions of the classification and general guidelines that apply to the entire classification. The complete guidelines can be found in Part I of *2010 ICD-10-CM (Draft)* by Buck, and chapter-specific guidelines that correspond to the chapters as they are arranged in the classification are provided. The official guidelines can also be downloaded from the link to the CMS website on the Evolve site.

Section II includes guidelines for selection of principal diagnosis for non-outpatient (inpatient) settings. Section III includes guidelines for reporting additional diagnoses in non-outpatient settings. Section IV is for outpatient coding and reporting.

Some (but not all) of the general coding guidelines are briefly discussed next. For more detailed information, consult the complete guideline section in the front of the coding manual or download the guidelines from the CMS website.

Codes from A00.0 through T88.9, Z00-Z99.89

The appropriate code or codes from A00.0 through T88.9, Z00-Z99.8 must be used to identify diagnoses, symptoms, conditions, problems, complaints, or other reasons for the encounter/visit. The following guidelines are provided to give the coder further direction in selecting the correct diagnostic code.

Signs and Symptoms

Codes that describe symptoms and signs, as opposed to a specific diagnosis, are acceptable for reporting purposes when a related definitive diagnosis has not been established (confirmed) by the healthcare provider.
Examples:
nausea, fatigue, cough, fever, vomiting
ICD-10-CM Chapter 18, Symptoms, Signs, and Abnormal Clinical and Laboratory Findings, Not Elsewhere Classified (codes R00.0-R99), contains many, but not all, codes for symptoms.

Conditions That Are an Integral Part of a Disease Process

Signs and symptoms recorded in the patient health record that are routinely correlated with a specific disease process should not be assigned as additional codes if they are symptoms of the definitive diagnosis, unless otherwise instructed by the classification. For example, symptoms such as cough and fever should not be recorded if the diagnosis is respiratory infection.

Conditions That Are Not an Integral Part of a Disease Process

When additional signs and symptoms exist that may not be associated routinely with a disease process, they should be coded separately when present. For example, if a patient presents with a sprained ankle and complains of chest pain, the chest pain should be coded separately because chest pain is not normally associated with ankle sprains.

Acute and Chronic Conditions

When a condition is described as both acute (subacute) and chronic, and separate subentries exist in the Index at the same indentation level, code both, and sequence the acute (subacute) code first. For example, locate the diagnosis "acute and chronic maxillary sinusitis" in the Index. The code for "acute" (J01.00) is sequenced first, and "chronic" (J32.0) is second.

Combination Codes

ICD-10-CM coding offers new features that provide increased detail and greater specificity, such as combination codes for conditions and common symptoms. A combination code is a single code used to classify two diagnoses or a diagnosis with an associated secondary process (manifestation). Combination codes are identified by referring to subterm entries in the Index and by reading the inclusion and exclusion notes in the Tabular. The combination code is assigned only when that code fully identifies the diagnostic conditions involved or when the Index so directs.

Examples:

I25.110 Arteriosclerotic heart disease of native coronary artery with unstable angina pectoris

K50.013 Crohn's disease of small intestine with fistula

K71.51 Toxic liver disease with chronic active hepatitis with ascites

Multiple coding should not be used when the classification provides a combination code that clearly identifies all of the elements documented in the diagnosis. When the combination code lacks necessary specificity in describing the manifestation or complication, an additional code should be used as a secondary code.

> ### 🕐 Stop and Think
>
> You note that the diagnosis in patient Lonnie Chadwick's medical record is "type 2 diabetes mellitus with mild nonproliferative diabetic retinopathic macular edema." Given that this is a combination of two diagnoses, a level of severity, and a physical manifestation of one of the diagnoses—type 2 diabetes mellitus, nonproliferative diabetic retinopathy, mild, and macular edema—assign the correct code. (*Hint:* All the possible combinations of types of diabetic retinopathy, severity, and presence or absence of macular edema are present under E11.3 Type 2 diabetes mellitus with ophthalmic complications.)

Late Effects (Sequelae)

As mentioned with the ICD-9 system, sequelae (the plural form of sequela) are late effects of injury or illness. As with the ICD-9 system, coding of late effects generally requires two codes with the condition or nature of the late effect sequenced first and the late effect code sequenced second. In ICD-10-CM, these codes appear at the end of each anatomical chapter.

Examples:

H59.032 Cystoid macular edema following cataract surgery (left eye)

K91.0 Vomiting following gastrointestinal surgery (digestive system)

Impending or Threatened Condition

Code any condition described at the time of discharge as "impending" or "threatened" as follows:

- If it did occur, code as confirmed diagnosis.
- If it did not occur, reference the Index to determine if the condition has a subentry term for "impending" or "threatened," and reference main term entries for "impending" and for "threatened."
- If the subterms are listed, assign the given code.
- If the subterms are not listed, code the existing underlying condition and not the condition described as impending or threatened.

Laterality

For bilateral sites, the last character of the 6-character diagnostic code indicates laterality (side of the body affected). An unspecified side code is also provided if laterality is not identified in the medical record. If no bilateral code is provided and the condition is bilateral, assign separate codes for both the left and the right side.

Examples:

C50.212 Malignant neoplasm of upper-inner quadrant of left female breast

H02.835 Dermatochalasis of left lower eyelid

L89.213 Pressure ulcer of right hip, stage III

Laterality codes are used frequently in the neoplasm and injury chapters.

> ### 📁 HIPAA Tip
>
> Version 5010 (the revised set of HIPAA transaction standards, adopted to replace Version 4010/4010A standards) accommodates the ICD-10 code sets and has an earlier compliance date than ICD-10 to ensure adequate testing time for the industry. This rule applies to all HIPAA-covered entities, including health plans, healthcare clearinghouses, and certain healthcare providers.

> ### ❓ What Did You Learn?
>
> 1. If a patient comes to the medical office with complaints of a fever of several days' duration and the cause cannot be determined, in what chapter of the ICD-10-CM would the appropriate code be found?
> 2. Coding of late effects generally requires two codes—the condition, or nature of the late effect, and the late effect itself. How are these two codes sequenced?
> 3. Which character of the diagnostic code indicates laterality?

DIAGNOSTIC CODING AND REPORTING GUIDELINES FOR OUTPATIENT SERVICES

Following is a brief outline of the coding guidelines for outpatient services. More detailed information can be found in the front of the ICD-10-CM manual under Section IV, ICD-10-CM Official Guidelines for Coding and Reporting. Although the conventions and general guidelines apply to all settings, coding guidelines for outpatient and provider reporting of diagnoses vary in many instances from guidelines for inpatient diagnoses. (Inpatient diagnoses are discussed in Chapter 18.) This is in recognition that the Uniform Hospital Discharge Data Set definition of **principal diagnosis** (condition established after study to be chiefly responsible for occasioning the admission of the patient to the hospital for care) applies only to inpatients in acute care, short-term care, long-term care, and psychiatric hospitals. Coding guidelines for inconclusive diagnoses (e.g., probable, suspected, rule out) were developed for inpatient reporting and do not apply to outpatients.

Selection of First-Listed Condition

In the outpatient setting, the term "**first-listed diagnosis**" (reason for the encounter) is now used instead of "principal diagnosis" and takes precedence over the outpatient guidelines. Diagnoses often are not established at the time of the initial encounter/visit. It may take several visits before the diagnosis is confirmed.

> **Key Note:**
>
> The coder should always begin the search for the correct code assignment in the Alphabetic Index. Never begin a search in the Tabular List because this can lead to coding errors, and never code directly from the Index.

Outpatient Surgery

When a patient presents for outpatient surgery (same-day surgery), code the reason for the surgery as the first-listed diagnosis, even if the surgery is not performed owing to a **contraindication** (an issue that makes a certain treatment or procedure inadvisable).

Observation Stay

If a patient is admitted for observation, assign a code for the medical condition as the first-listed diagnosis. When a patient presents for outpatient surgery and develops complications requiring admission to observation, code the reason for the surgery as the first reported diagnosis, followed by codes for the complications as secondary diagnoses.

Codes That Describe Symptoms and Signs

Codes that describe signs and symptoms are acceptable for reporting purposes when a diagnosis has not been confirmed by the provider. See Chapter 18, Symptoms, Signs, and Abnormal Clinical and Laboratory Findings Not Elsewhere Classified (Codes R00-R99) of ICD-10-CM.

Encounters for Circumstances Other than a Disease or Injury

ICD-10-CM provides codes to identify encounters for circumstances other than a disease or injury. Chapter 21, Factors Influencing Health Status and Contact with Health Services (Codes Z00-Z99.89), is provided to deal with occasions when circumstances other than a disease or injury are recorded as the diagnosis or problems.

Level of Detail in Coding

We learned earlier in this chapter how codes were constructed in the ICD-10-CM diagnosis coding process. If necessary, review the subsection entitled ICD-10-CM Code Structure before continuing.

Codes with 3, 4, or 5 Digits

ICD-10-CM is composed of codes with 3 to 7 digits. Codes with 3 digits are listed at the heading of a category of codes and may be subdivided further by the use of 4th, 5th, 6th, or 7th digits that provide greater specificity.

Use of Full Number of Digits

A 3-digit code is to be used only if it is not subdivided further. A code is invalid if it has not been coded to the full number of characters required for that code, including the 7th character extension, if applicable.

Code for Diagnosis, Condition, Problem, or Other Reason for Encounter/Visit

List first the ICD-10-CM code for the diagnosis, condition, problem, or other reason for encounter/visit shown in the medical record to be chiefly responsible for the services provided. List additional codes that describe any coexisting conditions. In some cases, the first-listed diagnosis may be a symptom when a diagnosis has not been confirmed by the healthcare provider.

Uncertain Diagnosis

Do not code diagnoses documented as "probable," "suspected," "questionable," "rule out," "working diagnosis" or other similar terms indicating uncertainty. Instead, code the condition to the highest degree of certainty for that encounter/visit, such as symptoms, signs, abnormal test results, or other reason for the visit.

Chronic Diseases

Chronic diseases treated on a continuing basis may be coded and reported as many times as the patient receives treatment and care for that particular condition.

Code All Documented Conditions That Coexist

Code all documented conditions that coexist at the time of the encounter/visit and require or affect patient care, treatment, or management. Do not code conditions that were previously treated and no longer exist. However, history codes (categories Z80-Z87) may be used as secondary codes if the historical condition or family history has an impact on current care or influences treatment.

Patients Receiving Diagnostic Services Only

For patients receiving diagnostic services only during an encounter/visit, sequence first the diagnosis, condition, problem, or other reason for the encounter/visit shown in the medical record to be chiefly responsible for the outpatient services provided during the encounter/visit. Codes for other diagnoses (e.g., chronic conditions) may be sequenced as additional diagnoses.

Patients Receiving Therapeutic Services Only

For patients receiving therapeutic services only during an encounter/visit, sequence first the diagnosis, condition, problem, or other reason for encounter/visit shown in the medical record to be chiefly responsible for the outpatient services provided during the encounter/visit. Codes for other diagnoses (e.g., chronic conditions) may be sequenced as additional diagnoses. An exception to this rule is when the primary reason for the admission/encounter is chemotherapy or radiation therapy where the appropriate Z code for the service is listed first and the diagnosis or problem for which the service is being performed is listed second.

Patients Receiving Preoperative Evaluations Only

For patients receiving preoperative evaluations only, sequence first a code from subcategory Z01.81-, Encounter for Pre-procedural Examinations, to describe the preoperative consultations. Assign a code for the condition to describe the reason for the surgery as an additional diagnosis. Code also any findings related to the preoperative evaluation.

Ambulatory Surgery

For ambulatory surgery, code the diagnosis for which the surgery was performed. If the postoperative diagnosis is known to be different from the preoperative diagnosis at the time the diagnosis is confirmed, select the postoperative diagnosis for coding because it is the most definitive.

Routine Outpatient Prenatal Visits

See Section I.C.15: Routine Outpatient Prenatal Visits in the guidelines.

Encounters for General Medical Examinations with Abnormal Findings

The subcategories for encounters for general medical examinations, Z00.0-, provide codes for encounters with and without abnormal findings. If a general medical examination results in an abnormal finding, the code for general medical examination with abnormal finding should be assigned as the first listed diagnosis. A secondary code for the abnormal finding should also be assigned.

Encounters for Routine Health Screenings

See Section I.C.21, Factors Influencing Health Status and Contact with Health Services, Screening.

🕐 Stop and Think

1. The diagnostic code found in Arnold Banneker's medical chart is E10.311. To assign this 6-digit code, what would his documented diagnosis have to read?
2. Football star Edwin McGovern has a diagnostic code of S52.012A. What does the "A" signify?
3. Doris Chambers' diagnostic code is C50.512. What is the diagnosis documented in her medical record?
4. Bernice Soledad is diagnosed with "age-related osteoporosis with current pathological fracture of the right shoulder, subsequent encounter for fracture with routine healing." What is the correct code for Beatrice's condition?
5. Ted Francis' record shows a diagnostic code of T43.1x1. What is the purpose of the "x" in this diagnosis code?

❓ What Did You Learn?

1. *True or false:* Coding guidelines for inconclusive diagnoses (e.g., probable, suspected, rule out) were developed for inpatient reporting and do not apply to outpatients.
2. Which chapter in the Tabular provides codes to deal with occasions when circumstances other than a disease or injury are recorded as reason for the encounter?
3. *True or false:* A code is invalid if it has not been coded to the full number of characters required for that code, excluding the 7th character extension, if applicable.
4. When a diagnosis is documented as "probable," "suspected," "questionable," or "rule out," what should be coded for that outpatient encounter/visit?
5. *True or false:* If a general medical examination results in an abnormal finding, the code for the abnormal finding should be assigned as the first-listed diagnosis.

HEALTH INSURANCE PORTABILITY AND ACCOUNTABILITY ACT AND CODING

Code sets for medical data are required for data elements in the administrative and financial healthcare transaction standards adopted under the Health Insurance Portability and Accountability Act (HIPAA) for diagnoses, procedures, and drugs. Under HIPAA, a code set is any set of codes used for encoding data elements such as tables of terms, medical concepts, medical diagnosis codes, or medical procedure codes.

Medical data code sets used in the healthcare industry include coding systems for

- diseases, impairments, other health-related problems, and their manifestations;
- causes of injury, disease, impairment, or other health-related problems;
- actions taken to prevent, diagnose, treat, or manage diseases, injuries, and impairments; and
- any substances, equipment, supplies, or other items used to perform these actions.

📁 HIPAA Tip

Although the HIPAA requirements apply only to electronic claims, to maintain consistency in claims processing, CMS has mandated that ICD-9-CM/ICD-10-CM requirements be applied to paper claims and electronic claims.

Code Sets Adopted as Health Insurance Portability and Accountability Act Standards

As of this writing, the following code sets have been adopted as the standard medical data code sets:

- ICD-9-CM, Volumes 1 and 2 (including *The Official ICD-9-CM Guidelines for Coding and Reporting*), as updated and distributed by HHS
- ICD-9-CM, Volume 3 Procedures (including *The Official ICD-9-CM Guidelines for Coding and Reporting*), as updated and distributed by HHS, for procedures or other actions taken for diseases, injuries, and impairments in hospital inpatients reported by hospitals
- National Drug Codes, as updated and distributed by HHS, in collaboration with drug manufacturers, for certain drugs and biological agents
- Codes on Dental Procedures and Nomenclature, as updated and distributed by the American Dental Association, for dental services
- The combination of CMS *Common Procedure Coding System* (HCPCS), as updated and distributed by HHS, and *Current Procedural Terminology,* Fourth Edition (CPT-4), as updated and distributed by the AMA, for physician services and other health-related services
- The HCPCS, as updated and distributed by CMS and HHS, for all other substances, equipment, supplies, or other items used in healthcare services

Students should be aware of and periodically check on the deadline for the implementation of ICD-10 codes, currently scheduled to go into effect in October 2014, by logging onto the CMS website at http://cms.gov/icd10/.

📁 HIPAA Tip

HIPAA-compliant claims cannot contain ICD-9 Volume 3 procedure codes on claims submitted by physicians' offices.

Implementation of ICD-10

Revisions have been made to the initial version of ICD-10-CM on the basis of the comments received from reviewers. An updated edition of ICD-10-CM became available in late 2003 for public viewing, and implementation was scheduled for 2010. In January 2009, this deadline was extended to October 1, 2013. As of this writing, this deadline was extended again to October 1, 2014. The final rule on the ICD-10-CM and the related ICD-10-PCS for inpatient hospital procedure coding was published in the January 16, 2009, *Federal Register* (link available on the Evolve site).

All billing systems and electronic health records software in use at every U.S. healthcare facility will have to be updated. Medical facilities considering converting to electronic health records should ensure that their systems can accommodate the changeover coming in 2014. Experts suggest that medical offices should begin planning for its implementation in 2012.

To prepare for the upcoming changes in diagnostic coding, the health insurance professional can download and view a version of the ICD-10-CM manual. For more information on this subject, visit the Evolve site.

❓ What Did You Learn?

1. Explain what a "code set" is under HIPAA.
2. List the standard code sets adopted by HIPAA.

IMPORTANCE OF LEARNING BOTH DIAGNOSTIC CODING SYSTEMS

As with the ICD-9-CM, accurate coding requires using the ICD-10-CM Official Guidelines for Coding and Reporting that contain information about the coding conventions. The additional digits in the ICD-10-CM codes offer more detailed and specific documentation. As a result, health insurance payers demand more specificity for claims being submitted for reimbursement.

Generally, because the Alphabetic Index and Tabular List are similar in both systems, the same method can be used to look up codes—locate the main diagnostic term in the Alphabetic Index and verify the code number to the "greatest specificity" in the Tabular List.

It is important that students learn the ICD-10-CM coding system while continuing to use ICD-9-CM because coders will need to access both sets of codes for a period of up to 2 years as the transition is made from one code set to the other. The CMS has developed the General Equivalence Mappings (GEMs), a crosswalk tool for all providers. Designed to serve as a link between the coding sets, the GEMs can help office personnel in converting systems, applications, reports and documents. Specifically, the GEMs can be used to convert databases from ICD-9-CM to ICD-10-CM.

Although the coding systems are similar, ICD-10-CM codes have been updated to reflect modern medicine and detailed medical terminology. Consequently, coding personnel may benefit from obtaining knowledge of advanced anatomy and physiology to have a better understanding of the ICD-10-CM coding system. Coding professionals recommend that health insurance professionals acquire additional training approximately 6 months before the October 1, 2014, compliance date. Remember to keep current by periodically consulting the CMS website for additional updates, or go to the Evolve site to find the link to sign up to receive automatic ICD-10 email updates.

What Did You Learn?

1. Explain why you think it is important for the health insurance professional to learn both the ICD-9 and the ICD-10 coding systems.

SUMMARY CHECKPOINTS

▶ Coding is a recognized process of transforming descriptions of a patient's disease process, disorder, or injury into universal numerical or alphanumerical formats that are understood by all healthcare entities.

▶ Basically, a diagnosis is the reason that brought the patient to the healthcare facility, such as a rash, sore throat, or chest pains. A final diagnosis after examination can be a much more precise statement.

▶ The U.S. healthcare system currently uses three major coding structures.
  • *International Classification of Diseases, 9th Revision, Clinical Modification* (ICD-9-CM) diagnosis codes (Volumes 1 and 2) are used in all clinical settings
  • ICD-9-CM procedure codes (Volume 3) are used in inpatient hospital settings
  • *Current Procedural Terminology, 4th revision* (CPT-4) codes used in physicians' offices and ambulatory payment classifications (APCs) are used by most providers for related services and procedures in the outpatient setting.

▶ The history of the ICD system dates back to the late 19th century in Europe. The first ICD system (ICD-1) was put into use in 1900. Since then, the ICD has been modified approximately once every 10 years with the exception of the 20-year period between the last two revisions—ICD-9 and ICD-10.

▶ Coding of healthcare data allows access to health records according to diagnoses and procedures for use in clinical care, research, and education and has many other common uses.

▶ Two primary concerns with the current ICD-9 system is the lack of specificity of the information expressed in the codes and the fact that it is running out of available code numbers in some chapters. Other issues that are addressed in ICD-10 include the use of full code titles, reflecting advances in medical knowledge and technology

▶ The Centers for Medicare and Medicaid Services (CMS) and the National Center for Health Statistics (NCHS), two departments within the U.S. Department of Health and Human Services (HHS), provide guidelines for coding and reporting using the ICD-9-CM and ICD-10-CM coding systems.

▶ The ICD-9-CM manual comprises three volumes: Volume 1, the Tabular List; Volume 2, the Alphabetic List; and Volume 3, Inpatient Procedural Coding. The first several pages of the manual consist of an introduction, providing a guide for using the ICD-9.

▶ Volume 2, the Alphabetic Index (typically presented before Volume 1, the Tabular List) contains three separate sections (indexes). The first section, the Index to Diseases, contains diagnostic terms for illnesses, injuries, and reasons for encounters with healthcare professionals. Within this section are two tables: the Hypertension Table and the Neoplasm Table. Section 2 contains the Table of Drugs and Chemicals, and Section 3 is the Alphabetic Index to External Causes of Injury and Poisoning.

▶ A diagnosis code in the ICD-9 structure consists of three to five characters, depending on whether a 3-digit, 4-digit, or 5-digit code best represents the patient's diagnosis.

▶ Main terms, printed alphabetically in boldface type in Volume 2, consist of diseases, conditions, nouns, adjectives, and eponyms. (Anatomic sites are not considered main terms in diagnostic coding.)

▶ Modifiers are words added to main terms that supply more specific information about the patient's clinical picture. Essential modifiers, part of a documented diagnosis, are indented under a main term that describes different anatomical sites, etiology, and clinical types. Nonessential modifiers are terms in parentheses immediately following a main term, but usually are not part of the listed diagnosis, that give alternative terminology to assist in locating the correct main term.

▶ ICD-9-CM coding conventions include abbreviations, punctuation, symbols, typefaces, footnotes, and other instructional notes, and each has a significant impact on the process of accurate coding. Conventions help accomplish the "ultimate" goal of diagnostic: To "code to the greatest level of specificity."

▶ Volume 1, (Tabular List) comprises 17 sections plus a section listing V codes (Supplementary Classification of Factors Influencing Health Status and Contact with Health Services) followed by the E codes (Supplementary Classification of External Causes of Injury and Poisoning). Five appendices, A through E, complete Volume 1.

▶ Three types of codes used in the main part of Volume 1: 3-digit codes, 4-digit codes, and 5-digit codes. Codes are organized first by category (3-digit codes), then by subcategory (4-digit codes), and finally by subclassification (5-digit codes). A 3-digit code must not be used if a 4-digit or 5-digit code describes the patient's diagnosis more precisely.

▶ The essential steps in accurate diagnostic coding are as follows:
  • Step 1—locate the diagnosis in the health record (or on the encounter form).
  • Step 2—determine the "main term" of the stated diagnosis.
  • Step 3—find the main term in the Alphabetic Index of the current version of ICD-9-CM.
  • Step 4—read and apply any notes or instructions contained in the Alphabetic Index. *Remember: Never code directly from the Alphabetic Index.*
  • Step 5—cross-reference the code found in the Alphabetic Index to the Tabular List
  • Step 6—read and be guided by conventions/symbols, footnotes, and cross-references.
  • Step 7—read the entire category, and code to the highest level of specificity.

▶ The ICD-10 coding system consists of two parts:
  ▶ ICD-10-CM is used for diagnosis in all healthcare settings.
  ▶ ICD-10-PCS is used for procedure coding in inpatient hospital settings only.

▶ Diagnostic coding under ICD-10-CM uses 3 to 7 digits. The first character is always an alphabetic letter, and all letters of the alphabet are used except the letter "U." (Alphabetic characters are not case sensitive.)

▶ The first step in diagnostic coding is to identify the main term of the diagnostic statement, which can typically be found in the patient's medical record. The coder must locate the main term in the Index. Main terms are listed alphabetically and can be diseases, conditions, adjectives, nouns, or eponyms. Anatomical sites are not considered main terms.

▶ After locating the main term, any essential or nonessential modifiers are noted. Essential modifiers are indented alphabetically under the main term, and they must be included in the diagnostic statement. Nonessential modifiers do not have to be a part of the listed diagnosis.

▶ Scan the main term entry (and applicable essential modifiers) for any instructional or cross-referencing notes (e.g., *see, see also*).

▶ Select the most appropriate code, and verify the selected code by cross-reference to the Tabular List. Never code directly from the Alphabetic Index.

▶ If a code that requires a 7th character is not 6 characters long, a placeholder "X" must be used to fill in empty characters. The 7th character is used only in Chapters 13, 15, 18, 19, and 20.

▶ Before attempting to assign a code to a given diagnosis, the coder should be familiar with instructional notes and conventions used in ICD-10-CM and what they mean.

▶ Codes that describe symptoms and signs, as opposed to a specific diagnosis, are acceptable for reporting purposes when a related definitive diagnosis has not been confirmed by the provider.

▶ For bilateral sites, the final character of the 6-character diagnostic code indicates laterality.

▶ In the outpatient setting, the term "first-listed diagnosis" (reason for the encounter) is used instead of "principal diagnosis" and takes precedence over the outpatient guidelines.

▶ For ambulatory surgery, code the diagnosis for which the surgery was performed.

▶ Always use the most recent ICD-10-CM coding manual.

▶ Code sets for medical data are required data elements in the administrative and financial healthcare transaction standards adopted under HIPAA for diagnoses, procedures, and drugs.

▶ It is important that students learn the ICD-10-CM coding system while continuing to use ICD-9-CM, because coders will need to access both sets of codes for a period of up to 2 years as the transition is made from one code set to the other.

⟳ CLOSING SCENARIO

Park Chalmers found this introductory chapter on ICD-10 coding extremely interesting. Park thought he needed a "structured" approach to learning, and the clear-cut steps to coding enhanced his ability to comprehend the process. After completing the chapter on ICD-10 coding, Park decided that his search for a challenging and meaningful career might be over. With a career in coding, he could realize both of his goals—a challenging career and an opportunity to work in the field of medicine. Although becoming a health insurance professional was not the same as becoming a physician, the anticipation of becoming an expert in insurance and coding spurred Park on, and he already was looking forward to the next chapter.

⊖ WEBSITES TO EXPLORE

For live links to the following websites, please visit the Evolve site at
http://evolve.elsevier.com/Beik/today

For the 2012 ICD-9-CM Official Guidelines for Coding and Reporting, log on to
http://www.findacode.com/pdf.html?id=2012-icd-9-cm-guidelines

For more information about the HIPAA standardized code sets, search
http://cms.hhs.gov and http://aspe.hhs.gov/admnsimp/faqcode.htm#codesetsadopted

The American Association of Medical Assistants (AAMA) website provides information about coding in the medical office and details about various educational workshops pertaining to this subject
http://www.aama-natl.org

For information on becoming a certified professional coder, log on to the American Academy of Professional Coders website at
http://www.aapc.com

The American Health Information Management Association website also provides information on becoming a certified professional coder at
http://www.ahima.org

ICD-9 Internet access for diagnostic coding is available at
http://www.eicd.com/EICDMain.htm

To learn the history and development of ICD, log on to
http://www.who.int/classifications/icd/en/HistoryOfICD.pdf

Extensive information on the ICD-10 system can found on the CMS website by logging on to
http://www.cms.gov/ICD10/11b1_2011_ICD10CM_and_GEMs.asp#TopOfPage

For additional information on ICD-10, follow the World Health Organization web link to
http://www.who.int/classifications/icd/en/

To read an overview of the ICD system, log on to
https://www.cms.gov/ContractorLearningResources/Downloads/ICD-10_Overview_Presentation.pdf

ICD-10 and HIPAA compliance can be viewed at
http://www.vips.com/index_hipaa.cfm?page=hipaa

Find "CMS PowerPoint: Basic Introduction to ICD-CM and ICD-CM-PCS" at
http://www.audiology.org/practice/coding/Documents/ICD-10%20Basic%20Introduction%200310.pdf

Find the PowerPoint presentation "Ten Rules to Follow to Get from ICD-9 to ICD-10" at
http://www.icd10prepared.com/content/PDF/Focus%20Topic_Mapping%20Rules.pdf

For a free ICD-10 download, go to www.cms.gov/icd10

Author's Note: Websites change frequently. If any of these URLs is unavailable, use applicable guide words in your Internet search to acquire additional information on the various subjects listed.

REFERENCES AND RESOURCES

Benefits of ICD-10. Available at http://www.healthcareitnews.com/blog/9-benefits-icd-10.

CMS Code Tables and Index. Available at http://www.cms.gov/ICD10/11b1_2011_ICD10CM_and_GEMs.asp#TopOfPage..

History of the development of the ICD. Available at http://www.who.int/classifications/icd/en/HistoryOfICD.pdf.

ICD-10-CM Book. Available at http://www.icd10codebooks.com/codes/icd10cm.html.

ICD-10-CM: General organization. Available at http://www.losalcodersnetwork.com/10.02.19.pdf.

ICD-10-CM Primer. Available at http://library.ahima.org/xpedio/groups/public/documents/ahima/bok1_038084.hcsp?dDocName=bok1_038084.

ICD-10-CM: 2011 release. Available at http://www.cdc.gov/nchs/icd/icd10cm.htm#10update.

ICD-10 Transition. Available at http://www.ahip.org/content/ShowFileContent.aspx?loadfile=D%3A%5CAHIPUploadedFiles%5CCMSFiles%5CICD10IntroFactSheet2010.04.09.pdf&filename=ICD10IntroFactSheet2010.04.09.pdf&mimetype=application%2Fpdf&doctitle=Fact+Sheet+%E2%80%93+ICD10+Introduction.

CHAPTER 13

Procedural, Evaluation and Management, and HCPCS Coding

Chapter Outline

I. Overview of Current Procedural Terminology (CPT) Coding
   A. Purpose of CPT
   B. Development of CPT
II. Three Levels of Procedural Coding
III. CPT Manual Format
   A. Introduction and Main Sections
   B. Category II Codes
   C. Category III Codes
   D. Appendices A through N
   E. CPT Index
      1. Main Terms
      2. Modifying Terms
      3. Code Layout
   F. Symbols Used in CPT
   G. Modifiers
   H. Unlisted Procedure or Service
   I. Special Reports
IV. Conventions and Punctuation Used in CPT
   A. Importance of the Semicolon
   B. Section, Subsection, Subheading, and Category
   C. Cross-Referencing with *See*
V. Basic Steps of CPT coding
VI. Evaluation and Management (E & M) Coding
   A. Vocabulary Used in E & M Coding
   B. Documentation Requirements
   C. Three Factors to Consider
   D. Key Components
      1. History
      2. Examination

      3. Medical Decision Making
   E. Contributing Factors
   F. Prolonged Services
VII. Subheadings of Main E & M Section
   A. Office or Other Outpatient Services
   B. Hospital Observation Services
   C. Hospital Inpatient Services
   D. Consultations
   E. Emergency Department Services
   F. Critical Care Services
   G. Nursing Facility Services
VIII. E & M Modifiers
IX. Importance of documentation
   A. E & M Documentation Guidelines: 1995 versus 1997
   B. Deciding Which Guidelines to Use
X. Overview of HCFA Common Procedure Coding system (HCPCS)
   A. HCPCS Level II Manual
      1. Index of Main Terms
      2. Table of Drugs
   B. Modifiers
   C. Appendices
XI. National Correct Coding Initiative (NCCI)
XII. Health Insurance Portability and Accountability Act (HIPAA) and HCPCS Coding
   A. Crosswalk
XIII. *Current Procedural Terminology, 5th Edition* (CPT-5)

CHAPTER OBJECTIVES

After completion of this chapter, the student should be able to:
1. Discuss the purpose and development of the CPT-4 manual.
2. Name and describe the three levels of procedural coding.
3. Explain the format of Current Procedural Terminology (CPT).
4. Interpret the conventions and punctuation used in CPT.
5. List the basic steps in CPT coding.

↻ OPENING SCENARIO

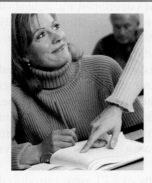

Park Chalmers found that ICD-10-CM coding met his needs for a chance at a challenging career and his desire to work in the medical field. He hoped that he would also find CPT coding to his liking. Melanie Sanders, another student in Park's medical insurance class, had struggled with diagnostic coding, and she confessed to Park that the chapter on CPT intimidated her. "If I don't get this coding stuff," Melanie confided to Park, "I'm going to have to drop the course." Melanie is not interested in becoming a professional coder—her career goal is to work in the clinical side of medical assisting. "I don't know why I have to know this stuff anyway," she tells Park, "I won't have to deal with coding once I've finished the program."

"Being familiar with all facets of administrative work in the medical office, including billing, insurance, and coding, makes you more employable," Park reminded her. "For instance, if you and one other applicant are competing for a job, and you know how to code, but the other applicant doesn't, you'd have the edge. If you stick with it, I'll help you," Park promised.

Park gave Melanie an important tip: "The secret to coding is in its structure. There is a very systematic method for finding the appropriate code," he explained. "The most important thing is to follow the steps outlined in the chapter and never code from the Alphabetic Index alone." Encouraged by Park's positive outlook toward coding and his pledge to help her, Melanie decided to give coding a second chance. With Park's help, she determined that perhaps she could understand CPT coding well enough to pass the course.

6. Outline the important rules and regulations for Evaluation and Management (E & M) coding.
7. Discuss the subheadings of the main E & M section.
8. Explain the use of E & M modifiers.
9. List the general principles of medical record documentation.
10. Provide an overview of the HCFA Common Procedure Coding System (HCPCS).
11. Explain the rationale of the National Correct Coding Initiative (NCCI).
12. Discuss the relationship of the Health Insurance Portability and Accountability Act (HIPAA) and HCPCS
13. Research and review CPT-5.

Physicians' Current Procedural Terminology, 4th Edition (CPT-4)
referral
section
see
special report

stand-alone code
subheading
subjective information
subsection
unit/floor time

CHAPTER TERMS

adjudication
category
Category II codes
Category III codes
code set
concurrent care
consultation
counseling
CPT-5
critical care
crosswalk
emergency care
established patient
Evaluation and
    Management
    (E & M) codes
face-to-face time

HCFA Common Procedure
    Coding System (HCPCS)
HCPCS codes
Health Care Financing
    Administration (HCFA)
indented codes
inpatient
key components
Level I codes
Level II codes
Level III codes
main terms
modifiers
modifying terms
new patient
observation
outpatient

OVERVIEW OF CURRENT PROCEDURAL TERMINOLOGY (CPT) CODING

The ***Physicians' Current Procedural Terminology, 4th Edition*** (CPT-4), is a manual containing a list of descriptive terms and identifying codes used in reporting medical services and procedures performed and supplies used by physicians and other professional healthcare providers in the care and treatment of patients. Current Procedural Terminology (CPT) was first developed and published by the American Medical Association (AMA) in 1966. The CPT system is governed by the CPT editorial panel, a group of individuals (made up mostly of physicians representing various specialties of medicine) who have the authority to make final decisions regarding changes and updates with regard to the content of CPT.

Because medicine is constantly changing, the AMA publishes an updated version of the CPT manual every year. It is important that the health insurance professional use the most recent edition of CPT when coding professional procedures and services for claims submissions to avoid rejected claims or incorrect claim **adjudication** (the process of deciding how an insurance claim is paid).

In 1983, CPT was adopted as part of the **Health Care Financing Administration (HCFA)** Common Procedure Coding System (HCPCS). With this adoption, HCFA (now called the Centers for Medicare and Medicaid Services [CMS]) mandated the use of HCPCS (pronounced "hick picks") to report services for Part B of the Medicare Program. In October 1986, HCFA also required state Medicaid agencies to use HCPCS in the Medicaid Management Information System. In July 1987, as part of the Omnibus Budget Reconciliation Act, HCFA required the use of CPT for reporting outpatient hospital surgical procedures. Today, in addition to use in federal programs (Medicare and Medicaid), CPT is used extensively throughout the United States as the preferred system of coding and describing healthcare services.

In 2000, the CPT **code set** was designed by the U.S. Department of Health and Human Services as the national coding standard for physicians and other healthcare providers to report professional services and procedures under the Health Insurance Portability and Accountability Act (HIPAA). The CPT code set must be used for all financial and administrative healthcare transactions that are transmitted electronically.

Today, not only Medicare and Medicaid but also most managed care and other insurance companies base their reimbursements on the values established by the CMS. As with ICD-10-CM diagnostic coding, it is important that the health insurance professional have a thorough understanding of CPT coding to facilitate accurate claims completion for maximal reimbursement. CPT codes are used instead of a narrative description in claim submission to describe what services or procedures were provided or what supplies were used during the patient encounter.

📁 HIPAA Tip

Under HIPAA, a code set is any set of codes used for encoding data elements, such as tables of terms, medical concepts, medical diagnosis codes, or medical procedure codes. Code sets for medical data are required for data elements in the administrative and financial healthcare transaction standards adopted under HIPAA for diagnoses, procedures, and drugs.

Purpose of CPT

The purpose of CPT coding is to provide a uniform language that accurately describes medical, surgical, and diagnostic services, serving as an effective means for reliable nationwide communication among physicians, insurance carriers, and patients. CPT codes are also used by most third-party payers and government agencies as a record of the activities of an individual healthcare provider.

Development of CPT

As mentioned previously, the AMA developed and published the first CPT in 1966. This first edition contained primarily surgical procedures with limited sections on medicine, radiology, and laboratory procedures.

The second edition was published in 1970 and presented an expanded system of terms and codes to designate diagnostic and therapeutic procedures in surgery, medicine, and other specialties. At that time, the 5-digit coding system was introduced, replacing the former 4-digit classification. Another significant change was a listing of procedures relating to internal medicine.

The third and fourth editions of CPT were introduced later in the 1970s. The fourth edition, published in 1977, presented significant updates in medical technology. Also, a system of periodic updating was introduced to keep pace with the rapidly changing medical environment.

❓💬 What Did You Learn?

1. What is CPT?
2. What is the purpose of CPT?
3. Why were CPT codes developed?
4. Who publishes CPT-4?
5. How often is CPT updated?

THREE LEVELS OF PROCEDURAL CODING

HCFA Common Procedure Coding System (HCPCS) codes are descriptive terms with letters or numbers or both used to report medical services and procedures for reimbursement. As discussed earlier, the codes provide a uniform language to describe medical, surgical, and diagnostic services. **HCPCS codes** are used to report procedures and services to government and private health insurance programs, and reimbursement is based on the codes reported. A code, in place of a narrative description, can summarize the services or supplies provided when billing a third-party payer. HCPCS codes are grouped into three levels, as follows:

Level I codes contain the AMA Physicians' CPT codes. These are 5-digit codes, accompanied by descriptive terms, used for reporting services performed by healthcare professionals. Level I codes are developed and updated annually by the AMA.

Level II codes consist of the HCPCS National Medicare Codes used to report medical services, supplies, drugs, and durable medical equipment not contained in the Level I codes. These codes begin with a single letter, followed by 4 digits. Level II codes supersede Level I codes for similar encounters, Evaluation and Management (E & M) services, or other procedures and represent the portion of procedures involving supplies and materials. National Level II Medicare Codes are not restricted to Medicare as their title may suggest. An increasing number of private insurance carriers are encouraging—and some are even requiring—the use of HCPCS National Codes. HCPCS Level II codes are in a separate manual from Level I codes (CPT). Level II codes are developed and updated annually by the CMS and their contractors.

Level III codes were developed by Medicaid state agencies, Medicare contractors, and private insurers for use on a local level to identify services for which there was no Level I or Level II code to avoid use of a "miscellaneous or not otherwise classified" code. Medicare referred to Level III codes as "local" codes. In August 2000, HIPAA directed CMS to adopt uniform standards for coding systems to be used for reporting all healthcare transactions, eliminating Level III local codes. The elimination of local codes was postponed, however, until December 31, 2003, after which only Level I and II codes could be used.

🗀 HIPAA Tip

The combination of HCPCS and CPT-4 (including codes and modifiers) is the HIPAA-adopted standard for reporting physician services and other healthcare services on standard transactions.

💬 What Did You Learn?

1. What are HCPCS codes?
2. List the three levels of HCPCS codes.

CPT MANUAL FORMAT

Introduction and Main Sections

Similar to the ICD-10-CM manual, CPT-4 is made up of several sections beginning with an introduction, identified by lowercase Roman numerals. The main body of the manual follows the introduction and is organized in six sections. Within each section are subsections with anatomical, procedural, condition, or descriptor subheadings. Table 13-1 lists the CPT sections and their number range sequence. The listed procedures and services and their identifying 5-digit codes are presented in numerical order except for the E & M section. Because E & M codes are used by most physicians for reporting key categories of their services, this section is presented first.

Five-digit CPT codes may be defined further by modifiers to help explain an unusual circumstance associated with a service or procedure. Appropriate coding modifiers are crucial to getting claims paid promptly and for the correct amount. Missing or incorrect modifiers are among the most common reasons that claims are denied by payers. It is easy to get confused on how to use modifiers correctly, especially because, similar to CPT codes, they are constantly changing. The most important thing to remember when using modifiers

TABLE 13-1	CPT Section Numbers and Their Sequence
SECTION TITLE	**NUMBERING SEQUENCE**
Evaluation and Management	99201-99499
Anesthesiology	00100-01999, 99100-99140
Surgery	10021-69990
Radiology (including Nuclear Medicine and Diagnostic Ultrasound)	70010-79999
Pathology and Laboratory	80047-89398
Medicine (except Anesthesiology)	90281-99199, 99500-99607

Modifier-22 is used to indicate that there was "something unusual about the procedure, it took longer than usual, or it was harder than usual. The only way you'll get consideration for additional payment is if you use the modifier and have good documentation."

Modifier-59 is used to indicate that a procedure or service was distinct or independent from other services performed on the same day (e.g., not normally reported together) but are appropriate under the circumstances, as documented.

Fig. 13-1 Examples of correct modifier use.

is that the health record must contain adequate documentation to support the modifier (Fig. 13-1). Modifiers are discussed in more detail on page 278.

When coding procedures, it is important always to have the most recent edition of the CPT book available to look up current modifier codes. (Modifiers are listed in Appendix A at the back of the CPT manual.) Also, it is advisable for healthcare providers and their billing staff to read Medicare (and other) coding newsletters and attend coding workshops periodically to keep up to date.

Each main section of the CPT is preceded by guidelines specific to that section. These guidelines define terms that are necessary to interpret correctly and report the procedures and services contained in that section. The health insurance professional should read and study these guidelines before attempting to assign a code.

Category II Codes

Category II codes are supplemental tracking codes, intended to be used for performance measurement. Category II codes provide a method for reporting performance measures. They are intended to facilitate the collection of information about the quality of care delivered by coding numerous services or test results that support performance measures that have been agreed on as contributing to good patient care. Category II codes are alphanumeric, consisting of 4 digits followed by the letter "F" (e.g., 0503 F—Postpartum care visit [Prenatal]). The use of Category II codes is optional, and they should not to be used as a substitute for Category I codes. Category II codes follow the six sections listed in the main body of the CPT manual.

Category III Codes

Immediately following the Category II codes are the **Category III codes** (Fig. 13-2). Category III codes were established by the AMA as a set of temporary CPT codes for emerging technologies, services, and procedures for which data collection is necessary to substantiate widespread use or for the approval process of the U.S. Food and Drug Administration (FDA). To be eligible for a Category III code, the procedure or service must be involved in ongoing or planned research. If a Category III code has not been proposed and accepted into the main body of CPT (i.e., Category I codes) within 5 years, it is archived, unless a demonstrated need for it develops.

In the introduction of the CPT manual, users are instructed not to select a code that merely approximates the service provided. The code should identify the service performed accurately. In some instances, Category III codes may replace temporary local codes (HCPCS Level III) assigned by carriers and intermediaries to describe new procedures or services. If a Category III code is available, it must be used instead of an *unlisted* Category I code. The use of the unlisted code does not offer the opportunity for collection of specific data. Category III codes are updated semiannually in January and July, and new codes are posted on the AMA website.

Appendices A through N

As with ICD-10-CM, CPT-4 contains several appendices, which follow the Category III codes. These appendices and their contents are as follows:

Appendix A—Modifiers
Appendix B—Summary of Additions, Deletions, and Revisions
Appendix C—Clinical Examples
Appendix D—Summary of CPT Add-On Codes
Appendix E—Summary of CPT Codes Exempt from Modifier -51
Appendix F—Summary of CPT Codes Exempt from Modifier -63
Appendix G—Summary of CPS Codes That Include Moderate (Conscious) Sedation
Appendix H—Alphabetic Index of Performance Measure by Clinical Condition by Topic
Appendix I—Genetic Testing Code Modifiers
Appendix J—Electrodiagnostic Medicine Listing of Sensory, Motor, and Mixed Nerves
Appendix K—Products Pending FDA Approval
Appendix L—Vascular Families
Appendix M—Summary of Crosswalked Deleted CPT Codes
Appendix N—Summary of Resequenced CPT Codes

0072T	total leiomyomata volume greater or equal to 200 cc of tissue
	Sunset January 2015
	➔ *CPT Assistant* Mar 05:1, 5, Dec 05:3; *CPT Changes: An Insider's View* 2005
	(Do not report 0071T, 0072T in conjunction with 51702 or 77022)
0073T	Compensator-based beam modulation treatment delivery of inverse planned treatment using 3 or more high resolution (milled or cast) compensator convergent beam modulated fields, per treatment session
	Sunset January 2015
	➔ *CPT Assistant* Mar 05:1, 6, May 05:7, Nov 09:3; *CPT Changes: An Insider's View* 2005
	(For treatment planning, use 77301)
	(Do not report 0073T in conjunction with 77401-77416, 77418)
0075T	Transcatheter placement of extracranial vertebral or intrathoracic carotid artery stent(s), including radiologic supervision and interpretation, percutaneous; initial vessel
	Sunset January 2015
	➔ *CPT Assistant* May 05:7; *CPT Changes: An Insider's View* 2005

Fig. 13-2 Example of Category III codes. (From American Medical Association: CPT 2011, Standard Edition. Chicago, 2010, American Medical Association.)

CPT Index

Main Terms

In the CPT manual, the index is presented last. As with ICD-10-CM, the CPT index is organized by **main terms** (Fig. 13-3). Each main term can stand alone, or it can be followed by up to three modifying terms. There are four primary classes of main term entries, as follows:

1. Procedure or service (e.g., colonoscopy, anastomosis, debridement)
2. Organ or other anatomical site (e.g., fibula, kidney, nails)
3. Condition (e.g., infection, pregnancy, tetralogy of Fallot)
4. Synonyms, eponyms, and abbreviations (e.g., ECS, Pean operation, Clagett procedure)

🕐 Stop and Think

Surgeon Milford Tramen saw Patrick Lovell, a 34-year-old Illinois farmer, in his office on February 19 for the repair of an injury to the patient's mouth. The presenting problem in the medical record documents that the patient was "kicked in the mouth while vaccinating hogs." The surgeon stitched up the 3.4-cm cut, and the nurse administered a tetanus shot. What would be the main term for the procedure performed by the surgeon?

Modifying Terms

As mentioned previously, each main term can stand alone or be followed by up to three **modifying terms** (Fig. 13-4). Modifying terms are indented under the main term; in some cases, unindented anatomical sites are listed alphabetically first, and modifying terms are indented under them.

```
Colonna Procedure
  See Acetabulum, Reconstruction

Colonography
CT Scan . . . . . . . . . . . . . . . . . . . . . . . . . . . .
    Diagnostic . . . . . . . . . . . . . . . .74261-74262
    Screening . . . . . . . . . . . . . . . . . . . . . .74263

Colonoscopy
Biopsy . . . . . . . . . . . . . . . . . . . . . .45380, 45392
Collection Specimen . . . . . . . . . . . . . . . .45380
    via Colotomy . . . . . . . . . . . . . . . . . . .45355
Destruction
    Lesion . . . . . . . . . . . . . . . . . . . . . . . . .45383
    Tumor . . . . . . . . . . . . . . . . . . . . . . . . .45383
Dilation . . . . . . . . . . . . . . . . . . . . . . . . . .45386
Hemorrhage Control . . . . . . . . . . . . . . . .45382
Injection
    Submucosal . . . . . . . . . . . . . . . . . . . .45381
```

Fig. 13-3 Example of main terms. (From American Medical Association: CPT 2011, Standard Edition. Chicago, 2010, American Medical Association.)

```
Denervation
Hip
    Femoral . . . . . . . . . . . . . . . . . . . . . .27035
    Obturator . . . . . . . . . . . . . . . . . . . . .27035
    Sciatic . . . . . . . . . . . . . . . . . . . . . . . .27035

Denervation, Sympathetic
  See Excision, Nerve, Sympathetic

Denis-Browne Splint . . . . . . . . . . . . .29590

Dens Axis
  See Odontoid Process

Denver Developmental
Screening Test . . . . . . . . . . . . .96101-96103

Denver Krupic Procedure
  See Aqueous Shunt, to Extraocular Reservoir

Denver Shunt
Patency Test . . . . . . . . . . . . . . . . . . . . . .78291

Denver-Krupin Procedure . . . . . . .66180

Deoxycorticosterone
  See Desoxycorticosterone

Deoxycortisol . . . . . . . . . . . . . .80436, 82634

Deoxyephedrine
  See Methamphetamine

Deoxyribonuclease
Antibody . . . . . . . . . . . . . . . . . . . . . . . . .86215

Deoxyribonuclease I
  See DNAse

Deoxyribonucleic Acid
Antibody . . . . . . . . . . . . . . . . . . .86225-86226
Extraction . . . . . . . . . . . . . . . . . .83890-83891

Depilation
  See Removal, Hair

Depletion
Plasma . . . . . . . . . . . . . . . . . . . . . . . . . .38214
Platelet . . . . . . . . . . . . . . . . . . . . . . . . .38213
T-Cell . . . . . . . . . . . . . . . . . . . . . . . . . . .38210
Tumor Cell . . . . . . . . . . . . . . . . . . . . . . .38211
```

Fig. 13-4 Example of main term with modifying terms. (From American Medical Association: CPT 2011, Standard Edition. Chicago, 2010, American Medical Association.)

For example, in Fig. 13-4, "Hip" is listed under the main term "Denervation" (in **bold**), after which three indented modifying terms are listed. All modifying terms should be examined closely, because these subterms often have an effect on the selection of the appropriate procedural code.

Code Layout

A CPT code can be displayed in one of the following three ways:

1. Single code (Proetz therapy, nose 30210)
2. Multiple codes (prolactin 80418, 80440, 84146)
3. Range of codes (prostatotomy 55720-55725)

Symbols Used in CPT

The CPT manual uses several symbols that help guide the health insurance professional in locating the correct code. Accurate procedural coding cannot be accomplished without understanding the meaning of each of these symbols (Table 13-2). These symbols are listed on the inside front cover of the CPT manual.

TABLE 13-2	Symbols Used in CPT Manual
SYMBOL	**EXPLANATION**
Bullet (●)	A bullet (●) before a code means the code is new to the CPT book for that particular edition
Triangle (▲)	A triangle (▲) means the description for the code has been changed or modified since the previous revision of the CPT book
Horizontal triangles (►◄)	Horizontal triangles (►◄) placed at the beginning and end of a descriptive entry indicate that it contains new or revised wording
Plus sign (+)	Add-on codes are annotated by a plus sign (+)
⊘	This symbol is used to identify codes that are exempt from the use of modifier -51
➲	Reference to *CPT Assistant, Clinical Examples in Radiology and CPT Changes* book
⚡	The lightning bolt indicates codes for vaccines that are pending FDA approval
⊙	This symbol is used to identify codes that include conscious (moderate) sedation
○	The open circle symbol indicates a reinstated or recycled code
#	The pound sign (#) indicates an out-of-numerical sequence code

Modifiers

Modifiers are important to ensuring appropriate and timely payment. A health insurance professional who understands when and how to use modifiers reduces the problems caused by denials and expedites processing of claims.

A modifier provides the means by which the reporting healthcare provider can indicate that a service or procedure performed has been altered by some specific circumstance, but its definition or code has not been changed. The judicious application of modifiers tells the third-party payer that this case is unique. By using appropriate modifiers, the office may be paid for services that are ordinarily denied. In addition, modifiers can describe a situation that, without the modifier, could be considered inappropriate coding.

Modifiers are not universal; they cannot be used with all CPT codes. Some modifiers may be used only with E & M codes (e.g., modifier -24 or modifier -25), and others are used only with procedure codes (e.g., modifier -58 or modifier -79). Check the guidelines at the beginning of each section for a listing or description of the modifiers that may be used with the codes in that section. Appendix A of the CPT manual contains a list of modifiers and their use.

HIPAA Tip

HIPAA does not mandate the use of modifiers. According to the adopted HIPAA implementation guide, use of modifiers is not required. Their usage is "situational," meaning that the use of a modifier is required only when a modifier clarifies or improves the reporting accuracy of the associated procedure code.

Unlisted Procedure or Service

Coders must understand the appropriate use of unlisted CPT codes. Unlisted codes are used for services that may be performed by physicians or other healthcare professionals that are not represented by a specific Category I (CPT) code. At the end of each subsection or subheading in question, a code is provided under the heading "other procedures," which typically ends in "-99." In the surgery section, note the "other procedures" code 39499 at the end of the "mediastinum" subsection. This code would be used for any unlisted procedures of the mediastinum.

Important note: Unlisted procedure codes should be assigned only if no other, more specific CPT code is available. If there is a Category III code that appropriately describes the procedure, it should be used instead of an unlisted code.

Special Reports

When a rarely used, unusual, variable, or new service or procedure is performed, many third-party payers require a **special report** to accompany the claim to help determine the appropriateness and medical necessity of the service or procedure. Items that should be addressed in the report, if applicable, include

- a definition or description of the service or procedure;
- the time, effort, and equipment needed;
- symptoms and final diagnosis;
- pertinent physical findings and size;
- diagnostic and therapeutic services;
- concurrent problems; and
- follow-up care.

What Did You Learn?

1. List the six main sections of CPT.
2. What is the purpose of the guidelines that appear at the beginning of each main section of CPT?
3. What are Category III codes?
4. Name the first five appendices in the CPT manual and what is contained in each.
5. What are the four primary classes of main term entries?
6. What is the function of a modifier?

CONVENTIONS AND PUNCTUATION USED IN CPT

There are two types of CPT codes: stand-alone and indented. The terminology of a **stand-alone code** is complete in and of itself. It contains the full description of the procedure without additional explanation. However, some procedures do not contain the entire written description. These are known as **indented codes**. Indented codes refer to the common portion of the procedure listed in the preceding entry, and correct code selection requires careful attention to the punctuation in the description.

Importance of the Semicolon

In the CPT, the semicolon is used to separate main and subordinate clauses in the code descriptions. This method was adopted to save space in the manual where a series of related codes are found. CPT code "38100 splenectomy; total (separate procedure)" is a stand-alone code. The code immediately following it, 38101, is indented and reads "partial (separate procedure)." The semicolon after splenectomy in code 38100 becomes part of the indented code 38101. The full description of code 38101 in effect would read "splenectomy; partial (separate procedure)." See Fig. 13-5 for an example of a stand-alone code followed by an indented code used in the previously mentioned example.

Section, Subsection, Subheading, and Category

Codes in the tabular section of CPT are formatted using four classifications: section, subsection, subheading, and category. Locate the code "51020" in the Tabular list. At the top left (page 272, 2011 edition), note the code range on that particular page (50972 through 51610), followed by the words "Surgery/Urinary System." "Surgery" is the **section**,

Hemic and Lymphatic Systems

Spleen

Excision

38100	Splenectomy; total (separate procedure) ➲ *CPT Assistant* Jul 93:9, Summer 93:10
38101	partial (separate procedure) ➲ *CPT Assistant* Summer 93:10
+ 38102	total, en bloc for extensive disease, in conjunction with other procedure (List in addition to code for primary procedure) ➲ *CPT Assistant* Summer 93:10

Fig. 13-5 Example of a stand-alone code followed by an indented code. Note the use of the semicolon, as described in the text above. (From American Medical Association: CPT 2011, Standard Edition. Chicago, 2010, American Medical Association.)

and "Urinary System" is the **subsection**. Just below, in large (red), bold font, note the word "Bladder." This is the **subheading**. Immediately under "bladder" is the word "incision," which indicates the **category** (Fig. 13-6).

Cross-Referencing with *See*

When searching for the correct main term, the word *see* is frequently encountered. *See* is used as a cross-reference term in the CPT Alphabetic Index and directs the coder to an alternative main term (Fig. 13-7).

🗨 What Did You Learn?

1. Explain the significance of the semicolon in CPT coding.
2. How is a stand-alone code different from an indented code?
3. What does the cross-referencing term *see* indicate?

BASIC STEPS OF CPT CODING

CPT coding is a structured process, and it is important for the health insurance professional to follow a few basic steps so that the correct code is identified and assigned.

1. *Identify the procedure, service, or supply to be coded.* These are typically found on the encounter form, in the patient record, in the data in the computerized accounting software, or on the ledger card. A procedure example is "excision of cervical stump, vaginal approach with anterior repair."

2. *Determine the main term.* The index is located at the back of the CPT manual. Main terms are in boldface type and are listed alphabetically with headings located in the top right and left corners, similar to a dictionary (Fig. 13-8). For the purpose of review, main terms are organized by four primary classes of main entries: a procedure or service; an organ or other anatomical site; a condition; or a synonym, eponym, or abbreviation. Subterms (if applicable) are indented under main terms. In this example, the main term is "excision."

3. *Locate the main term in the Alphabetic Index, and note the code or codes.* For example, if the procedure is "excision of cervical stump, vaginal approach with anterior repair," the coder first would locate "excision" in the Alphabetic Index. Under the main term "Excision" (in bold), locate the anatomical site "cervix" listed alphabetically, paying attention to the indented modifying terms. Adjacent to "vaginal approach," note the code range of 57550-57556. *Reminder! Do not select the final code from the Alphabetic Index alone.*

4. *Cross-reference the single code, multiple codes, or code range numerically in the tabular section of the manual.* In the tabular list, code 57550 lists the main terminology of this procedure, and the indented code (after the semicolon) "with anterior and/or posterior repair" becomes an

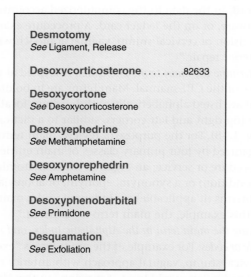

		Section	Subsection
50972—51610		Surgery /	Urinary System

50972   with ureteral catheterization, with or without dilation of ureter
→ *CPT Assistant* Oct 01:8

50974   wtih biopsy
→ *CPT Assistant* Oct 01:8

50976   with fulguration and/or incision, with or without biopsy
→ *CPT Assistant* Oct 01:8

50980   with removal of foreign body or calculus
→ *CPT Assistant* Oct 01:8

Subheading —[**Bladder**

Category —[**Incision**

51020   Cystotomy or cystostomy; with fulguration and/or insertion of radioactive material

51030   with cryosurgical destruction of intravesical lesion

51040   Cystostomy, cystotomy with drainage

51045   Cystotomy, with insertion of ureteral catheter or stent (separate procedure)

Fig. 13-6 Section of Tab List illustrating section, subsection, subheading, and category. (From American Medical Association: CPT 2011, Standard Edition. Chicago, 2010, American Medical Association.)

Desmotomy
See Ligament, Release

Desoxycorticosterone 82633

Desoxycortone
See Desoxycorticosterone

Desoxyephedrine
See Methamphetamine

Desoxynorephedrin
See Amphetamine

Desoxyphenobarbital
See Primidone

Desquamation
See Exfoliation

Fig. 13-7 Example of *see* used as a cross-reference. (From American Medical Association: CPT 2011, Standard Edition. Chicago, 2010, American Medical Association.)

integral part of the complete procedural description and must be included. (Refer to the subheading "Importance of the Semicolon.")

5. *Read and follow any notes, special instructions, or conventions associated with the code.*

6. *Determine and assign the appropriate code.* In this procedure example, the correct code would be 57555.

Before assigning an indented code, refer to the stand-alone code above it. Read the words that *precede* the semicolon, ensuring that the combined description (the portion of the stand-alone code *up* to the semicolon *plus* the wording included in the indented description) corresponds to the documented procedure or service.

What Did You Learn?

1. What is the first step in CPT coding?
2. What factors should be considered before assigning an indented code?

Arm, Upper	Artery, Coronary

Fig. 13-8 Example of header words at top of page in CPT manual. (From American Medical Association: CPT 2011, Standard Edition. Chicago, 2010, American Medical Association.)

EVALUATION AND MANAGEMENT (E & M) CODING

The **Evaluation and Management (E & M) codes** (99201 through 99499) are found at the beginning of the CPT manual. E & M codes deal with *what the healthcare provider does* during the time spent with the patient, rather than merely with the amount of time spent. The E & M section of the CPT is divided into broad categories, including office visits, hospital visits, and consultations. Most of the categories are divided further. There are two subcategories of office visits (new versus established patients) and two categories of hospital visits (initial versus subsequent visits).

The subcategories list codes that describe differing levels of service provided, ranging from low levels of service to higher and more intense levels of service. Initially, these codes were based on highly subjective factors that were applied inconsistently among carriers. In 1992, new, uniform national criteria were established to determine the appropriate level code to be used. Under these criteria, every visit regardless of location must include at least two of the following three components—history, examination, and medical decision making—depending on the category of service.

E & M codes represent the services provided directly to the patient during an encounter that do not involve an actual procedure. If a patient has an appointment in the office, only the office visit receives an E & M code. If any procedures are done (e.g., a urinalysis or an electrocardiogram), those procedures receive a CPT code. E & M codes are designed to classify services provided by a healthcare provider and are used primarily in outpatient settings. E & M codes are technically CPT codes (Level I HCPCS); however, they are referred to as E & M instead of CPT to distinguish between E & M services and procedural coding (Fig. 13-9). The level of service code selected for an office visit is given a numerical level (1 to 5). The code level assigned depends on the complexity of the history, examination, and medical decision making and usually is not affected by the time the provider spends with the patient. The range of codes for office or other outpatient services is 99201 to 99205 for new patients and 99211 to 99215 for established patients. A specific distinction between new and established patients is associated with E & M coding. The exact definitions are discussed in the next section.

Vocabulary Used in E & M Coding

To understand E & M coding more fully, the coder must become acquainted with several terms, as follows:

- **New patient**—an individual who has not received any professional services from the physician or another physician of the same specialty who belongs to the same group practice regardless of location of service *within the past 3 years.* (See the "Decision Tree for New vs. Established Patients" flow chart in the CPT-4 manual.)
- **Established patient**—an individual who has been treated previously by the healthcare provider (or one in the same group practice and of the same specialty), regardless of

location of service, within the past 3 years. If the provider saw the patient for the first time in a hospital, and that individual comes to the office for a follow-up visit after discharge, the individual is considered an established patient to the practice because health record documentation was generated from the hospital visit.

- **Outpatient**—a patient who *has not* been officially admitted to a hospital but receives diagnostic tests or treatment in that facility or a clinic connected with it.
- **Inpatient**—a patient who *has* been formally admitted to a hospital for diagnostic tests, medical care and treatment, or a surgical procedure, typically staying overnight.
- **Consultation**—when the attending healthcare provider recommends that the patient see another physician (often a specialist) for a problem usually associated with one major body system. A family practitioner may advise a patient who presents with a suspicious mole to see a dermatologist.

Note: Do not confuse a consultation with a referral. A consultation is usually a one-time visit; the attending physician (or provider) retains control of the patient's healthcare, and the consultation ends when the consulting provider renders his or her opinion. With a **referral**, the original provider relinquishes total care of the patient to the provider to whom the patient has been referred.

- **Counseling**—a discussion with the patient or the patient's family or both. Counseling typically includes one or more of the following:
  - Discussing diagnostic test results, impressions, or recommended studies
  - Discussing prognosis
  - Explaining the risks or benefits of recommended treatment or instruction for management of care
  - Performing patient or family teaching
- **Concurrent care**—when a patient receives similar services (e.g., hospital visits) by more than one healthcare provider on the same day.
- **Critical care**—the constant attention (either at bedside or immediately available) by a physician in a medical crisis.
- **Emergency care**—care given in a hospital emergency department.

Stop and Think

Tom Galliger was in the Air Force for 4 years. During that time, he did not see Dr. Boker, his physician in his hometown of Gaithersville. Dr. Boker's office policy is to place any inactive files on microfilm after 2 years of inactivity. After Tom finished his tour of duty, he returned home to Gaithersville. Soon after returning home, he sprained his ankle hiking in the mountains and subsequently scheduled an appointment with Dr. Boker. Would Tom be considered a new or established patient?

Evaluation and Management

Office or Other Outpatient Services

The following codes are used to report evaluation and management services provided in the physician's office or in an outpatient or other ambulatory facility. A patient is considered an outpatient until inpatient admission to a health care facility occurs.

To report services provided to a patient who is admitted to a hospital or nursing facility in the course of an encounter in the office or other ambulatory facility, see the notes for initial hospital inpatient care (page 14) or initial nursing facility care (page 24).

For services provided by physicians in the emergency department, see 99281-99285.

For observation care, see 99217-99220.

For observation or inpatient care services (including admission and discharge services), see 99234-99236.

——————— *Coding Tip* ———————

Determination of Patient Status as New or Established Patient

Solely for the purposes of distinguishing between new and established patients, **professional services** are those face-to-face services rendered by a physician and reported by a specific CPT code(s). A new patient is one who has not received any professional services from the physician or another physician of the same specialty who belongs to the same group practice, within the past three years.
An established patient is one who has received professional services from the physician or another physician of the same specialty who belongs to the same group practice, within the past three years.

In the instance where a physician is on call for or covering for another physician, the patient's encounter will be classified as it would have been by the physician who is not available.

CPT Coding Guidelines, Evaluation and Management, Definitions of Commonly Used Term, New and Established Patient

New Patient

99201   **Office or other outpatient visit** for the evaluation and management of a new patient, which requires these 3 key components:

- A problem focused history;
- A problem focused examination;
- Straightforward medical decision making.

Fig. 13-9 Portion from E & M coding section. (From American Medical Association: CPT 2011, Standard Edition. Chicago, 2010, American Medical Association.)

Documentation Requirements

Because the level of the E & M codes is based on the complexity of the history, examination, or medical decision making performed during the visit, the key to reimbursement is being able to prove the level of complexity of the performed services. The only valid source of proof is the documentation in the patient's medical record.

Coding E & M services should be based on the extent of documentation in the patient's medical record (Fig. 13-10). The criteria for E & M services must be well understood by the treating provider and documented in the record. Each record needs to show elements of the history, such as the chief complaint (CC); history of present illness (HPI), including location, severity, frequency, and duration; the review of systems (ROS); and past, family, and social history (PFSH). The physical examination should list all systems or organs examined. Medical decision making should discuss the number of options or diagnoses considered in the decision, the amount of data or complexity of data reviewed, and the risk to the patient of the decision made.

⭐ Imagine This!

Vancil Allen, a 73-year-old white man, was admitted to the hospital with chest pain and shortness of breath after a minor automobile accident. His cardiologist, Dr. Walters, was the admitting physician. While hospitalized, Vancil complained of severe pain in his right lower back. Further examination revealed a kidney stone. Subsequently, Dr. Tomi, a urologist, was called in to take over the care of Vancil's kidney problems.

Three Factors to Consider

The health insurance professional must determine three factors that would direct him or her to the proper category in the E & M coding section:

1. Place of service (where the service was provided)
   Physician's office
   Hospital
   Emergency department
   Nursing home
   Other
2. Type of service (the reason the service was rendered)
   Office visit
   Consultation
   Admission
   Newborn care
3. Patient status (type of patient)
   New patient
   Established patient
   Outpatient
   Inpatient

For example, Cindy Carlson recently moved to Jackson City because of a job transfer. Shortly after arriving in Jackson City, Cindy sprained her ankle while jogging in the park. She scheduled an appointment with Dr. Allen Schubert, a family practitioner, for medical treatment. In this scenario,

- the place of service would be the physician's office,
- the type of service would be an office visit, and
- the patient status would be "new" because Cindy has never been seen in Dr. Schubert's office before.

6/10/20XX

HX: This 27-year-old white male presents to the clinic today for chief complaint of an abrasion on the right knee following a fall yesterday. According to the patient, he had this soft tissue lesion before the fall; and when he fell, he basically abraded the lower half of the lesion. He is here for reevaluation and possible excision of the lesion.

PAIN ASSESSMENT: Scale 0-10, one.
ALLERGIES: DEMEROL
CURRENT MEDS: None

PE: NAD. Ambulatory. Appears well.
VS: BP: 120/74   WT: 150#
RIGHT KNEE EXAMINATION: The patient has a tibial prominence and just above that, there is what appears to be a 1.5-cm epidermal inclusion cyst with an abraded area inferiorly. There is mild erythema and serous drainage but no purulence. There is no appreciable edema. Just lateral to that lesion is a small superficial abrasion. The knee examination was totally within normal limits.

IMP: Epidermal inclusion cyst measuring 1.5 to 2 cm of the right knee, traumatized with abrasion

PLAN: The patient was empirically started on Keflex 500 mg 1 p.o. b.i.d. He was given instructions on home care and is to follow up this week for excision of the lesion. Routine follow-up as noted. RTN PRN.

Frederick Mahoney, MD

Fig. 13-10 Sample documentation.

After the first three factors have been established, the next step is to determine the three key components of the encounter.

Key Components

The health insurance professional must establish what level of service the patient received. Levels of service are based on the following three **key components**:
- History
- Examination
- Complexity of medical decision making

All three key components must be met or exceeded for new patients; only two must be met for established patients.

History

A patient history is **subjective information**. The essentials of the history are based on what the patient tells the healthcare provider in his or her own words. An experienced health insurance professional should be able to identify the various elements and levels of a history by reading the clinical notes entered into the health record. There are four levels of history taking: problem focused, expanded problem focused, detailed, and comprehensive. The health insurance professional should study the E & M Services Guidelines in the front of the CPT manual to become familiar with the key components for choosing the appropriate level of E & M service.

Examination

The second component in determining the correct E & M level is the patient examination. As with history taking, there are four levels, or detailed intensities, involved in a patient examination: problem focused, expanded problem focused, detailed, and comprehensive. The extent of the examination performed depends on clinical judgment and the nature of the presenting problem or problems (also referred to as the chief complaint or CC).

Medical Decision Making

The last of the three key components is medical decision making. The level of medical decision making is determined by weighing the complexity involved in the healthcare provider's assessment of and professional judgment regarding the diagnosis and care of the patient. In determining the complexity of decision making, the health insurance professional must consider the following three elements:
1. How many diagnostic and treatment options were considered
2. The amount and complexity of data reviewed
3. The amount of risk for complications, morbidity, or mortality

Contributing Factors

In addition to the three key components in assigning an E & M code, contributing factors sometimes enter into the picture. Contributing factors help the healthcare provider determine the extent of the three key components (history, examination, and medical decision making) necessary to treat the patient effectively. These contributing factors are as follows:
1. *Counseling:* Services are provided to the patient or family that include the following:
   Impressions and recommended diagnostic studies
   Discussion of diagnostic results
   Prognosis
   Risks and benefits of treatment
   Instructions
2. *Coordination of care:* A healthcare provider often must arrange for other services to be provided to a patient, such as being admitted to a long-term care facility or home healthcare.
3. *Nature of presenting problem:* The presenting problem (frequently called the *chief complaint*) guides the healthcare provider in determining the level of care necessary to diagnose the problem accurately and treat the patient effectively. There are five types of presenting problems:
   Minimal—Services typically are provided by a member of the medical staff other than the physician, but

a physician must be on the premises when the service is rendered. This type may be used only if the patient does not see the physician. *Example:* A 10-year-old girl comes in for an injection based on charted orders by the physician. A medical assistant gives the injection.

Self-limiting—Problem runs a definite or prescribed course, is transient in nature, and is not likely to affect the health status of the patient permanently. *Example:* A patient with a sore throat is examined.

Low severity—Risk of morbidity is low, and there is little to no risk of mortality without treatment. The patient is expected to recover fully without functional impairment. *Example:* A 16-year-old boy comes in with a case of severe acne.

Moderate severity—There is moderate risk of morbidity or mortality without treatment and an increased probability of prolonged functional impairment without treatment. *Example:* A 40-year-old woman with a 3-month history of severe, recurrent headaches undergoes an initial evaluation.

High severity—A patient has a high to extreme risk of morbidity or mortality without treatment and a high probability of severe, prolonged functional impairment without treatment. *Example:* A 10-year-old girl presents with severe coughing fits with wheezing that affect her sleep and other activities.

The healthcare provider should document the complexity of the patient's presenting problem in the health record. The health insurance professional must identify the words that correctly indicate the type of presenting problem.

4. *Time:* Time is measured in two ways in E & M coding:

Face-to-face time—This is the time the healthcare provider spends in direct contact with a patient during an office visit, which includes taking a history, performing an examination, and discussing results.

Unit/floor time—This includes time the physician spends on bedside care of the hospitalized patient and reviewing the health record and writing orders.

Note: Time is not considered a factor unless 50% of the encounter is spent in counseling. Time is never a factor for emergency department visits.

Time typically is noted in the E & M section in statements such as the one located under code 99203 shown in Fig. 13-11.

⭐ **Imagine This!**

Dr. Markov is asked to see a 56-year-old factory worker for dyspnea related to cirrhosis of the liver and ascites. Dr. Markov spends 60 minutes on the unit reviewing the chart and interviewing and examining the patient and an additional 20 minutes writing notes and conferring with the attending physician. Most (more than 50%) of Dr. Markov's interaction with the patient was related to eliciting the patient's values and goals of care, clarifying his understanding of his diagnosis and prognosis, giving information, and counseling. There were some specific suggestions about the use of morphine to relieve the patient's dyspnea. For this initial consultation in the hospital that lasted 80 minutes, you would choose E & M code 99254.

99203   **Office or other outpatient visit** for the evaluation and management of a new patient, which requires these 3 key components:

- **A detailed history;**
- **A detailed examination;**
- **Medical decision making of low complexity.**

Counseling and/or coordination of care with other providers or agencies are provided consistent with the nature of the problem(s) and the patient's and/or family's needs.

Usually, the presenting problem(s) are of moderate severity. Physicians typically spend 30 minutes face-to-face with the patient and/or family.

➔ *CPT Assistant* Winter 91:11, Spring 92:14, 24, Summer 92:1, 24, Spring 93:34, Summer 93:2, Fall 93:9, Spring 95:1, Summer 95:4, Fall 95:9, Jul 98:9, Sep 98:5, Feb 00:11, Aug 01:2, Apr 02:14, Oct 04:10, Feb 05:9, Apr 05:1, 3, Jun 05:11, Dec 05:10, May 06:1, Jun 06:1, Oct 06:15, Apr 07:11, Sep 07:1, Mar 09:3, Aug 09:5, Dec 09:9

Fig. 13-11 Example from E & M Section showing how time is noted. (From American Medical Association: CPT 2011, Standard Edition. Chicago, 2010, American Medical Association.)

Prolonged Services

When considering the applicable E & M coding level for a patient encounter, the health insurance professional looks at the history, examination, and medical decision making. Occasionally, the amount of time the healthcare provider spends face to face with the patient exceeds the usual length of service associated with the corresponding level in the inpatient or outpatient setting (Fig. 13-12). When this happens, this extra time is reported in addition to other physician services. The reason for the extra time spent must be documented.

Total Duration of Prolonged Services	Codes(s)
less than 30 minutes	Not reported separately
30-74 minutes (30 minutes - 1 hr. 14 min.)	99354 X 1
75-104 minutes (1 hr. 15 min. - 1 hr. 44 min.)	99354 X 1 AND 99355 X 1
105 or more (1 hr. 45 min. or more)	99354 X 1 AND 99355 X 2 or more for each additional 30 minutes

—— *Coding Tip* ——

Reporting Service of Less than 30 Minutes

Prolonged service of less than 30 minutes total duration on a given date is not separately reported because the work involved is included in the total work of the evaluation and management codes.

CPT Coding Guidelines, Evaluation and Management, Prolonged Physician Service with Direct (Face-to-Face) Patient Contact

Fig. 13-12 Example of extra time scenario. (From American Medical Association: CPT 2011, Standard Edition. Chicago, 2010, American Medical Association.)

What Did You Learn?

1. Explain the difference between a new and established patient.
2. How does an outpatient differ from an inpatient?
3. What are the three factors to consider before assigning an E & M code level?
4. Name the three key components in E & M coding.
5. What is subjective information?
6. Name the four contributing factors that assist the coder in assigning an E & M code.

SUBHEADINGS OF MAIN E & M SECTION

Following the Office or Other Outpatient Services codes of the main E & M section are additional subheadings. The codes in these various subheadings are used to report services provided to patients who are admitted to a hospital or nursing facility as a result of an encounter in the physician's office or other ambulatory facility.

Office or Other Outpatient Services

The first subheading under the main E & M section deals with reporting professional services provided in the physician's office or in an outpatient or other ambulatory facility. (An individual is considered an outpatient unless he or she has been formally admitted to a hospital.) In this section, codes are differentiated between "new" and "established" patients. As mentioned, codes for new patient services are 99201 through 99205, and codes for established patients are 99211 through 99215. As the codes increase numerically, the patient's problem becomes more complex or life-threatening or both. For new patients, all three key components (history, examination, and medical decision making) must be met or exceeded; however, only two must be met for established patients (Table 13-3).

Hospital Observation Services

Outpatient **observation** services are short-term services provided in a hospital, including the use of a bed and periodic monitoring by the hospital staff. Observation services are defined as any services that are considered reasonable and necessary to evaluate a patient's illness to determine the need for possible admission to the hospital as an inpatient. When patients are considered "observation status," they receive the same level of care and personal attention as they would receive had they been admitted to the hospital as an inpatient. Initial observation care codes for new or established patients are 99218 through 99220. Subsequent observation care codes are 99224 through 99226. Code 99217 is used to report all services provided to a patient on discharge from "observation status" if the discharge is on other than the initial date of observation status.

When observation status services are initiated at another site, such as the emergency department, physician's office, or nursing facility, all E & M services provided by the supervising physician in conjunction with initiating the "observation status" are considered part of the observation care, if performed on the same day, and should not be reported separately. It is important that office policies and procedures for reporting observation care services be reviewed and updated annually.

TABLE 13-3	Elements Needed to Substantiate Code Choice			
LEVELS OF E & M SERVICE	**PROBLEM FOCUSED**	**EXPANDED PROBLEM FOCUSED**	**DETAILED**	**COMPREHENSIVE**
History	Presenting problem (CC)	Presenting problem (CC)	Presenting problem (CC)	Presenting problem (CC)
	Brief HPI	Brief HPI	Extended HPI	Extended HPI
		Problem-focused ROS	Extended ROS	Complete ROS
			Pertinent PFSH	Complete PFSH
Examination	Limited to affected body area or organ system	Limited to affected body area or organ system and related organ systems	Extended to all affected body areas and any related organ systems	Multisystem examination or examination of complete single organ system
Medical decision making	Straightforward	Low	Moderate	High
Diagnosis and management	0-1 element	2 elements	3 elements	>3 elements
Data	0-1 element	2 elements	3 elements	>3 elements
Risk	Minimal	Low	Moderate	High

⭐ Imagine This!

Billy Marshall, a 6-year-old boy, was brought to the emergency department after a fall from a jungle gym at the school playground. Billy did not lose consciousness; however, he complained of headache and his teacher reported an episode of vomiting. Billy was admitted for 24-hour observation to rule out head injury.

Hospital Inpatient Services

Hospital inpatient services include services provided to hospital inpatients and patients in a "partial hospital" setting. To report E & M services provided to hospital inpatients, use the following codes:

- *Initial hospital care:* The codes in this category are for reporting services provided only by the admitting physician. Other physicians providing initial inpatient E & M services should use consultation or subsequent hospital care codes, as appropriate.
- *Subsequent hospital care:* The codes in this category are for reporting inpatient E & M services provided after the first inpatient encounter (for the admitting physician) or for services (other than consultative) provided by a physician other than the admitting physician. A hospitalized patient may require more than one visit per day by the same physician. Group the visits together, and report the level of service on the basis of the total encounters for the day. Third-party payers vary in their requirements for reporting this service.
- *Observation or inpatient care services (including admission and discharge services):* The codes in this category are used

to report observation or inpatient hospital care services provided to patients admitted and discharged on the same date of service. (See previous section on Hospital Observation Services.)

- *Hospital discharge services:* These codes are used for reporting services provided on the final day of a multiple-day stay.

Time is the controlling factor for assigning the appropriate hospital discharge services code. Total duration of time spent by the physician (even if the time spent is not continuous) should be documented and reported. These codes include final examination, discussion of hospital stay, instructions to caregivers, preparation of discharge records, prescriptions, and referral forms, if applicable.

Consultations

By definition, a physician may not bill for a consultation unless another physician formally requests his or her opinion about the patient's present or future course of treatment. In addition, the consulting physician must communicate that opinion in either a letter or a dictated report. The patient's medical record should include the request by the physician who initiated the consultation and any information (letter, report, or dictation) that was communicated back to this physician.

If a specialist has a patient transferred to his or her care and is going to assume ongoing responsibility for a portion of the patient's care, this is a referral, and office visit or hospital visit codes, not consultation codes, should be used. An example would be a referral from another oncologist for ongoing treatment because of patient choice or geographic transfer.

There are two consultation subheadings in E & M coding:

- Office or other outpatient (new or established patient)
- Inpatient (new or established patient)

These two subheadings define the location where the consultation was rendered—physician's office or other ambulatory facility, codes 99241 through 99245, or inpatient hospital, codes 99251 through 99255. Only one initial consultation is reported by a consultant for the patient on each separate admission. Any subsequent service is reported with applicable codes from Subsequent Hospital Care codes 99231 to 99233 or Subsequent Nursing Facility Care codes 99307 to 99310. A follow-up consultation includes monitoring the patient's progress, recommending management modifications, or advising on a new plan of care in response to the patient's status.

As of January 1, 2010, Medicare stopped recognizing consultation codes (99241 through 99255) as valid codes for payment. This is a significant change in Medicare policy, and some experts predict other large carriers (e.g. Blue Cross Blue Shield, Aetna, Humana) to adopt the same policy for uniformity, although none has to date. The following example can be used as a guideline for coding what previously would have been coded as a consultation visit.

Example: Surgeon Justin Lang sees Medicare patient Olive Bodkins in his office for a consultation for another provider in the area. Ms. Bodkins is a new patient (one who has not been seen in the previous 3 years by the surgeon or a billing partner); Dr. Lang will bill the consultation as a new patient visit at the appropriate level (1 through 5) using CPT codes 99201 through 99205. If Ms. Bodkins was an established patient (one who was seen during the previous 3 years by the surgeon or a billing partner), Dr. Lang would bill the consultation as an established patient visit at the appropriate level (1 through 5) using CPT codes 99211 through 99215.

🕐 Stop and Think

Dr. Toledo, a family practitioner, has been treating patient Alma Cahill for a rash on her face; however, the medication Dr. Toledo has prescribed is not helping the problem, and the rash is spreading to the neck. With Alma's approval, Dr. Toledo makes an appointment with Dr. Farmer, a dermatologist, for continued treatment of the rash. Is this a consultation or a referral?

Emergency Department Services

E & M codes 99281 through 99288 are used for new and established patients who have been treated in an emergency department that is part of a hospital. To qualify, the facility must be available for immediate emergency care 24 hours a day for patients not on "observation status."

The single code, 99288, for the subheading "Other Emergency Services" is used in physician-directed emergency care and advanced life support when the physician is located in a hospital emergency or critical care department and is in two-way voice communication with ambulance or rescue personnel outside the hospital. The physician directs the performance of necessary medical procedures.

Critical Care Services

The direct delivery of medical care by a physician to a critically ill or critically injured patient is referred to as critical care. A critical illness or injury acutely impairs one or more vital organ systems such that there is a high probability of imminent or life-threatening deterioration in the patient's condition. Critical care involves high-complexity decision making to assess, manipulate, and support vital system failure or to prevent further life-threatening deterioration of the patient's condition. Examples of vital organ system failure include, but are not limited to, central nervous system failure, circulatory failure, shock, renal failure, hepatic failure, metabolic failure, and respiratory failure. Critical care services are discussed in depth in the E & M section of the CPT manual.

Nursing Facility Services

The Nursing Facility Services category of E & M services includes codes for services provided to new or established patients in nursing facilities (NFs) (formerly referred to as skilled nursing facilities [SNFs], intermediate nursing facilities [ICFs], or long-term care facilities [LTCFs]). There are two major subcategories of nursing facilities: Initial Nursing Facility Care (codes 99304 through 99306) and Subsequent Nursing Facility Care (codes 99307 through 99310).

Nursing Facility Discharge Services codes 99315 (30 minutes or less) and 99316 (more than 30 minutes) are used to report the total duration of time spent by a physician for the final patient discharge from the nursing facility. This time includes a final examination of the patient; discussion of the nursing facility stay; instructions given to relevant caregivers for continuing care; and preparation of discharge records, prescriptions, and referral forms, as applicable.

Other Nursing Facility Services code 99318 is used to report an annual nursing facility assessment visit on the required schedule of visits if an annual assessment is performed. Refer to the CPT-4 coding manual for additional E & M categories and details on reporting services in these categories.

❓ What Did You Learn?

1. What does "observation status" mean in E & M coding?
2. List the two consultation subheadings in E & M coding.
3. What level of decision making must be used to assess critical care?
4. What services are typically included in the Nursing Facility Discharge Services category?

E & M MODIFIERS

Before assigning a final E & M code, it is important to check for potential modifiers that should be assigned to report an altered service or procedure (e.g., an unusual or special circumstance that affects the service or procedure). Attaching modifiers to codes provides additional information regarding the services performed. Leaving off a needed modifier can result in denial of payment. Modifiers used most often with the codes in the E & M section are 24, 25, 32, 52, and 57. (See Appendix A in the CPT manual for a complete list of modifiers and their use.)

> ### ❓ What Did You Learn?
>
> 1. What is the function of a modifier?
> 2. Why is it important to attach a needed modifier to a code?
> 3. Where are modifiers found in the CPT manual?

IMPORTANCE OF DOCUMENTATION

Health record documentation is required to record pertinent facts, findings, and observations about a patient's health history, including past and present illnesses, examinations, tests, treatments, and outcomes. The health record chronologically documents the care of the patient and is an important element contributing to high-quality care.

The appropriately documented health record facilitates

- the ability of the physician and other healthcare professionals to evaluate and plan the patient's immediate treatment and to monitor the patient's healthcare over time,
- communication and continuity of care among physicians and other healthcare professionals involved in the patient's care,
- accurate and timely claims review and payment,
- appropriate utilization review and quality of care evaluations, and
- collection of data that may be useful for research and education.

An appropriately documented health record can reduce many of the challenges associated with claims processing and may serve as a legal document to verify the care provided, if necessary. Fig. 13-13 shows a list of the top 10 coding and billing errors.

---

1. No documentation for services billed.
2. No signature or authentication of documentation.
3. Always assigning the same level of service.
4. Billing of consult vs. outpatient office visit.
5. Invalid codes billed due to old resources.
6. Unbundling of procedure codes.
7. Misinterpreted abbreviations.
8. No chief complaint listed for each visit.
9. Billing of service(s) included in global fee as a separate professional fee.
10. Inappropriate or no modifier used for accurate payment of claim.

Fig. 13-13 Top 10 coding and billing errors.

E & M Documentation Guidelines: 1995 versus 1997

In addition to the guidelines found in the CPT manual, HCFA (now CMS) published two sets of documentation guidelines. The first set of guidelines became effective in 1995, and the second set became effective in 1997. The goal was to develop and refine a way to assign a "score" accurately for each level of medical services in the E & M categories. The guidelines specifically identify the elements that must be documented in the medical record to support a particular level of service and a workable method to determine the level of medical decision making. Briefly, the 1995 guidelines are applicable to all medical and surgical services and in all settings. The 1997 guidelines, in addition to incorporating the 1995 guidelines, focus on specialists and outline each component of a typical E & M service. Box 13-1 provides an outline of the general principles to which healthcare practices must adhere when structuring medical records in accordance with the 1995 and 1997 guidelines. For further information on the 1995 and 1997 guidelines visit the Evolve site.

Deciding Which Guidelines to Use

Although it is acceptable to use either the 1995 or the 1997 E & M documentation guidelines, it is unacceptable to use them interchangeably on the same document. An extended history may be documented under the 1997 guidelines by identifying three chronic or inactive conditions and the current status of those conditions. The 1995 guidelines do not permit this documentation practice. Under the 1995 guidelines, an extended history requires documentation of at least four HPI elements. The HPI elements include *location, quality, severity, duration, timing, context, modifying factors,* and *associated signs/symptoms*.

> ### ❓ What Did You Learn?
>
> 1. Name three ways a well-documented health record contributes to high-quality healthcare.
> 2. What is the principal difference between the 1995 E & M documentation guidelines compared with the guidelines published in 1997?
> 3. Which set of guidelines does CMS prefer a medical office to use?

OVERVIEW OF HCFA COMMON PROCEDURE CODING SYSTEM (HCPCS)

HCPCS is a coding system that is composed of Level I (CPT) codes, Level II (national) codes, and formerly Level III (local) codes. HCPCS codes are mandated by CMS (formerly HCFA) for reporting services on Medicare claims and are required by most state Medicaid offices. To review,

Box 13-1

General Principles of Medical Record Documentation Using 1995 and 1997 Guidelines

1. The medical record should be complete and legible.
2. The documentation of each patient encounter should include:
   a. reason for the encounter and relevant history, physical examination findings, and prior diagnostic test results;
   b. assessment and clinical impression or diagnosis;
   c. plan for care; and
   d. date and legible identity of the observer.
3. If not documented, the rationale for ordering diagnostic and other ancillary services should be easily understood.

4. Past and present diagnoses should be accessible to the treating or consulting physician.
5. Appropriate health risk factors should be identified.
6. The patient's progress, response to and changes in treatment, and revision of diagnosis should be documented.
7. The CPT and ICD-10-CM codes reported on the health insurance claim form or billing statement should be supported by the documentation in the medical record.

Level I (CPT) codes are composed of 5 digits that describe the service, procedure, or test. CPT codes are developed and maintained by the AMA with annual updates. Level II (national) codes are 5-digit alphanumeric codes consisting of one alphabetical character (a letter between A and V) followed by 4 digits. HCFA (now CMS) created Level II codes to supplement CPT, which does not include codes for nonphysician procedures such as ambulance services; durable medical equipment, prosthetics, orthotics, and supplies (DMEPOS), and administration of injectable drugs. Level II codes are developed and maintained by CMS with quarterly updates and are a standard component of electronically transmitted claims.

Although thousands of medical products are described by Level II codes, no product brand names are included in the code descriptions. The presence of a Level II code indicates only that the product or service is available within the larger medical system; it does not guarantee payment. Individual payers develop their own reimbursement rules and criteria related to Level II codes, which differ from payer to payer. Following are examples of Level II codes:

A4615—Cannula, nasal

E0147—Walker, heavy duty, multiple braking system, variable wheel resistance

J2250—Injection, midazolam hydrochloride (Versed), 1 mg

If both a CPT code and HCPCS Level II code are available for the service provided, CMS requires that the HCPCS Level II code be used. Medicare has specific requirements for reporting Part B physician office services. These requirements are published in the *Medicare Claims Processing Manual*, Pub. 100-04, available on the CMS website.

HCPCS Level II Manual

HCPCS Level II codes are organized into 17 sections (Fig. 13-14). The D codes, which include dental procedure codes D0000 through D9999, represent a separate category of codes from the Current Dental Terminology (CDT-4)

- **A Codes:** Transportation Services Including
  - Ambulance
  - Medical and Surgical Supplies
  - Respiratory Durable Medical Equipment, Inexpensive and Routinely Purchased
  - Administrative, Miscellaneous and Investigational
- **B Codes:** Enteral and Parenteral Therapy
- **C Codes:** Hospital Outpatient Prospective Payment System (OPPS)
- **E Codes:** Durable Medical Equipment
- **G Codes:** Temporary Codes for Professional Services Procedures
- **H Codes:** Alcohol and/or Drug Services
- **J Codes:** Drugs Administered Other Than Oral Method
- **K Codes:** Temporary Codes for Durable Medical Equipment
- **L Codes:** Orthotic Procedures
- **M Codes:** Medical Services
- **P Codes:** Pathology and Laboratory Tests
- **Q Codes:** Temporary Codes
- **R Codes:** Domestic Radiology Services
- **S Codes:** Temporary National Codes
- **T Codes:** National Codes for State Medicaid Agencies
- **V Codes:** Vision/Hearing/Speech-Language Pathology Services

Fig. 13-14 Sections of HCPCS Level II (national) codes.

code set, which is copyrighted and updated by the American Dental Association. (Although HCPCS publishers may develop their own format, conventions, and supplemental information, they typically use the same basic formats and conventions.)

Index of Main Terms

The first main section of the HCPCS coding manual is an index of main terms, arranged in alphabetical order similar to Level I CPT-4 codes (Fig. 13-15). The index is followed

---

A

Abarelix, J0128 x
Abatacept, J0129
Abciximab, J0130
Abdomen
  dressing holder/binder, A4462
  pad, low profile, L1270
Abduction **control, each,** L2642
Abduction restrainer, A4566
Abduction **rotation bar, foot,** L3140-L3170
AbobotulinumtoxintypeA, J0586
Absorption **dressing,** A6251-A6256
Access, site, occlusive, device, G0269
Access **system,** A4301

Aide (Continued)
  bath/toilet, E0160-E0162, E0235, E0240-E0249
  services, G0150-G0156, G0179-G0181, S5180,
    S5181, S9122, T1021, T1022
Air bubble detector, dialysis, E1530
Air **Fluidized bed,** E0194
Air **pressure pad/mattress,** E0186, E0197
Air **travel and nonemergency transportation,** A0140
Alarm
  not otherwise classified, A9280
  pressure, dialysis, E1540
Alatrofloxacin **mesylate,** J0200
Albumin, **human,** P9041, P9042
Albuterol
  all formulations, inhalation solution,
    concentrated, J7610, J7611

Fig. 13-15 Example page from HCPCS Index. (Data from U.S. Department of Health and Human Services, Centers for Medicare and Medicaid Services.)

by the 17 alphabetized sections. Level II codes are located in the index using similar guidelines as CPT-4 codes, as follows:
- Identify the service or procedure performed. *Example:* A patient is provided with a nonprogrammable implantable infusion pump (ambulatory) for chemotherapy treatment.
- Identify the main term, and locate the term in the index. In our example, the main term would be "pump." Note in the index that pump is followed by a list of indented subterms, so find "implantable infusion." Tentative codes would be E0782 and E0783.
- Locate these codes in the applicable section of the alphanumeric list, and compare the code description with the service provided.
- Eliminate any codes that do not appropriately describe the service provided. In our example, E0783 would be incorrect because it describes a "programmable" pump.
- Check for symbols, notes, and footnotes that clarify code selection further, and review their definitions and other coverage guidelines that apply. In our example, code E0782 cannot be used in a skilled nursing facility setting. The coding resource may provide a note or symbol to identify this exclusion from Medicare coverage.
- Determine whether any modifiers should be used.
- Assign the appropriate code. In our example, E0783 is the correct code.

Table of Drugs

The Level II (national) code manual also contains a table of drugs, which the health insurance professional should use to locate appropriate drug names that correspond with the generic names listed in the J code subsection.

Modifiers

As with CPT-4, HCPCS Level II code sets contain modifiers. Modifiers in HCPCS Level II are alphabetical or alphanumeric. They are used to indicate that a service or procedure that has been performed has been altered by some specific circumstances but not changed in its definition or code. The HCPCS manual contains a complete list of modifiers and their meaning.

Appendices

Similar to CPT-4, the HCPCS coding manual contains several appendices:
- Appendix A—Select Internet Only Manuals (IOM)
- Appendix B—2010 Physician/Provider Payment Edits
- Appendix C—2010 Hospital Outpatient Prospective Payment System Edits
- Appendix D—General Correct Coding Policies for National Correct Coding Initiative Policy Manual for Medicare Services

(*Author's Note:* All HCPCS references are taken from *2011 HCPCS Level II Coding Manual*, Professional Edition, by Carol S. Buck, published by Saunders, 2011.)

What Did You Learn?

1. How are HCPCS Level II codes structured?
2. What do "J" codes represent in HCPCS coding?
3. What is the function of an HCPCS Level II code modifier?

NATIONAL CORRECT CODING INITIATIVE (NCCI)

The National Correct Coding Initiative (NCCI) is a system developed by the CMS to promote national correct practices to minimize coding errors that lead to incorrect payment on Medicare Part B claims. NCCI focuses on edits of services billed by the same provider, beneficiary, and date of service. It is based on coding conventions in the AMA CPT manual, national and local policies, coding guidelines from national societies, and analysis of Medicare medical and surgical practices. NCCI edits serve two purposes: (1) to ensure that the most comprehensive group of codes are billed rather than the component parts and (2) to edit two codes that cannot reasonably be performed together on the basis of either the definition or anatomical considerations.

The CMS updates the NCCI policy manual annually for Medicare services. Edits have been incorporated by Medicare carriers for physicians and by Medicare intermediaries for the Hospital Outpatient Prospective Payment System and the Outpatient Code Editor.

The Affordable Care Act requires all state Medicaid programs to incorporate "NCCI methodologies" in their claims processing systems by March 31, 2011. To view the most recent update on NCCI, visit the Evolve site.

HEALTH INSURANCE PORTABILITY AND ACCOUNTABILITY ACT (HIPAA) AND HCPCS CODING

One HIPAA requirement is that procedure coding be standardized. In October 2003, the Secretary of the Department of Health and Human Services authorized CMS, under the HIPAA legislation, to maintain and distribute HCPCS Level II codes. In addition, CMS was to establish uniform national definitions of services, codes to represent services, and payment modifiers to the codes. In August 2000, the *Federal Register* published regulations (65 FR 50312) to implement this HIPAA mandate. As reported earlier in this chapter, this regulation called for the elimination of Level III local codes by October 2002. The deadline was extended, however, to give contractors and providers an opportunity to identify unapproved codes and modifiers and to crosswalk them to temporary codes or permanent national codes. The final date for the use of any unapproved Level III codes was December 31, 2003, after which only Level I and Level II codes could be used.

Crosswalk

A **crosswalk** is a procedure by which codes used for data in one database are translated into the codes of another database, making it possible to relate information between or among databases. In coding, a crosswalk is a "link" that refers to a relationship between a medical procedure (CPT code) and a diagnosis (ICD code). Medicare uses CPT/ICD crosswalks to validate or substantiate medical necessity under Local Coverage Determinations/Local Medicare Review Policy. Third-party payers also establish crosswalk tables for validating and auditing medical claims. In brief, physicians dealing in Medicare Part B claims are paid by CPT procedure codes, not diagnoses. To validate proper coding (e.g., the reason for the procedure), providers must specify a diagnosis. If the diagnosis does not support the procedure, the claim may not get paid.

? What Did You Learn?

1. What does HIPAA require of HCPCS coding?
2. Which level of HCPCS codes did HIPAA eliminate?
3. What is a crosswalk?

CURRENT PROCEDURAL TERMINOLOGY, 5TH EDITION (CPT-5)

The **CPT-5** project is an ongoing effort by the AMA to make improvements in the structure and processes of CPT codes to reflect the coding demands of the current healthcare system and to address challenges presented by HIPAA. Ideally, this updated version would improve existing CPT features and correct deficiencies in the current CPT-4 coding system. It was originally intended for the transition into the changes proposed for CPT-5 to be gradual, and all improvements and modifications were to occur through the traditional CPT Editorial process. The project was supposed to be completed in 2003; however, at the present time, it is unclear when these codes will be implemented nationwide. As planned, CPT-5 codes would still be 5-digit codes, similar to the current CPT-4 codes, because one of the HIPAA directives stated that computer systems must be able to handle 6-digit specificity for alphanumeric diagnosis codes and alphanumeric CPT codes.

For more information on CPT-5, visit the Evolve site.

? What Did You Learn?

1. What organization is developing CPT-5?
2. Name two things CPT-5 is predicted to accomplish.

SUMMARY CHECKPOINTS

▶ The purpose of CPT is to provide a uniform language accurately describing medical, surgical, and diagnostic services, serving as an effective means for reliable communication among physicians, third-party payers, and patients nationwide.

▶ CPT was developed and published by the AMA in 1966. Originally, it contained mainly surgical procedures, with limited sections on medicine, radiology, and laboratory procedures. The second edition, published in 1970, expanded codes to designate diagnostic and therapeutic procedures in surgery, medicine, and other specialties. In 1970, the 5-digit system was introduced, replacing the former 4-digit codes, and internal medicine procedures were added.

▶ The CPT manual begins with an introduction, followed by six sections in the main body of the manual. Category III codes follow the main section, after which there are 14 appendices—A through N. The CPT index of main terms appears at the back of the manual.

▶ The CPT manual uses coding conventions and symbols that help guide the health insurance professional in locating the correct code. Accurate procedural coding cannot be accomplished without understanding the meaning of each of these conventions and symbols.

▶ The semicolon is used to separate main and subordinate clauses in the CPT code descriptions. The complete description listed *before* the semicolon applies to that code plus any additional succeeding, indented codes. The complete description *after* the semicolon applies only to that code.

▶ The basic steps for CPT coding are as follows:
  • Step 1—identify the procedure, service, or supply to be coded.
  • Step 2—determine the main term.
  • Step 3—locate the main term in the Alphabetic Index, and note the code.
  • Step 4—cross-reference the single code, multiple codes, or the code range numerically in the tabular section of the manual.
  • Step 5—read and follow any notes, special instructions, or conventions associated with the code.
  • Step 6—determine and assign the appropriate code.

▶ A new patient is a patient who has not received any professional services from the physician or another physician of the same specialty, regardless of location, who belongs to the same group practice within the past 3 years.

▶ An established patient is a patient who has been treated previously by the healthcare provider, regardless of location of service, within the past 3 years. If the provider saw the patient for the first time in a hospital and the patient comes to the office for a follow-up visit after discharge, the patient is considered an established patient to the practice because health record documentation was generated from the hospital visit.

▶ The three key components that establish the level in E & M coding are as follows:
  • *History*—subjective information based on four elements: presenting problem (in the patient's own words), HPI, ROS, and PFSH. The four levels of history are (1) problem focused, (2) expanded problem focused, (3) detailed, and (4) comprehensive.
  • *Examination*—deals with the degree to which the healthcare provider examines various body areas and organ systems that are affected by the presenting

problem. Four levels of examination exist: (1) problem focused, (2) expanded problem focused, (3) detailed, and (4) comprehensive.
  • *Medical decision making*—determined by weighing the complexity involved in the healthcare provider's assessment of and the professional judgment made regarding the diagnosis and care of the patient. The three elements considered are how many diagnostic and treatment options are considered; the amount and complexity of data reviewed; and the amount of risk for complications, morbidity, or mortality. Medical decision making has four levels: (1) straightforward, (2) low complexity, (3) moderate complexity, and (4) high complexity.

▶ Besides the previously mentioned three key components, the four contributing factors that may affect the level of E & M coding are:
  • Counseling
  • Coordination of care
  • Nature of presenting problem—minimal, self-limiting, low severity, high severity
  • Time

▶ Time can be measured two ways in E & M coding:
  • *Face-to-face time*—time the physician spends in direct contact with the patient during an office visit, which includes taking a history, performing an examination, and discussing results.
  • *Unit/floor time*—time the physician spends on patient bedside care and reviewing the health record and writing orders.

▶ The 1995 documentation guidelines are applicable to all medical and surgical services and in all settings. The 1997 guidelines, in addition to incorporating the 1995 guidelines, focus on specialists and outline each component of a typical E & M service.

▶ HCPCS is a coding system that is composed of Level I (CPT) codes, Level II (national) codes, and formerly Level III (local) codes. CPT codes are composed of 5 digits that describe procedures and tests. Level II (national) codes are 5-digit alphanumeric codes that describe pharmaceuticals, supplies, procedures, tests, and services.

▶ HCFA created Level II codes to supplement CPT, which does not include codes for nonphysician procedures such as ambulance services, durable medical equipment, specific supplies, and administration of injectable drugs. If a CPT code and HCPCS Level II code for the service are provided, CMS requires that the HCPCS Level II code be used. NCCI is a system developed by CMS to promote national correct practices in an effort to minimize coding errors that lead to incorrect payment on Medicare Part B claims.

▶ Because HIPAA requires standardized procedure coding, CMS required healthcare providers and contractors to eliminate any unapproved local procedure or modifier codes. To accomplish this, medical offices were to crosswalk unapproved local procedure and modifier codes to a temporary or permanent national code. All other unapproved local codes were to be deleted by October 16, 2002. (This deadline was subsequently extended to December 31, 2003.)

▶ The CPT-5 project is an ongoing effort by the AMA to make improvements in the structure and processes of CPT codes to reflect the coding demands of the current healthcare system and to address challenges presented by HIPAA. There is no set date for the transition to the CPT-5 coding system.

CLOSING SCENARIO

Park and Melanie have finished the chapter on CPT coding. Although they agree it was more challenging than the chapter on ICD-10-CM coding (particularly the E & M coding), Melanie believes that Park's help was extremely beneficial. She is now convinced that she will finish the course on time and with an acceptable grade. Meanwhile, Park still believes that coding is the right career move for him.

He has researched the websites at the end of the chapter to learn all he can about coding. He has even located a website bulletin board where practicing coders write in questions and answers on coding issues. After he finishes the medical insurance course, Park plans to take a coding course over the Internet. He is looking forward to continuing his pursuit of a career in coding.

WEBSITES TO EXPLORE

- For live links to the following websites, please visit the Evolve site at
  https://evolve.elsevier.com/Beik/today
- Access AMA at
  http://www.ama-assn.org
- CPT coding guidelines and conventions can be found at
  http://www.ama-assn.org/resources/doc/psa/admin-simp-cpt-wp.pdf
- Access Medicare Learning Network (Medlearn) at
  http://www.cms.hhs.gov/medlearn
- To visit CMS, log on to
  http://www.cms.hhs.gov
- To visit U.S. Department of Health and Human Services, log on to
  http://www.hhs.gov
- Access National Correct Coding Initiative at
  http://www.cms.gov/NationalCorrectCodInitEd/
- HCPCS General Information is available at
  http://www.cms.gov/MedHCPCSGenInfo/
- Access Documentation Guidelines (1995) at
  http://www.cms.gov/MLNProducts/Downloads/1995dg.pdf
- Access Documentation Guidelines (1997) at
  http://www.cms.gov/MLNProducts/Downloads/MASTER1.pdf
- Access National Correct Coding Initiative (NCCI) and Additional Edits at
  http://www.ncdhhs.gov/dma/provider/ncci.htm
- GEM Factsheet is available at
  http://www.cms.hhs.gov/MLNProducts/downloads/ICD-10_GEM_factsheet.pdf

- Access CPT-5 at
  http://www.ama-assn.org/ama1/pub/upload/mm/362/cat3-codes-first-10-yrs.pdf

Author's Note: Websites change frequently. If any of these URLs is unavailable, use applicable guide words in your Internet search to acquire additional information on the various subjects listed.

REFERENCES AND RESOURCES

American Medical Association: *Current Procedural Terminology, CPT (2007) Standard Edition,* Chicago, 2007, AMA Press.

American Medical Association: *HCPCS, 2005,* Chicago, 2005, AMA Press.

Buck CJ: *Step-by-Step Medical Coding,* ed 5, Philadelphia, 2004, Saunders.

Covell A: *Coding Workbook for the Physician's Office,* Clifton Park, NY, 2003, Delmar/Thomson Learning.

Davis JB: *CPT and HCPCS Coding Made Easy! A Comprehensive Guide to CPT and HCPCS Coding for Health Care Professionals,* Downer's Grove, IL, 2000, PMIC.

Fordney MT: *Insurance Handbook for the Medical Office,* ed 11, St Louis, 2010, Saunders.

HSS: *Understand the Three CPT Code Categories.* Available at http://health-information.advanceweb.com/Editorial/Content/Editorial.aspx?CC=42599.

Rowell JC, Green MA: *Understanding Health Insurance, A Guide to Professional Billing,* ed 7, Clifton Park, NY, 2004, Delmar/Thomson Learning.

U.S. Health and Human Services, Centers for Medicare and Medicaid Services: *Medicare Claims Processing Manual: Physician/Nonphysician Practitioners, Section 30.6.8.* Available at http://www.aishealth.com/.

The Patient

Chapter Outline

I. Patient Expectations
   A. Professional Office Setting
   B. Relevant Paperwork and Questions
   C. Honoring Appointment Times
   D. Patient Load
   E. Getting Comfortable with the Healthcare Provider
   F. Privacy and Confidentiality
   G. Financial Issues
II. Future Trends
   A. Aging Population
   B. Internet as a Healthcare Tool
   C. Patients as Consumers
III. Health Insurance Portability and Accountability Act (HIPAA) Requirements
   A. Authorization to Release Information
   B. HIPAA and Covered Entities
   C. HIPAA Requirements for Covered Entities
      1. HIPAA Transaction 5010
      2. Proposed Changes to the CMS-1500 Form
   D. Patient's Right of Access and Correction
   E. Accessing Information through Patient Authorization
   F. Accessing Information through De-identification
IV. Billing Policies and Practices
   A. Assignment of Benefits
   B. Keeping Patients Informed
   C. Accounting Methods

   1. "One-Write" or Pegboard Accounting System
   2. Electronic Patient Accounting Software
   D. Electronic Medical Records
V. Billing and Collection
   A. Billing Cycle
   B. Arranging Credit or Payment Plans
      1. Self-Pay Patients
      2. Establishing Credit
   C. Problem Patients
VI. Laws Affecting Credit and Collection
   A. Truth in Lending Act
   B. Fair Credit Billing Act
   C. Equal Credit Opportunity Act
   D. Fair Credit Reporting Act
   E. Fair Debt Collection Practices Act
VII. Collection Methods
   A. Collection by Telephone
      1. Timetable for Calling
      2. Selecting Which Patients to Call
   B. Collection by Letter
VIII. Billing Services
IX. Collection Agencies
X. Small Claims Litigation
   A. Who Can Use Small Claims
   B. How the Small Claims Process Works

CHAPTER OBJECTIVES

After completion of this chapter, the student should be able to:
1. List and discuss various patient expectations.
2. Name two future trends in the patient-practice relationship.
3. Explain various regulations in the Health Insurance Portability and Accountability Act (HIPAA) that affect patient billing.
4. Outline appropriate patient billing policies and practices.
5. Discuss billing and collection strategies in healthcare practices.
6. List federal regulations affecting credit and collection.

OPENING SCENARIO

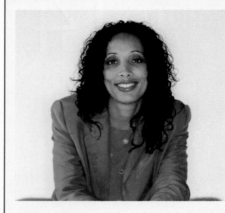

Callie Foster enrolled in the health insurance program not only because it offered interesting and challenging career opportunities but also because of an incident she had recently experienced. Callie had had ear pain for several days, so she called for an appointment at an ear, nose, and throat (ENT) clinic. Callie took time off work to drive the 30 miles to Dr. Susan Dayton's clinic. When she arrived and signed in at the front desk, the medical receptionist asked for her insurance card; however, after searching in vain through her pockets and purse, Callie said she must have left it at home. "Then," said the receptionist brusquely, "you will have to reschedule. Dr. Dayton does not see patients who do not have insurance." Before Callie could confirm the fact that she had coverage through her employer, the receptionist turned away, ignoring her protests. Callie ended up in the emergency department later that day with a ruptured eardrum.

This experience was upsetting, and Callie wants to find out what patients typically expect when they visit a healthcare office. She firmly believes that all members of the healthcare team should learn how to empathize and listen to what patients have to say. Callie was convinced that there is no excuse for impolite behavior and harsh treatment in a healthcare office.

Scott Tanner is a classmate of Callie Foster. Scott is interested in credit law and collections. Scott wants to learn about the small claims process; his parents own rental units and occasionally experience problems collecting rents. Scott and Callie look forward to having their questions answered in Chapter 14.

7. Explain two conventional collection methods.
8. Assess the benefits of a billing service.
9. Compare the advantages and disadvantages of using a collection agency.
10. Outline the steps involved in the small claims litigation process.

CHAPTER TERMS

accounts receivable
alternate billing cycle
assignment of benefits
billing cycle
collection agency
collection ratio
daily journal
defendant
de-identified
disbursements journal
Equal Credit Opportunity Act
Fair Credit Billing Act
Fair Credit Reporting Act
Fair Debt Collection
  Practices Act
general journal
general ledger

HIPAA-covered entities
meaningful use
"one-write" systems
patient information form
patient ledger
payroll journal
plaintiff
protected health
  information (PHI)
self-pay patient
small claims litigation
surrogates
treatment, payment,
  or (healthcare)
  operations (TPO)
Truth in Lending Act

PATIENT EXPECTATIONS

When patients visit a healthcare practice, they bring something with them that may not be obvious to the healthcare team. Besides sore throats, broken legs, or heart palpitations, they bring a set of expectations with them. These expectations were created by previous experiences with other healthcare providers, the media, and the opinions of friends and family. If the healthcare provider and office staff members are oblivious to those expectations, the entire practice risks being perceived as cold and unfeeling. If the healthcare staff is successful in meeting or exceeding these expectations, the patient is likely to be pleased with the care he or she receives.

The first step in creating a good patient-staff relationship begins when the individual telephones for an appointment. How this encounter is handled can have a lasting impression on how the patient perceives the entire practice, including the healthcare providers. If the rapport between the physicians and the medical team is strained and uneasy, patients sense this and are likely to feel tension also. The bottom line is that overlooking patients' needs and expectations can be costly to the practice. Without patients, there is no practice.

It is also important to be up-front with office policies and procedures. When patients are sick or hurting, they usually do not feel up to questioning the medical staff about their policies or procedures. They usually are reacting from their physical symptoms, and their lack of questions or interest is caused by the fear of the unknown. Some conditions can be frightening, such as a burning chest pain or a breast lump. It is the responsibility of the medical staff to find out what patients' expectations are by asking questions. Being open with patients, anticipating their concerns, and creating an environment in which patients feel they can discuss their needs safely are comforting and affirming.

Patient expectations vary from office to office. The following are some issues to consider when evaluating new patient protocol.

Professional Office Setting

When individuals walk into a hardware or clothing store, they are looking for physical items—tangible things they can pick up, examine, and put into their shopping cart. If they are unhappy with the hammer or sweater purchased, they can voice a complaint or return the item for a refund. Most services offered by a healthcare facility are considered to be intangible—individuals cannot see or feel them. When individuals buy intangible services, they compensate by looking for **surrogates**, or substitutes to put their mind at ease. Surrogates that patients look for in a healthcare office may be the office location, size, and layout and staff enthusiasm. The color of the walls and the appearance of the reception area can affect a new patient's initial judgment about the quality of care that particular office provides. A shabby reception room suggests shabby care.

Relevant Paperwork and Questions

A substantial amount of paperwork typically must be completed and many questions need to be answered when seeing a healthcare provider for the first time. Besides being brief and of high quality, paperwork should seem relevant to the reason the patient is there. Personal questions such as whether a patient smokes or drinks, how many pregnancies a female patient has had, and whether a patient is divorced or widowed, should be asked privately out of hearing from office staff members and other patients. It also might be necessary to explain how these forms and questions relate to the individual's care and treatment.

Honoring Appointment Times

Time is a valuable commodity, and staying on schedule communicates respect for the patient's time. Because the encounter may be a new experience for a patient, when he or she phones for an appointment, time-management experts recommend that the medical receptionist explain approximately how long an initial visit will take and what to expect. If the healthcare provider gets behind schedule, which occurs frequently, patients can become annoyed, glancing at their watches, shifting in their seats, and looking at the receptionist expectantly for explanations. Out of courtesy, the receptionist should keep the patient advised as to the length of delay and the reason for the delay. The patient might be told, "Dr. Miller has been delayed because of an emergency, so you may have to wait another 10 or 15 minutes." The patient should be kept apprised of the anticipated time he or she will be seen: "Dr. Miller has just left the hospital and will be here in approximately 10 minutes." If it looks like the wait is going to be lengthy, the receptionist should offer to reschedule the patient's appointment or, if it is practical for the specific situation, ask if the patient has a brief errand to run. Many individuals today believe that their time is equally as valuable as the physician's, especially if they have taken time off work for their appointment.

⭐ Imagine This!

Jennifer Cooper had a 2 PM appointment with Dr. Shirley Bennet, a gynecologist. She arrived about 10 minutes early, as the receptionist recommended when she made the appointment. After completing all the necessary new patient forms, the receptionist advised Jennifer that Dr. Bennet had been called out on an emergency cesarean section and would be about a half hour late. The staff gave Jennifer the options of waiting or rescheduling. Jennifer, already having waited nearly 2 weeks for an opening in Dr. Bennet's schedule, chose to stay. Dr. Bennet kept the reception staff informed periodically as to how things were progressing, and this information was quickly and quietly passed on to Jennifer. Additionally, she was offered a choice of coffee or a cold soda. The reception room atmosphere was comfortable with pleasant background music and had an assortment of recent issues of magazines to browse through. Although Jennifer ended up waiting nearly 45 minutes for her appointment with Dr. Bennet, she did not become irritated or impatient because she was kept apprised of Dr. Bennet's schedule and was treated courteously by the staff.

⭐ Imagine This!

Lurvis Burke, a civil engineer with a consulting engineering firm, took time out of his busy schedule to visit a cardiologist for a routine stress test, recommended by his family physician. Lurvis had a 9 AM appointment with Dr. Harlan Solomon and arrived shortly before his appointment time, filled out the new patient paperwork, and sat down to wait. Two hours later, his name was called and a member of the medical staff ushered him to an examination room without a word. When Dr. Solomon entered the examination room where Lurvis was waiting, he found an angry patient who informed him that he did not appreciate the long wait and that he considered his time just as important as the physician's. Lurvis vowed not to return to Dr. Solomon's office in the future. Compare this patient's experience with that of Jennifer Cooper.

🕐 Stop and Think

Reread the "Imagine This!" scenario featuring Lurvis Burke. Do you think Mr. Burke is justified in his decision not to return to this office? How would you have handled this situation if you were the front desk receptionist?

Patient Load

A new patient often draws conclusions about the competency of the healthcare provider and the entire healthcare team by observing how many others are waiting in the reception area. If the reception area is empty when the patient enters, he or she may think, "Why aren't there more people here? Maybe this doctor isn't very good." To avoid this negative reaction, some experts suggest scheduling new patients during a time when the practice is busiest. This can be a workable solution as long as it does not result in a longer wait for established patients.

★ Imagine This!

Juanita Lindo, the medical receptionist for Anthony Park, a neurosurgeon, informed new patients when scheduling appointments that Dr. Park preferred reserving an ample amount of time for the encounter. The physician allowed a half hour before the examination, an hour for the examination, and a half hour after to answer all questions and ensure the patient and family members were comfortable and well informed as to their options before leaving his office. When a patient arrived for an appointment, he or she was already aware of how long the encounter would take, explaining the absence of a reception room full of waiting patients.

Getting Comfortable with the Healthcare Provider

It is human nature for patients to want to like their physicians as much as respect them. Perceptive patients expect their physicians to reveal enough information about themselves so that they can identify with them. The physician and staff members do not need to discuss their personal lives with patients, but sharing some personal information promotes a good provider-patient relationship and often tends to relieve anxiety if the physician and staff members compare a personal experience that is relevant to what the patient is experiencing.

★ Imagine This!

Dottie Shrike visited Dr. Forrest Carpenter, her family practitioner, for treatment of an episode of anxiety and mild depression after being fired from her job as a teacher's aide. Dr. Carpenter, attempting to alleviate some of Dottie's angst, related a story about an experience he had had before becoming a physician. He was working for a trucking firm and had lost his job because of noncompliance with company policy. He was young then, like Dottie, and the experience left him feeling humiliated and vulnerable. Relating this story to Dottie allowed her to feel as if he really understood her problem, reinforcing the provider-patient relationship.

Privacy and Confidentiality

If the medical professional wants patients to reveal their personal health-related problems, patients must feel confident that this information will be kept private and confidential. If patients who are waiting in the reception room hear the front desk staff talking about other patients, it can lead them to believe that their own information will be treated casually, too. The office staff must make every effort possible to assure patients that any personal information they divulge will be held in the strictest confidence. When making and receiving telephone calls, staff members should speak quietly or close the glass partition (which is recommended by Health Insurance Portability and Accountability Act [HIPAA] regulations) so that conversations do not carry into the reception area. Also, the entire medical staff should be cautioned when talking among themselves or to patients in examining rooms. Walls are often thin, allowing voices to carry into adjacent rooms.

Financial Issues

Most patients have an idea of what their medical care and treatment should cost before they make an appointment. Some patients even do "comparison shopping." Although many patients may be embarrassed or uneasy discussing fees, especially ahead of time, it is good business practice to discuss the financial ramifications of the healthcare encounter. Most physicians prefer to leave the subject of fees to their reception staff. When a new patient telephones for an appointment and explains his or her condition or symptoms that prompted the call, giving the individual a range of what the initial fee would be is considered appropriate. Healthcare consumers expect the cost of their healthcare to be addressed up-front.

⏱ Stop and Think

Mary Ellen Brown calls Dr. Bennet's office for an appointment. She explains that she is new in the area and is looking for a "good OB-GYN" because she thinks she may be pregnant. What kind of information might the medical receptionist give Mrs. Brown?

💬 What Did You Learn?

1. Besides their health problems, what do patients bring with them to the healthcare office?
2. List four issues that affect patient expectations.
3. Why is a clean, well-kept reception room important?
4. What is the rationale of explaining policies and fees up-front to patients?

FUTURE TRENDS

Most healthcare experts agree that healthcare today bears little resemblance to healthcare a decade ago. The United States is faced with a rapidly changing healthcare environment, and individuals who are involved in the healthcare field must identify and anticipate future trends—from new technology to changing directions and demographics.

Aging Population

Over the next 30 years, as the baby boomer generation ages, the number of Americans older than age 65 will increase considerably. Healthcare facilities will need to be prepared to handle a growing volume of elderly patients; these elderly patients will have different medical needs than young adult or pediatric patients. Healthcare staff members should be aware of, or even specially trained in, particular skills for interacting with this demographic faction. Many local medical organizations or community colleges offer continuing education courses in the care and treatment of elderly patients.

Internet as a Healthcare Tool

The Internet offers access to a lot of relevant, quality healthcare information. Websites deliver large amounts of healthcare knowledge to consumers, allowing them to form their own opinions and expectations. Individuals are involved in the relatively new process of self-education that was not possible before the advent of the Internet. Websites can help individuals find physicians and hospitals that offer certain procedures; other websites offer lifestyle advice plus educational details and references for a multitude of health conditions.

Internet tools that can be used to reach the computer-oriented consumer can help healthcare facilities serve patients better. Some successful online patient-centered topics include

- physician-patient communication,
- online scheduling (e.g., examinations, procedures),
- online billing services,
- physician biographies, and
- procedural information.

It is predicted that patients in the future will rely more and more on the Internet, and healthcare providers will have to adapt their practices to meet these state-of-the-art electronic requirements.

> ⭐ **Imagine This!**
>
> Greg Manning was diagnosed with prostate cancer, and the options his physician gave him held a high probability of impotence, which was unacceptable to Greg. He logged onto the Internet and began an extensive search for possible alternatives. He found a clinic in another state where the medical staff offered a relatively new, noninvasive procedure that was highly successful in patients with similar malignancies. Greg traveled to the clinic and met with the staff physicians to discuss the procedure. Greg was happy with the alternative they presented and subsequently underwent the new procedure successfully.

Patients as Consumers

As evidenced by the increase in medical news on television and in advertising, radio broadcasts, periodicals, and Internet sites, the healthcare industry must acknowledge a new type of patient—one who is more educated, more aware of choices, and more likely to take an active part in his or her own healthcare decisions. Experts say that patients should be considered "consumers," rather than "patients." Today, Americans are exposed to a vast amount of medical information on a daily basis through various media outlets. Some of this information can be misleading and confusing. Whether or not patients are correctly informed, however, healthcare providers are expected to take the time to satisfy patients' questions about diagnosis, treatment, and therapy options.

A new set of healthcare consumer essentials has been developed that experts believe should become mandatory for any healthcare facility that endeavors to provide patient-centered service. These essentials include

- choice,
- control (self-care, self-management),
- shared medical decision making,
- customer service, and
- information.

Similar to other types of consumers, patients today are likely to switch healthcare plans or healthcare providers if they believe they are not getting the quality service they desire.

> ❓ **What Did You Learn?**
>
> 1. List three things that affect future trends in the healthcare office.
> 2. How might the Internet change the future of healthcare?
> 3. Name three medical services that currently are being offered over the Internet.
> 4. List four healthcare consumer imperatives that experts claim should be mandatory for patient-centered services.

HEALTH INSURANCE PORTABILITY AND ACCOUNTABILITY ACT (HIPAA) REQUIREMENTS

HIPAA has had a big impact on healthcare, in particular, where confidentiality is concerned. What is contained in a patient's health record has always been confidential—dating back to the wording of the Hippocratic Oath. However, HIPAA has refined the rules of confidentiality for covered entities in a much more comprehensive way.

Authorization to Release Information

The release of any information contained in a patient's health record to a third party, with certain exceptions, is prohibited by law. Civil and criminal penalties exist for the unauthorized release of such information. A healthcare provider can be allowed to release confidential information from an individual's health records only with the consent of the individual or the person authorized to give consent for that individual. However, patient consent is not required if the information is used or disclosed for **treatment, payment, or healthcare operations (TPO)**.

HIPAA and Covered Entities

HIPAA is a federal law designed to protect the privacy of individuals' health information. A major component of HIPAA addresses this privacy by establishing a nationwide federal standard concerning the privacy of health information and how health information can be used and disclosed. This federal standard generally preempts all state privacy laws except for laws that establish stronger protections. HIPAA privacy laws became effective on April 14, 2003.

HIPAA requires all employees and staff (including volunteers) at healthcare facilities to sign a confidentiality agreement to protect patients' privacy. To view an example Confidentiality Agreement, visit the Evolve site.

HIPAA-covered entities consist of healthcare providers, health plans (including employer-sponsored plans), and healthcare clearing houses (including billing agents). These covered entities must comply with HIPAA rules for any health information of identifiable individuals. Health information that is protected under HIPAA is referred to as individually identifiable health information or, more commonly, **protected health information (PHI)**. PHI refers not only to data that are explicitly linked to a particular individual but also health information with data items that reasonably could be expected to allow individual identification. PHI includes medical records, medical billing records, any clinical or research databases, and tissue bank samples. HIPAA regulations allow researchers to access and use PHI when necessary to conduct research. However, HIPAA affects only research that uses, creates, or discloses PHI that will be entered into the medical record or will be used for healthcare services, such as TPO. Covered entities generally are unable to communicate or transfer PHI to non-covered entities (who do not come under HIPAA rules) without violating HIPAA.

Potential identifiers that can link information to a particular individual include obvious ones, such as name and Social Security number. A more comprehensive list of potential PHI identifiers can be found on the Evolve site.

Note: The covered entity may assign a code or other means of identification to allow de-identified information, if it later = becomes necessary to reidentify the information. When the identifiable elements are removed, the information is, under most circumstances, considered **de-identified**.

HIPAA Tip

Covered entities such as health plans, healthcare providers, and claims clearinghouses must comply with HIPAA rules. Other businesses may comply voluntarily with the standards, but the law does not require them to do so.

HIPAA Requirements for Covered Entities

HIPAA Transaction 5010

The Administrative Simplification Act requires all physicians, providers, and suppliers who bill Medicare carriers, fiscal intermediaries, Medicare administrative contractors (MACs) for Parts A and B, and durable medical equipment MACs for services provided to Medicare beneficiaries to submit claims electronically with certain exceptions. With the adoption of the new ICD-10 diagnosis codes (discussed in Chapter 12), the Accredited Standards Committee X12 Version 4010/4010A1 that was adopted in 2000 (and modified in 2003) will become obsolete, because they cannot accommodate the expanded format of the ICD-10 code sets.

The Centers for Medicare and Medicaid Services (CMS) introduced a new version of standards, called the HIPAA 5010 Transaction Standards. As a prerequisite for implementing the new ICD-10 codes by 2013, claims and certain administrative transactions must be submitted electronically using the X12 Version 5010 Standards by June 30, 2012. Failure to implement these changes by the specified date could result in penalties. The 5010 Standards impact the data that are transmitted via the 837P, which is the electronic data set equivalent to the paper CMS 1500 (08/05) form.

It is important that covered entities and the health insurance professionals who work for them are aware of, understand, and help plan for the changes that the HIPAA 5010 Transaction Standards present. New software systems and maybe even revisions in billing procedures in use before this date may be needed to become compliant.

For more detailed information on the HIPAA 5010 Transaction, visit the Evolve site.

It is important that health insurance professionals keep abreast of these and other potential changes involving electronic claims transactions. The CMS website is a good resource for keeping up-to-date.

Proposed Changes to the CMS-1500 Form

As noted in Chapter 5, as a result of the conversion to the 5010 Standards, the National Uniform Claims Committee (NUCC) proposed certain data reporting revisions in the Version 005010 837 professional electronic claim transaction that could affect the paper CMS-1500 form. After considering several options for completely revising the form, the NUCC decided to make "minor changes" to the existing form. Also, a revised NUCC 1500 Reference Instruction Manual is being developed for the revised form when it officially takes effect. For a list of the proposed changes and to view a mock-up of the "cleaned" form, log onto the NUCC website at http://www.nucc.org/. Health insurance professionals should keep up-to-date with these potential changes to the 1500 form by periodically logging on to the NUCC website.

Patient's Right of Access and Correction

The HIPAA privacy rules provide for the patient's right to correct or amend his or her medical record. Although HIPAA rules limit this right by reasonable protections for the covered entity who controls the protected information, a patient has a right to ask for corrections or amendments to his or her medical record and to place an explanation into the record if that request is denied. The privacy notice that a medical practice gives to patients must specify how they should make requests to amend their records (e.g., in writing). The practice may refuse such a request for several reasons, including that the patient's record is accurate and complete. However, the patient has the right to appeal. If the practice agrees to amend the patient's record, it must notify the individual and others to whom the information was provided that the record has been amended. However, the rules do not include a requirement that incorrect information be removed from the record; rather, it should be labeled as corrected, and the correction should be appended.

HIPAA provides a limited public policy exception for PHI disclosure involving public health issues, judicial and administrative proceedings, law enforcement purposes, and others as required by law. To learn more about what HIPAA requires of covered entities, visit the Evolve site.

Update: A federal rule, proposed by the Department of Health and Human Services in 2011, would require hospitals, physicians' offices, and insurance companies to advise a patient, if requested, of anyone who has accessed the patient's electronic medical record (EMR). Under this proposed rule, healthcare-related businesses must list everyone in their firms—from physicians to data-entry clerks—who has accessed a patient's EMR and when. To keep up-to-date on this proposed rule, visit the Evolve site.

> **📁 HIPAA Tip**
>
> Basic patient rights under HIPAA include the following:
> 1. Right to notice of privacy practices (NOPP)
> 2. Right to access to PHI
> 3. Right to an accounting of how PHI has been disclosed outside normal patient care channels
> 4. Right to request an amendment or correction to PHI

Accessing Information through Patient Authorization

HIPAA states that when an authorization to release information (Fig. 14-1) is required from a patient, it must include the following elements:

- A description that identifies the information in a specific and meaningful fashion
- The name of the person authorized to make the requested use or disclosure
- The name of the person to whom the covered entity may make the requested use or disclosure
- A description of each purpose of the requested use or disclosure
- An expiration date or event that relates to the purpose of the use or disclosure
- A statement of the individual's right to revoke the authorization in writing and the exceptions to the right to revoke, with a description of how the individual may revoke the authorization
- A statement that information used may be subject to additional disclosure by the recipient and no longer be protected by this rule
- Signature of the individual and date signed
- A description of a representative's authority to act for an individual if the authorization is signed by a personal representative of the individual.

> **📁 HIPAA Tip**
>
> Uses and disclosures not requiring patient consent include:
> 1. To carry out treatment, payment, or healthcare operations (TPO)
> 2. For public health, health oversight, judicial or administrative proceedings, coroners and medical examiners, and law enforcement

Accessing Information through De-identification

Covered entities can release de-identified health information without patient authorization. PHI can be de-identified through a general deletion of specific identifiers, such as name, address, telephone number, Social Security number, medical record number, and any other of the 18 elements that may identify a patient. To release the information without

Standard Authorization to Use or Disclose Protected Health Information (PHI)

Section A: The individual for whom this authorization is being requested. Please complete the following:

Name: First _____ M ____ Last _____   Group # _____   Identification # _____

Social Security Number _____   Date of Birth _____

Address _____   City _____   State ____ ZIP ____

Area Code & Telephone Number _____   E-mail Address (if available) _____

Section B: Please place an "X" in the box next to each category of specific Protected Health Information to disclose. (You may mark as many boxes as appropriate.)

☐ Any and All Information about my CHIP Coverage   ☐ Claims   ☐ Premium Payment/Billing History

☐ Eligibility and Enrollment   ☐ Other (describe): _____

Section C: Describe the reason for the release or request of information.

☐ At my request   ☐ Other (describe): _____

Section D: Who will provide this information?

Name   CHIP and its Plan Administrator

Address   400 W. Monroe, Suite 202

Anytown, IL 08095

Relationship   Health Plan

Section E: Who will receive this information?

Name _____

Address _____

Relationship _____

Section F: Please place an "X" in the box next to the date or event that describes when your authorization will expire. (Please mark only one box.)

☐ Upon Revocation   ☐ 1 year after my death   ☐ 1 year after my CHIP coverage ends

☐ A specific date: _____ Month Day Year   ☐ Other (describe): _____

Section G: I understand that:

- This authorization will expire on the date or event listed in Section F above.
- This authorization is voluntary.
- Payment, enrollment or eligibility for benefits for my health care will not be affected if I do not sign this form.
- I may revoke this authorization at any time by notifying in writing the company/individual listed in Section D from providing the PHI identified in this authorization, but if I do revoke this authorization, it won't have any affect on any actions the Comprehensive Health Insurance Plan took before they received the revocation.
- Information disclosed as a result of this authorization may no longer be protected by federal privacy laws and may be disclosed by the company or individual receiving the information.
- I should retain as my copy one of the duplicate authorization forms I received.

Section H: Signature.

I hereby authorize the use or disclosure of the Protected Health Information as described in Section B pertaining to the Individual listed in Section A.

Signature of Individual or Individual's Personal Representative _____   Date: month/day/year _____

Section I: If Section H is signed by a Personal Representative, please complete the information below:

Personal Representative's Name _____   Relationship to Individual _____

Personal Representative's Address _____   City _____   State ____ ZIP ____

Personal Representative's Area Code & Telephone Number _____   Personal Representative's E-mail Address (if available) _____

TPAuth Rev 6.03   Page 1 of 1 (See Instructions on Next Page)   Standard Authorization–CHIP

Fig. 14-1 HIPAA-approved release of information form.

patient authorization, the covered entity cannot have actual information that could be used alone or in combination with other information to identify an individual. For more detailed information on de-identification of PHI, visit the Evolve site.

Stop and Think

What information in the following documentation should be removed to de-identify this patient?

Frasier, Eric
DOB 1/13/1977
Patient #12112
6/10/20XX

History: Eric presents to the clinic today for chief complaint of an abrasion on the right knee following a fall yesterday. According to the patient, he has had this soft tissue lesion for some time, and when he fell, he abraded the lower half of the lesion. He is here for reevaluation and possible excision of the lesion.

Pain assessment: Scale 0 to 10, 1
Allergies: Meperidine (Demerol)
Current medications: None
Physical examination: NAD; ambulatory; appears well
Vital signs: Blood pressure 120/74 mm Hg; weight 150 lb
Right knee examination: The patient has a tibial prominence, and just above that, there is what appears to be a 1.5-cm epidermal inclusion cyst with an abraded area inferiorly. There is mild erythema and serous drainage but no purulence. There is no appreciable edema. Just lateral to the lesion is a small superficial abrasion. The knee examination was normal.

IMP: Epidermal inclusion cyst measuring 1.5 to 2 cm of the right knee, traumatized with abrasion

Plan: The patient was empirically started on cephalexin (Keflex) 500 mg 1 p.o. b.i.d. He was given instructions on home care and is to follow up this week for excision of the lesion. Routine follow-up as noted. Return as needed.

Frederick Mahoney, MD
Friendly Family Clinic

Note: To see a list of 18 patient identifiers, visit the Evolve site.

What Did You Learn?

1. What are the three entities that are covered under HIPAA?
2. List at least six elements that make a patient health record identifiable.
3. How does a patient health record become de-identifiable?
4. Name three exceptions to the confidentiality rule.

BILLING POLICIES AND PRACTICES

Although specific billing policies and procedures differ from one practice to another, the goals are similar. Many healthcare facilities anticipate that the patient will pay for services or procedures the same day they are rendered. If the patient has insurance, most offices collect a partial payment (copay) or coinsurance—typically 10% to 25% of the fee—on the day of the visit. If the patient does not have insurance, he or she may be expected to pay in full at the time of the visit or make payment arrangements if the office policy allows this option. Some third-party carriers indicate the amount of copay the patient must make on the face of the insurance identification card. Medical facilities are in business to make a profit; procedures and policies should be in place to protect the financial success of the practice.

Assignment of Benefits

An **assignment of benefits** is an arrangement by which a patient requests that his or her health insurance benefit payments be made directly to a designated person or facility such as a physician or hospital. When new patients come to the healthcare office, they are typically requested to fill out a form providing name, address, employer, and health insurance information. Usually at the bottom of the page is a place for the patient's signature or, in the case of a minor or mentally handicapped individual, the signature of a parent or legal guardian. This form is commonly referred to as the **patient information form**.

On many patient information forms, in addition to the authorization to release information, there is nomenclature above the patient's signature that provides for the assignment of benefits, authorizing this transfer of payment from the insured to the healthcare provider. Sometimes the assignment of benefits is a separate document. It is common for a healthcare provider to refuse to see a patient unless this assignment of benefits is signed, or unless payment is made up-front. Infrequently, a health insurance contract may include a clause that prohibits the assignment of benefits. If the insurance contract disallows it, the carrier does not have to honor a patient's assignment of benefits. The only exception is if there is a state law mandating it, such as in Florida and Louisiana. If assignment is prohibited, the benefit payment goes directly to the patient or contract member.

Many healthcare providers participate in a health maintenance organization, a preferred provider organization, or some similar organization. These practitioners are referred to as participating providers. When a provider is a participating provider, assigning benefits on the CMS-1500 form or on the patient information form is unnecessary because there is a contractual agreement between the provider and the third-party carrier that payment automatically is sent directly to the provider. That is one of the benefits to becoming a participating provider.

Keeping Patients Informed

It is important that patients understand the patient accounting policies and procedures of the healthcare practice, such as

- approximately how much the medical service or procedure will cost,
- when patients are expected to pay for services, and
- if the practice is willing to submit claims to insurance carriers.

Discussing professional fees with patients is an important step that requires a sensitive and balanced approach by the health insurance professional. Patients should not be intimidated or offended when discussing fees and payment policies; however, the health insurance professional should ensure that patients are clear about their responsibilities. Most patients appreciate having billing information presented clearly and matter-of-factly, yet always in a pleasant and courteous manner. The healthcare office staff should encourage patients to ask questions about their bills or the payment or insurance process. Many offices have printed materials available such as an informational brochure for stating or reinforcing the financial policies and procedures of the practice. This written information can be helpful in collecting fees.

Establishing sound billing practices is important in a healthcare office. Although medical practitioners are dedicated to the health and well-being of their patients, they are ultimately running a business for the purpose of making a profit. Keeping accurate financial records is just as important as keeping accurate patient health records.

The ultimate goal in healthcare office billing is reimbursement or payment for the medical services provided to patients. A satisfactory collection ratio (the total amount collected divided by the total amount charged) can be challenging at times. Some healthcare offices display a sign that payment for services rendered is expected on the day services are provided. In other words, patients are expected to pay as they go, just as retail stores expect customers to pay for a tube of toothpaste or a can of soup at the time of purchase.

The receptionist should request payment on the day of the visit, either before or after the encounter is concluded. Experts consider this the most effective payment policy. Patients who put off paying for their services are historically more difficult to collect from. It is common practice for the receptionist to ask for a particular percentage—often 20%—of the current charge; 20% is a common coinsurance amount.

> ### 🕐 Stop and Think
>
> The accounts receivable total of Dr. David Barclay's office was $231,500 for the first quarter of the year. If $173,625 of this amount was successfully collected, what would be Dr. Barclay's collection ratio for this quarter?

Accounting Methods

There is a good chance that the office where the health insurance professional finds employment uses a computerized patient accounting system for financial records. This is not always the case, however, and the health insurance professional should be aware of how paper accounting records are generated and maintained. A typical paper method of accounting includes a series of journals and ledgers such as the following:

A **daily journal** (or day sheet) (Fig. 14-2) is a chronological record of all patient transactions including previous balances, charges, payments, and current balances for that day.

A **disbursements journal** (Fig. 14-3) is a listing of all expenses paid out to vendors such as building rent, office supplies, and salaries. Some offices maintain a separate **payroll journal** (Fig. 14-4) for wages and salaries.

A **general journal**, the most basic of journals, is a chronological listing of transactions. It has a specific format for recording each transaction. Each transaction is recorded separately and consists of

- a date,
- all accounts that receive a debit entry (these are typically listed first with an amount in the appropriate column),
- all accounts that receive a credit entry (these are indented and listed next with an amount in the appropriate column), and
- a clear description of each transaction.

A **general ledger** is the core of the practice's financial records. The general ledger constitutes the central "books" of an accounting system; every transaction flows through the general ledger. These records remain as permanent tracking of the history of all financial transactions from day 1 of the life of a practice. The general ledger can be used to prepare a range of periodic financial statements such as income statements and balance sheets.

A **patient ledger** (Fig. 14-5) is a chronological accounting of activities of a particular patient (or family) including all charges and payments. The entire group of patient ledgers is referred to as the **accounts receivable**.

"One-Write" or Pegboard Accounting System

Paper accounting systems, such as "one-write" or "write-it-once" systems, have been widely used in physicians' offices over the years. **"One-write" systems** (Fig. 14-6) (also known as the pegboard system) were a practical method of accounting for medical practices before computers and patient accounting software became widely available. These systems were considered efficient because, through the use of shingled documents with carbon strips, they captured information at the time the transaction occurred on multiple documents, eliminating the need for recopying the data, which can lead to errors. A few businesses (i.e., small rural clinics, dentists, and veterinarians) still use a one-write system because of its low cost, simplicity, and versatility. One-write systems are inexpensive and easy to learn.

	PLACE FIRST PEG HERE	DATE	PROFESSIONAL SERVICE	FEE	PAYMENT	ADJUST-MENT	NEW BALANCE	OLD BALANCE	PATIENT'S NAME

JOURNAL OF DAILY CHARGES, PAYMENTS & DEPOSITS

	DATE	PROFESSIONAL SERVICE	FEE	PAYMENT	ADJUST-MENT	NEW BALANCE	OLD BALANCE	PATIENT'S NAME
1								
2								
3								
4								
5								
6								
7								
8								
9								
10								
11								
12								
13								
14								
15								
16								Totals this page
17								Totals previous page
18								Totals to date

COLUMN A   COLUMN B   COLUMN C   COLUMN D   COLUMN E

MEMO _____

DAILY - FROM LINE 31

ARITHMETIC POSTING PROOF	
Column E	$
Plus Column A	
Sub-Total	
Minus Column B	
Sub-Total	
Minus Column C	
Equals Column D	

MONTH - FROM LINE 31

ACCOUNTS RECEIVABLE PROOF	
Accts. Receivable Previous Day	$
Plus Column A	
Sub-Total	
Minus Column B	
Sub-Total	
Minus Column C	
Accts. Receivable End of Day	

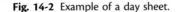

Fig. 14-2 Example of a day sheet.

Electronic Patient Accounting Software

Most healthcare offices are now computerized and use some type of electronic patient accounting software program. Previous barriers to computerization have been largely overcome by the introduction of cost-effective and user-friendly systems for the management of clinical records and appointments. Computerized patient billing software typically includes accounts receivable, appointment scheduling, insurance billing, and practice management modules.

Computerized patient accounting typically begins with inputting the demographic patient data (i.e., name, address, birth date) and creating a patient "account" within the software program. When all patient data have been entered into the system, patient lists and many other documents can be generated in several ways. A list of patient appointments by day and by provider and an encounter form for each one can be printed. When the patient encounter is concluded, the health insurance professional inputs the information from

FEBRUARY 2012

DATE	DESCRIPTION	CHECK NUMBER	AMOUNT	PER CAPITA	RENT	PHONE	OFFICE SUPPLIES	POSTAGE	OFFICERS' EXPENSE	NEWS LETTER
1-FEB	ABC Realty	291	475.00		475.00					
1-FEB	AFT	292	2,301.60	2,301.60						
1-FEB	State Fed	293	1,288.60	1,288.60						
1-FEB	Central Labor Council	294	75.60	75.60						
1-FEB	Bell Telephone	295	131.00			131.00				
7-FEB	State Fed	296	1,828.60	1,828.60						
21-FEB	Sue Smith, Sec'y	297	50.00						50.00	
28-FEB	Mary Jones, Petty Cash	298	18.50				16.00	2.50		
			6,168.90	5,494.40	475.00	131.00	16.00	2.50	50.00	0.00

Fig. 14-3 Sample cash disbursements journal.

Date	Employee	Hourly Rate	Regular Hours	Overtime Hours	Net Pay	Check Number	Federal Withholding	OASI	Insurance	Retirement	Other	Gross Pay	Fund	Account

Fig. 14-4 Payroll journal.

the encounter form including date, diagnosis code, procedure code, and charges. Also, any payments can be posted to the computer program. A current copy of the patient ledger can be printed and given to the patient as a statement or receipt. Appointments can be scheduled, deleted, and adjusted within the accounting system. Periodic statements, aging reports, and CMS-1500 claim forms can be generated.

The computer program performs all phases of the accounting process quickly and accurately. However, any system, whether computerized or manual, is only as good as the individual who inputs the information. Accuracy is crucial. A backup system is also crucial in case of power fluctuations or failure. Without a dependable backup system, all electronic data could be lost as a result of electrical problems or human error. Daily backups should be made and stored in a fireproof vault to prevent loss of patient records.

Electronic Medical Records

An EMR (also referred to as an electronic health record) stores a patient's health history and medical information in electronic format rather than on paper, eliminating the need for bulky files and space-consuming storage facilities. With an EMR, healthcare providers and other clinical staff

Westview General Practitioners Office
600 W Maple Road, Building 5000, Suite 301
Bridgeton, OR 63145-2099

STATEMENT TO:

JOHN Q. PUBLIC
1212 WEST PACIFIC LANE
SAN DIEGO, CA 99999

- -
TEAR OFF AND RETURN UPPER PORTION WITH PAYMENT

DATE 2012	PROFESSIONAL SERVICE	FEE	PAYMENT	ADJUST-MENT	NEW BALANCE
4/21	OV Level 2	125 00			125 00
4/21	ROA CK #555		25 00		100 00
4/22	XYZ Ins. submitted				
5/18	XYZ CK #010111A		100 00		—0—

Westview General Practitioners Office, 600 W Maple Road,
Building 5000, Suite 301, Bridgeton, OR 63145-2099

Fig. 14-5 Sample patient ledger card.

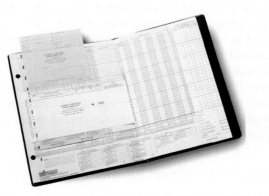

Fig. 14-6 Front office "one-write" (pegboard) billing example. (Courtesy Bibbero Systems, Inc., Petaluma Calif. [800] 242-2376; Fax [800] 242-9330; www.bibbero.com.)

members enter essential patient data—physicians' orders, prescriptions, and other important information—directly into a computer using a highly secure network. This process allows for better coordination of patient care through immediate access to secure data.

Recent Congressional legislation established a program that provides incentives to physicians and hospitals who use certified EMR technology in a meaningful manner, referred to as "meaningful use." **Meaningful use** incentives seek to encourage widespread EMR adoptions and ensure healthcare providers are using EMRs properly in their day-to-day operations. The goals are to reduce medical errors, improve overall patient care, and save money. EMRs are discussed in more detail in Chapter 16.

BILLING AND COLLECTION

Individuals who work in healthcare offices claim that collecting past due accounts is one of the least pleasant aspects of the job. Healthcare practices that maintain a high collection ratio say that the most effective way to collect money is to establish a formal financial policy that is clear to patients and that is enforced by healthcare staff members. Patients need to know that it is important to pay in full and on time, and the medical staff needs to know what is expected of them. The health insurance professional sometimes must take a firm stand, and the situation can become uncomfortable. An assertive approach to account collection does not have a negative effect on developing good rapport with patients. A collection policy that is fair and clear to patients and staff members results in fewer misunderstandings (Fig. 14-7).

Following is a list of suggestions that some healthcare practices use to aid their financial success. These items are often included in the practice's policy manual.

- Have a written payment and credit policy. Give a copy to each patient, and discuss it with him or her. Ensure that each point is understood.
- Do not ignore overdue bills. The older the bill, the more uncollectible it becomes. Begin a plan of action as soon as the account becomes 30 days old.
- Rebill promptly. Some experts suggest rebilling every 15 days, rather than the traditional 30 days. Stamp or place a sticker on the second statement with the words "Second Notice."
- Telephone or write a letter. This action can be effective if the second statement does not get a response from the patient.
- Do not apologize when telephoning or writing about delinquent bills. Simply ask the customer to write a check today for the full amount owed. If the patient is agreeable and the practice has the capability, immediate payment can be taken over the phone using a credit or debit card.
- Be pleasant and courteous. There is never a reason to get into an argument, even if the patient becomes hostile. Listen patiently to what the individual has to say without interrupting; try to be understanding.
- Ask for the full amount, not just a partial payment. If a patient owes $500, ask for the full $500. If the patient says he or she will send a partial payment, ask what the exact amount will be and what date the payment will be sent. Do not accept vague statements such as, "I'll send you something in a couple of days." Also, ask for a precise date when the remainder of the bill will be paid.
- Negotiate the terms but not the amount. If you believe the patient truly has a problem paying, offer to work out a payment plan, but do not make this offer right away; do this only as a last resort. Also, always adhere to the office policy when negotiating terms.
- Use the services of a small claims court. If patient promises are not kept or if the account ages past a certain time period (e.g., 60 days, depending on office policy), small claims litigation is an alternative.

Stop and Think

You notice that Theodore Simpson's account balance is $365, and he has not made a payment for 45 days. Office policy is to telephone patients 15 days after the last statement has been sent. How will you handle this? Create a telephone scenario of your conversation with Mr. Simpson.

Billing Cycle

Sending statements to patients on a regular basis is necessary to maintain cash flow for the practice and an acceptable collection ratio. Every healthcare office has its own routine for sending statements. Typically, statements are mailed every 30 days. This process is called a **billing cycle**. In large practices, one 30-day mass billing for all patients is a cumbersome task. Such facilities often use an **alternate billing cycle**—a billing system that incorporates the mailing of a partial group of statements at spaced intervals during the month. With an alternate billing cycle, the breakdown of accounts is frequently determined by an alphabetical list of last names or by account numbers. For example, patients with last names ending in "A" through "F" would be sent statements on the first of the month, patients with last names ending with "G" through "L" would receive statements on the 10th day of the month, and so forth. One advantage to an alternate billing cycle is that cash flow is distributed throughout the entire month, whereas billing only once a month generates a large amount of receipts at one time. No one specific method is considered best for all healthcare practices. Each practice must establish its own system that works well.

Note: If the patient has valid insurance coverage, it is important to make sure that the insurance carrier was billed appropriately and if the claim was denied before sending statements asking for the full amount.

Arranging Credit or Payment Plans

The cost of some medical treatments or procedures can be thousands of dollars, and the patient might not have adequate insurance coverage (or may have no insurance at all)

Payment Policy

Thank you for choosing our practice! We are committed to the success of your medical treatment and care. Please understand that payment of your bill is part of this treatment and care.

For your convenience, we have answered a variety of commonly asked financial policy questions below. If you need further information about any of these policies, please ask to speak with a Billing Specialist or the Practice Manager.

How May I Pay?
We accept payment by cash, check, VISA, Mastercard, American Express and Discover.

Do I Need A Referral?
If you have an HMO plan with which we are contracted, you need a referral authorization from your primary care physician. If we have not received an authorization prior to your arrival at the office, we have a telephone available for you to call your primary care physician to obtain it. If you are unable to obtain the referral at that time, you will be rescheduled.

Which Plans Do You Contract With?
Please see attached list.

What Is My Financial Responsibility for Services?
Your financial responsibility depends on a variety of factors, explained below.

Office Visits and Office Services

If you have:	You are Responsible for:	Our staff will:
Commercial Insurance Also known as indemnity, "regular" insurance, or "80%/20% coverage."	Payment of the patient responsibility for all office visit, x-ray, injection, and other charges at the time of office visit.	Call your insurance company ahead of time to determine deductibles and coinsurance. File an insurance claim as a courtesy to you.
Medicare HMO	All applicable copays and deductibles at the time of the office visit.	File the claim on your behalf, as well as any claims to your secondary insurance.
Workers' Compensation	If we have verified the claim with your carrier No payment is necessary at the time of the visit. If we are not able to verify your claim Payment in full is requested at the time of the visit.	Call your carrier ahead of time to verify the accident date, claim number, primary care physician, employer information, and referral procedures.
Workers' Compensation (Out of State)	Payment in full is requested at the time of the visit.	Provide you a receipt so you can file the claim with your carrier.
Occupational Injury	Payment in full is requested at the time of the visit.	Provide you a receipt so you can file the claim with your carrier.
No Insurance	Payment in full at the time of the visit.	Work with you to settle your account. Please ask to speak with our staff if you need assistance.

Fig. 14-7 Payment policy. (Courtesy Karen Zupko & Associates.)

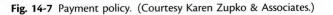

to pay the medical fees. Many healthcare facilities offer patient financing plans, which allow patients to get treatments or procedures and pay for them in periodic installments—similar to buying a car. A comprehensive range of plan options that offer low, or at least manageable, monthly payments to fit almost every budget is available in healthcare facilities across the United States.

Self-Pay Patients

Some patients may have inadequate health insurance coverage or no insurance at all. These are referred to as **self-pay patients**. Just because patients are self-pay does not mean they would deliberately try to avoid paying their bills. Some individuals who do not carry health insurance are still able to pay their medical bills in a timely manner.

As mentioned previously, the patient should be provided with the policies and expectations of the healthcare practice early on in the encounter. Under most state laws, full payment for medical services is due and payable at the time the service is provided. However, healthcare providers often take the initiative to temper this mandate as they see fit.

When a patient completes the patient information form, and there is no insurance listed, the health insurance professional should inquire about the reason. It is possible that the insurance section was overlooked. If the patient has no insurance, it is prudent to inquire tactfully how the patient intends to pay for the service. Some healthcare offices ask the patient whether or not he or she has insurance when the appointment is made and, if not, the patient must make at least a partial payment in advance.

Ideally, the practice should have an established credit plan for self-pays because it is mandatory that every patient be treated equally. Equally as important, the healthcare office cannot refuse to see an established patient because of an outstanding debt. There is a procedure, however, whereby (if carried out within the confines of the law) a healthcare provider can terminate the patient-provider relationship. This procedure involves sending a certified letter to the patient, with a return receipt to confirm the patient received the letter, communicating the fact that the patient can no longer be treated (for whatever reason spelled out in the letter), and giving the patient a specified amount of time to find alternative care. Following this structured method of notifying the patient that the practice will no longer accept him or her as a patient and spelling out the reason why limit the practice's liability in the event of legal action brought by the patient accusing the practice of "abandonment."

Establishing Credit

When patients cannot make payment in full, credit is sometimes arranged, and a payment plan is established (Fig. 14-8). Some medical facilities offer a credit arrangement whereby the patient can pay the fee, interest-free, in several installments. Other medical facilities allow more flexibility for self-paying patients by offering an installment plan with interest rates lower than most major credit cards.

An installment payment plan of more than four payments comes under the federal Truth in Lending Act of 1968, Regulation Z. Regulation Z applies to each individual or business that offers or extends consumer credit if the following four conditions are met:
1. The credit is offered to consumers.
2. Credit is offered on a regular basis.
3. The credit is subject to a finance charge (i.e., interest) or must be paid in more than four installments according to a written agreement.
4. The credit is primarily for personal, family, or household purposes.

The Truth in Lending Act of 1968 and Regulation Z are discussed in more detail later.

Problem Patients

Sometimes the health insurance professional may know or have reason to believe that it will be difficult to collect fees from a particular patient. A policy should be in place for "problem" patients such as these or for patients who, for whatever reason, "send up a red flag." Following are some suggestions to maximize collection success from problem or questionable patients:
• Contact a local credit bureau to find out if the patient is creditworthy.

---

5   Financial Arrangements

Payment is expected at time of service.

For your convenience, we offer the following methods of payment. Please check the option which you prefer.

_____ Cash

_____ Personal Check

_____ Credit Card   _____ Visa   _____ Mastercard

_____ I wish to make arrangements with an office manager today.

Late Charges

I realize that failure to keep this account current may result in you being unable to provide additional services except for emergencies or where there is prepayment for additional services. In the case of default on payment of this account, I agree to pay collection costs and reasonable attorney fees incurred in attempting to collect on this amount or any future outstanding account balances.

Thank you for filling out this form completely.
The information you have provided will help us serve your healthcare needs more effectively and efficiently.
If you have any questions at any time, please ask – we are always happy to help.

Fig. 14-8 Sample of financial arrangement plan.

- Discuss the credit policy with the patient before the encounter, and establish a payment that is affordable for the patient.
- Have the patient sign a written agreement.
- Ask the patient to make a down payment of at least 20%.
- Arrange with the patient and his or her bank for automatic withdrawals if the patient has an account where that is a viable option.
- Charge interest (if that is practice policy) or a "carrying fee" to give the patient added incentive to make regular payments and pay off the balance promptly.

Note: Even if the practice does not charge interest, if it is mutually agreed that the account will be paid off in more than four payments, the practice by law must provide the patient with a copy of the Truth in Lending Law.

- Arrange to have payments automatically deducted each month on a presigned credit card form.
- Do not allow the payments to extend past the treatment program, or 12 months, whichever is the shorter time.
- Provide the patient with a self-addressed, stamped, return envelope in each bill.

Keep a copy of the signed agreement on file so that the office staff can refer to the agreement for specific monthly payments or fees for missed payments. Most healthcare offices keep these agreements in a separate file rather than in the patient's health record.

When setting up payment arrangements, be considerate but firm. The health insurance professional should explain the payment plan clearly, emphasizing that payments must not be missed and that the payment must be received on or before the due date.

For more tips on medical collection procedures, visit the Evolve site.

> **? What Did You Learn?**
>
> 1. List five things a healthcare practice can do to aid in its financial success.
> 2. Explain how an alternate billing cycle can be used.
> 3. What is meant by a self-pay patient?
> 4. Name the four conditions that must be met under Regulation Z when a business extends credit.

LAWS AFFECTING CREDIT AND COLLECTION

Because healthcare offices typically extend credit to their patients, they need to comply with federal consumer credit laws. It is important that the health insurance professional become acquainted with collection laws. The relevant federal laws dealing with consumer credit are introduced in this section.

Truth in Lending Act

The **Truth in Lending Act** helps consumers of all kinds. It requires the person or business entity to disclose the exact credit terms when extending credit to applicants and regulates

how the business advertises consumer credit. The following items must be disclosed to a consumer who buys on credit:
- The monthly finance charge
- The annual interest rate
- When payments are due
- The total sale price (the cash price of the item or service, plus all other charges)
- The amount of any late payment charges, and when they will be imposed

Fair Credit Billing Act

The **Fair Credit Billing Act** (FCBA) sets guidelines for disputing what a consumer believes to be an error on his or her credit card statement. The FCBA applies only to accounts considered to be open-end accounts, such as credit card accounts and charge accounts issued by department stores. The FCBA does not apply to installment loans. The FCBA would apply to medical practices if the practice allows patients to pay with credit cards. In addition to advising how to handle billing disputes, the FCBA requires that the entity granting credit tell consumers (in periodic mailings) what their rights are.

Equal Credit Opportunity Act

The **Equal Credit Opportunity Act** states that a business entity may not discriminate against a credit applicant on the basis of race, color, religion, national origin, age, sex, or marital status. The Equal Credit Opportunity Act does allow freedom to consider legitimate factors in granting credit, such as the applicant's financial status (earnings and savings) and credit record. Despite the prohibition on age discrimination, a consumer who has not reached the legal age for entering into contracts can be rejected.

Fair Credit Reporting Act

The **Fair Credit Reporting Act** deals primarily with credit reports issued by credit reporting agencies. It is intended to protect consumers from having their eligibility for credit damaged by incomplete or misleading credit report information. The law gives consumers the right to a copy of their credit reports. If they see an inaccurate item, they can ask that it be corrected or removed. If the business entity reporting the credit problem does not agree to a change or deletion, or if the credit bureau refuses to make it, the consumer can add a 100-word statement to the file explaining his or her side of the story. This statement becomes a part of any future credit report.

Fair Debt Collection Practices Act

The **Fair Debt Collection Practices Act** addresses abusive methods used by third-party collectors—bill collectors hired to collect overdue bills. Small businesses are more directly affected by state laws that apply directly to collection methods used by a creditor. The Fair Debt Collection Practices Act states that unless a debtor consents or a court order permits, debt collectors may not call to collect a debt

- at any time or place that is unusual or known to be inconvenient to the consumer (8 AM to 9 PM is presumed to be convenient);
- when the creditor is aware that the debtor is represented by an attorney with respect to the debt, unless the attorney fails to respond to the communication in a reasonable time period; and
- at work if the creditor is aware of the fact that the patient's employer prohibits such contacts. .

What Did You Learn?

1. List the five federal laws that affect credit and collection.
2. Generally, if a state law allows more time for the debtor to notify the creditor about a billing error than the federal statute does, which prevails?
3. What does the Equal Credit Opportunity Act address?
4. Name the three telephone limitations upheld by the Fair Debt Collection Practices Act.

COLLECTION METHODS

No matter how experienced, how resourceful, or how persuasive the health insurance professional or collection manager is, there always will be some bad debts in a healthcare practice. Two common methods healthcare offices use for collecting bad debts are collection by telephone and collection by letter.

Collection by Telephone

Collecting overdue accounts by phone is a job that many healthcare office employees would prefer not to do. It is so much easier to write a collection letter than to call a patient about a delinquent account, but the collection call is considered far more effective because patients usually respond more readily to a friendly voice than they do to a letter. Many offices have found that the collection call, when done correctly, is an inexpensive and effective collection technique. It costs money to continue sending statements and letters.

Making collection calls throughout the day with special emphasis from 5 PM to 8 PM is recommended whenever possible. Most offices report that more patients can be reached between 5 PM and 7 PM than at any other time during the day. The health insurance professional should be aware of the legal limits of telephone collection calls as spelled out in the Fair Debt Collection Practices Act. For more information on this act, see the listing in Websites to Explore.

Timetable for Calling

A workable telephoning timetable needs to be specific and must be followed consistently to get results. This may be one half of the list per week or per month, depending on the size of the practice. Random calling tends not to work as well.

Do not wait too long to get aggressive with collections. Many offices wait 4, 5, or 6 months before making the first collection call; such a policy yields a very low return. Collection specialists claim that calling closer to the time of service results in greater payoffs. The longer an account is left without follow-up calls, the less chance there is of collecting the fees.

Selecting Which Patients to Call

The next step is to select which patients to call. Some offices believe that it is not cost-effective to call accounts that are less than a certain amount (e.g., $30 to $45). A large practice with thousands of patient visits per month may not find it cost-effective to call accounts less than $100. Fig. 14-9 shows examples of typical conversation scenarios and how the health insurance professional might handle the situation.

Patient:	"The check is in the mail."
HIP:	"Thank you for mailing your check. What day did you mail it? What was the amount of the check and the check number?"
Patient:	"I don't pay the bills. Talk to my wife."
HIP:	"Mr. Hughes, you're our patient. That is why I'm calling you regarding the account."
Patient:	"I'll have to discuss it with my husband. He's at work right now."
HIP:	"May I call your husband at work and straighten this out? What is the phone number?"
Patient:	"I'll have to think about it and see if I can raise the money."
HIP:	"Mr. Hughes, credit was extended to you in good faith when it was needed. I'm sure you are a responsible person and want to meet your obligations."
Patient:	"I'm laid off work and can't pay anything now."
HIP:	"Mrs. Hughes, I'm sorry that you've been laid off. How long have you been out of work? Are you receiving unemployment compensation? Is your spouse working?"
Patient:	"But I can't pay all of it now."
HIP:	"We have a payment plan available, Mr. Williams, that will bring your account up-to-date without too much difficulty."

Fig. 14-9 Sample phone conversations. HIP, Health insurance professional.

Collection by Letter

Collecting delinquent accounts by letter has been successful for some healthcare practices. The timing and wording of written communications with patients should be based on numerous factors, including the size of the balance owing, the payment history of the patient, and the philosophy and policy of the practice.

When composing collection letters, be careful with the wording used so as not to anger or upset the patient. Be matter-of-fact and nonthreatening. Adopt the attitude that the patient has simply overlooked the bill and will make a payment because of this reminder letter. Fig. 14-10 shows examples of collection letters. These letters can be tailored to fit the particular needs of the practice and the patients.

Additional letters or phone calls can be added to extend the time between communications. The key is to stay in constant communication with overdue accounts, rather than adopting a "wait until tomorrow" attitude or assuming that the account will have to be written off or turned over for collection.

What Did You Learn?

1. Why might a telephone call be more effective in collecting delinquent accounts than a letter?
2. When should the healthcare practice make its first collection call?
3. What minimum amount warrants a telephone call?

Example Letter 1: Send when the account is past 30 days.	Example Letter 2: Send 15 days after letter #1 if no payment is made.
Dear Mrs. Williams: Your account balance of $340.50 is now overdue. Please send your payment to the above address at your earliest convenience. If you have questions, you can reach our bookkeeper at xxx-xxxx between 8 a.m. and 5 p.m. weekdays. Sincerely, XYZ Family Clinic	Dear Mrs. Williams: Despite several communications, we have not received payment for your overdue balance in the amount of $340.50. Your account is now seriously past due. Please send your payment to the above address or contact our bookkeeper at xxx-xxxx if you have questions. We will contact you by telephone if we do not hear from you within 7 days. Sincerely, XYZ Family Practice
Example Letter 3: Send 15 days after letter #2 if no payment is made.	**Example Letter 4:** Send 15 days after letter #3 if no payment is made.
Dear Mrs. Williams: We have made all reasonable attempts to work with you to reduce your seriously overdue balance with our clinic. You have not met the terms of the payment plan that we agreed upon. Professional services have been provided to your family in good faith, and payment of your account will protect your status as a family in good standing. We must hear from you within 15 days of the date of this letter. Our bookkeeper is available on weekdays between the hours of 8 a.m. and 5 p.m. Sincerely, XYZ Family Clinic	CERTIFIED MAIL RETURN RECEIPT REQUESTED Dear Mrs. Williams: You have failed to pay or satisfactorily reduce your severely delinquent balance despite our many efforts to work with you. Therefore, XYZ Family Clinic will no longer be providing medical care for you and your children. You should place your family under the care of another physician as soon as possible. You may contact XYZ Family Clinic or the County Medical Society for a referral to a new physician. When you have selected another physician, please send us a signed authorization so that we can provide a copy of your children's medical charts or a summary of its contents to your new physician. XYZ Family Clinic will remain available to treat your children for a short time, which will be no more than 30 days from the date of this letter. Please make the transfer to a new physician as soon as possible within that period. Sincerely, XYZ Family Clinic

Fig. 14-10 Sample letter series for delinquent accounts.

BILLING SERVICES

Some healthcare practices "outsource" their medical billing by hiring a separate professional medical billing service. A reputable medical billing service can provide comprehensive, cost-effective, HIPAA-compliant medical billing solutions for healthcare professionals nationwide. Medical billing services are typically organized and run by medical billing professionals who design, implement, and manage the accounts receivable portion of the healthcare practice. A well-run medical billing service can help a healthcare practice run more efficiently by eliminating staffing issues, undisciplined medical billing and collection processes, outdated medical billing systems, and archaic reporting tools that result in poor collection ratios. Billing services can perform multiple functions for the healthcare practice such as

- preparing and submitting insurance claims;
- providing data entry of patient demographics, insurance information, charges, payments, and adjustments;
- tracking payments from patients and third-party payers;
- producing practice management reports; and
- collecting delinquent accounts.

Usually, a computer, modem, and Internet access are all that is necessary to access a billing service's network, after which the medical facility can retrieve up-to-the-minute patient information and practice management reports at any time on a secure server. Many billing services are available locally and nationwide. With the advent of the Internet, a healthcare office can interact with a professional billing service anywhere in the United States. Care should be taken, however, when choosing a billing service. The service should be thoroughly researched and references checked out with several of their current customers.

What Did You Learn?

1. What is a billing service?
2. List five functions of a billing service.

COLLECTION AGENCIES

A **collection agency** is an organization that obtains or arranges for payment of money owed to a third party—in this case, a healthcare office. Many healthcare practices use collection agencies to help collect delinquent accounts. Collection agencies provide a service to businesses that

- are too small to have a collection department of their own,
- lack the expertise to collect delinquent accounts themselves,
- think a collection agency would get faster results, or
- simply do not want to deal with the hassle of collections.

Most collection agencies request at least 50% of the money they collect. Experts suggest that delinquent bills should be turned over for collection only when it is obvious that payment by any other means is a dead issue. When to go to a collection agency is a business decision made within each healthcare practice.

If the decision is made to turn delinquent accounts over to a collection agency, care should be taken when choosing the agency. Experts say that a credible collection agency should be a member of a national trade association, such as the Consumer Data Industry Association (formerly Associated Credit Bureaus) and American Collectors Association. These organizations provide all-important standards and training. When choosing a collector, choose one that specializes in collecting medical accounts. Also, use standard business practices such as talking with associates; checking references, credentials, and local professional or trade memberships; and touching base with state or local licensing authorities and perhaps the Better Business Bureau. In addition to checking references and credentials, the healthcare practice should ensure that the agency chosen

- employs trained, certified collectors who understand and abide by the Fair Debt Collection Practices Act and follow the requirements of state laws;
- is insured, licensed, and bonded; and
- is able to collect in other states.

HIPAA Tip

The HIPAA Privacy Rule does not require consent from a patient before turning in his or her account for collection. Covered providers still must be cautious when using PHI for collection purposes in determining just how much PHI is needed to accomplish the specific goal of satisfying their account receivables.

What Did You Learn?

1. What is a collection agency?
2. List four reasons a healthcare practice might hire a collection agency.
3. What two trade organizations do experts suggest contacting when choosing a collection agency?
4. Name three things to look for in a reputable collection agency.

SMALL CLAIMS LITIGATION

Small claims litigation is an alternative to turning accounts over for collection. Filing a small claims suit can be effective for a healthcare practice to collect delinquent accounts. Before making the decision to take a delinquent patient to small claims court, however, the cost should be weighed against the monetary gain. The cost of generating a small claims lawsuit is typically $30 to $50 for filing fees and another $20 to $100 for an enforcement officer or process server, so the account ideally should total enough to offset this expense. The process is administrated by the services at local county or district courts, but the individual initiating the small claims lawsuit must prepare the paperwork.

The small claims process is set up to make it easy for individuals or businesses to recover legitimate debts without using expensive legal advisors. The claim is usually heard by a judge in chambers (or, in some cases, an appointed arbitrator), with the parties presenting their sides in person. The individual or business entity that initiates the legal process must pay the initial costs such as filing and serving fees, but these fees can usually be recovered from the debtor if the case is won. Small claims suits can be for any amount of money up to a limiting threshold, which varies by state, usually $3000 to $5000; however, there is ongoing legislation in many states to increase these limits.

Who Can Use Small Claims

Generally, any person of legal age or any business entity can file a small claims lawsuit if there is a legitimate claim against someone who owes money and is refusing to pay. All that is necessary is proof that the debt exists. In the case of a healthcare office, this is usually some sort of written evidence such as a patient ledger. It is important that there is full and proper documentation. The most prolonged and expensive disputes generally result from inadequate paperwork and a lack of attention to detail.

Before a claim can proceed, the court expects the **plaintiff** (the party bringing the lawsuit) to have explored all other avenues of settlement. This means that the plaintiff should allow the other side (in this case, the patient) a "reasonable period of time" to make a payment before resorting to legal action.

How the Small Claims Process Works

The procedure starts with the plaintiff filling out a standard form, which outlines details about the claim and the various parties. The following information needs to appear on the form:
1. Name of the party being sued
2. Current address of that party
3. Amount of the plaintiff's claim
4. Basis, or proof, of the claim

The completed form is returned to the court office with the appropriate filing and serving fees. A copy of the form is "served" to the **defendant** (the party being sued), who may choose to pay the debt in full plus all accrued fees before the process goes any further. He or she also may dispute the claim in its entirety.

If the claim, or any part of it, is disputed, the matter goes to a court hearing where the evidence is heard in informal surroundings, usually around the table in a judge's chambers. The plaintiff and defendant are given an opportunity to introduce evidence, ask questions, and explain to the judge (or arbitrator) why judgment should be entered in his or her favor. The judge usually makes an immediate decision, and the parties involved get a full and final result on the day of the hearing. The judgment of the court is an official statement in the court's records that the defendant owes the plaintiff a certain amount of money with interest. The judgment must be enforced out of the defendant's assets. More simply put, if the judgment is in favor of the plaintiff, the defendant must pay immediately. If the defendant does not pay after judgment, the plaintiff can "attach," or gain ownership of the defendant's assets such as a paycheck, a bank account, or a car.

Small claims litigation can be successful, but it is time-consuming and can be costly if there are a lot of claims. If the healthcare practice has someone on staff who is able and willing to prepare all the proper documents and attend court hearings, this process can have positive results. Filing and serving fees can be far less than the typical 50% of the outstanding debt kept back by a collection agency.

What Did You Learn?

1. What was the initial intent of the small claims process?
2. What is a typical monetary threshold for a small claims suit?
3. What is the first step in initiating a small claims suit?
4. List the four elements of information that must appear on the small claims form.

SUMMARY CHECKPOINTS

▶ Patients typically come to a healthcare office expecting certain things such as the following:
- *Professional office setting*—Because patients cannot see and touch an intangible service such as healthcare, they look for substitutes to put their mind at ease, such as the office location, size, and layout and staff enthusiasm.
- *Relevant paperwork and questions*—Patients prefer paperwork to be brief, of high quality, and relevant to the encounter. Patients should be given reasons why these forms and questions are important to their care and treatment.
- *Honoring appointment times*—Time is a valuable commodity in everyone's life; if the schedule lags, the patient should be told the reason for the delay and offered alternatives to waiting.
- *Patient load*—Negative conclusions about the competency of the entire healthcare team can be offset by explaining to the patient why the reception room has no or few patients waiting.

- *Getting comfortable with the healthcare provider*—Sharing a relevant personal experience or information promotes a good provider-patient relationship and can relieve patient anxiety.
- *Privacy and confidentiality*—Patients must feel confident that any personal information they divulge would be kept private and confidential.
- *Financial issues*—Discuss financial issues and practice policies up-front with patients so that they know what to expect.

▶ Future trends in the patient-practice relationship include the following:
- *An aging population*—Over the next 30 years, the number of Americans older than age 65 will increase, and healthcare facilities should be prepared to handle an increasing volume of elderly patients.
- *Using the Internet as a healthcare tool*—Patients will rely more on the Internet, and healthcare providers will have to adapt their practices to meet these state-of-the-art electronic requirements.
- *Seeing patients as consumers*—Similar to other types of consumers, patients today are likely to switch healthcare plans or healthcare providers or both if they think they are not getting quality service.

▶ Any individual or any business involved in transferring data or carrying out transactions related to patient PHI is a HIPAA-covered entity. The law applies to three groups:
- *Healthcare providers*—Any provider of healthcare services or supplies who transmits any health information in electronic form in connection with a transaction for which standard requirements have been adopted
- *Health plans*—Any individual or group plan that provides or pays the cost of healthcare
- *Healthcare clearinghouses*—Any public or private entity that transforms healthcare transactions from one format to another

▶ Personally identifiable information includes information about an individual collected by the covered entity that could be used to identify the individual, regardless of the source of such information or the medium in which it is recorded (e.g., name, address, email address, telephone number, birth date, and Social Security number).

▶ When all identifiable elements are removed, the information under most circumstances is considered de-identified.

▶ Two common methods of accounting are used in healthcare facilities today:

- *"One-write" pegboard accounting system*—This system, made up of several accounting forms and carbonized shingled receipts, captures information at the time the transaction occurs with a single writing and eliminates the need for recopying the data.
- *Electronic patient accounting software*—A computer software program can perform all phases of the accounting process quickly and accurately. It allows the input of demographic data, creating a patient "account" from which many documents can be generated, such as a list of appointments by day and by provider and an encounter form for each. Appointments also can be scheduled, deleted, and adjusted within the accounting system. Periodic statements, aging reports, and insurance claims can be generated.

▶ Some things a healthcare practice might do to increase its financial success include, but are not limited to, the following:
- Establish a written credit policy.
- Discuss payment and practice policies up-front with patients.
- Bill promptly.
- Plan an action for bills more than 30 days old.
- Telephone (or send a letter) after the second statement.
- Use the services of a small claims court.

▶ Laws affecting credit and collection include
- the Truth in Lending Act,
- the Fair Credit Billing Act,
- the Equal Credit Opportunity Act,
- the Fair Credit Reporting Act, and
- the Fair Debt Collection Practices Act.

▶ The steps involved in small claims litigation are as follows:
- Acquire the proper forms from the local county or district court, along with instructions on how to fill them out properly.
- Include the following information on the original form: (1) the name of the defendant, (2) the current address of the defendant, (3) the amount of the plaintiff's claim, and (4) the basis of the claim.
- Attach documentation that provides proof that the money is owed.
- Return the completed form (and the required number of copies) to the court office with the appropriate filing and serving fees.
- Appear in court on the date indicated to substantiate the case.

CLOSING SCENARIO

Before Callie Foster completed Chapter 14, her goal was to learn how to be considerate, patient, and empathetic to patients because of a recent negative incident she had experienced at a healthcare office. Her confrontation had been very upsetting, and she firmly believed that no one should be treated so rudely. Callie thought that what other patients expect when they come to a healthcare office is what she herself expected when she went to Dr. Dayton's office. However, as she progressed through the chapter, it became obvious that although consideration, patience, and empathy are important during the actual patient-staff encounter, when it comes to collections, sometimes a fair but firm and pragmatic attitude is necessary.

Scott found the section on consumer credit laws especially interesting and informative. To him, the steps involved in the small claims litigation process were straightforward and manageable—a fair and economical way to collect outstanding accounts.

WEBSITES TO EXPLORE

- For live links to the following websites, please visit the Evolve site at
  http://evolve.elsevier.com/Beik/today
- For information on HIPAA regulations, go to
  http://www.hipaaadvisory.com/regs
- For more information on financial policies for healthcare offices, go to
  http://www.pcc.com/practmgmt/business/efficiency2.php
- For more information on laws regarding credit and collection, log on to
  http://www.ftc.gov/bcp/edu/pubs/consumer/credit/cre18.shtm
- For more information on fair debt collection, log on to
  http://www.fair-debt-collection.com
- For more information on the Consumer Data Industry Association, log on to
  http://www.cdiaonline.org/index.cfm
- For more information on the American Collectors Association, log on to
  http://www.debtmarketplace.com
- For more information on small claims procedures for individual states, log on to
  http://www.nolo.com/legal-encyclopedia/stateArticleGroup-31016.html

Author's Note: Websites change frequently. If any of these URLs is unavailable, use applicable guide words in your Internet search to acquire additional information on the various subjects listed.

REFERENCES AND RESOURCES

American Medical Association: *How to "HIPAA"—top 10 tips 2003 AMA.* Available at: http://www.ama-assn.org/ama1/pub/upload/mm/435/hipaa10tips-opt.pdf..

Burton B: *2004 Quick Guide to HIPAA for the Physician's Office,* Philadelphia, 2004, Saunders.

Centers for Medicare and Medicaid Services: *HHS modifies HIPAA code sets (ICD-10) and electronic transactions standards,* January 15, 2009. Available at: http://www.cms.hhs.gov/apps/media/press/factsheet.asp?Counter=3407.

Moynihan J: Preparing for 5010: internal testing of HIPAA transaction upgrades recommended by December 31, *J AHIMA* 81:22–26, 2010. Available at: http://library.ahima.org/xpedio/groups/public/documents/ahima/bok1_046274.hcsp?dDocName=bok1_046274.

Quinsey CA: Practice brief. A HIPAA security overview, *J AHIMA* 75:56A–556C, 2004.

Rules of spring: reviewing the upcoming regulations on HIPAA Privacy Rule modifications, *J AHIMA* 34–35, 2011.

CHAPTER 15

The Claim

Chapter Outline

I. Introduction
II. General Guidelines for Completing CMS-1500 Form
III. Keys to Successful Claims
  A. First Key: Collect and Verify Patient Information
  B. Second Key: Obtain Necessary Preauthorization and Precertification
  C. Third Key: Documentation
  D. Fourth Key: Follow Payer Guidelines
  E. Fifth Key: Proofread Claim to Avoid Errors
  F. Sixth Key: Submit a Clean Claim
  G. Rejected Claims versus Denied Claims
IV. Health Insurance Portability and Accountability Act (HIPAA) and National Standard Employer Identifier Number
V. Claim Process
  A. Step One: Claim Is Received
  B. Step Two: Claims Adjudication

C. Step Three: Tracking Claims
  1. Creating a Suspension File System
  2. Creating an Insurance Claims Register System
D. Step Four: Receiving Payment
E. Step Five: Interpreting Explanation of Benefits
  1. Troubleshooting Explanation of Benefits
  2. Downcoding
F. Step Six: Posting Payments
G. Time Limits
VI. Processing Secondary Claims
  A. Real-Time Claims Adjudication
VII. Appeals
  A. Incorrect Payments
  B. Denied Claims
  C. Appealing a Medicare Claim

CHAPTER OBJECTIVES

After completion of this chapter, the student should be able to:

1. Explain the rationale for understanding both paper and electronic claims submission.
2. Summarize the general guidelines for completing the CMS-1500 paper claim form.
3. List and explain the six keys to successful claims.
4. Determine the role of the National Standard Employer Identifier Number (EIN) in claims processing.
5. Identify and briefly explain the six steps of the claims process.
6. Outline the process for submitting secondary claims.
7. Discuss the process for appealing incorrect payments and denied claims.

CHAPTER TERMS

adjudication
appeal
birthday rule
clean claim
coordination of benefits
correct code initiative
downcoding
employer identification number (EIN)

explanation of benefits (EOB)
insurance claims register (log)
Medicare Secondary Payer claims
real-time claims adjudication (RTCA)
secondary claim
suspension file

OPENING SCENARIO

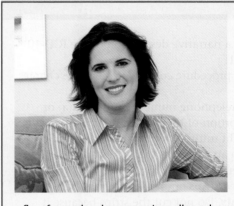

Zoey Edwards, confined to a wheelchair after an automobile accident at the age of 12, was looking for a career opportunity that allowed her to work out of her home. She noticed an article in a flyer from a local community college about a healthcare billing and insurance program. The article listed the career possibilities for graduates of this program, along with testimonials from several former students who had established successful home-based businesses in healthcare billing and insurance. Zoey decided that a career in this field might meet her needs. Through a state-of-the-art communications network and with the help of the student services staff at the college, Zoey was able to participate in classes from the comfort of her own home, traveling to campus only for major examinations.

Kristin Underwood was also looking for an opportunity to work at home and still care for her two preschool children. Kristin had a friend who worked as a health insurance professional in a local healthcare office, so she was aware of the challenges and rewards this career area offered. Kristin thought she had the personality traits and work ethic to make a home business successful, so she enrolled in a career school in her neighborhood and signed up for a healthcare insurance course.

INTRODUCTION

We learned in Chapter 5 that there are two basic methods for submitting health insurance claims—paper and electronic. We also learned that claims must be electronically submitted to a Medicare Administrative contractor, Durable Medical Equipment Medicare Administrative Contractor, or a fiscal intermediary from a provider's office or institution using a computer with software that meets electronic filing requirements as established by the Health Insurance Portability and Accountability Act (HIPAA) claim standard and by meeting Centers for Medicare and Medicaid Services (CMS) requirements. We also learned that there are limited exceptions to this mandate (see Chapter 5). In addition, more and more nongovernment payers are requiring claims to be submitted electronically.

Do these changes mean that the CMS-1500 (08/05) paper claim form will become obsolete and the health insurance professional does not need to learn the guidelines for completing it? This author doesn't think so. The National Uniform Claim Committee (NUCC) is proposing revisions to the CMS-1500 (08/05) paper claim form that would accommodate data reporting changes in the Version 005010 837 professional electronic claim transaction and other business needs. The time frame for when a revised form would be required is unknown as of this writing. Because some healthcare providers still use the CMS-1500 form, this chapter integrates information that applies to paper and electronic claim processing.

GENERAL GUIDELINES FOR COMPLETING CMS-1500 FORM

Steps for completing the universal CMS-1500 claim form for generic commercial carriers and the major payers—Medicaid, Medicare, and TRICARE/CHAMPVA—are available in Appendix B in the back of this textbook and on the Evolve site. Box 15-1 lists some general guidelines for preparing all paper claims. Earlier chapters also stressed the importance of strict adherence to payer-specific guidelines when preparing claims. In addition, the NUCC "1500 Health Insurance Claim Form Reference Instruction Manual for Version 08/05" provides detailed instructions, is updated periodically, and is available on the Evolve site. The NUCC instructions are intended to be a guide only, and the health insurance professional should follow specific federal, state, or other payer guidelines for more definitive claims completion instructions.

What Did You Learn?

1. What is the function of NUCC in relation to the paper CMS-1500 claim form?
2. Why should the health insurance professional learn how to complete paper claims?
3. List five important guidelines for submitting paper claims.

KEYS TO SUCCESSFUL CLAIMS

Claims processing involves many steps, and each step must be performed thoroughly and accurately to receive the maximum payment that the health record documentation substantiates. This process begins with the patient appointment and ends with the subsequent payment by the carrier. Understanding how this process works allows the health insurance professional to file claims properly, resulting in full and timely reimbursement. Fig. 15-1 illustrates the six "keys" to successful claims processing. Although these "keys" may appear applicable only to paper claims, most of them also apply to the electronic claims process.

Box 15-1

General Guidelines for Completing the CMS-1500 Form

- Use preprinted red and white CMS-1500 claim form only.
- Follow OCR guidelines.
- Submit claims that are legible using computer-generated or typed entries.
- Submit only six line items per claim. Do not compress two lines of information on one line.
- Send paper claims unfolded in large envelopes.
- Use standard fonts (preferably Courier) in 10-point or 12-point size.
- Type within each block and not outside the block. Characters out of alignment would cause the claim to be returned as misaligned.
- Follow payer guidelines regarding where to type the insurance carrier's name and address. Some carriers stipulate that the area to the right of the bar code be left blank.

- Do not submit a narrative description of the ICD-10 code in Item 21.
- Do not submit procedure codes with negative charges in Item 24d.
- Do not type a telephone number in the NPI(a) or NON-NPI(b) portion of the field in Item 33.
- Do not highlight information. Instead, underline information on attachments that you want to bring to the payer's attention.
- Remove pin-feed strips on pin-fed claims at the perforations only. Do not cut the strips because it may alter the document size.
- Do not tape, glue, or staple attachments to the CMS-1500 claim form. Do not tear, bend, or fold corners of the claim form with attachments.
- Attachments should be the same size as the paper claim form (8½ × 11 inches).

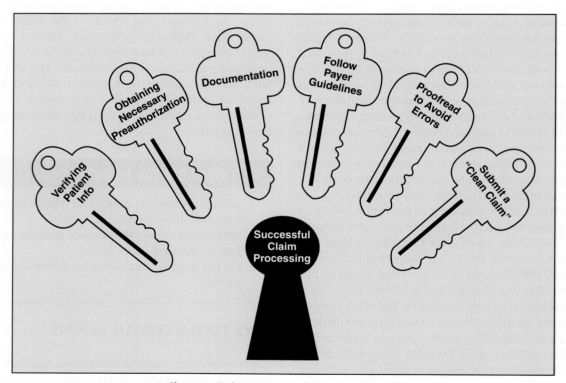

Fig. 15-1 Six keys to successful claims processing.

First Key: Collect and Verify Patient Information

Unless a patient visits the healthcare facility on a regular basis (e.g., weekly allergy shots or blood pressure checks), the health insurance professional should verify the patient's information each time he or she visits the office. New patients must complete a patient information form on the first visit. Established patients should be required to update the form at least annually because within a year's time the patient could have remarried, moved to a new address, changed jobs, or, most important to the health insurance professional, changed insurance companies. In addition to demographic data (e.g., name, address, age, gender), the patient information form should include basic items such as the insurance carrier's name, policy and group numbers (if applicable), the insured's name (if different from the patient), effective date of coverage, and any secondary insurance information. Some practices with a high volume of Medicare patients have a separate information form for Medicare patients.

After the patient information form is completed, the health insurance professional should check it over to ensure that the correct information has been entered in the required blanks and all information is legible. One key to successful claims submission is to have the patient provide as much information as possible, and the health insurance professional should verify this information.

In some situations, more than one insurer is involved. Such cases might occur when the patient and his or her spouse are covered under separate employer group plans or when the parents of a minor patient are divorced, and each parent has his or her own insurance policy. In the case of the latter, if the primary carrier is not designated on the information form, the health insurance professional should obtain this information from the parent who accompanies the child to the office.

In addition to the standard demographic and insurance questions asked on the patient information form, many healthcare practices include a section (often at the bottom of the form) for the patient to sign a release of information and an assignment of benefits. Other practices use separate forms for these functions. Although HIPAA law says it is unnecessary for treatment, payment, or (healthcare) operations (TPO), most healthcare facilities request that patients sign and date a valid release of information before they submit an insurance claim. Most facilities also require that patients sign an assignment of benefits, authorizing the insurance carrier to send payment directly to the healthcare provider.

Verifying a patient's current insurance coverage (e.g., enrollment and copays) is one of the most important administrative duties of the health insurance professional. Accurate verification has a direct impact on the promptness and correctness of claim payments. Many third-party payment delays are caused by inaccurate verification on the part of the practitioner's office or missed information at the time of the verification. Many insurance companies offer online services for providers to exchange eligibility and benefits information on their patients electronically. After obtaining a complete and accurate patient information form, the health insurance professional should make a photocopy of the patient's insurance identification (ID) card and place it in an easily accessible location in the patient's health record, such as inside the front cover. Many insurance ID cards also have information on the back. The health insurance professional should always check the back of the card for information and make a photocopy of it as well.

HIPAA Tip

Patients have certain rights and protections against the misuse or disclosure of their health records. All patients should receive a Notice of Privacy Practices that informs individuals of their rights and of the legal duties of the healthcare practice with respect to protected health information.

⭐ Imagine This!

Shirley Gibson, a health insurance professional for Westlawn Family Medical Center, updates all demographic and insurance information when patients come to the office for an appointment. Additionally, she checks to ensure that the release of information and assignment of benefits forms are signed, dated, and current. After the patient completes the new information form, Shirley checks it for accuracy and legibility. If two insurance companies are listed, she asks the patient which is primary. In some cases, Shirley has to call either the employer or the insurance carrier to verify which is the primary carrier. "It is important for smooth, efficient, and timely claims processing to have all information current and accurate before the claim is prepared for submission," Shirley says. "It is surprising," she adds, "how much people move around, change jobs, and change insurers these days."

Second Key: Obtain Necessary Preauthorization and Precertification

The health insurance professional should be familiar with the rules regarding preauthorization and precertification. Some third-party payers reject certain types of claims if they do not know about and approve the services beforehand. Services that most often require preauthorization or precertification include inpatient hospitalizations, new or experimental procedures, and certain diagnostic studies. Emergency services typically do not need prior authorization, but they often require some type of follow-up with the insurance company—typically within 24 to 48 hours. Although the front office staff of the provider often provides this service, it is ultimately the patient's responsibility to know when and how to notify the insurance company for preauthorization or precertification; however, the health insurance professional should advise the patient when this process is necessary to avoid rejected claims. Also, if the patient is incapacitated in any way, the health insurance professional or a member of the healthcare staff should notify the patient's insurer to acquire the necessary preauthorization. Telephone numbers for contacting the carrier are usually on the back of the patient's ID card. Fig. 15-2 shows the back of an insurance ID card with a toll-free number to call

IMPORTANT PHONE NUMBER INFORMATION

For pre-admission certification, OB and emergency admissions call 1-800-558-xxxx.

To locate a participating provider call 1-800-810-xxxx or access BlueCard website @ www.bcbs.com.

Providers - Please submit all claims to your local Blue Cross and Blue Shield Plan.

Pharmacists - Pharmacy Benefits Manager (PBM) is AdvancePCS. For assistance call 1-800-600-xxxx.

Wellmark Blue Cross and Blue Shield of Iowa, an independent licensee of the Blue Cross and Blue Shield Association.

Fig. 15-2 Back of insurance ID card.

when precertification is necessary. Some carriers issue a "prior authorization" number, which should be indicated in Block 23 of the CMS-1500 form.

Reminder: Medicare (fee-for-service) does not need prior authorization to provide services.

Stop and Think

Helen Rigdon was admitted as an inpatient to Memorial East Hospital after a visit to the emergency department for a bleeding ulcer. After Helen was discharged, she received an EOB from her insurance carrier stating that they were denying the claim because there had been no preauthorization for the hospital admission. In this case, whose responsibility was it to contact the insurance company to obtain the required preauthorization?

Third Key: Documentation

It is the healthcare provider's responsibility to document appropriate comments in the patient's health record. Each entry must indicate clearly the history, physical examination, and medical decision making for the patient. The provider also fills out an encounter form, indicating the proper procedure codes (CPT or HCPCS level II) and diagnosis codes (ICD-10-CM) to describe the patient's condition and the services that were rendered. These codes should be checked before transferring to the claim because some practitioners when in a hurry may indicate the wrong ones. The health insurance professional places the appropriate diagnosis codes, procedure codes, charges, and any other pertinent information in the proper boxes on the claim. Whether claims are submitted on paper or in electronic format, each required field on the claim helps to determine if it is "clean." Claims that are not clean are returned for more information or are denied. It is important that the claim show the exact diagnosis that is documented in the health record.

Fourth Key: Follow Payer Guidelines

As pointed out in previous chapters, some major payers (Medicaid, Medicare, Blue Cross and Blue Shield, TRICARE/CHAMPVA) have slightly differing guidelines for completing the CMS-1500 claim form. The health insurance professional must obtain the most recent guidelines from each of these major payers to complete the claim exactly to their specifications.

Fifth Key: Proofread Claim to Avoid Errors

Claims are frequently rejected or denied. Being aware of some common mistakes can help the health insurance professional avoid delays, denials, or rejections. With paper claims, it is good practice first to proofread the claim carefully when it is completed, paying particular attention to code entries and dollar amounts. Make sure the claim is dated and the proper signature is affixed. When the claim is completed and signed, make a photocopy for the file. Box 15-2 lists some common errors that cause a claim to be rejected or denied.

Sixth Key: Submit a Clean Claim

The most important process in the healthcare insurance cycle is submitting a clean claim to the third party payer. A clean claim means that all of the information necessary

Box 15-2

Common Errors Made on Claims

- Patient's insurance ID number is incorrect
- Patient information is incomplete
- Patient/insured name and address do not match the insurer carrier's records
- Physician's EIN, provider number, NPI, or Social Security number is incorrect or missing
- There is little or no information regarding primary or secondary coverage
- Physician's (or authorized person's) signature has been omitted
- Dates of service are incorrect or do not correlate with information from other providers (e.g., hospital, nursing homes)
- The fee column is blank, not itemized, and not totaled
- The CPT or ICD-10 codes are invalid, or the diagnostic codes are not linked to the correct services or procedures
- The claim is illegible
- Preauthorization/precertification was not obtained before services were rendered

for processing the claim has been entered on the claim form, and the information is correct. Clean claims are usually paid in a timely manner. Paying careful attention to what information should be entered in each field helps produce clean claims. Refer to Appendix B at the back of the book for examples of completed claims.

Stop and Think

Silver River Medical Center has a higher than average number of rejected paper claims. The billing and insurance staff consists of four health insurance professionals; each individual handles approximately 50 to 55 claims per day. Many of the claims are rejected or denied because of simple errors—transposed numbers, misspelled patient names, incorrect charges, or the provider signature has been omitted. What might the billing/insurance staff do to resolve this problem?

What Did You Learn?

1. Why is it important to update the patient information form with each patient visit?
2. What is the result of failing to obtain preauthorization or precertification for certain procedures such as inpatient hospitalization?
3. Whose responsibility is it to document appropriate comments in the health record?
4. What is a "clean claim"?

Rejected Claims versus Denied Claims

A claim that does not successfully pass through the adjudication process to the payment system is rejected. Examples of why a claim is rejected include provider not found, member not found, incorrect address was used, or more than one rendering provider submitted a claim. A claim that is denied was passed through to a payment system but was not payable for numerous reasons including, but not limited to, member ineligible, benefit not covered, or benefit maximum has been met. A rejected claim must be researched differently than a denied claim. Questions regarding rejected claims should be directed to the carrier or clearinghouse. Questions regarding denied claims should be directed to the carrier's customer service department.

HEALTH INSURANCE PORTABILITY AND ACCOUNTABILITY ACT (HIPAA) AND NATIONAL STANDARD EMPLOYER IDENTIFIER NUMBER

The Secretary of the Department of Health and Human Services (HHS) requires that the **employer identification number (EIN)** assigned by the Internal Revenue Service

(IRS) be used as the employer identifier standard for all electronic healthcare transactions as required by HIPAA. The ruling requires the following:

- Health plans must accept the EIN on all electronic transactions that require an employer identifier.
- Healthcare clearinghouses must use the EIN on all electronic transactions that require an employer identifier.
- Healthcare providers must use the EIN on all transactions, wherever required, that are electronically transmitted.
- Employers must disclose their EIN when requested to do so by an entity that conducts standard electronic transactions requiring that employer's identifier.

An EIN consists of 9 digits with the first 2 digits separated by a hyphen (e.g., 00-1234567). The IRS assigns EINs to employers, who can obtain an EIN by submitting IRS Form SS-4 (Application for Employer Identification Number). Business entities that pay wages to one or more employees are required to have an EIN as their taxpayer identifying number; most employers already have an EIN assigned to them.

In May 2002, the HHS issued a final rule to standardize the identifying numbers assigned to employers in the healthcare industry by using the existing EIN (this EIN should appear in Block 25 of the CMS-1500 form with a space replacing the hyphen). Most covered entities were to have been in compliance with the EIN standard by July 30, 2004. Although small healthcare facilities were allowed an additional year to comply, all providers should now be in compliance.

What Did You Learn?

1. What is the format of an EIN?
2. How does a provider acquire an EIN?

CLAIM PROCESS

After a claim has been received by a third-party payer, it is reviewed, and the carrier makes payment decisions. This process is referred to as **adjudication**. If the claim is clean, it continues on through several more steps to the reimbursement process, and, ideally, the insurance carrier pays up to the allowed amount (according to the patient's policy) for the services that have been billed. However, the carrier can reduce payment or deny the claim completely. If any information is missing, or if there are errors on the claim, the process is stopped, and the claim is returned to the healthcare office where it originated. Fig. 15-3 is a flow chart that illustrates how a paper claim progresses through the various steps after it is received at the payer's facility. The steps discussed in the following sections and listed in Fig. 15-4 are for a paper claim. (The steps for processing an electronic claim are discussed in Chapter 16.)

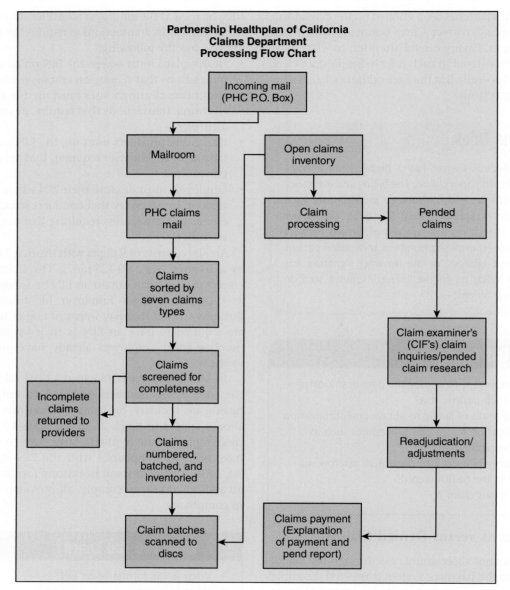

Fig. 15-3 Claims department processing flow chart.

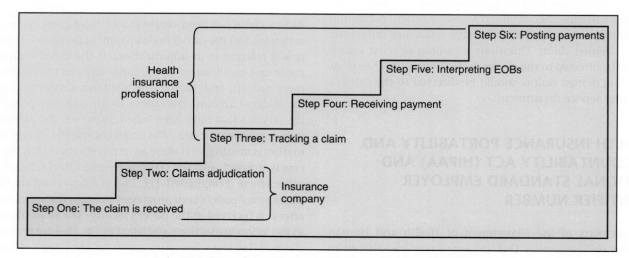

Fig. 15-4 Steps of the claim process. EOBs, explanation of benefits.

Box 15-3

General Guidelines for Optical Character Recognition Scanning

- Use only the original preprinted red and white CMS-1500 claim form. This form is designed specifically for OCR systems. The scanner cannot read black-and-white (copied, carbon, faxed, or laser printer–generated) claim forms.
- Do not use red ink pens, highlighters, sticky notes, stickers, correction fluid, or tape anywhere on the claim form. Red ink or highlighter would not be picked up in the scanning process and would black out information.
- Do not write or use stamps or stickers that say "Rebill," "Tracer," or "Second Submission" on the claim form.
- Use standard fonts that are 10 to 12 characters per inch. Do not mix character fonts on the same claim form.

- Do not use italics or script. Handwritten entries should be avoided.
- Use upper case (capital letters) for all alpha characters.
- Do not use punctuation marks, slashes, dashes, or any special characters anywhere on the claim form.
- Use black printer ribbon, ink-jet, or laser printer cartridges. Ensure that ink is not too light or faded.
- Ensure that all claim information is entirely contained within the proper field on the claim form and on the same horizontal plane. Misaligned data would delay processing and may be missed.
- If corrections need to be made, reprinting the claim is preferred. Correction fluid should not be used.

Step One: Claim Is Received

When the insurance carrier receives the claim, it is dated, and the claim is processed through an optical character recognition (OCR) scanner. If any attachments accompanied the claim, the practice name, provider/group number, address, and telephone number should appear on each attached document. Providing this information on each attachment helps prevent claim denial in case the attachments get separated from the claim during the adjudication process. Box 15-3 lists the general guidelines for OCR scanning.

Step Two: Claims Adjudication

After the data are entered into the payer's computer system, if the claim is clean, it is approved and proceeds on to be paid. However, it first must pass through a series of edits to verify the patient's coverage and eligibility and check for medical necessity, exclusions, preexisting conditions, and noncovered services contained in the patient's policy. If the claim requires additional information, the insurer contacts the healthcare practice or the patient. In the case of a paper claim, this contact usually is accomplished by mail, but it also can be by telephone. If the claim is not clean, it is rejected and returned to the provider.

When a claims error is discovered that could result, or already has resulted, in inaccurate reimbursement, a corrected claim should be prepared and submitted. The health insurance professional should mark the corrected claim as a "corrected billing" and "not a duplicate claim." It also is advisable to include a note describing the error, plus any additional documentation necessary to support the correction. Some practices use a claims correction form (Fig. 15-5) for submitting corrected claims. The form is filled out, attached to a corrected claim, and resubmitted to the payer.

HIPAA Tip

HIPAA has developed a transaction that allows payers to request additional information to support claims. This transaction uses Logical Observation Identifiers Names and Codes (LOINC) to request the clinical information that is required to process healthcare claims.

Step Three: Tracking Claims

The healthcare practice should have a mechanism in place for tracking claims. Typically, it takes a paper claim 4 to 6 weeks to complete the entire claims process; however, this time varies by carrier and geographic location. Sometimes a claim may be clean, but a question arises, which results in a delay. Carefully tracking the progress of claims alerts the health insurance professional to the claims that remain unpaid past the normal payment time.

At the end of a set time period, if the claim is not paid and no communication has been received explaining the delay, the health insurance professional should follow up on the claim. Many offices use a form similar to the one in Fig. 15-6 for claims follow-up. If the medical facility uses computerized patient accounting software, this is typically a built-in function.

Claim Correction Form

Physician offices are encouraged to submit claims electronically. This form should be used in situations where the provider cannot submit corrected claims electronically or where electronic submissions would not adequately address the issue.

Submitted To:

Plan/Payer Name: _____ Date Submitted: _____

Plan/Payer Address: _____

City _____ State: _____ Zip: _____

Telephone: (_____) _____ Fax: (_____) _____ E-mail: _____

Patient Name: _____ D.O.B.: _____
       First   M.I.   Last

Subscriber Name: _____ Date of Service: _____

Policy #: _____ Group #: _____ Original Claim #: _____

Submitted From:

Provider Name: _____ TIN or ID #: _____

Contact: _____ Telephone: (_____) _____ Ext. _____

Fax: (_____) _____ E-mail: _____

THE FOLLOWING WAS CORRECTED ON THIS CLAIM:

❑ The patient's policy/group number was incorrect. The correct number(s) are shown above.

❑ The correct CPT code is _____ instead of _____

❑ Wrong date of service was filed. The correct date is _____

❑ Visits were denied based on the diagnosis given. Proper diagnosis code is _____ instead of _____

❑ Visit: ❑ Procedure: denied as over carrier's utilization limits. Please see attached letter to justify extensions of these limits.

❑ Carrier indicated that the patient is covered by another plan that is Primary. This is incorrect. Patient indicates you are Primary.

❑ The secondary carrier is: _____ ❑ There is no secondary carrier.

❑ The procedure was denied as medically not necessary. Documentation to support the medical necessity of this service is attached.

❑ Our clerk: ❑ Carrier's clerk: failed to enter correct number of times (units) procedure was performed. Correct units are as follows:

     D.O.S.: _____ Code: _____ Units: _____ Charge Total $: _____

❑ Multiple Surgical Procedures:

     ❑ Carrier failed to approve any procedure at 100%.   ❑ Carrier approved incorrect procedure at 100%.

     Carrier should have approved code _____ @ 100%/50% instead of _____

     Carrier should have approved code _____ @ 100%/50% instead of _____

     Carrier should have approved code _____ @ 100%/50% instead of _____

❑ Modifiers should be attached to code(s)

	Code	Code			Code	Code
❑ -50	_____	_____		❑ -51	_____	_____
❑ -58	_____	_____		❑ -59	_____	_____
❑ -79	_____	_____		❑ -GA	_____	_____
❑ __	_____	_____		❑	_____	_____

❑ The following E/M visit was denied as included in the global surgical fee. In fact, the service was a significant separately identifiable service provided above and beyond the procedure and submitted with appropriate E/M modifier. Please reconsider with attached documentation:

     Code: _____ with modifier(s): ❑ -24 ❑ -25   Charge $: _____

❑ UPIN information for code _____ was omitted. Physician name: _____ UPIN: _____

❑ Plan specific provider I.D. omitted. The I.D. # is _____

❑ CLIA number was omitted. The CLIA number is _____

❑ The place of service was incorrect. The place of service should be _____

❑ The service was rendered at the physician's physical location listed in Box 32 of the claim form.

❑ Failed to attach EOB from Primary carrier. The EOB is attached to this form.

❑ Failed to enter correct information on indicated line of claim form.

     Line #: _____ Correct Information: _____

❑ Other reason for claim correction: _____

❑ Comment: _____

June 2003

Fig. 15-5 Example of a claims correction form.

Prompt Payment Tracking Form

Information Checklist

Please provide copies of the following:

- ❑ The claim form submitted to insurance company
- ❑ Electronic claim receipt if applicable
- ❑ Correspondence from the insurance company (EOBs, requests for additional information, etc.)
- ❑ Details of written/oral contacts with insurance company regarding this claim
- ❑ Other pertinent information

Note: Mark out all confidential patient information, such as name, date of birth or social security number.

Practice/Physician Information (complaint by)

Name: _____

Address: _____

City, Zip _____

Phone: _____ Fax: _____

E-Mail: _____

Insurance Company and Claim Information

Original Submission Date: _____

Company: _____

Phone: _____

Date(s) of Services: _____

Claims Rep (if known): _____

Submitted via: ❑ Paper   ❑ Electronic

Action by Insurance Company

Date of Initial Response from Ins. Co.: _____

❑ Denied   ❑ Requested Additional Information   ❑ Reduced Payment   ❑ Other (see attached)

Insurance Company Response: _____

_____

_____

Current Status of Claim: _____

_____

_____

Fig. 15-6 Example of a claims tracking form.

⭐ Imagine This!

Laurence Benson visits his family physician, Dr. Myron Peters, yearly for annual wellness examinations. Every 3 years, Dr. Peters orders an electrocardiogram for Laurence as part of his routine examination. Normally, Laurence's insurance carrier, XYZ Health Indemnity, pays within 2 to 3 weeks. It is Dr. Peters' office policy to send a statement to the patient if the insurance carrier does not pay within 60 days. When Laurence received an overdue statement, he called Dr. Peters' office and asked the health insurance professional to check into the matter. When she did, she was told that the claim was "pending" because the individual who reviewed it saw something on the attached electrocardiogram that required further assessment by the medical review committee, but the committee was "bogged down" with a backlog of claims to review.

🕐 Stop and Think

Reread Imagine This! concerning Dr. Peters. How might Dr. Peters' health insurance professional modify her routine to avoid future problems similar to the one experienced by Mr. Benson?

Creating a Suspension File System

For offices filing paper claims, some sort of claims tracking system such as a **suspension file** is recommended. A suspension file is a series of files set up chronologically and labeled according to the number of days since the claim was submitted. Claims in a file labeled "current" might be 30 days or less; a second series might be labeled "claims over 30 days," and so forth. Another type of follow-up system that works well is one in which claims are filed according to the date they are submitted.

Claim copies should be removed systematically as they are finalized. Paid claims can be filed in a permanent folder or binder, under each major payer. If payment has not been received, some sort of follow-up procedure can be initiated. Claims follow-up should be given a high priority and become a regularly scheduled part of the health insurance professional's work week.

Experienced health insurance professionals who deal with Medicare and Medicaid carriers recommend making inquiries in writing or using the forms specifically created for follow-up. Inquiries to commercial carriers often are handled more efficiently by a telephone call. If a claim has been rejected for a simple reason, without notification, a quick phone call is time well spent. In the case of resubmission, always attach a note with the date, the contact person's name, and a description of the conversation.

Keep a copy of all correspondence as documented proof of response.

Creating an Insurance Claims Register System

An alternative to the suspension file is to record claims information on a columnar form known as an **insurance claims register** or **log** (Fig. 15-7). When a claim is submitted, the health insurance professional records the filing date, the patient's name and chart number, the name and address of the payer, and the amount billed. As payments are received, the original copy of the claim form is removed from the follow-up file and compared with the explanation of benefits (EOB). The amount paid is recorded in the applicable column along with any difference from the amount billed as shown on the log sheet. Any notations, such as "claim sent to review" or "claim rejected for additional information," should be recorded in the status column along with the date the notice was received. If a claim is resubmitted, that date should be recorded on the log as well.

Step Four: Receiving Payment

The insurer sends the payment for services and the EOB—sometimes called a **remittance advice (RA)**—back to the provider's office. (Whether or not there is a payment, there is always an EOB or RA.) If the practice submits claims electronically, the EOB or RA also may be in an electronic format. Each EOB should be checked thoroughly to ensure that the payment is consistent with the fee schedule or contracted amount from the insurance company (Table 15-1). Claims that have been denied or rejected for any reason or that have been reduced in payment should be reviewed to determine the source of the denial or payment reduction. A decision must be made whether to pursue the claim further.

Step Five: Interpreting Explanation of Benefits

The **explanation of benefits (EOB)** is the document sent by the insurance carrier to the provider and the patient explaining how the claim was adjudicated. The EOB is the key to knowing how much of the claim was paid, how much was not, and why—in other words, adjudicated. Sometimes understanding what this document means can be challenging. Every payer has a different EOB format. The EOB has a unique vocabulary, such as "applied to deductible," "above usual and customary," "patient copay," and "allowable." Codes are often used, and the health insurance professional must determine what each code means. Deciphering the EOB language and codes reveals the following:

- Date received
- Date processed
- Amount of billed charges
- Charges allowed by the carrier

INSURANCE CLAIMS REGISTER

Filing Date	Chart Number	Patient's Name	Name & Address Where Claim Submitted	Amount Billed	Amount Paid	Difference	Status or Comment
10/6	1221	Matthew Kramer	First Insurance 1st Avenue Newark, NJ 12345	$525			10/21 busy 10/30 busy 11/6 busy
10/6	1350	Luke Myers	Better Insurance 3rd Avenue New York City, NY 02110	$1200	$700	$500	Requester Review 10/30
10/6	1098	Christi Wilson	County Farm Ins 6th Avenue New Era, IA 45678	$125	$50	$75	$75 deductible. Bill Patient
10/6	1352	Rose Larson	Last Insurance 7th Avenue New Hope, MS 56789	$1500	0		Sent to Medical Review 10/30

Fig. 15-7 Example of an insurance claims register.

- How much of the claim was applied to patient deductible
- How much of the patient's annual deductible has been met
- Why a service was reduced or denied

Knowing how to read the EOB is important because it aids in collecting full reimbursement including any balance owed by the patient. Fig. 15-8 shows an EOB from a commercial insurance company and an explanation of what each code means.

Troubleshooting Explanation of Benefits

As discussed earlier, an EOB explains the outcome of the claim that was submitted for payment processing. If the payment was reduced or rejected, the EOB itemizes the reason. By reading the EOB and following the instructions, the health insurance professional can analyze the situation. If an error has been made on the claim and it is correctable, it should be done so in a timely manner. If it is believed that the insurance carrier made the error, it should be reported to the carrier immediately.

Initially, there are several things to evaluate when looking over an EOB that indicates no payment or a reduced payment. The first thing is to compare the totals billed on the EOB and the CMS-1500 form. If they do not match, it is a good indication that the insurer missed a procedure. If the totals match, but the number of line items (actual procedure codes performed) do not, more than likely the insurer bundled one procedure into another, without listing them as "duplicate."

TABLE 15-1	Common Payment Errors
RESULT	**REASON**
A service is reduced	The adjudicator may have downcoded the claim for lack of documentation
	CPT code was converted to a relative value scale code that did not directly correlate with CPT
Reimbursement is made at a much reduced rate	Possibly a data entry error. Compare the CPT code submitted with the code paid
Low reimbursement	Precertification was not completed
	Insufficient documentation to establish medical necessity
Multiple units are paid as one unit	The insurer "missed" a number in the unit column
Reimbursement for a procedure or service suddenly decreases	This could mean a recalculation of the allowable fee or an error. Phone the payer
Payment is not received	Claim is lost or "caught in the system." Begin your inquiry
Multiple procedures were not paid	The insurance company either ignored the additional procedures or lumped them in with the primary procedure

Republished with permission of Ingenix. Copyright © 2007.

The odds are that if a claim is reduced or rejected, the problem lies with the provider's office. However, this is not always the case, and the health insurance professional should be vigilant in analyzing the EOB. One billing professional suggests keeping copies of sample EOB files for procedures the medical practice performs regularly for each payer. A payment discrepancy would stand out when compared with the sample EOB file. This "example" file can be used for appealing claims as long as all patient identification is deleted.

⭐ Imagine This!

Dr. Edwin Carter, a podiatrist, performed three arthroplasties on Priscilla Fortune's toes at $500 each procedure. When the EOB was received, the total charge was $1500, but there were only two codes of 28285 listed. This meant that Ms. Fortune's insurance carrier had bundled two of the procedures into one, but the fee schedule was considered for only one. To clear things up, Wayne Thomas, Dr. Carter's health insurance professional, had to contact the insurer and explain that there were three distinct procedures performed on three individual toes and not two, as the carrier had assumed.

Downcoding

Downcoding by an insurance company occurs when claims are submitted with outdated, deleted, or nonexistent CPT codes. When this happens, the payer assigns a substitute code it thinks best fits the services performed. Often the healthcare practice does not agree with the choice because the substituted code results in a lesser payment. Similar problems occur when an insurer's payment system is based on CPT codes and a relative value scale code is submitted that does not directly translate to CPT. When these claims are reviewed by a claims adjuster, he or she assigns a valid CPT code. Coding accurately and knowing which coding systems payers use help to avoid these downcoding problems. (See Chapter 17 for more information on the relative value scale.)

If the claims adjuster changes a valid procedure code that was submitted on the claim, the health insurance professional should contact the claims adjuster and ask for the reason. If the contact is by mail, documentation that supports the code submitted should be included. In some cases, a procedure is denied because the insurer states that it is considered "integral to the main procedure." In other cases, a modifier that was submitted on the claim was dropped or the claim was subject to a **correct code initiative** edit. Correct code initiative edits are the result of the National Correct Coding Initiative, which develops correct coding methods for CMS. The edits are intended to reduce overpayments that result from improper coding. If the denial was due to a correct code initiative edit, documentation supporting why the procedure was distinct and not related to another procedure must be submitted. For more information on the National Correct Coding Initiative, visit the Evolve site. ⊜

Step Six: Posting Payments

After the EOB has been reconciled with the patient's account, the health insurance professional (or other staff member) posts the payment received from the insurance carrier to the patient ledger and bills the patient for any applicable outstanding copayments or deductible amounts. Participating providers cannot balance bill, but nonparticipating providers for commercial claims are allowed to bill the patient for any balance the insurance carrier does not pay. It is against the law to waive Medicare copayments unless financial hardship has been established and documented. Fig. 15-9 illustrates a payment entry on a patient ledger. (*Note:* Contractual adjustments are discussed in Chapter 17.)

Time Limits

As stated previously, claims should be submitted to the insurance carrier as soon as possible, ideally within 30 days or sooner of the conclusion of treatment. Claims for patients who receive ongoing treatment typically are submitted on a periodic basis—every 15 to 30 days, depending on the policy of the healthcare practice. Most third-party payers have time

EXPLANATION OF BENEFITS

EMPLOYEE BENEFIT PLAN ADMINISTRATION SERVICES

EMPLOYER/GROUP NAME	SOUTHEAST IOWA SCHOOLS		DATE PREPARED	08–06–XX
PLAN/LOCATION NUMBER	10000000 14008020 02		SOCIAL SECURITY I.D. NUMBER	
EMPLOYEE/MEMBER NAME	BEIK JANET I		CONTROL #	8470.0
PATIENT NAME	BEIK JANET I		EOB #	9808060048

JANET I BEIK
545 IOWA CITY RD
SOMEWHERE IA 00506

SOUTHEAST IOWA SCHOOLS
SOMEWHERE IA 00506

PROVIDER NAME and TYPE OF SERVICE	DATES FROM/THRU	AMOUNT CHARGED	AMOUNT COVERED	EXPL. CODE	COVERED AT 100 %	COVERED AT %	COVERED AT %
HAYS, ANDERSON, DIAGNOSTIC LABORATORY	06–22–XX	15.00	15.00	099 514	15.00		
ADJUSTMENTS TO BENEFITS	TOTAL →	15.00	15.00		15.00		
			Less Deductible				
			Balance		15.00		
			Benefit %		AT 100%	AT %	AT %
			Plan Benefits		15.00		
			Total Benefit		15.00		

099   THIS PREFERRED PROVIDER ACCEPTS THE "AMOUNT COVERED" AND HAS AGREED NOT TO
099   BILL PATIENTS FOR MORE THAN DEDUCTIBLES, COPAYS & NONCOVERED CHARGES.
514   THIS WORKSHEET WAS PROCESSED BY JENNIFER

DEDUCTIBLE SATISFIED: 1000.00

PAYMENTS HAVE BEEN ISSUED TO THE FOLLOWING BASED ON ABOVE EXPENSES.

HAYS, ANDERSON   15.00

Fig. 15-8 Example of explanation of benefits.

limits for when claims can be submitted to be considered for payment. The time limit for each of the major carriers discussed in this book is addressed in the corresponding chapters.

Most third-party payers do not pay a claim if the time limit for claim submission has been exceeded. Not all payers deny late claims but instead levy a fine or penalty because of lateness or "past timely filing" status. The time limit in which to file a claim varies from carrier to carrier and often depends on various circumstances such as the following:

- Whether the provider of the services participates (or is contracted) with the insurer
- Whether the provider of services does not participate (or is not contracted) with the insurer
- The method in which the claim was submitted for payment (i.e., electronic or paper)

STATEMENT

Westlake Medical Clinic
2604 Spindle Center
Cherokee, XY 23133
231-555-1212

Stanley P. Grady
1234 Old Colony Road
Calamus City, XY 23232

DATE	REFERENCE	DESCRIPTION	CHARGES	CREDITS PYMNTS.	CREDITS ADJ.	BALANCE
20XX		BALANCE FORWARD ⟶				26 00
1/10	Stanley	99214, ROA	135 00	8 00		153 00
3/21	Stanley	99214, ROA	135 00	8 00		280 00
5/18	Stanley	99214, ROA	135 00	8 00		407 00
5/20		XYZ Ins. Claim				
6/24		XYZ Ins. Ck 319116		324 00		83 00
6/24		Contr. Adj XYZ			50 00	33 00

B40BC-2   PLEASE PAY LAST AMOUNT IN BALANCE COLUMN ⟶

Fig. 15-9 Example of a patient ledger card with entries.

- The type of provider who is billing for services (e.g., physician, hospital)
- When coordination of benefits apply

Generally, an insurer allows a maximum of 1 year from the date of service for submitting a claim; however, some commercial carriers allow 180 days. If there is any question about time limits, the health insurance professional should contact the carrier. It is a good idea to include time limits for each major payer in the same file containing their claims submission guidelines.

Most insurance companies also have a time limit for filing appeals. The time limit varies from carrier to carrier, and it is important that the health insurance professional keep this information on file so that it is readily available when and if needed.

The health insurance professional should establish a routine for completing and submitting insurance claims (e.g., the end of every week, the 15th and 30th of each month). How often claims are submitted varies depending on

- the size of the practice;
- office staffing;
- the type of claim (e.g., workers' compensation, Supplemental Security Income, Medicare);
- how the claims are submitted (electronically or paper);
- whether claims are sent directly or a clearinghouse is used; and
- the major carriers involved.

What Did You Learn?

1. What is typically the first thing that happens to a claim when it is received by the insurer?
2. If the insurer determines a claim is "unclean," what happens to it?
3. Name the two suggested methods for tracking claims.
4. List four common payment errors.
5. Why is it important for the health insurance professional to know how to interpret EOBs?

Imagine This!

Maise Smyth is employed as a billing and insurance clerk for a family practice physician, Dr. Isaac Finnes, at the Gulf Coast Medical Clinic. Dr. Finnes sees approximately 25 patients a day. The clinic is not yet computerized, so all of the claims are submitted on paper. To accomplish this challenging workload, Maise has set up a routine for submitting preparation. At the end of each day, she sorts the health records by insurer name. Following is Maise's schedule for claims preparation:

    Monday—Blue Cross and Blue Shield
    Tuesday—Medicare and Medicaid
    Wednesday—TRICARE/CHAMPVA
    Thursday—Magna Insurance (a major carrier in the area)
    Friday—all miscellaneous carriers/claims follow-up

By the end of the day on Friday, all claims for patients seen that week have been prepared and submitted. Because there are only a few miscellaneous carriers, Maise has time on Friday afternoon to do any necessary claims tracking.

PROCESSING SECONDARY CLAIMS

Occasionally, patients may be covered under two insurance plans. In this situation, the health insurance professional may have to prepare and submit a primary claim and a **secondary claim**. The insurer who pays first is the primary payer, and that payer receives the first claim. The insurance company who pays after the primary carrier is referred to as the secondary insurer. This second carrier receives a claim after the primary carrier pays its monetary obligations.

As previously stated, the health insurance professional must determine which coverage is primary and which is secondary. If it is not immediately obvious which payer is primary, the health insurance professional should first ask the patient. If the patient does not know, a telephone call to one of the insurance companies should answer the question quickly and easily. If there is a second insurance policy,

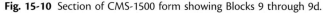

9. OTHER INSURED'S NAME (Last Name, First Name, Middle Initial)
GARCIA SAM T

a. OTHER INSURED'S POLICY OR GROUP NUMBER
123456

b. OTHER INSURED'S DATE OF BIRTH			SEX	
MM	DD	YY		
11	03	1978	M [X]	F [ ]

c. EMPLOYER'S NAME OR SCHOOL NAME
ACME DRYGOODS INC

d. INSURANCE PLAN NAME OR PROGRAM NAME
CERTIF EMPLOYEE BENEFITS

Fig. 15-10 Section of CMS-1500 form showing Blocks 9 through 9d.

it is important to check "yes" in Block 11d on the CMS-1500 form and complete Blocks 9 through 9d (Fig. 15-10).

Occasionally, a patient and spouse (or parent) are covered under two separate employer group policies, resulting in what is referred to as **coordination of benefits**. When a coordination of benefits situation exists, the health insurance professional should

• verify which payer is primary and which is secondary, and
• send a copy of the EOB from the primary payer along with the claim to the secondary carrier (if the EOB is not included, the claim is likely to be rejected or delayed pending coordination of benefits determination).

The rule of thumb for dependent children covered under more than one policy is as follows: The payer whose subscriber has the earlier birthday in the calendar year is generally primary. This is referred to as the **birthday rule**. In the case of divorce, the birthday rule may not apply. The custodial parent's policy may be primary, depending on the legal arrangement ordered by the court.

Medicare Secondary Payer claims are claims that are submitted to another insurance company before they are submitted to Medicare. When a Medicare beneficiary has other insurance coverage that is primary to Medicare, the other insurer's payment information must be included on the claim that is submitted to Medicare; otherwise, Medicare may deny payment for the services. The health insurance professional should check the current guidelines of the specific payer in question when a secondary policy is involved. See Chapter 9 for more information on submitting Medicare Secondary Payer claims.

Stop and Think

Fran and Ted Washburn and their two children have been coming to Gulf Coast Clinic on a regular basis for nearly 2 years. Shortly before the last office visit, Fran and Ted divorced; Ted changed jobs and moved to a different address in a nearby town. Fran and Ted are both employed, and each is covered under a separate employer group policy. Ted's date of birth is 09/06/65 and Fran's is 08/16/66. Which parent's policy should be considered primary?

Real-Time Claims Adjudication

Real-time claims adjudication (RTCA) is a means of electronic communication that allows instant adjudication of an insurance claim including the third-party insurer's payment, adjustment, and patient responsibility. RTCA typically reduces the time frame of claims submission to adjudication from the traditional 2 to 6 weeks to just a few seconds.

Healthcare providers are becoming increasingly concerned about the impact consumer-directed healthcare plans and high-deductible plans have on their ability to collect timely payment from their patients. Because these plans require patients to pay more out-of-pocket costs, some providers believe collecting payment from patients may become increasingly difficult. Many payers are asking providers not to collect copays at the time of service, the reason being that any attempt to collect at the time of service may create credit balances or patient dissatisfaction. RTCA enables a provider to bill for services before the patient leaves the office and to receive a fully adjudicated response back from the insurer at the time of service. With this technology, the provider can send out the inquiry and receive and print the response, displaying total and allowable charges and the patient's responsibility (coinsurance, deductible, and copayment). Providers can be certain of the amount the patient should pay at the time of service.

> ### 💬 What Did You Learn?
>
> 1. What is a secondary claim?
> 2. What document typically must accompany a secondary claim?
> 3. Explain what is meant by the "birthday rule."
> 4. What is the benefit of RTCA to healthcare providers?

APPEALS

An **appeal**, as defined in insurance language, is the process of calling for a review of a decision made by a third-party carrier. In many instances, providers of service and patients have the right to appeal a rejected insurance claim or a payment made that the provider or patient (or both) believes is incorrect.

Incorrect Payments

Before appealing a payment or a claim, whether with Medicare or a private commercial insurer, the health insurance professional should notify the insurer in writing that there has been an error. Many payers have a set time limit for claim appeals and often print it on their EOB.

A basic rule for appealing a claim is to include a copy of the original claim, EOB or RA, and any additional documentation necessary to provide evidence for the appeal.

Cover letters are also effective for appeals and provide the claims reviewer all of the necessary information regarding the reason for the appeal. If the payer does not respond to an appeal, the health insurance professional can pursue other alternatives, such as contacting the state's insurance commissioner and sending a clear, well-documented account of the discrepancy. See Websites to Explore at the end of this chapter for links to individual state insurance departments.

Denied Claims

If the health insurance professional believes a claim has been wrongly denied, an appeal can be filed. The appeal process differs from carrier to carrier; however, appeals generally must be in writing and initiated within a specified number of days—usually 30 to 60. The appeal letter should identify the claim and the reason the health insurance professional believes the claim should be approved.

The appeal is usually sent directly to the carrier with any written comments, documents, records, or other information relating to the claim, even if such information was not submitted with the original claim. The carrier typically reviews the appeal within 30 calendar days. Sometimes the insurance carrier's review committee allows the provider (or their representative) to present the case in person or over the telephone, which allows the individual or committee members conducting the review to ask questions to clarify the reason why the provider (or the provider's representative) thinks the claim is valid. The outcome of the appeal is determined, and the provider is notified verbally or in writing of the decision. This decision is usually final; however, some carriers allow second-level or third-level appeals. The health insurance professional should consult guidelines of individual carriers regarding the steps to take when initiating an appeal.

If the claim remains unpaid after all levels of appeal are exhausted, there are still some options open. If there have been repeated problems with a particular carrier, the state insurance commission can be contacted, and the problem case can be outlined in a letter. A second option is to file a complaint with HIPAA. Also, it may be important to get the patient involved because he or she often can make helpful contributions.

> ### 📁 HIPAA Tip
>
> HIPAA provides an online health plan complaint form so that healthcare providers and their staff members can report administrative and payment disputes with health insurers and third-party payers. The form is designed to collect information from physicians on health plan and third-party payer noncompliance with the provisions of the HIPAA Transaction and Code Set Standards.

Appealing a Medicare Claim

Participating providers, suppliers, and patients have the right to appeal any decision about Medicare services regardless of whether the patient is enrolled in original Medicare, a Medicare managed care plan (Medicare Part C), or a Medicare prescription drug plan (Medicare Part D). (Providers and suppliers who do not accept assignment on claims typically have limited appeal rights.) The type of Medicare coverage dictates the specific appeal filing process. The five levels of the Medicare appeals process are discussed at length in Chapter 9. Detailed information on the Medicare appeals process can also be found on the Evolve site.

📁 HIPAA Tip

According to HIPAA privacy regulations, documents relating to uses and disclosures, authorization forms, business partner contracts, notices of information practice, responses to a patient who wants to amend or correct his or her information, the patient's statement of disagreement, and a complaint record must be maintained for 6 years.

❓ What Did You Learn?

1. What can the health insurance professional do if he or she believes a claim has been wrongly denied?
2. If a payer does not respond to an appeal, what alternative does the health insurance professional have?
3. True/False—A Medicare claim cannot be appealed if the provider is PAR.

SUMMARY CHECKPOINTS

▶ It is recommended that the health insurance professional learn the general guidelines to completing the CMS-1500 claim form.

▶ The six keys to successful claims are as follows:
- *Verify patient information*—It is important to keep patient information and a signed release of information current to generate clean claims, process them expeditiously, and minimize claim delay or denial because of misinformation. Also, if there is a second insurance carrier, primary status must be determined.
- *Obtain necessary preauthorization and precertification*—Most insurance carriers have a rule that when a patient is to be hospitalized or undergo certain procedures or diagnostic studies, preauthorization or precertification must be acquired beforehand. If this is not done, the claim is likely to be denied. (Medicare does not require preauthorization for medically necessary services.)
- *Documentation*—The healthcare provider must document accurate and appropriate information in the patient's health record to substantiate the procedures and diagnoses listed on the claim form.
- *Follow payer guidelines*—Because every third-party payer has slightly different guidelines for completing and submitting claims, the health insurance professional should create and maintain a file for each payer's current guidelines and follow those guidelines to the letter when preparing claims.
- *Proofread the claim to avoid errors*—It is important to proofread paper claims carefully before submitting them. Most errors that result in denial are simple mistakes such as typos, transpositions, or omissions, resulting from carelessness and failure to double check each entry on the claim form.
- *Submit a clean claim*—The ultimate goal in the healthcare insurance process is to submit a clean claim, meaning all of the necessary, correct information appears on the claim. Clean claims typically are processed quickly.

▶ The claim process includes several steps:
- When the claim is received by the third-party payer, the claim is dated, attachments (if any) are confirmed, and the claim is processed through an OCR scanner.
- The claim passes through a series of edits and is compared with the patient's policy to verify coverage, eligibility, medical necessity, exclusions, preexisting conditions, and noncovered services. If the claim is "clean," it is approved and proceeds on for payment, if payment is due. If there is a problem with the claim, the provider is notified by mail or by telephone.
- At the end of a set time period, if a claim is not paid and no communication has been received explaining the delay, it needs to be followed up. The healthcare facility should have a mechanism in place for tracking claims so that no claim "falls through the cracks." This tracking mechanism could be a suspension filing system or an insurance claims log system.
- Whether or not a payment is made against a claim, there is always an EOB. Each EOB should be checked to ensure no error has been made by the insurance carrier. If the claim is denied or there has been a payment reduction, a decision must be made whether or not to appeal.
- Interpreting the EOB is key to understanding how the claim was adjudicated. Accurately deciphering an EOB aids in collecting full reimbursement, including any balance owed by the patient.
- After the EOB has been reconciled, the payment is posted to the patient's account ledger. Participating providers of commercial claims cannot balance bill beyond deductibles and copayments; nonparticipating

providers can balance bill. Medicare copayments cannot be waived, unless a financial hardship case has been established.

▶ Time limits for submitting claims vary with insurance carriers; however, most allow 1 year after the date of service. It is important to follow specific payer guidelines because some demand claims submission within 90 days. The health insurance professional should endeavor to file all claims in a timely manner for the benefit of the practice and the patient.

▶ The most important consideration with patients who are covered under more than one insurance policy is to establish which one is primary. After that, complete the claim for the primary carrier, checking "yes" in Block 11d on the CMS-1500 form and completing Blocks 9 through 9d. Usually, the process for sending a claim to the second-ary carrier is to include the EOB from the primary carrier with the claim. It is important to check the guidelines of the secondary carrier for submission rules.

▶ The first step in appealing a denied claim (or a claim where the payment has been reduced) is to notify the insurance carrier. Most payers have time limits for appealing claims and for submitting claims. The health insurance professional should check the payer-specific guidelines for appealing claims. If all efforts of appeal are exhausted without success and the health insurance professional is certain the claim is valid, a remaining option is to contact the state insurance commissioner's office.

▶ The Medicare program has a multilevel appeals process to allow providers and patients to challenge the determination on a claim.

CLOSING SCENARIO

Zoey and Kristin feel confident that what they have learned about healthcare billing and filing insurance claims will give them a solid foundation for an "at-home" career. Learning the keys to successful claims was an important concept in the overall health insurance process. If a claim was not clean, the bottom line was that submitting it was a waste of time, effort, and money for all parties involved. Understanding what happens to a claim after it reaches the payer's office was also interesting and enlightening for these two students. Until now, where the claim went after it left the healthcare office and what was done with it were basically mysteries to them, and the term "adjudication" was simply another perplexing word with ambiguous meaning. After completing Chapter 15, the entire claim process and meaning of adjudication became clear.

After reviewing Chapter 9 and researching the websites that provided in-depth information regarding the multilevel Medicare appeals process, the women realize that appealing Medicare claims can be an interesting learning experience well worth their effort. Overall, Zoey and Kristin know they are on their way to an exciting and rewarding home career.

WEBSITES TO EXPLORE

For live links to the following websites, please visit the Evolve site at

http://evolve.elsevier.com/Beik/today

• For more information on HIPAA, log on to
http://www.cms.gov/HIPAAGenInfo/

• For general information on claims processing, log on to
http://www.ama-assn.org

• For links to individual state insurance offices, log on to
http://www.naic.org/state_web_map.htm

• To learn more about the Medicare appeals process, check the following websites
http://www.cms.hhs.gov

http://www.medicare.gov
http://www.cms.hhs.gov/medlearn

Author's Note: Websites change frequently. If any of these URLs is unavailable, use applicable guide words in your Internet search to acquire additional information on the various subjects listed.

REFERENCES AND RESOURCES

Humana: *Real-Time Claims Adjudication.* Copyright 2009. Available at: http://www.humana.com/providers/tools/claims/rtca.asp.

What Is the Medicare Appeal Process? Available at: http://www.ehow.com/how-does_5477080_medicare-appeal-process.html#ixzz1PvQWoniW.

CHAPTER 16

The Role of Computers in Health Insurance

Chapter Outline

I. Introduction
II. Impact of Computers on Health Insurance
III. Role of Health Insurance Portability and Accountability Act (HIPAA) in Electronic Transmissions
IV. Electronic Data Interchange
   A. History of Electronic Data Interchange
   B. Benefits of Electronic Data Interchange
V. Electronic Claims Process
   A. Methods Available for Filing Claims Electronically
   B. Enrollment
   C. Electronic Claims Clearinghouse
   D. Direct Data Entry Claims
   E. Clearinghouse versus Direct
   F. Advantages of Filing Claims Electronically
VI. Medicare and Electronic Claims Submission
VII. Additional Electronic Services Available
   A. Electronic Funds Transfer
   B. Electronic Remittance Advice
   C. Role of Computers in Transitioning to ICD-10 Diagnostic Coding System
VIII. Electronic Medical Record
   A. Combination Records
   B. Digital Imaging Hybrid
   C. Potential Issues
   D. Future of Electronic Medical Records
   E. Privacy Concerns of Electronic Medical Records
   F. Federal Funding for Electronic Medical Record Trials and "Meaningful Use"

CHAPTER OBJECTIVES

After completion of this chapter, the student should be able to:

1. Explain how computers have impacted health insurance.
2. Discuss the role of the Health Insurance Portability and Accountability Act (HIPAA) in electronic transmissions.
3. Provide a brief history of electronic data interchange, and explain its benefits.
4. Identify the various aspects of the electronic claims process.
5. Provide a brief outline of Medicare electronic claim submission procedures.
6. List and describe additional electronic services available to the health insurance professional.
7. Describe an electronic medical record (EMR) and the two types of EMR hybrids.
8. List potential issues of EMRs.
9. Discuss the future of EMRs, including privacy concerns for patients.
10. Explain how federal funding for EMR trials relates to "Meaningful Use."

CHAPTER TERMS

Administrative Simplification and Compliance Act (ASCA)
billing services
clearinghouse
code sets
combination records
digital imaging hybrid
direct data entry (DDE)
electronic data interchange (EDI)
electronic funds transfer (EFT)
electronic media claim (EMC)
electronic medical record (EMR)

electronic remittance advice (ERA)
enrollment process
General Equivalence Mappings (GEMs)
identifiers
meaningful use
privacy standards
security standards
small provider of services
small supplier
telecommunication
unusual circumstances

⟳ OPENING SCENARIO

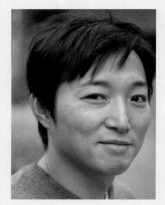

Student Ellie Farnsworth has an associate's degree in computer technology. She enrolls in the medical insurance course to be able to apply her computer skills to medical billing and health insurance claims. Ellie realizes that HIPAA has changed the face of not only electronic claims transmission but also world healthcare in general. Ellie wonders why so much emphasis is being placed on HIPAA. "Every chapter talks about HIPAA," Ellie complains. "It's like we eat, sleep, and drink HIPAA."

Benji Yutsuki is also computer literate. He understands the vulnerability of electronic transmissions but agrees with Ellie that there is a lot to understand with HIPAA. "My aunt works in a medical office, and she said they call it the 'HIPAA hippo,'" he says with a laugh. Benji tries to convince Ellie to be patient, however. "I believe HIPAA is more important than we might think," Benji adds, "especially as far as patients and the general public are concerned."

After the two students discuss HIPAA and how this act affects electronic healthcare transactions, they agree that it is in their best interest to attempt to understand why it was created and its importance to healthcare in general.

INTRODUCTION

Computers have influenced every area of society, particularly medicine, which depends on computers as much or perhaps more than any other type of business. Most healthcare facilities use computers in some part of their day-to-day operations. Some systems are basic and perform just a few simple tasks; others are quite sophisticated, incorporating multiple locations and off-site data storage. Computers have changed record keeping in a way that no other advancement has. Many patient records are stored on computer systems; the computer files are backed up, and secured to protect them in the event of computer failure. The medical field depends on computers to keep track of financial records as well. It is very important that patient records and financial information are kept highly secured so that no one can access these data without proper authority. This chapter focuses on the role of computers in medicine, specifically their impact on the health insurance claims and billing processes.

IMPACT OF COMPUTERS ON HEALTH INSURANCE

In the past, it was unusual to find a medical office where computers were used for patient accounting and insurance claims submission. As the age of technology advanced, however, the use of computers became more widespread. From a health insurance perspective, computers are now used for
- enrolling an individual in a health plan,
- paying health insurance premiums,
- checking eligibility,
- obtaining authorization to refer a patient to a specialist,
- processing claims,
- electronic medical records (EMRs), and
- notifying a provider about the payment of a claim.

However, as computer technology advanced, it became clear that the health information being transmitted through computers and the Internet had to be monitored, and laws were needed to protect the security of health information and the privacy of individuals. The U.S. government, under Health Insurance Portability and Accountability Act (HIPAA) regulations, now mandates that all healthcare information that is electronically transmitted follow specific rules and guidelines to provide this needed security and protection.

ROLE OF HEALTH INSURANCE PORTABILITY AND ACCOUNTABILITY ACT (HIPAA) IN ELECTRONIC TRANSMISSIONS

One of the main reasons Congress enacted HIPAA was to reform health insurance and simplify healthcare administrative processes. The intent of the HIPAA **Administrative Simplification and Compliance Act (ASCA)** was to improve the administration of Medicare by taking advantage of the efficiencies gained through electronic claims submission. Provisions of this act require healthcare providers, health plans, and healthcare clearinghouses to use certain standard transaction formats and code sets for the electronic transmission of health information. These requirements also apply to healthcare providers who transmit health information in electronic form in connection with the transactions covered in the rule. As usage of electronic transmissions of healthcare information increased, privacy and security regulations were adopted to enhance the privacy protections and security measures directed at health information.

One of the goals of ASCA was to reduce the number of forms and methods of completing claims and other payment-related documents and to use a universal identifier for providers of healthcare. Another goal was to increase the use and efficiency of computer-to-computer methods of exchanging standard healthcare information. The five specific areas of administrative simplification addressed by HIPAA are as follows:

- **Electronic data interchange (EDI)** is the electronic transfer of information in a standard format between two entities. EDI allows business entities to exchange information and transact business in a rapid and cost-effective way. Transactions included within HIPAA consist of standard electronic formats for enrollment, eligibility, payment and remittance advice (RA), claims, health plan premium payments, health claim status, and referral certification and authorization.
- **Code sets** include data elements used to document uniformly the reasons why patients are seen and procedures or services provided to them during healthcare encounters. HIPAA adopted specific code sets for diagnosis and procedures to be used in all healthcare transactions. HCPCS (Ancillary Services/Procedures), CPT-4 (Physicians' Procedures), CDT (Dental Terminology), ICD-10-CM diagnoses codes for physicians, ICD-10-PCS for inpatient hospital procedures, and NDC (National Drug Codes) codes are the adopted code sets for procedures, diagnoses, and drugs.
- **Identifiers** are the numbers used in the administration of healthcare to distinguish individual healthcare providers, health plans, employers, and patients. These identifiers must be used in all transactions, as required by the HIPAA standard. Over time, identifiers are intended to simplify the administrative processes such as referrals and billing, improve accuracy of data, and reduce costs.
- **Security standards** need to be developed and adopted for all health plans, clearinghouses, and providers to follow and to be required at all stages of transmission and storage of healthcare information to ensure integrity and confidentiality of the records at all phases of the process, before, during, and after electronic transmission.
- **Privacy standards** are intended to define what are appropriate and inappropriate disclosures of individually identifiable health information and how patient rights are to be protected.

ASCA made it compulsory for all Medicare claims to be submitted electronically effective October 16, 2003, with certain exceptions (see section on Medicare and Electronic Claims Submission later in this chapter). These electronic claims are to be in a format that complies with the appropriate standard adopted for national use. ASCA allowed extra time for medical facilities to implement and test HIPAA-compliant software.

❓ What Did You Learn?

1. Name five things that computers are used for in relation to health insurance.
2. List the five specific areas of administrative simplification addressed by HIPAA.

ELECTRONIC DATA INTERCHANGE

EDI may be most easily defined as the replacement of paper-based documents with electronic equivalents. More specifically, EDI is the exchange of documents in standardized electronic form, between business entities, in an automated manner, directly from a computer application in one facility to an application in another. EDI offers the prospect of easy and inexpensive communication of information throughout the healthcare community. In the case of insurance claims, EDI is the electronic exchange of information between the provider's office and a third-party payer.

History of Electronic Data Interchange

The early applications of what later became known as EDI can be traced back to the 1948 Berlin Airlift, where the task of coordinating air-freighted consignments of food and other consumables (which arrived with differing manifests and languages) was assisted by creating a standard shipping manifest. Electronic transmission began during the 1960s, initially in the transportation industries, when standardization of documents became necessary, and the U.S. Transportation Data Coordinating Committee (TDCC) was formed to coordinate the development of translation rules among four existing sets of industry-specific standards. A further step toward standardization came with the creation of standards for the American National Standards Institute (ANSI), which gradually extended and replaced the standards created by the TDCC. To see a timeline of EDI, visit the Evolve site or use the words "History and Timeline of EDI" in your search engine.

Benefits of Electronic Data Interchange

EDI leads to faster transfer of data, fewer errors, instant document retrieval, and less time wasted on exception handling, resulting in a more streamlined communication process. Benefits of EDI can be achieved in such areas as inventory management, transport, and distribution; administration and cash management; and, in this case, transmission of healthcare information data. EDI offers the prospect of simple and inexpensive communication of structured information throughout the healthcare community.

📂 HIPAA Tip

HIPAA has set standards for the electronic transmission of healthcare data. As of October 16, 2003, any healthcare service provider has the option of sending client medical billing data electronically to a health plan (or payer), but if so, the data must be in a HIPAA-compliant format. The health plan must be able to receive and process the data and respond electronically, likewise in a HIPAA-compliant format.

ELECTRONIC CLAIMS PROCESS

We learned in Chapter 5 that there are two basic methods for submitting health insurance claims—using the universal CMS-1500 paper claim and submitting claims electronically. Also, with few exceptions, ASCA prohibits payment of services or supplies that a provider did not bill to Medicare electronically. This section discusses various aspects of electronic claims processing.

Methods Available for Filing Claims Electronically

The electronic claims process incorporates the use of EDI. There are three ways to submit claims electronically:

1. **Direct data entry (DDE)** (also called *carrier direct*)—accomplished using practice management software to submit electronic claims directly from the provider's office to a specific carrier via a modem. (Practice management software must support this function.)
2. **Clearinghouse**—the provider sends claims to a clearinghouse using **telecommunications**. The claim information is entered and edited for errors. The clearinghouse sorts the claims by payer and transmits them to the various insurance companies using the specific formats required by each.
3. **Billing service**—a company files claims on the provider's behalf for a fee, usually a per-claim charge. The provider supplies the billing service the necessary claims documentation that the billing service keys into a computer and submits to the appropriate third-party payer electronically. Billing services typically offer other services, such as keeping current with rapidly changing Medicare and insurance laws.

To send claims electronically, the medical practice needs a computer, modem, and HIPAA-compliant software.

Enrollment

Whether the medical practice chooses to use a clearinghouse or submit claims directly to the insurance carrier, it needs to go through an **enrollment process** before submitting claims. The enrollment process typically involves completing and returning EDI setup requirement forms. This process is necessary so that the business that receives the claims can create a compatible information file about the practice in its computer system and process claims. Most government and many commercial carriers require enrollment. Some also require that the practice sign a contract before sending any claims. The enrollment process typically takes several weeks to complete, and providers are typically required to submit "test" claims before the conversion from paper claims can be completed. The biggest obstacle to getting set up for electronic claims processing is the time that it takes for approval from state, federal, and, in some cases, commercial or health maintenance organization carriers.

Electronic Claims Clearinghouse

As mentioned previously, an electronic claims clearinghouse is a business entity that receives claims from several medical facilities and consolidates them so that one transmission containing multiple claims can be sent to each insurance carrier. More specifically, a clearinghouse serves as an intermediary between medical practices and the insurance companies, facilitating the electronic exchange of information between the facilities.

A clearinghouse works as follows. When claims are received from providers/suppliers, they are edited and validated to ensure they are error-free and checked for completeness. If an error is discovered or information is missing, the issuing facility is notified that there is a problem with a claim. Often, the claim can be corrected quickly and resubmitted to the clearinghouse, eliminating the costly delay associated with mailing back an incorrectly submitted paper claim. If the claim is clean, the clearinghouse translates the data elements into a format that is compatible with the format required by the target insurance carrier. (The data are not changed, but the order in which they are presented may be changed to accommodate the sequence required by the claims processing software system of a particular insurance company.) When reformatted, the data are sent electronically (usually overnight) to the target insurance company for processing. The insurance company prepares an explanation of benefits (EOB) or a RA, which is sent electronically to the clearinghouse. The data are reformatted (back into the original format) and transmitted back to the originating medical facility. Fig. 16-1 is a flow chart of electronic claims transmission through a clearinghouse.

Medical Billing Flow Chart

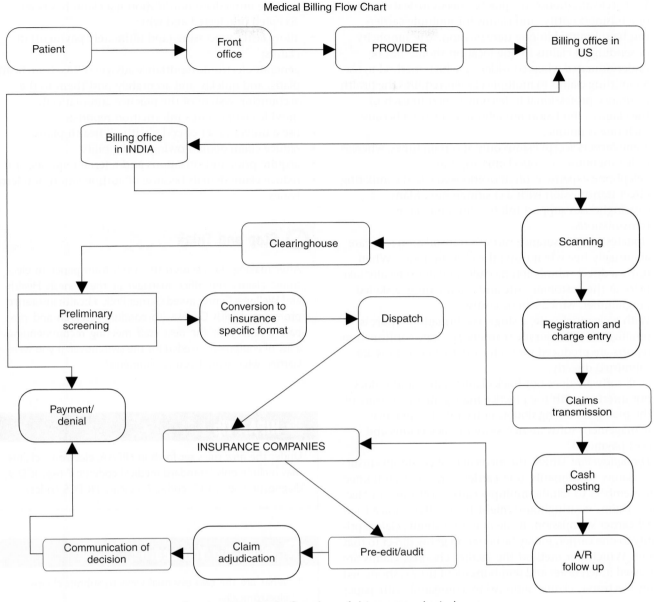

Fig. 16-1 Example of a flow chart of claim sent to clearinghouse.

Direct Data Entry Claims

Submitting claims directly to an insurance carrier, referred to as DDE claims, is a little more complex. As with a claims clearinghouse, most government carriers and many commercial carriers require enrollment before submitting DDE claims electronically. The medical facility also needs software from each insurance carrier to which it will be submitting claims. Most carriers have their own software or can recommend someone who supports direct transmissions within range of the medical facility. With direct data entry, the health insurance professional can log onto the website of a specific insurance carrier (e.g., TRICARE) and key claims directly into their system. The most common direct claims submission method is done by creating a "print image" file of the insurance claim and using the direct claims software to

send the claims to the insurance carrier; however, the method used in DDE claims can vary from carrier to carrier.

Clearinghouse versus Direct

When deciding which method is better for a medical facility to use—a clearinghouse or direct to the carrier—there are several things to consider:

- Submitting claims directly to the carrier is normally the less expensive method if the practice submits claims primarily to one carrier. However, if the practice submits claims electronically to multiple carriers, it may be more expensive than using a clearinghouse. If the direct method is chosen, the practice needs to enroll and become compatible with the software of each carrier to which claims are submitted.

- With a clearinghouse, the practice needs to deal with only one business entity, and claims for multiple carriers can be submitted in one transmission. The simplicity of sending all claims to one location should not be underestimated when considering which method to use. Submitting claims to multiple carriers requires the health insurance professional to become expert in each of the claims submission modules that are used because each one is unique.
- Some carriers accept claims only at certain times, whereas a clearinghouse accepts claims any time.
- Telephone expense is often overlooked when comparing direct transmission with a clearinghouse. Many clearinghouses support toll-free lines for claims transmissions.
- Updates to an insurance carrier's transmission software are usually free when using the clearinghouse. When using a direct submission module, updates typically take place at the customer's site and often require a skilled programmer, which can be costly.
- With a clearinghouse, a single confirmation report is produced for all insurance carriers. Separate confirmation reports are produced for each carrier where claims are submitted directly.
- DDE software does not track claims status, and it does not interface with the practice management software of the practice, making double entry into the practice management software necessary to track claims and post payments.

The bottom line: Unless the medical facility submits insurance claims to primarily one carrier and has well-trained staff members to handle multiple carrier software, an electronic claims clearinghouse might be a better choice than direct carrier submission. If the practice submits claims primarily to one carrier, it may be better off going direct to that carrier. Whichever method the facility chooses, claims are processed much faster and reimbursement time is shortened using electronic claims submission compared with paper claims.

🕐 Stop and Think

Fairview Geriatric Care Center sees only patients on Medicare. Hattie Carmichael, the health insurance professional at Fairview, must make a recommendation at the next staff meeting whether to submit claims through a clearinghouse or use DDE. Which method of claims submission do you think Hattie should choose?

Advantages of Filing Claims Electronically

There are numerous advantages to filing claims electronically. EDI transmissions typically
- result in faster, more efficient claim submissions with fewer errors;

- provide immediate notification if a claim has been accepted or rejected and why;
- allow faster processing (and ultimately payment) of claims;
- generate electronic remittance advices (ERAs) from health plans, and quickly and accurately post them to the accounting system of the practice automatically;
- provide claims status information reports;
- use a universal set of codes with all health plans;
- reduce claim denials owing to eligibility;
- acquire prior authorizations and referral requests; and
- reduce claim denials because of authorization or referral issues.

🕐 Stop and Think

After making the decision to switch from paper to electronic claims, the office manager at the Genesis Health and Wellness Center asked Garner Polk, a health insurance professional with Genesis, to conduct research and prepare a report for the next staff meeting recommending a list of equipment needed for the switchover. If you were Garner, what would you recommend?

📁 HIPAA Tip

Under the new rules set forth in HIPAA, electronic claims may include only "standard medical code sets" (e.g., ICD-9 diagnostic codes, CPT codes, Medicare HCPCS codes).

❓ What Did You Learn?

1. What are the two essential ways to submit claims electronically?
2. Name the process that needs to be completed before sending claims electronically.
3. How does the claims clearinghouse process work?
4. When might direct carrier submission be a better choice than a clearinghouse?
5. List five advantages of filing claims electronically.

MEDICARE AND ELECTRONIC CLAIMS SUBMISSION

Congress enacted ASCA to improve the administration of the Medicare program by taking advantage of the efficiencies to be gained through electronic claim submission or **electronic media claims (EMCs)**. The Department of Health and Human Services (HHS) published the final "rule" for the electronic submission of Medicare claims mandated under ASCA. With certain exceptions, ASCA required that all claims sent to the Medicare program on or after October 16, 2003, be submitted electronically.

When billing electronically, disbursement time is greatly reduced. The payment floor for paper claims is 28 days, which means that when a clean claim (one that does not require external development) is submitted, the provider/beneficiary will be eligible to receive payment on the 29th day. In comparison, electronic claims have a 13-day payment floor, which means that clean claims are eligible for payment on the 14th day. With this faster turnaround time, follow-up time is minimized.

Electronic claims submission is required only for initial Medicare claims, including initial claims with paper attachments, submitted for processing by the medical fiscal intermediary or carrier that serves the physician, practitioner, facility, supplier, or other healthcare provider. The rule does not require any other transactions (e.g., changes, adjustments, or appeals to the initial claim) to be submitted electronically.

Claims submitted via DDE are considered to be electronic claims for purposes of the rule. In addition, claims transmitted to a Medicare contractor using the free or low-cost claims software issued by Medicare fee-for-service plans are also electronic claims for purposes of the rule. Exceptions to the electronic claims submission requirement under the rule are as follows:

- The entity has no method available for submitting claims electronically. Three situations fall into this category:
  1. Roster billing of vaccinations covered by the Medicare program
  2. Claims for payment under Medicare demonstration projects
  3. Claims where more than one plan is responsible for payment before Medicare
- The entity submitting the claim is a small provider of services or small supplier. A **small provider of services** is a hospital, critical access hospital, skilled nursing facility, comprehensive outpatient rehabilitation facility, home health agency, or hospice program with fewer than 25 full-time equivalent employees. A **small supplier** is a physician, practitioner, facility, or supplier with fewer than 10 full-time equivalent employees.
- The Secretary of HHS finds that a waiver of the electronic submission requirement is appropriate because of unusual circumstances. **Unusual circumstances** exist in any one of the following situations:
  1. Submission of dental claims
  2. A service interruption in the mode of submitting the electronic claims that is outside of the control of the submitting entity but only for the period of the interruption and subject to the specific requirements set forth under the rule
  3. On demonstration to the satisfaction of the Secretary of HHS that other extraordinary circumstances exist that preclude the submission of electronic claims

Other than these exceptions, ASCA states that no payment may be made under Parts A or B of the Medicare program for claims submitted in nonelectronic form. Entities that fail to comply with the rule may be subject to claim denial, overpayment recovery, and applicable interest on overpayments. HHS does not intend to broaden these limited exceptions.

To keep up-to-date on Medicare's electronic claims submission requirements, visit the Evolve site.

Stop and Think

Margaret Turner, a family practice physician, runs a health clinic in Flint County, which is located in a rural area of the Midwest. Besides herself, Dr. Turner employs a physician assistant, a registered nurse, a laboratory technician, two full-time medical assistants, and a part-time bookkeeper. Dr. Turner hires a private billing service (which has 16 full-time employees) to handle all of the clinic's billing and insurance claims. Based on the HHS rule, does Dr. Turner's facility qualify as an exempt entity?

Imagine This!

Clark Emmerson, a health insurance professional with Loveland Health Center, sends all of the center's insurance claims to RapidServ Clearinghouse. RapidServ performs an edit check on each claim and redistributes them in batches to the appropriate carrier. On one particular batch, a computer error resulted in the employer identification number being left off the claims. RapidServ caught the error, corrected it, and sent the claims on without having to return them to Clark for completion.

What Did You Learn?

1. To what entities is the HHS final rule applicable?
2. To what types of claims does the rule not apply?
3. Give an example of an "unusual circumstance" for which waiver of electronic submission might apply.

ADDITIONAL ELECTRONIC SERVICES AVAILABLE

In addition to submitting claims electronically, several other electronic services are available to the health insurance professional for streamlining the insurance claims submission process.

Electronic Funds Transfer

Electronic funds transfer (EFT) is a system whereby data representing money are moved electronically between accounts or organizations. In the case of insurance claims, when claims are submitted electronically, many carriers transfer the payments directly into the provider's bank account rather than mailing a check, making the funds instantly usable. There are several advantages to receiving insurance payments via EFT rather than paper checks. EFT

- reduces the amount of paper;
- eliminates the risk of paper checks being lost or stolen in the mail;
- saves time and hassle of going to the bank to deposit checks; and
- speeds funds to the provider's bank account, where they can be used or can start earning interest immediately, whereas paper checks can take up to a week to process.

To enroll in the Medicare direct deposit program or the direct deposit program of another carrier, all the provider needs to do is contact the specific payer and ask for an EFT enrollment form, fill it out, and mail it back. To help ensure the validity of deposit information, the form must have original signatures (no copies, facsimiles, or stamped signatures) and include a copy of a canceled or voided check for the bank and the account in which the provider wants the monies to be deposited. Fig. 16-2 shows a typical form used to authorize EFT.

Electronic Remittance Advice

In addition to EFT, Medicare and other carriers offer an **electronic remittance advice (ERA)**. An ERA allows the provider's office to receive EOBs or RAs electronically. With ERA, payments can be posted automatically to patient accounts, allowing the health insurance professional to update accounts receivable much more quickly and accurately than if he or she had to post the payments manually. Fig. 16-3 is an example form authorizing the carrier to transmit an RA electronically.

If a medical facility chooses to receive a Medicare ERA, it first needs to have its computer system programmed. A programmer needs the most recent Centers for Medicare and Medicaid Services (CMS) ANSI specifications (available on the CMS website). When a practice begins receiving payment reports electronically, the practice may choose to discontinue receiving the paper copy.

The electronic capabilities of many third-party payers and clearinghouses include periodic claim status reports (Fig. 16-4), which give a detailed list of claims that have to be paid, are pending, or have been denied. These reports can be hard copies or electronic through the practice software.

Role of Computers in Transitioning to ICD-10 Diagnostic Coding System

On January 1, 2012, standards for electronic healthcare transactions changed from Version 4010/4010A1 to Version 5010. These electronic healthcare transactions include functions such as claims, eligibility inquiries, and RAs. In contrast to Version 4010/4010A1, Version 5010 accommodates

the ICD-10 codes and must have been in place before the changeover to ICD-10 to allow adequate Version 5010 testing and implementation time. If providers did not conduct electronic transactions using Version 5010 as of June 30 2012, delays in claim reimbursement may result.

The conversion from the ICD-9 diagnostic coding system to the ICD-10 system no doubt will be challenging because the number of codes is increasing from roughly 14,000 in the ICD-9 system to nearly 70,000 in ICD-10. To handle this monumental task, computers will definitely be involved. The National Center for Health Statistics, CMS, American Health Information Management Association, American Hospital Association, and 3 M Health Information Systems have put together some **General Equivalence Mappings (GEMs)**. GEMs is a computerized tool that can be used to convert data from ICD-9 to ICD-10—referred to as forward mapping—and back to ICD-9—referred to as backward mapping. The mapping process with GEMs is not exact, owing to the extent of more specific diagnostic wording used in the ICD-10 codes, and is not a substitute for learning how to use the ICD-10-CM and ICD-10-PCS coding manuals. GEMs is available as a download from the Internet. To read or download this document, visit the Evolve site.

When coding claims, it is considered more efficient and accurate to work from the patient health record documentation and then select the appropriate codes from the coding manual. However, with the movement to EMRs, the healthcare provider often chooses the code, after which professional certified coders review the documentation and make suggestions for possible changes.

What Did You Learn?

1. What occurs when funds are transmitted electronically?
2. List two advantages of EFT.
3. What is one advantage of receiving an RA electronically compared with a paper RA?
4. Discuss the function and use of GEMs.

ELECTRONIC MEDICAL RECORD

An **electronic medical record (EMR)** is an electronic file wherein a patient's health information is stored in a computer system. Synonymous terms for EMR include EPR (electronic patient record), EHR (electronic health record), and CPR (computerized patient record).

The use of EMRs to store patient health information is becoming increasingly prevalent in today's healthcare environment. The information contained in EMRs varies greatly in type—ranging from simple and routine clinical data to sophisticated medical images. An EMR typically includes the following components:

- *Patient's history*—including past encounters, medications, procedures, referrals, and vital statistics

Electronic Funds Transfer (EFT) Form

Please choose one of these options:

☐ Elect EFT payments ☐ Change EFT information ☐ Terminate EFT payments

Name of Brokerage Firm: _____

Name of Broker: _____

Business Address: _____

City: _____ State: _____ Zip Code: _____

Phone Number: _____

Please attach a voided check, if available. When providing the Account and Routing/Transit Numbers, please refer to the series of numbers located at the bottom of your check and insert those numbers located between the symbols shown. For your reference, please see the sample check on the reverse side of this form.

Type of Account: ☐ Business Account   or   ☐ Personal Account   *(check one)*
                 ☐ Checking   or   ☐ Savings   *(check one)*

Name(s) on Account: _____
Please list all names that appear on the account

Account Number: ⑆ _____ ⑈

Name of Financial Institution: _____

City: _____ State: _____

Routing/Transit Number: ⑆ ☐ ☐ ☐ ☐ ☐ ☐ ☐ ☐ ⑆

<u>IMPORTANT NOTE:</u> It is the applicant's responsibility to ensure that the information provided on this form is complete and accurate. _____ will not be responsible and shall be held harmless for errors made in EFT payments that are a result of inaccurate or incomplete information provided on this form. In no event and under no circumstances will _____ liability exceed the amount of the EFT payments in question.

_____   _____
Signature of Account Owner   Date   Signature of Brokerage Firm Authorized Representative   Date

_____   _____
Print Name   Print Name

_____   _____
Title   Title

To protect the privacy of your financial information, please do not fax or e-mail completed forms. Please mail your signed and completed forms to the following address: **Health Care, Inc., Treasury Department, 93 Fourth Street, Anytown, MA 09080**

For Internal Use Only:	Vendor ID #

Fig. 16-2 Example of an electronic funds transfer form.

Authorization for Electronic Transmission of AHCCCS Fee-For-Service Remittance Advice

I Hereby request and authorize the AHCCCS Administration to transmit my Fee-For-Service Remittance Advice via the Internet to the electronic mail (email) address listed below. I understand that I will no longer receive a paper copy of my Remittance Advice once I begin receiving my Remittance Advice electronically.

I understand that although my Remittance Advice will be transmitted electronically, my reimbursement check(s) will continue to be delivered by the U.S. Postal Service to the pay-to address(es) on file with the AHCCCS Administration Provider Registration Unit.

I understand that it is my responsibility to notify the AHCCCS Administration Provider Registration Unit in writing of any change in my email address.

Provider/Group Name: _____

AHCCCS Provider Identification Number: _____

Street Address: _____

City: _____ State: _____ ZIP Code: _____

Telephone: ( ) _____ Fax: ( ) _____

Name of Contact Person: _____

Email address: _____

Signature of Provider
or Authorized Representative: _____

Date: _____

Mail this form to: AHCCCS Provider Registration Unit
MD 8100
701 E. Jefferson St.
Anytown, XY 85034

or

Fax this form to: AHCCCS Provider Registration Unit
(602) 256-xxxx

Please allow 10 working days for implementation of this change.

Fig. 16-3 Example authorization for an electronic remittance advice.

Fig. 16-4 Example of an electronic claims status information advice.

• *Transaction capability*—such as ordering of laboratory tests, medical procedures, and prescriptions
• *Administrative functionality*—including invoice generation, payment requests, payer documentation compliance, and clinical research data compilation

There are obvious benefits to be gained from being able to store, ask questions of, and exchange medical information electronically among various healthcare sites. With the advances in technology, some professional offices and hospitals use electronic media to save money and space. However, not all offices are ready to change completely over to electronic files. Options are to use one of two types of hybrid medical records.

Combination Records

Combination records allow the amount of paper records to be reduced because some of the documents are stored electronically and some are kept in paper form. Any type of record that can be created electronically, such as chart notes, test results, and prescription records, are stored as electronic records for easy access. Other documents that were originally created on paper—consent forms and correspondence—are kept in paper form. It is up to each office to determine which records are kept on paper and which are kept in electronic form.

Digital Imaging Hybrid

If the goal of a healthcare office is to migrate completely to an EMR system, a **digital imaging hybrid** may be a good choice. For this type of medical record keeping, many of the documents are maintained in their paper form, but to save space and time when trying to locate a specific record, the paper documentation is scanned and digitally filed into a computer system. In some cases, the paper documentation may be disposed of, or the office may choose to store the

physical documents offsite in case they are needed in the future.

Although storing medical records electronically saves space and allows for easier access to the healthcare staff, some professionals worry about the possibility of an electrical outage, viruses, hacking, or other computer issues. If such a problem occurs, no one would be able to access the electronic records. For this reason, some providers are uncomfortable with transferring completely to an electronic system. Using a hybrid system provides the best of both worlds—keeping the paper records just in case, but providing the easy access of an electronic system. For more information on hybrid records, visit the Evolve site.

Potential Issues

Two of the major disadvantages that some professionals see with changing over to an EMR system are the cost and the amount of time it takes to transfer records. They may be concerned that the transition would disrupt the quality of care they can provide for their patients or concerned about the cost of purchasing, setting up, and maintaining the system and the potential need for additional staff. However, if the transition is planned carefully, it can be a smooth process. The use of a hybrid system allows a facility to take its time transferring records. All records for new patients can be immediately entered into the electronic system; records for established patients can be transferred as each patient is seen or through a gradual, systematic process.

Another issue is that there are many EMR systems on the market. The idea of streamlining patient care across the United States can be achieved only when a single system is used because two or more systems may be incompatible. For example, if a hospital uses a different EMR system than nearby healthcare providers whose patients use that facility, records may not be available to the hospital, or vice versa—from the hospital to the provider. Although EMRs may reduce office paperwork, they may not coordinate care between several treating physicians, pharmacies, and allied health workers if different systems are used by each group.

Finally, there is the issue of security of EMRs, which must be completely confidential. Hackers ultimately may be able to penetrate EMRs despite security precautions, and they may release confidential information to others or use it fraudulently. This possibility has both providers and patients worried about how safe and confidential EMRs really are.

One of the most significant activities of the healthcare industry is information management. Because of the enormous amount of patient data in existence, computer technology can be an extremely useful tool for the healthcare industry. There are obstacles to overcome, however, because computerized patient medical records are used universally in the healthcare environment.

⭐ Imagine This!

The computer system in the Fairview Geriatric Care Clinic was damaged during an electrical storm. Hattie Carmichael, the health insurance professional, had made a tape backup, so no data were lost. However, the computer technical support staff informed her that it would be a week or more before the system would be up and running again. Because this qualified as an "unusual circumstance," Hattie informed InfoData, the local Medicare B carrier, that she would be submitting paper claims while the computer was not functional.

Future of Electronic Medical Records

The ultimate goal in healthcare is an intercommunicative EMR system, in which an emergency department physician in Florida can treat a vacationing heart patient from the Midwest effectively by "pulling up" his EMR on a computer. If and when this goal is reached, clinicians would be able to access a more timely and complete picture of a patient's clinical history, allowing physicians to make better informed healthcare decisions for patients. To be effective, however, the EMR system would have to integrate data from several sources through a linked collection of records and message capabilities. The system also would have to provide decision support such as reminders, alerts, and clinical pathway information. The EMR must serve as the provider's primary source of information including orders and test results. With this approach, all the user needs to be fully operational are a browser, an Internet service provider, and a personal computer.

If an EMR system is to provide a comprehensive solution for a contemporary practice environment, it should streamline workflow efficiency, improve adherence to treatment standards, provide detailed financial practice analysis, enhance patient education and interaction, and optimize compliance with regulatory and managed care guidelines. Claims submission, physician referrals, patient records, and scheduling information are among the pieces of administrative data that providers could send through a secure central processing hub. This technology would guarantee that data transactions comply with all regulations mandating the privacy of medical data transfer and would allow a non–Web-enabled application to run centrally over an Internet connection. The software could be operated as though it were local on the remote user's computer.

The advantages of this process would be considerable. Users could employ a handheld device, PC, or laptop to input medical record information into a file held on a proprietary server. Some large medical centers already offer such services to their physician groups. This service allows patients in an emergency to inform the emergency department physician where to find their charts or laboratory reports on the Internet.

Privacy Concerns of Electronic Medical Records

As previously mentioned, both providers and patients want assurances that data transferred electronically would not become vulnerable and would not fall into the wrong hands. To address this, the American Medical Association in collaboration with microchip maker Intel have introduced an encrypted identification code that can keep Internet transactions private and patients' rights protected. As consumers explore online EMR possibilities and begin to trust that online healthcare can be kept as confidential as banking accounts, the market can explore its full potential, and providers can realize its benefits.

Federal Funding for Electronic Medical Record Trials and "Meaningful Use"

Until the American Recovery and Reinvestment Act (ARRA) of 2009 was passed, healthcare providers were expected to take the full risk of investing in high-priced EMR systems. Because of the potential for government payers, such as Medicare, to realize significant cost savings if providers adopted EMR systems, the Health Information Technology for Economic and Clinical Health (HITECH) Act (part of the ARRA 2009 economic stimulus package) came up with an incentive program to encourage more physicians to adopt an EMR system.

To receive the EMR stimulus money, healthcare providers must show "meaningful use" of an EMR system. **Meaningful use** describes the use of health information technology that, ideally, would lead to improvements in healthcare and further the goals of information exchange among professionals. The first step in achieving meaningful use is to invest in a certified EMR system after which providers must be able to demonstrate that it is being used to meet federal requirements.

To become "meaningful users," providers must demonstrate that they are using certified EMR technology in ways that can be measured significantly in both quantity and quality. The three main components of meaningful use are

- the use of a certified EMR in a meaningful manner, such as electronic prescriptions;
- the use of certified EMR technology for electronic exchange of health information to improve quality of health care; and
- the use of certified EMR technology to submit clinical quality and other measures.

The meaningful use of EMR incentives is projected to

- improve care coordination,
- reduce healthcare disparities,
- engage patients and their families,
- improve population and public health, and
- ensure adequate privacy and security.

Initially, this incentive program does not invoke penalties; however, physicians who do not adopt an EMR by 2015 will be penalized 1% of Medicare payments, increasing to 3% over 3 years. As of this writing, there are no penalty provisions for Medicaid.

HHS released final rules on how healthcare providers can qualify for monetary incentives to put EMRs into operation beginning in 2011. For more information on this topic, visit the Evolve site.

📁 HIPAA Tip

HIPAA compliance security standards mandate safeguards for physical storage and maintenance, transmission, and access to individual health information. The standards apply not only to the transactions adopted under HIPAA but also to all individual health information that is maintained or transmitted. HIPAA gives organizations the flexibility to choose the best security solutions to meet the security and privacy mandates.

💬 What Did You Learn?

1. What are EMRs?
2. Explain the two options of hybrid medical records.
3. What are two important concerns regarding EMRs?

SUMMARY CHECKPOINTS

▶ The age of technology has had a great impact on health insurance. Many functions that were previously performed manually are now done faster and with fewer errors using a computer. Processing claims electronically is one of the biggest changes the computer has brought to claims processing. Advanced technology has also created a concern for the security of privacy of health information.

▶ The five areas of administrative simplification addressed by HIPAA are as follows:
  • *Electronic data interchange (EDI)*—electronic transfer of information in a standard format between two entities. Transactions included within HIPAA consist of standard electronic formats for enrollment, eligibility, payment and RA, claims, health plan premium payments, health claim status, and referral certification and authorization.
  • *Code sets*—data elements used to document uniformly the reasons why patients are seen and procedures or services provided to them during healthcare encounters. HIPAA adopted the following specific code sets: HCPCS (Ancillary Services/Procedures), CPT-4 (Physicians' Procedures), CDT (Dental Terminology), ICD-10-CM for physician diagnoses, ICD-10-PCS for inpatient hospital procedures, and NDC (National Drug Codes).

  • *Identifiers*—numbers that HIPAA requires to be used in the administration of healthcare to distinguish individual healthcare providers, health plans, employers, and patients.
  • *Security standards*—required for all health plans, clearinghouses, and providers to follow at all stages of transmission and storage of healthcare information to ensure integrity and confidentiality of the records at all phases of the process, before, during, and after electronic transmission.
  • *Privacy standards*—to define what are appropriate and inappropriate disclosures of individually identifiable health information and how patient rights are to be protected.

▶ EDI is the exchange of documents in standardized electronic form, between business entities, in an automated manner, directly from a computer application in one facility to an application in another. The essential elements of EDI include the following:
  • *Electronic transmission medium* such as magnetic tapes and disks
  • *Structured, formatted messages based on agreed standards* or set of rules
  • *Fast delivery* of electronic documents from sender to receiver
  • *Direct communication* between applications

▶ A clearinghouse acts as an intermediary between the medical facility and the insurance carrier. A clearinghouse receives claims from several medical facilities, checks the claims for errors or omissions, consolidates the claims, and transmits them (usually in batches) to individual insurance carriers.

▶ Advantages of submitting claims electronically include, but are not limited to, the following:
  • Faster, more efficient claim submissions, with fewer errors
  • Immediate claim status notification
  • Quicker processing (and ultimately faster payment) of claims
  • Fast and accurate posting of ERAs automatically to the practice's accounting system
  • Use of universal code sets with all health plans
  • Reduction of claim denials because of eligibility, authorization, or referral issues

▶ HHS published the final "rule" for electronic submission of Medicare claims mandated under ASCA. With certain exceptions, ASCA requires that all claims sent to the Medicare Program on or after October 16, 2003, be submitted electronically. This rule is applicable only to providers, practitioners, and suppliers who submit claims under Part A or Part B of Medicare.

▶ Other electronic services available to the health insurance professional include the following:

- *EFT* allows data representing money to be moved electronically from one bank account to another. In the case of insurance, reimbursement to providers in the form of EFTs is instantaneous, allowing funds to be immediately available to the medical practice.
- *ERA* allows Medicare and other carriers to transmit the explanation of benefits or RA to the provider electronically, and payments can be posted directly into patient accounts automatically.
- *EMR* is an electronic file stored in a computer or other electronic medium containing a patient's health information.

▶ The future of EMRs looks promising. More and more medical facilities are replacing their manual record-keeping systems with electronic systems, and although the initial expense can be sizable, the improved efficiency of EMRs and the capability of integrating multiplatform environments tip the scale in favor of EMRs. There are some concerns, however, including possible breaches in the privacy and confidentiality of protected health information.

CLOSING SCENARIO

Now that they are finished with the chapter, Ellie and Benji realize that as health insurance professionals, they will no doubt receive and transmit protected health information on a daily basis. With the advent of HIPAA, patients will depend on people like them more than ever to ensure that their health information remains confidential and secure. By understanding and implementing the HIPAA administrative and technical requirements, health insurance professionals can assure patients that their electronic claims will be processed in a timely manner and private health information will be safeguarded. Ellie and Benji realize that one of the important reasons HIPAA was created was to protect the privacy and security of healthcare information that is electronically transmitted; they also realize the importance of HIPAA to healthcare in general.

WEBSITES TO EXPLORE

- For live links to the following websites, please visit the Evolve site at
  http://evolve.elsevier.com/Beik/today
- Guides providing formats for data exchanged by healthcare entities (CMS-1500 08/05, UB04, ADA-94, and proprietary forms) may be obtained at
  http://www.wpc-edi.com/hipaa
- For more information on individual code sets, browse
  http://cms.hhs.gov
  http://www.cms.hhs.gov/ElectronicBillingEDITrans/
- Official versions of National Data Communications files are available at
  http://www.physiciansnews.com/cover/505.html

Author's Note: Websites change frequently. If any of these URLs is unavailable, use applicable guide words in your Internet search to acquire additional information on the various subjects listed.

REFERENCES AND RESOURCES

AHIMA e-HIM Work Group on Health Information in a Hybrid Environment 2003: *The complete medical record in a hybrid electronic health record environment.* Available at: http://www.ahima.org.

Amatayakul M: Make your telecommuting program HIPAA compliant, *J AHIMA* 73:16A–16C, 2002.

Bonewit-West K: *Computer Concepts and Applications for the Medical Office,* Philadelphia, 1993, Saunders.

Davis N, LaCour M: *Introduction to Health Information Technology,* Philadelphia, 2002, Saunders.

Fordney MT: *Insurance Handbook for the Medical Office,* Philadelphia, 2002, Saunders.

Gylya BA: *Computer Applications for the Medical Office,* Philadelphia, 1997, FA Davis.

Hagland M: Electronic record, electronic security, *J AHIMA* 75:18–22, 2004.

Keller C, Valerius J: *Medical Insurance,* Columbus, Ohio, 2002, Glencoe/McGraw-Hill.

Moisio M: *Guide to Health Insurance Billing,* Albany, NY, 2001, Delmar.

Quinsey CA, Brandt MD: *AHIMA practice brief: information security–an overview,* Chicago, 2003, AHIMA.

Rowell J, Green M: *Understanding Health Insurance,* Albany, NY, 2004, Delmar.

Sabri EH, Gupta AP, Beitler MA: *Purchase Order Management Best Practices,* Fort Lauderdale, Fla, 2006, J Ross Publishing.

Sanderson SM: *Computers in the Medical Office,* Columbus, Ohio, 1998, Glencoe/McGraw-Hill.

Sanderson SM: *Patient Billing, Using MediSoft Advanced,* Columbus, Ohio, 2002, Glencoe/McGraw-Hill.

The Impact of Computers on a Medical Practice. Available at: http://www.ehow.com/facts_5732616_impact-computers-medical-practice.html#ixzz1Q0tNSHkZ.

Wagner M: *U.S. Allocates $1.2 Billion for Electronic Medical Records,* 2009, Information Week. Available at: http://www.informationweek.com/news/healthcare/EMR/showArticle.jhtml?articleID=219400954.

CHAPTER 17

Reimbursement Procedures: Getting Paid

Chapter Outline

I. Understanding Reimbursement Systems
  A. Types of Reimbursement
    1. Fee-for-Service
    2. Discounted Fee-for-Service
    3. Prospective Payment System
    4. Relative Value Units
    5. Managed Care Organizations
    6. Capitation
II. Medicare and Reimbursement
  A. Medicare Prospective Payment System
  B. How the Medicare Prospective Payment System Works
    1. Acute Inpatient Prospective Payment System
    2. Outpatient Prospective Payment System
    3. Skilled Nursing Facility Prospective Payment System
    4. Home Health Prospective Payment System
    5. Inpatient Rehabilitation Facility Prospective Payment System
    6. Inpatient Psychiatric Facility Prospective Payment System
    7. Long-Term Care Hospital Prospective Payment System
    8. Medicare Advantage Program (Centers for Medicare and Medicaid Services Hierarchical Condition Category)
III. Other Systems for Determining Reimbursement
  A. Relative Value Scale
  B. Resource-Based Relative Value Scale
  C. Diagnosis-Related Groups
    1. How Diagnosis-Related Groups Work
    2. Assigning a Diagnosis-Related Group to a Patient
    3. Calculating Diagnosis-Related Group Payments
  D. Ambulatory Payment Classifications
  E. Resource Utilization Groups
IV. Transition of Medicare to Resource-Based Relative Value Scale
  A. Setting Medicare Payment Policy
  B. Medicare Inpatient Hospital Prospective Payment System
  C. Medicare Long-Term Care Hospital Prospective Payment System
V. Additional Prospective Payment Systems
  A. Home Health Prospective Payment System
  B. Inpatient Rehabilitation Facility Prospective Payment System
  C. Significance of Reimbursement Systems to the Health Insurance Professional
VI. Peer Review Organizations and Prospective Payment Systems
VII. Understanding Computerized Patient Accounting Systems
  A. Selecting the Right Billing System
  B. Managing Transactions
    1. Posting and Tracking Patient Charges
    2. Processing Payments
    3. Insurance Carrier Adjustments (Contractual Write-offs)
  C. Generating Reports
    1. Accounts Receivable Aging Report
    2. Insurance Claims Aging Report
    3. Practice Analysis Report
VIII. Health Insurance Portability and Accountability Act and Practice Management Software

OPENING SCENARIO

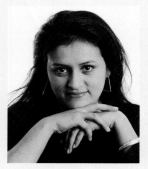

Dave Brown does not understand why it is important for a health insurance professional to learn about reimbursement systems and patient accounting systems. In his opinion, the important content in this course is the information regarding completing and submitting insurance claims forms. When that is mastered, he is prepared to start a successful medical billing career—or is he?

Janetta Karlowski has a different opinion. She had been working as a billing and insurance clerk in a medical office for the past 4 years and enrolled in the course because she did not know enough about these systems, and this lack of information was holding her back. "Reimbursement systems are constantly changing, and new ones are being added," she told Dave. "Granted, they may be complicated and confusing, but you have to stay on top of things to really do the job right or you'll find yourself being replaced by someone who is better educated."

Dave is still skeptical as he looks over the objectives. PPS, APCs, RUGs, DRGs—it's like alphabet soup. How can anyone make sense of all these acronyms? "We'll work together," Janetta tells him, "and we'll get through this chapter together. We've come this far; we can't quit now." She realized this information was more advanced than the previous chapters, and perhaps she should not have criticized Dave for being skeptical of its relevance to the average medical billing and insurance clerk. After 4 years of experience, however, Janetta is convinced that knowledge is power, and the more you know about your specialty, the better your chances are for advancement and higher pay.

CHAPTER OBJECTIVES

After completion of this chapter, the student should be able to:
1. List and explain the various types of reimbursement.
2. Discuss the Medicare prospective payment system (PPS) and how it works.
3. Outline the various systems for determining reimbursement: relative value scale (RVS) resource-based relative value scale (RBRVS), diagnosis-related groups (DRGs), ambulatory payment classifications (APCs), and resource utilization groups (RUGs).
4. Summarize the transition of Medicare to RBRVS.
5. Describe additional PPS.
6. Discuss responsibilities of peer review organizations as they relate to PPS.
7. Identify the various functions that most patient accounting software systems can perform.
8. List the advantages of practice management software that is compliant with the Health Insurance Portability and Accountability Act (HIPAA).

CHAPTER TERMS

accounts receivable aging report
activities of daily living (ADLs)
ambulatory payment classifications (APCs)
average length of stay (ALOS)
balance billing
business associate
capitation
case-mix adjustment
comorbidity
contractual write-off
cost outliers
covered entity
diagnosis-related group (DRG)
discounted fee-for-service
disproportionate share
DRG grouper
fee-for-service
geographic practice cost index (GPCI)
home health prospective payment system
inpatient rehabilitation facility prospective payment system (IRF PPS)
labor component
long-term care hospital prospective payment system (LTCH PPS)
managed care organizations (MCOs)
nonlabor component
peer review organization (PRO)
per diem rates
principal diagnosis
prospective payment system (PPS)
reimbursement
relative value scale (RVS)
residential healthcare facility
resource utilization groups (RUGs)
resource-based relative value scale (RBRVS)
short-stay outlier
skilled nursing facility (SNF)
standardized amount
Tax Equity and Fiscal Responsibility Act (TEFRA)
usual, customary, and reasonable (UCR)

UNDERSTANDING REIMBURSEMENT SYSTEMS

To understand fully the entire health insurance picture and how fees are established, the health insurance professional should be aware of the various reimbursement systems, their structure, and how they affect health insurance in general. Understanding reimbursement systems is important in making the most of payment opportunities. Current reimbursement systems are based on five elements that impact the dollar amount paid:
• Third-party payer
• Healthcare setting/provider
• Coding system (ICD/CPT)
• Data set used
• Encoder, grouper, and data entry software used

Because reimbursement systems can be challenging, every healthcare facility ideally should assign someone the responsibility of being the "reimbursement expert." The health insurance professional might fit this role best, and he or she should be prepared to take on this responsibility. The rules are constantly changing with the frequent introduction of new payment formulas, and it takes diligence and dedication to keep current with these changes. Small adjustments in the payment rates can make a big difference in practice income. The following sections describe the various types of reimbursement and their fee structures.

Types of Reimbursement

From an insurance standpoint, the term **reimbursement** means payment to the insured for a covered expense or loss experienced by or on behalf of the insured. More specifically in health insurance, reimbursement is a payment made to a provider or to a patient in exchange for the performance of healthcare services. There are several different types of reimbursement in the healthcare office. Table 17-1 lists common types of reimbursement.

Fee-for-Service

As we learned in Chapter 4, **fee-for-service** is a system of payment for healthcare services whereby the provider charges a specific fee (typically the **usual, customary, and reasonable [UCR]** fee) for each service rendered and is paid that fee by the patient or by the patient's insurance carrier. UCR is a fee amount an insurance carrier will accept based on the prevailing charges made by physicians in a similar specialty for a particular service or procedure within a specific community or geographic area.

Discounted Fee-for-Service

When a healthcare provider offers services at rates that are lower than UCR fees, that arrangement is called discounted fee-for-service. A typical example of **discounted**

fee-for-service is when a healthcare provider is a participating provider with a preferred provider organization (PPO) and charges patients enrolled in the PPO lower rates in return for certain amenities from the PPO. (See Chapter 7 for details about PPOs.)

Prospective Payment System

A third type of reimbursement is the **prospective payment system (PPS)**. With a PPS, reimbursement is made to the healthcare provider on the basis of predetermined factors (e.g., patient category or type of facility) and not on individual services. PPS is Medicare's system for reimbursing Part A inpatient hospital costs. The amount of payment is determined by the assigned **diagnosis-related group (DRG)**. PPS rates are set at a level intended to cover operating costs for treating a typical inpatient in a given DRG. DRGs are discussed in more detail later in this chapter.

The Centers for Medicare and Medicaid Services (CMS) uses a separate PPS for reimbursement to acute inpatient hospitals, home health agencies, hospice, hospital outpatient care, inpatient psychiatric facilities, inpatient rehabilitation facilities, long-term care hospitals (LTCH), and skilled nursing facilities (SNFs). Payments for each hospital are adjusted for differences in area wages, teaching activity, care to the poor, and other factors. PPS and DRGs are discussed in more detail later. To see related links for more detailed information about each specific PPS, visit the Evolve site.

Relative Value Units

Many insurance companies reimburse on a fee schedule that is based on relative value units (RVUs). More and more practices are also converting to a provider fee schedule that is based on RVUs. With the use of computers for medical billing, attaching RVUs to each procedure in the system provides the advantage of having a logical explanation for patients who inquire about the cost of their procedure (e.g., "the procedure is valued at 10 RVUs, and our conversion factor is $70 per RVU"). Patients tend to understand and accept this more readily than explaining what a UCR fee is (e.g., "$700 is what the average charge is for physicians in the same specialty in our area"). Additionally, when procedure codes are attached to an RVU, when the practice finds it necessary to increase its charges, the practice merely increases the conversion factor, rather than go into each procedure in the computer system and reset the charge amount. RVUs are discussed in more detail later in the chapter.

Managed Care Organizations

Managed care organizations (MCOs) vary greatly in their policies and procedures for reimbursement, and laws vary significantly from state to state. Individual MCO contracts have specific restrictions and requirements, and contracts may have rate reductions and discounts of certain types of care (e.g., telephone consultations). Referral processes typically require prior authorization, and billing procedures with MCOs are often complex.

TABLE 17-1	Comparison of Reimbursement Methods
REIMBURSEMENT TYPE	**EXPLANATION**
Fee-for-service	Services or procedures are paid as charged from physician's fee schedule
Discounted fee-for-service	Services or procedures are paid at insurers' contracted rates
PPS	Flat-rate reimbursement based on predetermined factors such as diagnoses, procedures, or a combination of both
Capitation	Payment is based on a fixed, per capita amount for each person served without regard to the actual number or nature of services provided

Capitation

Capitation is a method of payment for healthcare services in which a provider or healthcare facility is paid a fixed, per capita amount for each individual to whom services are provided without regard to the actual number or nature of the services provided to each individual patient. Capitation is a common method of paying physicians in health maintenance organizations (HMOs).

❓ What Did You Learn?

1. Define reimbursement.
2. List the basic types of reimbursement.
3. Explain the difference between fee-for-service and discounted fee-for-service.
4. _____ is a common method of reimbursement in health maintenance organizations.

MEDICARE AND REIMBURSEMENT

The **Tax Equity and Fiscal Responsibility Act (TEFRA)** enacted by Congress in 1982 provided for limits on Medicare reimbursement that applied to stays in long-term acute care hospitals. After TEFRA was passed, the fee-for-service–based payment system was replaced with a PPS.

Initially, only Medicare patients were included in the PPS. Later, Medicaid patients were added on a state-by-state basis. As mentioned, with the PPS, a predetermined payment level is established primarily on the basis of a patient's diagnoses and services performed, and the hospital receives a set payment. If money spent to care for a patient is less than the PPS payment, the healthcare facility is allowed to keep the extra money and makes a profit on the care provided. However, if the money spent to care for a patient is more than the PPS payment, the healthcare organization loses money in caring for the patient.

Medicare presently has three primary reimbursement systems:

- *Prospective payment*—a system of predetermined prices that Medicare uses to reimburse hospitals for inpatient and outpatient services and SNFs, rehabilitation hospitals, and home health services.
- *Fee schedules*—consisting of price lists that Medicare uses to reimburse healthcare providers for the services they provide and other healthcare providers for items and services that are not "bundled" into PPS, such as clinical laboratory tests, durable medical equipment, and some prosthetic devices.
- *Medicare Advantage* (Medicare Part C)—Medicare's managed care program in which Medicare pays a set fee to managed care plans to provide care for Medicare beneficiaries.

⭐ Imagine This!

Four different patients visit Dr. Carson Inglewood, a family practice physician, for symptoms of influenza. Dr. Inglewood's charge for an office visit is $50. Tony, a 22-year-old college student, has a commercial policy through the university that accepts fee-for-service charges. Emma, a 36-year-old bank teller, belongs to a PPO that Dr. Inglewood has contracted with at 10% discounted fee-for-service charges. Umberto, a 42-year-old factory worker, has healthcare coverage with a capitated health maintenance organization. Eunice, a 67-year-old retired teacher, is on Medicare. All four are established patients. Ellen McIntyre, Dr. Englewood's health insurance professional, verifies the individual adjusted charges as follows:

Tony—$50 (UCR fee)

Emma—$45 (10% discount)

Umberto—$10 (capitation fee per patient per month)

Eunice—$34.50 (Medicare's fee schedule allowed amount)

Medicare Prospective Payment System

Congress adopted the PPS to regulate the amount of resources the federal government spends on medical care for elderly and disabled individuals. The Social Security Amendments of 1983 mandated the PPS for acute hospital care for Medicare patients. The system was intended to encourage hospitals to modify the way they deliver services. Congress had the following four chief objectives in creating the PPS:

1. To ensure fair compensation for services rendered and not compromise access to hospital services, particularly for those who are seriously ill.
2. To ensure that the process for updating payment rates would account for new medical technology, inflation, and other factors that affect the cost of providing care.
3. To monitor the quality of hospital services for Medicare beneficiaries.
4. To provide a mechanism through which beneficiaries and hospitals could resolve problems with their treatment.

Congress gave primary authority for implementing the PPS to the Centers for Medicare and Medicaid Services (CMS). As a federal entity, CMS sets guidelines and rules that impact the entire insurance industry, and everyone must follow these guidelines and rules. Congress also assigned responsibilities to outside, independent organizations to ensure that the medical profession, hospital industry, and Medicare beneficiaries had the opportunity to provide input on the creation and implementation of the system.

Under the Medicare PPS, hospitals are paid a set fee for treating patients in a single DRG category, regardless of the actual cost of care for the individual. The DRG system is an inpatient classification structure based on several factors including principal diagnosis, additional diagnosis, surgical factors, age, sex, and discharge status. DRGs are discussed in more detail later.

In addition to payment adjustments for differences in area wages, teaching activity, care to the poor, and other factors, hospitals may receive additional payments to cover extra costs associated with atypical patients—patients whose stays are either considerably shorter or considerably longer than average (referred to as **cost outliers**) in each DRG.

Stop and Think

Referring to the scenario in Imagine This! concerning Dr. Inglewood's practice, what is your reaction to the variation in adjusted charges for the four patients being seen in the same office for the same condition? Do you think it is reasonable that Tony's insurer must pay the full $50, whereas Medicare allows only $34.50 for Eunice's visit?

How the Medicare Prospective Payment System Works

In a PPS, payment levels are set ahead of time, or prospectively, and are intended to pay the healthcare provider for a particular group of services. The established payment rate for all services that a patient in an acute care hospital receives during an entire stay is based on a predetermined payment level that is selected on the basis of averages. This means that some providers' actual costs would be above the average payment and some would be below. Whatever the case, the provider receives only the preset amount, regardless of whether actual costs are more or less.

CMS has developed several variations of payment systems from the initial PPS currently being used by Medicare and other third-party payers in the United States. Following are brief definitions of these various CMS PPS structures.

Acute Inpatient Prospective Payment System

The inpatient prospective payment system (IPPS) is the Medicare PPS used for acute care hospital inpatient stays. Under IPPS, each case is categorized into a DRG with a payment weight assigned to it based on the average resources used to treat patients in that particular DRG. Medicare publishes a final rule with revisions to IPPS every year for the upcoming fiscal year, which goes into effect on October 1—the beginning of the federal government's fiscal year.

Outpatient Prospective Payment System

The outpatient prospective payment system (OPPS) is the Medicare PPS used for hospital-based outpatient services and procedures. Under OPPS, payment is based on the assignment of ambulatory payment classifications (APCs) and reimburses a predetermined amount by procedures performed. Medicare publishes revisions to OPPS annually for the upcoming fiscal year that go into effect on January 1 of the following year.

Skilled Nursing Facility Prospective Payment System

The skilled nursing facility prospective payment system (SNF PPS) is a per diem reimbursement system for all costs (routine, ancillary, and capital) associated with covered SNF services furnished to Medicare beneficiaries. Per diem rates are a hospital's all-inclusive daily rates as calculated by department.

Home Health Prospective Payment System

The home health PPS is the reimbursement system developed by CMS to cover home health services provided to Medicare beneficiaries. Medicare pays home health agencies a predetermined base payment. The payment is adjusted for the health condition and care needs of the beneficiary and for the geographic differences in wages for home health agencies across the United States. The adjustment for the health condition, or clinical characteristics, and service needs of the beneficiary is referred to as the **case-mix adjustment**.

Inpatient Rehabilitation Facility Prospective Payment System

The inpatient rehabilitation facility (IRF) PPS is the reimbursement system developed by CMS to cover inpatient rehabilitation services provided to Medicare beneficiaries. The IRF PPS uses the patient assessment instrument to assign patients to case-mix groups according to their clinical status and resource requirements.

Inpatient Psychiatric Facility Prospective Payment System

The inpatient psychiatric facility PPS is a per diem PPS based on 15 DRGs.

Long-Term Care Hospital Prospective Payment System

The PPS for LTCHs classifies patients into diagnostic groups based on clinical characteristics and expected resource needs of inpatient stays in LTCHs (defined as hospitals with an average length of stay greater than 25 days). The patient classification groupings are called LTC-DRGs—they are the same DRGs used under the hospital inpatient PPS.

Medicare Advantage Program (Centers for Medicare and Medicaid Services Hierarchical Condition Category)

The Medicare Advantage program employs a CMS hierarchical condition category (HCC) risk assessment payment model. This capitation payment model is used to provide payment to managed care organizations (e.g., HMOs and PPOs) on behalf of Medicare beneficiaries. The CMS HCC risk assessment adjusts per-beneficiary capitation payments with a risk adjustment methodology using diagnoses to measure relative risk owing to health status. Select diagnostic codes are used to define disease groups, referred to as hierarchical condition categories, or HCCs.

CMS also develops fee schedules for specific providers and services such as physicians, ambulance services, clinical laboratory services, durable medical equipment, and supplies. You can read more about them on the CMS website at http://www.cms.gov/.

HIPAA Tip

HIPAA regulations do not mandate that all healthcare facilities become computerized.

What Did You Learn?

1. What congressional act provided for limits on Medicare reimbursements for stays in long-term acute care hospitals?
2. List the three primary reimbursement systems for Medicare.
3. Name the federal entity that sets guidelines and rules that impact the entire insurance industry.
4. T/F—Under the Medicare PPS, hospitals are paid a set fee for treating patients in a single DRG category based on the actual cost of care for the individual.
5. Define a "cost outlier."
6. Identify six types of prospective payment systems.

OTHER SYSTEMS FOR DETERMINING REIMBURSEMENT

Until the latter part of the 20th century, fee-for-service was the usual method of determining reimbursement in the United States. As the nation faced an increase in the elderly population and access to healthcare improved, the government enacted legislation to control the increasing cost of healthcare associated with these factors. Out of these federal laws, several new systems of reimbursement appeared (Table 17-2).

Relative Value Scale

The **relative value scale (RVS)**, first developed by the California Medical Association in the 1950s, is a method of determining reimbursement for healthcare services based on establishing a standard unit value for medical and surgical procedures. RVS compares and rates each individual service according to the relative value of each unit and converts this unit value to a dollar value. RVS units are based on average charges for a same or similar procedure of all healthcare providers during the time in which the RVS was established and published. The total relative value unit (RVU) consists of the following three components:

TABLE 17-2	Prospective Payment Systems Comparison	
TYPE OF SYSTEM	**APPLICABLE SETTING**	**REIMBURSEMENT BASED ON**
DRG	Acute care	Diagnosis and procedures
APC	Ambulatory care	Procedures, using diagnoses to verify medical necessity
RUG	Skilled nursing facilities	Minimum data set including activities of daily living index
HH PPS	Home health care	Outcome and assessment information set
IRF PPS	Inpatient rehabilitation facilities	Length of hospital stay and function-related group classification

APC, Ambulatory payment classifications; *DRG,* diagnosis-related groups; *HH PPS,* home health prospective payment system; *IRF PPS,* inpatient rehabilitation facility prospective payment system; *RUG,* resource utilization group.

1. A relative value for *physician work*
2. A relative value for *practice expense*
3. A relative value for *malpractice risk*

Example: For CPT code 29530 (strapping, knee), the physician work RVU is 0.57, the practice expense RVU is 0.41, and malpractice risk is 0.05.

According to the American Medical Association (AMA), the biggest challenge in developing an RVS-based payment schedule was overcoming the lack of any available method or data for assigning specific values to physicians' work. The Harvard University School of Public Health, in cooperation with CMS, conducted a study that led to the initial relative work values. This nationwide study surveyed physicians to determine the work involved in each of approximately 800 different medical services. More than half of the relative value estimates of almost 6000 services were based directly on findings from the Harvard study.

Values for new and revised procedures that appear in the Current Procedural Terminology (CPT) manual are included in the updated RVS each year. The AMA works in conjunction with national medical specialty societies to develop recommendations for CMS regarding values to be assigned to these new and revised codes.

Resource-Based Relative Value Scale

The Omnibus Budget Reconciliation Act of 1989 legislated a system to replace the UCR structure, which at that time was being used for the Medicare fee system. This new system, called the **resource-based relative value scale (RBRVS)**, was designed not only to address the increasing cost of healthcare in the United States but also to try to resolve the inequities between geographic areas, time in practice, and the current payment schedule. Also included in this new reimbursement system was the elimination of **balance billing**—the practice of billing patients for any balance left after deductibles, coinsurance, and insurance payments have been made.

At the base of this new system was the RVS discussed in the previous section. Similar to the RVS, there are three components of the RBRVS:

1. Total work (time, technical skill, mental effort, physical effort, judgment, and stress)
2. Practice costs
3. Malpractice costs

The six factors that compose "total work" are measured before, during, and after the specific service or procedure. Practice costs are defined as overhead costs, including office rent, nonphysician salaries, equipment, and supplies. Malpractice costs are based on the average professional liability premiums healthcare providers have to pay each year. (See Box 17-1.)

Diagnosis-Related Groups

The DRG system classifies hospital inpatient cases into categories with similar use of the facility's resources. This system is used as the basis to reimburse hospitals for inpatient services and was established to create an incentive for hospitals to operate more efficiently and more profitably. Under DRGs, a hospital is paid a predetermined, lump sum amount, regardless of the costs involved, for each Medicare patient treated and discharged. DRGs are organized into major diagnostic categories, which are based on a particular organ system of the body (e.g., musculoskeletal system, nervous system). Only one DRG is assigned to a patient for a particular hospital admission. Typically, one payment is made per patient, and that payment is based on the DRG assignment.

The DRG grouping is based on diagnoses, procedures performed, age, sex, and status at discharge. DRGs are used for reimbursement in the PPS of the Medicare and Medicaid healthcare insurance systems. DRGs adopted by CMS are defined by diagnosis and procedure codes used in the International Classification of Diseases (ICD) coding manual.

The history, design, and classification rules of the DRG system and its application in patient discharge data and updating procedures are published in the *DRG Definitions Manual* (CMS, U.S. Department of Health and Human Services [HHS]). Several refinements of DRGs and different national versions have been published. More detailed information about these different systems is available on the Internet using "DRG Definitions Manual" as search words.

> ⭐ **Imagine This!**
>
> Alvin Rictor, a 66-year-old construction worker, underwent a procedure at Mid-Prairie Acute Care Facility to reattach his severed left leg. The hospital's total incurred expense was $12,000 (e.g., staff time, operating room expenses, supplies, anesthesia); however, DRG 209 (major joint and limb reattachment procedures of lower extremity) was assigned, which reimbursed the hospital $9600. As a result, Mid-Prairie Acute Care Facility sustained a $2400 loss on Alvin Rictor's hospital stay.

How Diagnosis-Related Groups Work

A patient's DRG categorization depends on the coding and classification of the patient's healthcare information using the ICD coding system. The key piece of information is the patient's **principal diagnosis**—the reason for admission to the acute care facility. The primary procedure to be performed also plays an important part in assigning DRGs. In addition to the coding of the patient's principal diagnosis, the healthcare organization codes and submits information about comorbidities and complications. (A **comorbidity** is the presence of more than one disease or disorder that occurs in an individual at the same time.) Also taken into consideration is the patient's principal procedure and any additional operations or procedures done during the time spent in the hospital. The **DRG grouper** (a computer software program that takes the coded information and identifies the patient's DRG category) also considers the patient's age, gender, and discharge status. All this information together determines the DRG category, which sets the payment dollar amount for the acute inpatient hospital visit.

Assigning a Diagnosis-Related Group to a Patient

As discussed in the previous section, the principal diagnosis and principal procedure determine the DRG assignment. Other factors that may play a role in DRG assignment are secondary diagnoses, patient age, the presence or absence of complications or comorbidities, patient sex, and discharge status. Each DRG is assigned a relative weight and an **average length of stay (ALOS)**. Relative weights indicate the relative resource consumption for the DRG. ALOS is the predetermined number of days of approved hospital stay assigned to an individual DRG. Referring to the earlier example in Imagine This!, DRG 209 at Mid-Prairie Acute Care Facility has a relative weight of 2.0782 and ALOS of 5 days.

Calculating Diagnosis-Related Group Payments

Calculating DRG payments involves a formula that accounts for the adjustments discussed in the previous section. The DRG weight is multiplied by a **standardized amount**, which

---

> **Box 17-1**
>
> **Formula for Calculating Medicare Resource-Based Relative Value Scale**
>
> Work RVU × work GPCI
> + Practice expense (PE) RVU × PE GPCI
> + Malpractice expense (PLI) RVU × PLI GPCI
> ─────────────────────────────────
> = Total RVU × conversion factor = payment

is a figure representing the average cost per case for all Medicare cases during the year. The standardized amount is the sum of

- a **labor component**, which represents labor cost variations in different areas of the United States, and
- a **nonlabor component**, which represents a geographic calculation based on whether the hospital is located in a large urban or other area. The labor component is adjusted by a wage index.

If applicable, cost outliers, **disproportionate share** (payment adjustment to compensate hospitals for the higher operating costs they incur in treating a large share of low-income patients), and indirect medical education payments are added to the formula.

Ambulatory Payment Classifications

Ambulatory payment classifications (APCs) were put into effect in August 2000 for hospital outpatient services provided to Medicare beneficiaries. When CMS implemented the APC system, it changed the way hospitals are reimbursed for outpatient services. Before this system was put into practice, hospital outpatient services were based almost entirely on actual cost. Services provided under the hospital outpatient prospective payment system (OPPS) now are classified and paid according to APCs.

APCs are made up of CPT Level I and HCFA Common Procedure Coding System (HCPCS) Level II codes, which are divided into approximately 900 categories. Each APC is assigned a national payment rate that is based on the median cost for all services within the APC group. Hospitals can receive payment on one or more APC per encounter; however, if no payable HCPCS code is assigned to the claim, no payment is received.

APCs were developed from ambulatory patient groups (APGs), and the amount and type of resources used in outpatient visits are grouped into APC categories. Services in each APC have similar clinical characteristics, resource use, and cost. Under the APC system, providers receive fixed payments for individual services assigned to the various APC categories. Generally, CMS establishes a payment rate for each APC based on hospital cost data submitted annually to CMS. The APC payment rates are adjusted for geographic cost differences, and payment rates and policies are updated annually.

Since 2000, there have been numerous significant updates to the APC system as a result of the Medicare, Medicaid, and SCHIP Benefits Improvement and Protection Act of 2000; the Medicare Prescription Drug, Improvement, and Modernization Act of 2003; and the Deficit Reduction Act of 2005. An advisory panel reviews the APC groups and their associated weights periodically and advises the Secretary of HHS and CMS concerning the clinical integrity of the APC groups and their associated weights established under the Medicare hospital OPPS.

APC payments are made to hospitals when a Medicare outpatient is discharged from the emergency department or clinic or is transferred to another hospital (or other facility) that is not affiliated with the initial hospital where the patient received outpatient services. If the patient is admitted from a hospital clinic or emergency department, there is no APC payment, and Medicare pays the hospital under inpatient DRG methodology.

Health insurance professionals can stay informed of annual changes to the APC system through the annual updates that go into effect each January by logging on to the CMS website.

Resource Utilization Groups

The basic idea of **resource utilization groups (RUGs)** is to calculate payments to a skilled nursing facility (SNF) according to the severity and level of care needed by each resident under a Medicare Part A stay. SNFs are nursing homes that provide skilled nursing or skilled rehabilitation services or both to Medicare patients who need a level of medical care that cannot be provided in a custodial-type nursing home or in the patient's home.

When a patient is admitted to a **residential healthcare facility** or nursing home, the physician is required to prepare a written plan of care for treatment including rehabilitative therapy. Under this type of PPS, SNFs are required to classify residents into one of the RUGs-IV based on assessment data from the resident assessment, known as the minimum data set (MDS). The RUG-IV grouper represents a major change in long-term care, which includes new definitions of RUG groups, changes in therapy minutes and the ADL index.

CMS requires that an MDS be completed for each resident by a registered nurse, and each resident's RUG is based on the MDS. The MDS must be completed periodically during the resident's stay, as appropriate. There are more than 500 items on the MDS, and data from about a quarter of these items are used to determine the RUG—the payment rate for each resident covered in a Medicare Part A stay. CMS conducts oversight activities to monitor the accuracy of the MDS.

RUG categories are divided further into hierarchical groups on the basis of the patient's ability to perform **activities of daily living (ADLs)**. ADLs are behaviors related to personal care including bathing or showering, dressing, getting in or out of bed or a chair, using the toilet, and eating. A qualified registered nurse assessor places each patient into an RUG category by completing a patient review. Each RUG category is assigned a numeric value on the basis of the resources necessary to care for that type of patient, with a greater value assigned to categories that require more resources.

🕐 Stop and Think

Nathan Schnoor, an 84-year-old Medicare patient, was hospitalized at Bestcare Hospital for congestive heart failure. Medicare's ALOS for this DRG category was 21 days; however, at the end of this time, Nathan's condition had deteriorated. Bestcare staff informed Nathan's family that, under Medicare rules, he had to be discharged, and arrangements were made to transfer him to a nursing home. What are the ramifications of the Medicare PPS and the DRG structure in situations such as this?

TRANSITION OF MEDICARE TO RESOURCE-BASED RELATIVE VALUE SCALE

CMS implemented the Medicare RBRVS physician fee schedule in 1992. The Medicare RBRVS physician fee schedule replaced the Medicare physician payment system of "customary, prevailing, and reasonable" charges from which physicians were paid according to the provision of each service. The current Medicare RBRVS physician fee schedule is calculated using the "relative value" of a service provided (identified by a CPT code) and based on the resources the service consumes. The relative value of each service is based on three components: the amount of physician work that goes into the service, the practice expense associated with the service, and the professional liability expense to provide the service. The relative value of each service is multiplied by the geographic practice cost index (GPCI) (pronounced "gypsy") for each Medicare locality and then translated into a dollar amount by an annually adjusted conversion factor. The dollar amount resulting from this calculation is what Medicare will pay to provide that particular service. Many public and private payers, including Medicaid programs, have adopted components of the Medicare RBRVS for calculating physician reimbursement.

For more information on RBRVS and to learn more about how payments are calculated using the Medicare RBRVS formula, see Box 17-1 and visit the Evolve site.

Setting Medicare Payment Policy

Medicare payment rules are made by CMS, which is headquartered in Baltimore. However, the Medicare program is administered largely at the local and regional levels by private insurance companies that contract with CMS to handle day-to-day billing and payment matters. CMS also administers and oversees the Medicaid program.

Medicare Inpatient Hospital Prospective Payment System

The IPPS is the payment system whereby Medicare reimburses hospitals for providing inpatient care to beneficiaries. Under this system, which began in 1983, Medicare sets prices for more than 500 DRGs. The prospective payment fee, also referred to as the *DRG payment,* covers all hospital costs for treating the patient during a specific inpatient stay including the costs of all devices that are used. (Separate payment is made to physicians for the care they provide to patients during these inpatient admissions.) CMS adjusts DRG payments annually to reflect changes in hospital costs and changes in technology.

Medicare Long-Term Care Hospital Prospective Payment System

LTCHs are certified under Medicare as short-term acute care hospitals that have been excluded from the IPPS. For the purpose of Medicare payments, LTCHs are defined as having an average inpatient length of stay of greater than 25 days. Under the Medicare **long-term care hospital prospective payment system (LTCH PPS)**, patients who require hospital-level care for an average of 25 days or longer are classified into distinct diagnostic groups based on clinical characteristics and expected resource needs.

The LTCH PPS uses long-term care (LTC)-DRGs as a patient classification system. Each patient stay is grouped into an LTC-DRG on the basis of diagnoses (including secondary diagnoses), procedures performed, age, gender, and discharge status. Each LTC-DRG has a predetermined ALOS or the typical length of stay for a patient classified to the LTC-DRG. Under the LTCH PPS, an LTCH receives payment for each Medicare patient on the basis of the LTC-DRG to which that patient's stay is grouped. This grouping reflects the typical resources used for treating such a patient. Cases assigned to an LTC-DRG are paid according to the federal payment rate including adjustments. For more information on LTCH PPS, visit the Evolve site.

One type of case-level adjustment is a **short-stay outlier.** A short-stay outlier is an adjustment to the federal payment rate for LTCH stays that are considerably shorter than the ALOS for an LTC-DRG. Without this short-stay outlier adjustment, Medicare would pay an inappropriate amount for cases that did not receive a full episode of care at the LTCH. Cases qualify as a short-stay outlier when the length of stay is between 1 day and up to and including ⅚ of the ALOS for the LTC-DRG to which the case is grouped. A length of stay that exceeds ⅚ of the ALOS for the LTC-DRG is considered to have exceeded the short-stay outlier threshold. When a case exceeds the short-stay outlier threshold, Medicare pays a full LTC-DRG payment for that case. For more information on short-stay outliers, visit the Evolve site.

> 💬 **What Did You Learn?**
>
> 1. The current Medicare RBRVS physician fee schedule is calculated using the _____ _____ of a service provided (identified by a given CPT code) and based on the resources the service consumes.
> 2. T/F—Medicare payment rules are made by the AMA.
> 3. What is the IPPS used for?
> 4. Define a long-term care hospital.
> 5. A _____ is an adjustment to the federal payment rate for LTCH stays that are considerably shorter than the ALOS for an LTC-DRG.

ADDITIONAL PROSPECTIVE PAYMENT SYSTEMS

After the prospective payment reimbursement systems proved successful and showed adequate care for patients, new offshoots appeared as different types of healthcare became prevalent. Two of these are the home health PPS and IRF PPS.

Home Health Prospective Payment System

The Balanced Budget Act of 1997, as amended by the Omnibus Consolidated and Emergency Supplemental Appropriations Act (OCESAA) of 1999, called for the development and implementation of a prospective payment system (PPS) for Medicare home health services. The BBA put in place the interim payment system (IPS) until the PPS could be implemented. In 2000, the government began phasing in fixed payment for home health services, the **home health prospective payment system**. Determination of payment category depends on the Outcome and Assessment Information Set (OASIS). This data set includes coded information about the patient's diagnoses and functional status and information about the patient's outcome from services provided. In January 2011, there were more than 150 home health resource groups, and the home health agency receives a payment for each 60-day block of service.

An agency receives half of the estimated base payment for the full 60 days as soon as the fiscal intermediary receives the initial assignment. The agency receives the residual half of the payment at the close of the 60-day episode, unless there is an applicable adjustment to that amount. The full payment is the sum of the initial and residual percentage payments, unless there is an applicable adjustment. This split payment approach provides reasonable and balanced cash flow for home health agencies. Another 60-day episode can be initiated for patients with longer stays. Visit the Evolve site to learn more about the home health PPS.

Inpatient Rehabilitation Facility Prospective Payment System

In the Balanced Budget Act of 1997, Congress authorized CMS to implement a PPS for inpatient rehabilitation. CMS activated the **inpatient rehabilitation facility prospective payment system (IRF PPS)** in 2001. Reimbursement in the IRF PPS is based on information found in the IRF patient assessment instrument, which contains patient clinical, demographic, and other information and classifies the patient into distinct groups based on clinical characteristics and expected resource needs.

Reimbursement rates in IRF PPS are adjusted by an area wage index and updated for inflation. Payments are reduced for certain transfers and outliers, including cases with short stays, cases with interrupted stays, and cases when the patient dies during the stay. Payments are increased for IRFs in rural areas, for IRFs with a disproportionate share of low-income patients, and for certain high-cost cases. For more detailed information on the IRF PPS, visit the Evolve site.

Significance of Reimbursement Systems to the Health Insurance Professional

A good deal of information has just been presented on various reimbursement systems with a focus mainly on PPS. What does all this information mean to the health insurance professional, and why is it significant? Being a successful health insurance professional does not stop with knowing how to complete and submit insurance claims. To function well on the job, an individual should have a working knowledge of each of the systems discussed in this chapter, to what category of patients each applies, how each is structured, how fees are established within each system, and on what these fees are based. There is a direct correlation between knowledge and capability and job prospects. The more informed a health insurance professional becomes, the better his or her employment prospects and job advancement.

🕐 **Stop and Think**

Megan Trimble and Bob Shackler are seeking employment after completing a medical insurance and billing program at a career school in their vicinity. Megan did her best to learn all she could about the various reimbursement systems, whereas Bob, considering the information insignificant for his career goals, disregarded it. What advantages might Megan have over Bob in their search for successful employment as health insurance professionals?

PEER REVIEW ORGANIZATIONS AND PROSPECTIVE PAYMENT SYSTEMS

A **peer review organization (PRO)**, now more commonly referred to as a quality improvement organization, in this context is an agency typically composed of a group of practicing physicians and other healthcare professionals paid by the federal government to evaluate the services provided by other practitioners and to monitor the quality of care given to patients. PROs were established by TEFRA to review quality of care and appropriateness of admissions, readmissions, and discharges for Medicare and Medicaid patients. These organizations are held responsible for maintaining and lowering admissions rates and reducing lengths of stay, while ensuring adequate treatment. These organizations sometimes are called *professional standards review organizations*.

The basic responsibility of PROs is to ensure that Medicare hospital services are appropriate, necessary, and provided in the most cost-effective manner. PROs have considerable power to force hospitals to comply with HHS admission and quality standards. They may deny payment to hospitals where abusive practices are found and, in some instances, report such practices to HHS for further enforcement action. Congress required HHS to contract with PROs to monitor

- the validity of diagnostic information supplied by hospitals for payment purposes;
- the completeness, adequacy, and quality of care provided to Medicare beneficiaries;
- the appropriateness of admissions and discharges; and
- the appropriateness of care in outlier cases in which additional Medicare payments were made.

Not all PROs deal with healthcare. One of the largest and most complex PROs is the one used by the Internal Revenue Service to conduct audits through its Coordinated Examination Program. The Internal Revenue Service PRO, comprising teams of senior revenue agents and specialists including computer analysts, engineers, and economists, is the "watch dog" over the Coordinated Examination Program that audits taxpayers. For the purpose of relevancy, however, this section is limited to PROs as they apply primarily to government health programs such as Medicare and Medicaid.

UNDERSTANDING COMPUTERIZED PATIENT ACCOUNTING SYSTEMS

In addition to learning about the various reimbursement systems related to medical billing and insurance, a well-rounded health insurance professional should be knowledgeable about computerized patient accounting systems. Chapter 16 discussed electronic data entry and submitting insurance claims electronically. The healthcare office typically uses some kind of computerized patient accounting software. Reimbursement systems address the structure of various fee schedules and the structure and setting for each, whereas computerized patient accounting systems address receiving payment for professional services and report generation. Many different patient accounting systems are available today, and they all are capable of performing the following seven system functions:

1. Input and storage of patient demographic and insurance information
2. Transaction posting
3. Allocation of system control operations
4. Generating patient statements
5. Processing and submitting insurance claims
6. Managing and collecting delinquent accounts
7. Creating reports

Performing these seven functions in a systematic and timely manner is the key to effective and efficient patient accounting.

Chapter 14 suggested that a healthcare practice establish fair policies, practice sound accounting procedures, and maintain a well-trained staff. It is usually the responsibility of the physicians who run the practice to establish accounting policies and procedures of the practice. When the physicians have reached a consensus on these policies and procedures, they should meet with the staff and discuss how the procedures and policies are to be implemented and how to troubleshoot any potential problems that may arise. When a workable system has been established, the patient accounting policies and procedures should be documented. After this process is completed, it is a good idea for the staff to meet periodically to discuss suggested changes, updates, and revisions as needed. Finally, patients must be informed, verbally or through practice brochures, about all established practice policies and procedures.

Selecting the Right Billing System

To function efficiently and maximize collections, the healthcare practice should have a patient accounting system that fits its needs. When setting up a new healthcare practice or revamping an existing practice, after the policies and procedures have been established, the staff has been trained, and a method for informing patients has been established, the next step is selecting a patient accounting system that best fits the type of practice in question. Many factors need to be considered when deciding to purchase a new, or upgrade an old, software package to handle the billing needs of the practice. The professional staff should take the time to do some research when making this important decision because the capabilities of the billing system create the framework for a satisfactory cash flow into the practice. Some important initial questions should be asked of any potential billing software and hardware seller to ensure that the practice is dealing with a reputable firm. These questions include the following:

1. How long has the company been in business, and what is their history?
2. How long has the particular software package in question been on the market?
3. How many and what types of practices use their software?
4. Can client names be furnished for references?
5. Are software demo disks available?
6. What is the availability and accessibility of setup, training, and support for the software system?
7. What would it cost to get the system fully functional?
8. What hardware and networking requirements are recommended for optimal efficiency?

If the practice is upgrading from an older system, it is also important to find out if the new software would have the capability to import data from the previous billing system and, if so, what the cost for this service would be. In addition, it should be determined if such transfers would be successful, or is it likely that data sometimes would be lost or scrambled? In the case of the latter, it also would be necessary to know if the software company would furnish on-site technical support to "debug" the system.

The cost of a medical billing software system generally has no direct correlation with its capabilities or customer satisfaction ratings. Software packages range in cost from $5000 to $50,000 (and sometimes more), depending on the amenities that some companies offer in addition to their "basic package." Many medical billing software packages on the market today function well if managed by sufficiently trained personnel. It often takes several weeks of "trial and error" to get a new system running smoothly.

A few healthcare offices still depend solely on a manual patient accounting system such as the once popular "pegboard" method. However, offices that use a computerized billing system that functions well are convinced that the advantages far outweigh any disadvantages such as computer "glitches" and occasional "down time." Medical billing software systems available today have built-in capabilities that allow

- customized encounter form generation,
- appointment scheduling,
- electronic chart documentation,
- integrated test result reporting,
- creation and storage of multimedia patient documentation,

- electronic claims submission,
- electronic payment reconciliation,
- accounts receivable tracking, and
- internal collection modules.

All of these features provide efficiency, accountability, and oversight control that usually are impossible with a manual process. However, it is recommended that to achieve optimal results from any computerized patient accounting system, the staff should allow adequate time for training and establish a suitable framework for monitoring the system for HIPAA compliance. Most software companies provide training sessions to assist the staff in learning how to use the system.

Remember: Any computer system is only as good as the operators who input the data and have knowledge of the system's capabilities. To use its full potential, it is also important to learn how to use all of the options that the billing system is capable of performing.

> ### 📁 HIPAA Tip
>
> HIPAA does not require patients to sign consent forms before physicians, hospitals, or ambulances can share information for treatment purposes as long as it pertains to the same case.

Managing Transactions

A successful healthcare practice must maintain control over the many transactions required in the process of providing quality services to patients. Whether the healthcare office is computerized or not, there are numerous transactions to handle throughout the day, such as

- posting and tracking patient charges,
- processing payments (cash, checks, or electronic funds transfers), and
- making adjustments to patient accounts.

Posting and Tracking Patient Charges

The typical process for posting and tracking patient charges is as follows. After the patient has completed the encounter, the health insurance professional enters the charge for the procedure or service on the patient's account ledger from the encounter form. This can be done either manually or using the computerized patient accounting software. Fig. 17-1 illustrates a typical software program screen showing charges and payments for a patient.

Code libraries that integrate with CPT-4 and ICD-10-CM codes contained on peripheral electronic media (disk or CD-ROM) or that are integrated into the patient accounting software allow fast and accurate selection of applicable diagnostic and procedural coding. Most systems also allow the practice to set up specialty-specific or multiple "code sets" to streamline insurance submissions, assisting in billing the appropriate insurance carrier with the correct, carrier-specific codes. (*Note:* ICD-9 codes are to be used until September 30, 2013; however, this date may be extended.)

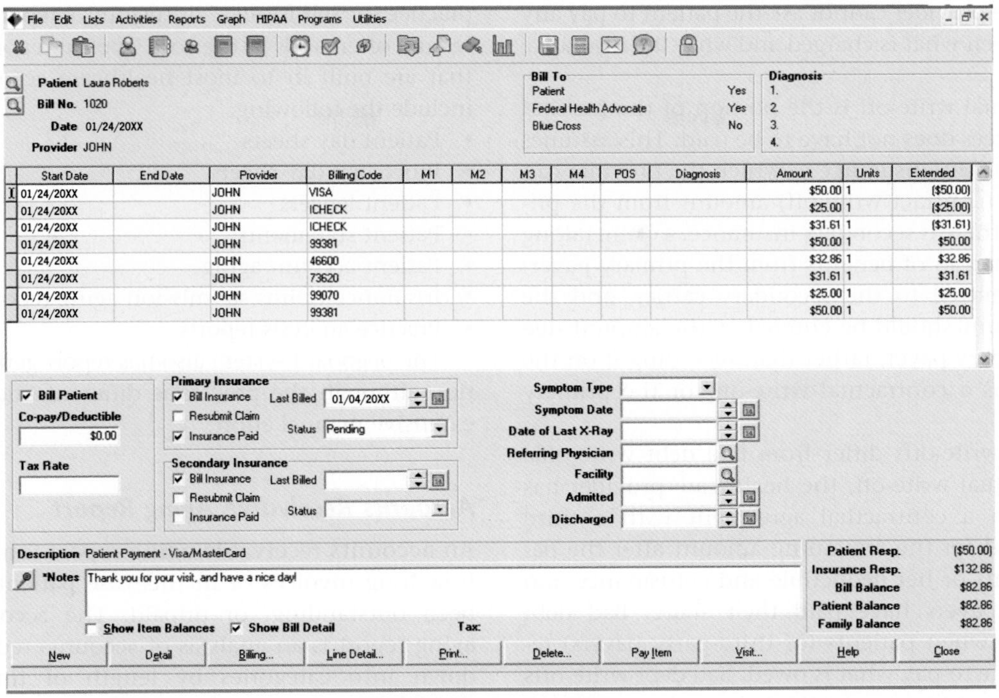

Fig. 17-1 Patient account.

Processing Payments

As with posting charges, all payments, whether they are in person, received in the mail, or electronic funds transfers, must also be posted to the patient's account. This task can be accomplished manually or by using the computerized patient accounting software. Fig. 17-2 shows how patient accounting software can track patient charges and remittance history.

Insurance Carrier Adjustments (Contractual Write-offs)

A **contractual write-off** is used when some kind of contract or agreement exists between the provider and an insurance carrier whereby the provider agrees to accept the payer's allowed fee as payment in full for a particular service or procedure. If the patient has paid the yearly deductible and

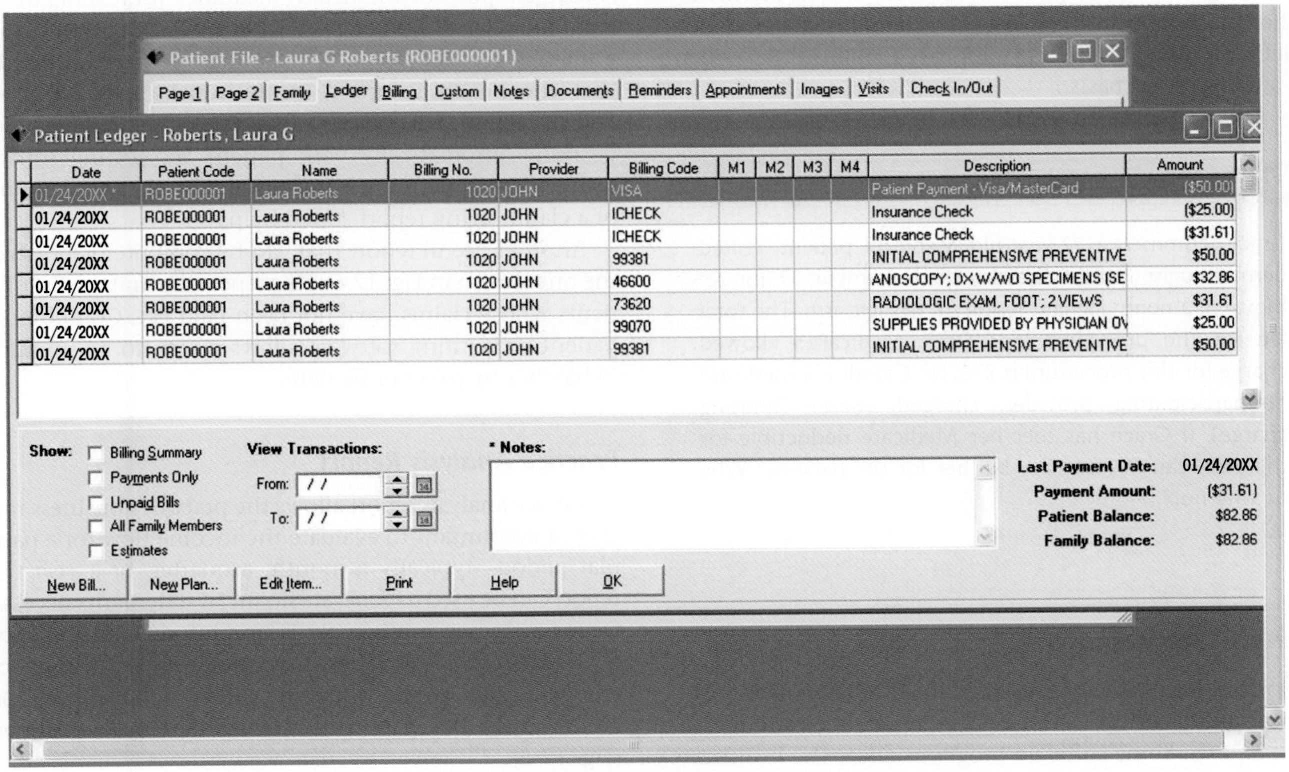

Fig. 17-2 Patient accounting software.

coinsurance, the provider cannot ask the patient to pay any difference between what is charged and what the insurance carrier allows.

The contractual write-off is the portion of the fee that the provider agrees does not have to be paid. This assumes there is no secondary insurance to which the provider can bill the unpaid (contract write-off) amount from the primary insurer. If there is secondary insurance, a claim (along with the explanation of benefits from the primary payer) should be submitted to the secondary carrier, and the remaining amount should be entered as the amount due from the secondary payer, rather than recording it on the patient ledger as a contractual write-off for the primary payer.

Contractual write-offs differ from bad debt write-offs. With a contractual write-off, the healthcare provider has agreed, through a contractual agreement with a third party, not to bill for the remaining amount after the patient has paid his or her deductible and coinsurance and all third-party payers have paid their share. Bad debt write-offs result when patients (or third-party payers) refuse or are unable to pay what is owed. Bad debt write-offs sometimes are used to zero out the balance for a patient's services when it has been determined that the account is uncollectible.

As discussed in Chapter 9, a Medicare nonparticipating (nonPAR) provider or supplier is one who has not signed a contract with Medicare. NonPARs not accepting assignment can charge beneficiaries no more than 115% of the Medicare allowance. In such cases, the beneficiary must pay the difference between the allowed amount and the limiting charge, and contractual write-offs do not apply. On unassigned claims, the Medicare payment is sent to the beneficiary rather than the healthcare provider. (NonPARs may choose whether to accept Medicare's approved amount as payment on a case-by-case basis.)

⏱ Stop and Think

Grace Plummer, a 72-year-old Medicare patient, visited dermatologist Harold Grassley on November 17 for removal of a nonmalignant lesion on her left arm. The total fee for the procedure was $125. Medicare's allowed charge for this procedure is $75. Dr. Grassley, a Medicare nonparticipating provider, charged $86.25 (limiting charge). If Grace has met her Medicare deductible for the year, can Dr. Grassley bill her for the balance? Why or why not?

Generating Reports

Reporting formats vary greatly with different software systems, but all software is capable of generating various standard reports. Some software programs allow the healthcare practice to "self-format" or customize reports; however, this feature often adds to the cost. Typical reporting capabilities that are built in to most healthcare accounting software include the following:

- Patient day sheets
- Procedure day sheets
- Patient ledgers
- Patient statements
- Patient account aging
- Insurance claims submission aging reports
- Practice analysis reports

The pegboard system also has report-generating capabilities, although the process is different and involves more extensive manual effort.

Accounts Receivable Aging Report

An **accounts receivable aging report** is a report showing how long invoices or in this case patient accounts have been outstanding, or unpaid. The accounts receivable aging report is an analysis of accounts receivables broken down into categories by length of time outstanding (Fig. 17-3).

When analyzing a patient accounts receivable aging report, the total money owed that is 120 days old and older should be small compared with the total accounts receivable. Most experts say that if 20% of the practice's unpaid revenues are 120 days old or older, steps should be taken to improve collections.

Insurance Claims Aging Report

A usable report for the health insurance professional is the insurance claims aging report. Chapter 15 discussed keeping a manual register or log of insurance claims submitted so that the health insurance professional can track claims and no claim "falls between the cracks." This process can be done automatically with patient accounting software using report-generating features. Fig. 17-4 shows an example of a claims aging report sorted by payer.

Another useful report that can be computer generated is the one shown in Fig. 17-5. This report illustrates a list of patients whose claims have not been paid yet. Computerized patient accounting software allows claims to be submitted in batches by payer or by date.

Practice Analysis Report

A practice analysis report allows the practice's business manager or accountant to evaluate the income flow for a particular period—typically a month, a quarter, or a year. This report can be used to generate financial statements necessary for tax purposes, profit analysis, and future planning. A typical practice analysis report furnishes a breakdown of total charges, categorized specialty charges, total patient payments, insurance payments, and contractual adjustments (Fig. 17-6).

Happy Valley Medical Clinic
Patient Aging by Date of Service
As of March 30, 20XX
Show all data where the Date From is on or before 3/30/20XX

Chart	Name		Current 0 - 30	Past 31 - 60	Past 61 - 90	Past 91 ---->	Total Balance
AGADW000	Dwight Again		130.00			86.00	216.00
Last Pmt: -200.00	On: 3/26/20XX	434-5777					
AUSAN000	Andrew Austin		165.00				165.00
Last Pmt: 0.00	On:	767-2222					
BRIJA000	Jay Brimley					445.00	445.00
Last Pmt: -30.00	On: 10/23/20XX	(222)342-3444					
BRISU000	Susan Brimley		8.00			32.00	40.00
Last Pmt: -30.00	On: 9/5/20XX	(222)342-3444					
CATSA000	Sammy Catera					71.00	71.00
Last Pmt: 0.00	On:	227-7722					
DOEJA000	Jane S Doe		15.00			79.00	94.00
Last Pmt: 0.00	On: 3/11/20XX	(480)999-9999					
JONSU001	Susan Jones					180.00	180.00
Last Pmt: 0.00	On:						
MARRO000	Roberto Marionellio					510.00	510.00
Last Pmt: 0.00	On:						
SIMTA000	Tanus J Simpson					456.00	456.00
Last Pmt: -10.00	On: 12/3/20XX	(480)555-5555					
SMIJO000	John Smith					1,095.00	1,095.00
Last Pmt: 0.00	On:						
WAGJE000	Jeremy Wagnew					-1.00	-1.00
Last Pmt: -22.00	On: 8/22/20XX	(121)419-7127					
YOUMI000	Michael C Youngblood					85.00	85.00
Last Pmt: 0.00	On:	(602)222-3333					
	Report Aging Totals		$318.00	$0.00	$0.00	$3,038.00	$3,356.00
	Percent of Aging Total		9.5 %	0.0 %	0.0 %	90.2 %	100.0 %

Fig. 17-3 Computer-generated accounts receivable report.

What Did You Learn?

1. List five functions most patient accounting software systems are capable of performing.
2. Name four important questions to ask a patient accounting software vendor.
3. What are three different ways a healthcare practice receives payment?
4. What is a "contractual write-off"?
5. List six different reports patient accounting software systems can generate.
6. What is the purpose of a practice analysis report?

HEALTH INSURANCE PORTABILITY AND ACCOUNTABILITY ACT AND PRACTICE MANAGEMENT SOFTWARE

Most healthcare practices today are computerized to some extent. The level of computerization may range from simple billing functions and patient scheduling to electronic healthcare records and entire practice management activities. HIPAA *does not* require healthcare practices to purchase computer systems. However, some experts claim that the installation of a HIPAA-compliant software system may help a practice reduce its administrative costs. Two of the principal areas of a physician's practice affected by HIPAA are the practice's billing software and practice management software.

HIPAA includes rules related to the format of electronic transactions; protection of patient's privacy; ensuring the security of patients' health information; and defining universal identifiers for individuals, healthcare providers, and employers. Compliance with two components of HIPAA, the Transactions and Code Set Standard (Transaction Standards) and the Privacy Standards, was required by October 2002 and April 2003.

According to the *Guide to Medical Practice Software* (see References and Resources at the end of the chapter), there are more than 1500 active practice management software vendors. With this in mind, two questions arise:

1. How does a healthcare practice evaluate its current software system for HIPAA compliance?

1500 A/R Aging All

SOFTAID DEMO DATA

03/19/20XX 16:11:34

Status Carrier Code	Claim ID	Last Bill	Current	31 to 60	61 to 90
CLAIM STATUS: PRIMARY					
AETNA OF CALIFORNIA–AETNA5					
CLOONEY, GEORGE 58698775501	135741	03/05/20XX	160.00	0.00	0.00
AETNA OF CALIFORNIA			**160.00**	**0.00**	**0.00**
HOME HEALTH AGENCY – AG					
CLOONEY, GEORGE 58698775501	135740	03/05/20XX	60.00	0.00	0.00
HOME HEALTH AGENCY			**60.00**	**0.00**	**0.00**
BLUE CROSS BLUE SHIELD OF FLOR–BCBS					
CLOONEY, GEORGE 59709885501	135735	03/01/20XX	160.00	0.00	0.00
CLOONEY, GEORGE 59709885501	135736	03/01/20XX	240.00	0.00	0.00
CLOONEY, GEORGE 59709885501	135738	03/10/20XX	80.00	0.00	0.00
CLOONEY, GEORGE 59709885501	135739	03/04/20XX	113.00	0.00	0.00
BLUE CROSS BLUE SHIELD OF FLOR			**593.00**	**0.00**	**0.00**
TOTAL: PRIMARY			**813.00**	**0.00**	**0.00**
CLAIM STATUS: SECONDARY					
MEDICAID–MCD					
CLOONEY, GEORGE 58698775501	135737	03/03/20XX	1,580.00	0.00	0.00
MEDICAID			**1,580.00**	**0.00**	**0.00**
TOTAL: SECONDARY			**1,580.00**	**0.00**	**0.00**

Current	31 to 60	61 to 90	91 to 120	> 120
2,393.00	0.00	0.00	0.00	0.00
100.00 %	0.00 %	0.00 %	0.00 %	0.00 %

Fig. 17-4 Claims aging report sorted by payer.

2. If a practice is in the market for a new software system, how should it evaluate various vendors in terms of HIPAA compliance?

It is important that the software vendor understands the requirements of the HIPAA Transaction Standards. The Transaction Standards has specified American National Standards Institute (ANSI) 5010 as the standard for electronic transactions including billing, payment, eligibility verification, and preauthorization. A physician must ensure the electronic claims sent to third-party payers are in this specific format. Whether a practice is evaluating its current computer vendor or shopping for a new one, it should ensure that the vendor is not only aware of the Transaction Standards but also able to speak intelligently about or show how their systems are compliant with the Transaction Standards.

Ensuring that the vendor can assist the practice in complying with the HIPAA Privacy Rule is also important. The Privacy Rule has imposed numerous requirements on healthcare providers and their practices. Before disclosing a patient's protected health information (PHI) except for the purposes of treatment, payment, or healthcare operations, a practice must obtain the written consent from the patient. A HIPAA-approved authorization form to release PHI is more detailed and specific than many generic authorizations and has a definite expiration date.

A computerized practice management system can alleviate potential administrative problems a healthcare practice may encounter in complying with the Privacy Rule with relative ease, often with just a few simple keystrokes or mouse clicks. Most practice management systems

Happy Valley Medical Clinic
Primary Insurance Aging

Date of Service	Procedure	Current 0 - 30	Past 31 - 60	Past 61 - 90	Past 91 - 120	Past 121 ---->	Total Balance

Aetna (AET00)   Erik (602)333-3333

SIMTA000   Tanus J Simpson   SSN:
Claim: 1   Initial Billing Date: 3/21/20XX   Last Billing Date: 10/30/20XX   Policy: GG93-GXTA   Group: 99999

12/3/20XX	43220	275.00					275.00
12/3/20XX	71040	50.00					50.00
12/3/20XX	81000	11.00					11.00
12/3/20XX	99213	50.00					50.00
	Claim Totals:	386.00	0.00	0.00	0.00	0.00	386.00

Claim: 15   Initial Billing Date: 10/30/20XX   Last Billing Date: 10/30/20XX   Policy: GG93-GXTA   Group: 99999

10/25/20XX	99213	60.00					60.00
10/25/20XX	90707	10.00					10.00
	Claim Totals:	70.00	0.00	0.00	0.00	0.00	70.00
	Insurance Totals:	456.00	0.00	0.00	0.00	0.00	456.00

Cigna (CIG00)   Bill S. Preston 234-5678

BRIJA000   Jay Brimley   SSN:
Claim: 16   Initial Billing Date: 10/26/20XX   Last Billing Date: 10/26/20XX   Policy: 98547377   Group: 12d

3/25/20XX	99214	55.00					55.00
3/25/20XX	97260	30.00					30.00
	Claim Totals:	85.00	0.00	0.00	0.00	0.00	85.00
	Insurance Totals:	85.00	0.00	0.00	0.00	0.00	85.00

U.S. Tricare (US000)

YOUMI000   Michael C Youngblood   SSN:
Claim: 17   Initial Billing Date: 10/26/20XX   Last Billing Date: 10/26/20XX   Policy: USAA236678   Group: 25BB

8/22/20XX	99213	60.00					60.00
8/22/20XX	97128	15.00					15.00
8/22/20XX	97010	10.00					10.00
	Claim Totals:	85.00	0.00	0.00	0.00	0.00	85.00
	Insurance Totals:	85.00	0.00	0.00	0.00	0.00	85.00

Report Aging Totals		$626.00	$0.00	$0.00	$0.00	$0.00	$626.00
Percent of Aging Total		100.0 %	0.0 %	0.0 %	0.0 %	0.0 %	100.0 %

Page 1

Fig. 17-5 List of patients whose claims have not been submitted yet.

Practice Analysis

Code	Description	Amount	Quantity	Average	Cost	Net
01	patient payment, cash	−8.00	1	−8.00		−8.00
02	patient payment, check	−15.00	1	−15.00		−15.00
03	insurance carrier payment	−154.00	2	−77.00		−154.00
04	insurance company adjustment	−10.00	1	−10.00		−10.00
06	OhioCare HMO Charge - $10	10.00	1	10.00		10.00
07	OhioCare HMO Charge - $15	15.00	1	15.00		15.00
29425	application of short leg cast, walking	30.00	1	30.00		30.00
50390	aspiration of renal cyst by needle	38.50	1	38.50		38.50
73510	hip x-ray, complete, two views	90.00	1	90.00		90.00
80019	19 clinical chemistry tests	80.00	1	80.00		80.00
84478	triglycerides test	50.00	2	25.00		50.00
90703	tetanus injection	20.00	1	20.00		20.00
92516	facial nerve function studies	125.00	1	125.00		125.00
96900	ultraviolet light treatment	23.50	1	23.50		23.50
99070	supplies and materials provided	20.00	1	20.00		20.00
99201	OF−new patient, problem focused	280.00	2	140.00		280.00
99211	OF−established patient, minimal	100.00	2	50.00		100.00
99212	OF−established patient, problem focused	200.00	5	40.00		200.00
99213	OF−established patient, expanded	300.00	3	100.00		300.00
99394	established patient, adolescent, per…	90.00	1	90.00	0.00	90.99

Total Procedure Charges	$1,472.00
Total Product Charges	$0.00
Total Inside Lab Charges	$0.00
Total Outside Lab Charges	$0.00
Total Insurance Payments	−$154.00
Total Cash Copayments	$0.00
Total Check Copayments	$0.00
Total Credit Card Copayments	$0.00
Total Patient Cash Payments	$0.00
Total Patient Check Payments	−$23.00
Total Credit Card Payments	$0.00
Total Deductibles	$0.00
Total Debit Adjustments	$0.00
Total Credit Adjustments	−$10.00
Total Medicare Debit Adjustments	$0.00
Total Medicare Credit Adjustments	$0.00
Net Effect on Accounts Receivable	$1,285.00

Fig. 17-6 Practice analysis report.

can provide various functions where PHI is concerned, such as

- tracking the date that the patient's consent to release PHI was obtained;
- maintaining electronic copies of the signed consent and authorization forms;
- tracking patient requests for restrictions on use and disclosure of PHI, whether the physician agreed to the request, and, if so, retaining a copy of the modified consent;
- tracking whether and when the consent was revoked by the patient; and
- tracking when patient authorizations were obtained, what they were obtained for, and their expiration dates.

The Privacy Standards provide that a patient may request an accounting of all disclosures made by a **covered entity** (which includes healthcare plans, healthcare providers,

and healthcare clearinghouses) within the preceding 6 years. The disclosure must include, among other items, the date, name and address (if available) of the person or entity that received the information, and a description of the PHI disclosed. Practice management software designed in compliance with HIPAA Privacy Standards makes all of this information available to the healthcare office by viewing the main "window" or connected "windows" related to that particular patient, rather than having to undertake a manual review of the hard copy in the patient's file.

A software vendor is *not required* to provide all of these services. However, it is in the best interest of the healthcare facility to partner with a vendor who is willing to work with the practice in achieving HIPAA compliance.

If a practice contracts with an entity considered a business associate, as described by the Privacy Standards, the practice should ensure that the agreement between them includes certain protections as defined in the Privacy Standards. HIPAA defines a business associate as an individual or corporate "person" who

- performs on behalf of the covered entity any function or activity involving the use or disclosure of PHI and
- is *not* a member of the covered entity's workforce.

This definition includes a requirement that the business associate use appropriate safeguards to prevent use of disclosure of PHI other than as provided in the agreement. If a healthcare practice finds that its current vendor is unable or unwilling to meet the HIPAA standards, it may be wise to begin shopping for a new vendor whose products and services can help the practice achieve HIPAA compliance.

📁 HIPAA Tip

Effective July 1, 2004, Medicare rejects electronic claims that have diagnosis codes, Zip Codes, or telephone numbers that are not HIPAA compliant. Medical facilities should ensure their billing systems are modified to generate electronic claims that pass Medicare HIPAA compliancy edits for diagnosis codes, Zip Codes, and telephone numbers.

⭐ Imagine This!

Dr. Agussi uses a computer system that prepares claim information in an electronic file to be submitted to a claims clearinghouse. After the system prepares the electronic file, Dr. Agussi's health insurance professional, Angela Peters, uploads the file to the software provided by the clearinghouse. Later, Angela downloads an electronic remittance file. Dr. Agussi's software reads this file and automatically posts payment information. Dr. Agussi receives maximum value for his computer software if the electronic claim file prepared by the computer system and the electronic remittance file provided by the clearinghouse are in standard ANSI format. This is possible only if Dr. Agussi's system and the clearinghouse accept and submit standard transactions.

Dr. Benton uses a computer system that prepares claim information in an electronic file to be submitted directly to the payer. Franklin Zetta, Dr. Benton's health insurance professional, dials into the payer's system and uploads the electronic file. Later, Franklin dials back into the payer's system and downloads an electronic remittance file. Dr. Benton's software reads this file and automatically posts payment information. Dr. Benton's system and the payer must support standard transactions because Dr. Benton and the payer are transacting directly with each other.

A healthcare office gets maximum value from patient accounting software or a practice management system if it is able to prepare, send, receive, and process ANSI standard electronic transactions.

❓💬 What Did You Learn?

1. To what four areas of patient accounting software do HIPAA rules relate?
2. Why is it important that a software vendor understand HIPAA requirements?
3. What requirements has HIPAA imposed on healthcare practices that relate to patient privacy?
4. Name the three categories that constitute covered entities.
5. List the two factors that define a business associate.

SUMMARY CHECKPOINTS

▶ There are four basic types of reimbursement:
- *Fee-for-service*—The healthcare provider charges a specific fee (typically the RVU multiplied by the current conversion factor) for each service rendered and is paid that fee by the patient or by the patient's insurance carrier.
- *Discounted fee-for-service*—Although providers typically charge all patients the same amount for the same service (except nonPAR Medicare providers), they accept reimbursement for services at lower rates than their usual fees under certain circumstances, such as when a provider contracts with a PPO. In a PPO with a discounted fee-for-service reimbursement structure, a PAR provider takes a contractual adjustment according to the PPO contract that results in a discount for member patients.
- *PPS*—The Medicare reimbursement system for inpatient hospital costs is based on predetermined factors and not on individual services. Rates are set at a level intended to cover operating costs for treating a typical inpatient in a given DRG. Payments for each hospital are adjusted for various factors such as differences in area wages, teaching activity, and care to the poor.
- *Capitation*—A common method of reimbursement used primarily by HMOs, the provider or healthcare facility is paid a fixed, per capita amount for each person enrolled in the plan without regard to the actual number or nature of services provided.

▶ PPS is a reimbursement system of predetermined prices that Medicare uses to reimburse hospitals for inpatient and outpatient services, SNFs, rehabilitation hospitals, and home health services. PPS rates are set at a level intended to cover operating costs for treating a typical inpatient in a given DRG.

▶ TEFRA, enacted by Congress in 1982, set limits on Medicare reimbursement that applied to stays in LTCHs. After TEFRA was passed, the fee-for-service–based payment system was replaced with the PPS. Congress adopted the PPS to regulate the amount of resources the federal government spends on medical care for elderly and disabled patients. The Social Security Amendments of 1983 mandated the PPS for acute hospital care for Medicare patients. The system was intended to encourage hospitals to modify the way they deliver services.

▶ DRG is a system of classifying hospital inpatient cases into categories with similar use of the facility's resources. Under this system, a hospital is paid a predetermined, lump sum amount, regardless of the costs involved, for each Medicare patient treated and discharged.

▶ APC is a system designed to explain the amount and type of resources used in an outpatient encounter. Under the APC system, Medicare pays hospitals for treating patients in outpatient clinics and physicians for treating patients in their offices. Each procedure or treatment has an APC code. Services in each APC are similar clinically in terms of the resources they require. A fixed payment rate is established for each APC.

▶ RUGs are used to calculate reimbursement in SNFs according to severity and level of care. Under the Medicare PPS, patients are classified into an RUG that determines how much Medicare would pay the SNF per day for that patient.

▶ The responsibilities of a PRO as they relate to the PPS include
   • evaluating services provided by practitioners and monitoring the quality of care given to patients;
   • ensuring that Medicare hospital services are appropriate, necessary, and provided in the most cost-effective manner;
   • monitoring the validity of diagnostic information supplied by hospitals for payment purposes;
   • ensuring that the care provided to Medicare beneficiaries is complete, adequate, and of good quality;
   • ascertaining the appropriateness of admissions and discharges; and
   • supervising the care in outlier cases in which additional Medicare payments were made.

▶ PROs have the ability to force hospitals to comply with HHS admission and quality standards.

▶ Patient accounting software systems have the capability of performing many functions including
   • input and storage of patient demographic and insurance information,
   • transaction posting,
   • allocation of system control operations,
   • generating patient statements,
   • processing and submitting insurance claims,
   • managing and collecting delinquent accounts, and
   • creating reports.

▶ A contractual write-off is the process of adjusting or canceling the balance owing (often through a provider's contract agreement with the insuring party) on a patient's account after all deductibles, coinsurance amounts, and third-party payments have been made.

▶ Advantages gained when a healthcare facility uses HIPAA-compliant software are:
   • Electronic claims are transmitted in the correct ANSI format.
   • Patient privacy is protected.
   • The security of patient health information is ensured.
   • Universal identifiers are defined for individuals, healthcare providers, and employers.
   • Potential administrative problems are alleviated with use of built-in privacy compliance functions.
   • Electronic records of patient consents and authorizations are tracked and maintained.

CLOSING SCENARIO

Dave breathed a sigh of relief as they finished the chapter. "Now that wasn't so bad, was it?" teased Janetta. Grudgingly, Dave admitted that all the acronyms eventually made sense, and he was glad he had stuck with it. Dave believed he had a good grasp on how fees are calculated for the various healthcare settings. Empowered with this information, he believed he would be much more versatile as a health insurance professional. The information on patient accounting systems was "right down his alley" because he viewed himself as a "computer guru." He and Janetta made a good team—she had helped him with the reimbursement issues, and he tutored her through the section on computerized office management. "This was great," exclaimed Janetta. "In a healthcare office everyone works as a team, and this was good practice." Dave and Janetta feel confident that they are ready for new challenges in the ever-changing world of medical billing and health insurance.

WEBSITES TO EXPLORE

- For live links to the following websites, please visit the Evolve site at
  http://evolve.elsevier.com/Beik/today
- To learn more about government acts regulating reimbursement systems, use "reimbursement systems" as your search words and log on to
  http://www.gpoaccess.gov/fr/index.html
- Obtain additional information on RVS from
  http://www.cdc.gov http://www.cms.hhs.gov
- For additional information on RBRVS, log on to
  http://www.ama-assn.org/ama/pub/category/10559.html
- For additional examples of calculating ALOS, visit the following website and key "average length of stay in hospitals" in the advanced search box; log on to
  http://www.dsf.health.state.pa.us/health
- For more information on the home health PPS, log on to
  http://www.cms.gov/HomeHealthPPS/

Author's Note: Websites change frequently. If any of these URLs is unavailable, use applicable guide words in your Internet search to acquire additional information on the various subjects listed.

REFERENCES AND RESOURCES

Belli P: *Reimbursement Systems: An Exploration of the Literature on Reimbursement Systems for Health Providers,* London, 2000, World Bank.

Böhm-Bawerk E: *Value and Price: An Extract,* ed 2, South Holland, Ill, 1973, Libertarian Press.

Center for Health Policy Research, American Medical Association: *The Impact of Medicare Payment Schedule Alternatives on Physicians,* Chicago, 1988, American Medical Association.

Hadley J, Berenson RA: Seeking the just price: constructing relative value scales and fee schedules, *Ann Intern Med* 106:461–466, 1987.

Hsaio WC, Braun P, Becker ER, et al: The resource-based relative value scale: toward the development of an alternative physician payment system, *JAMA* 258:799–802, 1987.

Hsiao WC, Braun P, Goldman P, et al: *Resource Based Relative Values of Selected Medical and Surgical Procedures in Massachusetts,* Boston, 1985, Final Report on Research Contract for Rate Setting Commission, Commonwealth of Massachusetts Harvard School of Public Health.

Hsiao WC, Stasson W: Toward developing a relative value scale for medical and surgical services, *Health Care Finance Rev* 1:23–38, 1979.

Karban K: CY 2011 changes to the hospital OPPS, *J AHIMA* 82(4): 54–56, 2011.

Kirchner M: Will this formula change the way you get paid? *Med Econ* 65:138–152, 1988.

Moorhead R: Here's what's wrong with the relative value scale, Presented at the 18th Annual Meeting of AAPS, Asheville, NC, October 12-14, 1961.

Orient JM: Physicians' pay targeted for "cost containment", *AAPS News* 43:1, 1987.

Sterling RB: *Guide to Medical Practice Software 2000,* Fort Worth, TX, 1999, Harcourt.

Vola A, Kallem C: A guide to US quality measurement organizations, *J AHIMA* 82(4):41–43, 2011.

CHAPTER 18

Hospital Billing and the UB-04

Chapter Outline

I. Hospital Versus Physician Office Billing and Coding
II. Modern Hospital and Health Systems
   A. Emerging Issues
III. Common Healthcare Facilities
   A. Acute Care Facilities
   B. Critical Access Hospitals
   C. Ambulatory Surgery Centers
   D. Other Types of Healthcare Facilities
      1. Subacute Care Facilities
      2. Skilled Nursing Facilities
      3. Intermediate Care Facilities
      4. Long-Term Care Facilities
      5. Hospice
      6. Home Health Agencies
IV. Legal and Regulatory Environment
   A. Accreditation
      1. The Joint Commission
      2. National Committee for Quality Assurance
      3. Accreditation Association for Ambulatory Health Care
      4. Utilization Review Accreditation Commission
   B. Professional Standards
   C. Governance
   D. Confidentiality and Privacy
   E. Fair Treatment of Patients
V. Common Hospital Payers and their Claims Guidelines
   A. Medicare
      1. Quality Improvement Organizations
      2. Keeping Current with Medicare
      3. Medicare Part A: Review
      4. What Medicare Part A Pays
      5. How Medicare Part A Payments Are Calculated
      6. Medicare Severity-Adjusted System
      7. IPPS 3-Day Payment Window
   B. Medicaid
   C. TRICARE
   D. CHAMPVA
   E. Blue Cross and Blue Shield
   F. Private Insurers
VI. National Uniform Billing Committee and the UB-04
   A. UB-04 Data Specifications
   B. 837I: Electronic Version of the UB-04 Form
      1. Data Layout of the 837I
VII. Structure and Content of the Hospital Health Record
   A. Standards in Hospital Electronic Medical Records
   B. Standard Codes and Terminology
VIII. Inpatient Hospital/Facility Coding
   A. ICD-9-CM (Volume 3) Codes for Inpatient Hospital Procedures
      1. Organization of ICD-9-CM Volume 3
      2. Classification of Procedures in ICD-9-CM Volume 3
   B. Code Sets Used for Inpatient Hospital/Facility Claims in ICD-10-PCS
      1. ICD-10-PCS
      2. Structure of ICD-10-PCS Codes
      3. Format of the ICD-10-PCS
      4. Selecting the Principal Diagnosis
   C. National Correct Coding Initiative
   D. Recent Rule Changes Affecting Hospital Billing
      1. The 72-Hour Rule
IX. Outpatient Hospital Coding
   A. Hospital Outpatient Prospective Payment System
   B. Ambulatory Payment Classification Coding
X. The Hospital Billing Process: Understanding the Basics
   A. Informed Consent
   B. Present on Admission (POA)
   C. Hospital Charges
      1. Hospital Charge Description Master
   D. Electronic Claims Submission (ECS)
   E. Health Information Management (HIM) Systems
   F. Payment Management
XI. HIPAA-Hospital Connection
XII. Billing Compliance
XIII. Career Opportunities in Hospital Billing
   A. Training, Other Qualifications, and Advancement
   B. Job Outlook

OPENING SCENARIO

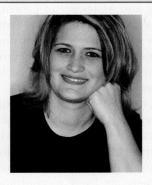

Brittany Weston has been employed as a health insurance professional in a two-physician practice for 5 years. Two years ago, she began taking evening classes at Deerfield Community College to become a health information technician. After graduating from Deerfield's accredited health information technician program, Brittany became eligible to take the registered health information technician (RHIT) examination. Passing this examination gives Brittany the right to use the credentials RHIT. Brittany is also required to obtain 20 continuing education hours every 2 years to maintain her credentials.

Brittany has now found new employment as an RHIT in the Health Information Management Department at Broadmoor Medical Center. One of the first things she learned during orientation at Broadmoor was the mission of the Health Information Management Department: total support of the facility's optimal standards for quality care and services through provision of quality information. The functions of Broadmoor's Health Information Management team support administrative processes, billing through classification systems, medical education, research through data gathering and analysis, utilization,

risk and quality management programs, legal requirements, data security, and release of information to authorized users.

Brittany realizes that her job duties as an RHIT will be different from and perhaps more challenging than those in her former occupation. These duties include the following:

- Compiling health information (e.g., reviewing, cataloging, and checking medical reports for completeness; organizing medical reports for placement in files; reviewing charts to ensure that all reports and signatures are present)
- Completing health information forms (e.g., preparing charts for new admissions, filling out forms, preparing requests for specific reports or certificates)
- Compiling and filling out statistical reports such as daily/monthly census, Medicaid days, admissions, discharges, and length of stay
- Filing reports in health records, recording information in logs and files
- Retrieving health information records from filing system
- Providing information from health records after determining appropriateness of request
- Coordinating health information records procedures with other departments

Brittany is looking forward to her new career as an RHIT. She hopes to return to the classroom eventually and acquire the necessary credentials in Health Information Management, which would allow her career aspirations to grow.

CHAPTER OBJECTIVES

After completion of this chapter, the student should be able to:

1. Differentiate between physician office and hospital billing and coding.
2. Explain the modern hospital system.
3. Identify common types of healthcare facilities.
4. Discuss the legal and regulatory environment of today's hospitals.
5. List common hospital payers and how to acquire their claims guidelines.
6. Describe the UB-04 and its relation to the National Uniform Billing Committee.
7. Discuss the structure and content of the hospital health record.
8. Outline the inpatient hospital/facility coding process.
9. Discuss outpatient hospital coding systems.
10. Summarize the hospital billing process.
11. Explain the HIPAA/hospital connection.
12. Provide a rationale for medical compliance.
13. Analyze the career opportunities in hospital billing.

CHAPTER TERMS

72-hour rule
accreditation
Accreditation Association for Ambulatory Health Care (AAAHC)
activities of daily living (ADLs)
acute care
acute care facility
acute condition
ambulatory payment classifications (APCs)
ambulatory surgery centers (ASCs)
benefit period
billing compliance
Blue Cross and Blue Shield member hospitals
case mix
charge description master
cost sharing
covered entity

Critical access hospital (CAH)
Defense Enrollment Eligibility Reporting System (DEERS)
diagnosis-related group (DRG)
electronic claims submission (ECS)
electronic medical record (EMR)
electronic remittance advice (ERA)
Emergency Medical Treatment and Labor Act (EMTLA)
emergency medical condition
exacerbation
form locators
for-profit hospitals
general hospital
governance
health information management (HIM)
hospice

hospital outpatient
  prospective payment
  system (HOPPS)
informed consent
intermediate care facilities
fiscal intermediaries
(The) Joint Commission
licensed independent
  practitioners
long-term care facilities
medical ethics
Medicare Severity-Adjusted
  (MS-DRG) System
multiaxial structure
National Committee for
  Quality Assurance (NCQA)
National Correct Coding
  Initiative (NCCI)
National Uniform Billing
  Committee (NUBC)
nonavailability statement
  (NAS)
outliers

palliative care
pass-throughs
per diems
pricing transparency
principal diagnosis
prospective payment system
  (PPS)
quality improvement
  organizations
registered health information
  technicians (RHITs)
respite care
skilled nursing facility (SNF)
subacute care unit
surrogate
swing bed
transaction set
UB-04
Utilization Review
  Accreditation Commission
  (URAC)
vertically integrated
  hospitals

HOSPITAL VERSUS PHYSICIAN OFFICE BILLING AND CODING

Everything that we have discussed so far in this textbook has applied to billing, coding, and insurance claims processing for physicians' offices and clinics. This last chapter presents some basic information and guidelines for billing, coding, and patient services in inpatient hospital facilities and other hospital-based healthcare. This chapter does not present enough detailed information to enable you become a hospital biller and coder; that amount of information would fill an entire separate textbook. Instead, this chapter provides an overview of the basics. If you find this information interesting, you may want to further explore a career in hospital billing or health information management.

MODERN HOSPITAL AND HEALTH SYSTEMS

The ideal modern hospital is a place where sick or injured individuals seek and receive care and, in the case of teaching hospitals, where clinical education is provided to the entire spectrum of healthcare professionals. Today's hospital provides continuing education for practicing physicians and increasingly serves the function of an institution of higher learning for entire neighborhoods, communities, and regions. In addition to its educational role, the modern hospital conducts investigational studies and research in medical sciences.

The construction of today's modern hospital is regulated by federal laws, state health department policies, city ordinances, the standards of private accrediting organizations such as The

Joint Commission, and national and local codes (e.g., building, fire protection, sanitation). These requirements safeguard patients' privacy and the safety and well-being of patients and staff. The popular ward concept of the mid-19th and early 20th centuries, in which multiple patients were housed in one common area, is no longer permissible. Today, hospitals have mainly semiprivate and private rooms. Although permissible in most states, four-bed rooms are the exception.

Beginning in the early 1990s, hospitals became part of the evolution toward **vertically integrated hospitals** (hospitals that provide all levels of healthcare) and other provider networks. It is predicted that inpatient care will gradually diminish with continued advances in medicine, and that hospitals, as we once knew them, are likely to continue downsizing. Simultaneously, ambulatory care in physicians' offices and clinics will increase. The hospital, particularly in comparison with its earliest days, will play a different role in the future as part of an integrated collection of providers and sites of care. For more information on the history of hospitals, refer to Websites to Explore at the end of this chapter.

Emerging Issues

A goal of the entire healthcare system is to reduce costs and, at the same time, be more responsive to customers, a trendy designation being given to today's healthcare consumers (i.e., patients). The elderly are the heaviest users of healthcare services, and the percentage of elderly individuals in the population is increasing significantly. Also affecting this scenario are the rapid advances in medical technology, often involving sophisticated techniques and equipment, that are making more diagnostic and treatment procedures available. Other emerging healthcare trends are as follows:

- Movement from hospital-based acute care to outpatient care
- Trend toward a more holistic, preventive, and continuous care of health and wellness
- Advent of Health Insurance Portability and Accountability Act (HIPAA) regulations addressing security and privacy of protected health information (PHI)
- Growing emphasis on security, especially in large public facilities, and the need to balance this with the desired openness to patients and visitors
- The increasing introduction of highly sophisticated diagnostic and treatment technology
- A shift to computerized patient information, e.g. electronic health records (EHRs)
- Emergence of **palliative care** (temporary relief of pain/symptoms without a cure—sometimes called comfort care) as a specialty

A link to the American Hospital Association (AHA) website, which provides the latest research and analysis of important and emerging trends in the hospital and healthcare field, can be found on the Evolve site.

⭐ Imagine This!

When Brittany was going through her orientation, the presenter, the soon-to-be-retired health information manager, told the new recruits about the "ward system," which existed in the large teaching hospital where she was first employed. There were two large wards on each floor—medical was on the third floor, surgical was on the fourth floor, and so forth. The ward on the west end of the third floor was Ward M3A; the ward on the east end was Ward M3B. Each of these wards was a large room with sometimes 30 beds. These beds were occupied by indigent or "state" patients, individuals who did not have insurance or the financial ability to pay for their healthcare. These patients wore dingy hospital gowns with their respective ward identification stenciled in large digits on the front so as to identify them if they wandered out of the ward.

Patients who had insurance or could pay for their care were housed on the second floor in private or semiprivate rooms and were attended by "staff" physicians. The patients in the wards were attended by medical students, interns, and residents who were overseen by staff physicians. The wards were not air-conditioned; they were crowded, malodorous, and noisy. Medical students acquired much of their medical education here, often at the expense of the patients.

The health information manager concluded, "Inpatient medical care as we know it today has improved 200-fold."

❓ What Did You Learn?

1. Describe a typical general hospital.
2. How are today's modern hospitals regulated?
3. What is meant by *vertically integrated hospital*?
4. List at least three emerging healthcare trends.

COMMON HEALTHCARE FACILITIES

The best-known type of healthcare facility is the **general hospital**, which is set up to handle care of many kinds of disease and injury. It may be a single building or a campus and typically has an emergency department to deal with immediate threats to health and the capacity to provide emergency medical services. A general hospital is usually the major healthcare facility in a region, with a large number of beds for intensive care and long-term care and specialized facilities for medical care, surgery, childbirth, and laboratories. Big cities may have several different hospitals of various sizes and facilities. Large hospitals are often called medical centers and usually conduct operations in virtually every field of modern medicine. Types of specialized hospitals include trauma centers; children's hospitals; seniors'

hospitals; and hospitals for dealing with specific medical needs such as psychiatric problems, pulmonary diseases, orthopedic procedures, and other specialized areas of care.

Some hospitals are affiliated with universities for medical research and the training of medical personnel. In the United States, many facilities are **for-profit hospitals**, meaning that their monetary income must be greater than expenses, whereas elsewhere in the world, most hospitals are nonprofit. Many hospitals have volunteer programs in which individuals (usually students and senior citizens) provide various ancillary services.

A medical facility smaller than a hospital is typically referred to as a clinic and is often run by a government agency or a private partnership of physicians. Clinics generally provide only outpatient services.

Acute Care Facilities

An **acute care facility** is what most individuals usually think of as a "hospital," although all services provided may not relate directly to an **acute condition** (condition in which a patient's medical state has become unstable). This facility is equipped and staffed to respond immediately to a critical situation.

An **acute care facility** can be defined as a facility offering inpatient, overnight care, and services for observation, diagnosis, and active treatment of an individual with a medical, surgical, obstetric, chronic, or rehabilitative condition requiring the daily direction or supervision of a physician. **Acute care** involves assessing and treating sudden or unexpected injuries and illnesses. Acute healthcare settings provide emergency care, sophisticated diagnostic tools, and surgical interventions and can provide patient care 24 hours a day, 7 days a week, 365 days a year. The staff consists of nurses, doctors, technicians, therapists, and other ancillary staff who have roles in caring for and/or supporting the patient.

After a patient is discharged from the hospital, two different claims typically are generated—one from the hospital for institutional charges and the other from the physician for his or her professional services. As we learned in earlier chapters, physician service claims are submitted to the patient's insurance carrier using an electronic claims submission process or the CMS-1500 paper form, if the provider qualifies. Hospital service claims are typically submitted electronically or by using a nationally recognized billing form called the UB-04 (short for uniform bill 2004), sometimes referred to as the CMS-1450 form.

Critical Access Hospitals

A **critical access hospital (CAH)** is one that is certified to receive cost-based reimbursement from Medicare. The Critical Access Hospital Program was created by the 1997 federal Balanced Budget Act as a safety net to guarantee Medicare beneficiaries access to healthcare services in rural areas. It was designed to allow more flexible staffing options required by the community, simplify billing methods, and create incentives to develop local integrated health delivery systems including acute, primary, emergency, and long-term care.

The reimbursement that a CAH receives is intended to improve financial performance, thereby reducing hospital closures. Each hospital must review its own situation to determine whether CAH status would be advantageous. CAHs are certified under a different set of Medicare Conditions of Participation (CoP) that are more flexible than those of acute care hospitals.

Ambulatory Surgery Centers

Ambulatory surgery centers (ASCs) are facilities where surgical procedures that do not require hospital admission are performed. They provide a cost-effective and convenient environment that may be less stressful than that offered by many hospitals. Particular ASCs may perform surgical procedures in a variety of specialties or dedicate their services to one specialty, such as eye care or orthopedic services.

An ASC treats only patients who already have seen a healthcare provider and who together have selected surgery as an appropriate treatment. All ASCs must have at least one dedicated operating room and the equipment needed to perform surgery safely and to ensure quality patient care. Physician offices and clinics that are not so equipped are not considered ASCs. Patients who elect to have surgery in an ASC arrive on the day of the procedure, undergo the procedure in a specially equipped operating room, and recover under the care of the nursing staff, all without a hospital admission.

ASCs are among the most highly regulated healthcare facilities in the United States. Medicare has certified more than 80% of these centers, and most states require ASCs to be licensed. These states also specify the criteria that ASCs must meet for licensure. States and Medicare survey ASCs regularly to verify that the established standards are being met. All accredited ASCs must meet specific standards that are evaluated during on-site inspections. In addition to state and federal inspections, many surgery centers go through a voluntary accreditation process conducted by peers. As a result, patients visiting an accredited ASC can be assured that the center provides the highest quality care.

Other Types of Healthcare Facilities

Many other types of healthcare facilities besides acute care hospitals and ASCs exist (Fig. 18-1). Following is a brief discussion of a few of the more familiar types.

Subacute Care Facilities

A **subacute care facility** is a comprehensive, highly specialized inpatient program designed for individuals who have experienced an acute event as a result of an illness, injury, or **exacerbation** (worsening) of a disease process. It specifies a level of maintenance care in which there is no urgent or

- Acute Care Facilities
- Ambulatory Surgical Centers
- Assisted Living Residences
- Assisted Living Residences: Residential Care Facilities—Mentally Ill
- Birth Centers
- Community Clinics and Emergency Centers
- Chiropractic Centers
- Community Mental Health Clinics Centers
- Comprehensive Outpatient Rehabilitation
- Designated Trauma Centers
- Free Standing End Stage Renal Disease Service
- Home/Community-Based Services: Adult Day Programs
- Home/Community-Based Services: Personal Care/Homemaker
- Home Health Agencies
- Hospices
- Hospitals (General, Psychiatric, Rehabilitation, Critical Access)
- Intermediate Care Facilities for Mentally Retarded
- Long-Term Care (Nursing Homes/Nursing Care) Facilities
- Physical Therapy: Outpatient
- Portable X-ray Services
- Residential Care Facilities—Developmentally Disabled
- Rural Health Clinics
- Skilled Nursing Facilities
- Sub-Acute Care Facilities
- Swing Bed Facilities

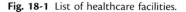

Fig. 18-1 List of healthcare facilities.

life-threatening condition requiring medical treatment. Subacute care may consist of long-term ventilator care or other procedures provided on a routine basis either at home or by trained staff at an SNF. This type of care often is seen as a bridge between the hospital's acute care units and facilities for patients who require ongoing medical care or who are still dependent on advanced medical technology.

In a subacute care facility, patients have the advantage of constant access to nursing care as they move toward recovery and return to their home, which acute care facilities typically do not provide. If the physician determines that recuperative care is required after an acute hospitalization, the patient may be transferred to a facility that specializes in subacute services; however, a stay in a subacute care facility is generally short term.

Skilled Nursing Facilities

An SNF is an institution or a distinct part of an institution that is licensed or approved under state or local law and is primarily engaged in providing skilled nursing care and related services as an SNF, extended care facility, or nursing care facility approved by The Joint Commission or the Bureau of Hospitals of the American Osteopathic Association (AOA), or otherwise determined by the health plan to meet the reasonable standards applied by any of these authorities.

Previously referred to as "nursing homes," SNFs have evolved in the services they provide. They offer 24-hour skilled nursing care; rehabilitation services such as physical, speech, and occupational therapy; assistance with personal care activities such as eating, walking, toileting, and bathing; coordinated management of patient care; social services; and activities. Some SNFs offer specialized care programs for patients with Alzheimer's disease or other illnesses or short-term **respite care** for frail or disabled individuals when family members require a rest from providing care in the home. Respite care services give individuals such as family members temporary relief from tasks associated with care-giving. A crucial element of an SNF is periodic reviews by the state or local department of social and health services.

⭐ Imagine This!

Broadmoor Respite Services offers a wide range of services to caregivers who require temporary relief from their responsibilities. These services include companion services, personal care, household assistance, and skilled nursing care to meet specific needs of patients with disabilities, patients with chronic or terminal illnesses, and elderly patients. Broadmoor Respite Services provides overnight, weekend, and longer stays for individuals with Alzheimer's disease or a related dementia so that a caregiver can have longer periods of time off. The facility provides meals, helps with activities of daily living, and provides therapeutic activities to fit the needs of residents in a safe, supervised environment.

Intermediate Care Facilities

Intermediate care facilities are designed for individuals with chronic conditions who are unable to live independently but who do not need constant intensive care. Intermediate care facilities provide supportive care and nursing supervision under medical direction 24 hours a day but do not provide continuous nursing care. They stress rehabilitation therapy that enables individuals to return to a home setting or to regain or retain as many functions of daily living as possible. A full range of medical, social, recreational and support services are also provided.

Long-Term Care Facilities

Long-term care facilities provide care for adults who are chronically ill or disabled and are no longer able to manage in independent living situations. Long-term care is the type of care that individuals may need when they no longer can perform **activities of daily living (ADLs)** by themselves, such as bathing, eating, and getting dressed. It also includes the kind of care an individual would need if he or she had a severe cognitive impairment such as Alzheimer's disease.

When we think of long-term care, we often think of nursing homes. Long-term care can be received in a variety of settings, however, including an individual's own home, assisted living facilities, adult day care centers, and hospice facilities. Long-term care does not refer to the medical care needed to get well from an illness or injury or to short-term rehabilitation from an accident or recuperation from surgery.

Hospice

Hospice is not a specific place; it is a facility or service that provides care for terminally ill patients and support to their families, either directly or on a consulting basis with the patient's physician. Emphasis is on symptom control and support before and after death. Hospice attempts to meet each patient's unique physical, emotional, social, and spiritual needs and the special needs of the patient's family and close friends. The goals of hospice are to keep the patient as comfortable as possible by relieving pain and other discomforting symptoms, to prepare for a death that follows the wishes and needs of the patient, and to reassure the patient and loved ones by helping them understand and manage what is happening. This support assists patients and families through the process of facing, understanding, and accepting death.

Home Health Agencies

Home health agencies provide a wide range of healthcare services that can be given in the patient's home. Home healthcare is usually less expensive and more convenient than, and can be just as effective as, care provided in a hospital or skilled nursing facility. In general, home healthcare includes part-time or intermittent skilled nursing care and other skilled care services, such as physical and/or occupational therapy and speech-language therapy services. Services may also include medical social services or assistance from a home health aide. A home healthcare agency typically coordinates the services ordered by the patient's physician orders.

❓ What Did You Learn?

1. Name three major types of healthcare facilities.
2. How does an acute care facility differ from a critical access hospital?
3. In what type of facility might an individual receive long-term care?
4. What is hospice?

LEGAL AND REGULATORY ENVIRONMENT

State and federal governments, accrediting organizations, employers, and healthcare plans have developed methods for ensuring quality in managed care plan systems. As physicians and healthcare consumers have become more aware of the need for protection against excessive containment of managed care costs, many state governments have enacted laws designed to protect patients' rights.

All acute care or general hospitals must be licensed by the particular state in which they are located to provide care within the minimum health and safety standards established by regulation and rule. The U.S. Department of Health and Human Services (HHS) enforces the standards by periodically conducting surveys of these facilities. Medicare pays for services provided by hospitals that voluntarily seek and are approved for certification by the Centers for Medicare and Medicaid Services (CMS). CMS contracts with HHS to evaluate compliance with the federal hospital regulations by periodically conducting surveys of these agencies.

A hospital may seek accreditation by nationally recognized accrediting agencies such as The Joint Commission or the AOA. Surveys conducted by The Joint Commission and AOA are based on guidelines developed by each of these organizations.

The federal **Emergency Medical Treatment and Labor Act (EMTLA)** was enacted by Congress as part of the Consolidated Omnibus Budget Reconciliation Act of 1985. This act states that member hospitals must respond to an individual's **emergency medical condition** (defined as the onset of a health condition that requires immediate medical attention) by determining the nature of the condition. If an emergent condition exists, it must be treated to the best of the facility's ability regardless of ability to pay. Patients can then be transferred as appropriate after the condition has been stabilized.

EMTLA applies to virtually all hospitals in the United States with the exception of the Shriners' Hospitals for Children and many military hospitals. Its provisions apply to all patients—not just to Medicare beneficiaries.

🕐 Stop and Think

After a fall from his bicycle on his way home from school, Bobby Thaddeus, an 8-year-old boy, complained of pain in his right arm. His mother, fearing his arm might be fractured, brought Bobby to Meadville Hospital's emergency department. The emergency staff at Meadville refused to treat the child, advising Bobby's mother to take him to their family practitioner for treatment. A spokesman at Meadville defended the hospital's policy, stating that it was put in place to curb misuse of emergency department services. Nonemergencies overloaded staff and facilities with routine medical problems that could be handled as well elsewhere. When routine injuries and illnesses were brought to the emergency department, they cause delayed treatment of true emergencies. Do you agree with the hospital's policy? Why or why not? Was Meadville violating the Emergency Medical Treatment and Active Labor Act in refusing to treat Bobby's injury?

Accreditation

Accreditation is a voluntary process through which an organization is able to measure the quality of its services and performance against nationally recognized standards. It is the process by which a private or public agency evaluates and recognizes (certifies) an institution—in this case, hospitals—as fulfilling applicable standards. The Joint Commission evaluates whether hospitals, nursing homes, and managed care organizations meet certain specified requirements. The **Accreditation Association for Ambulatory Health Care (AAAHC)** and the **National Committee for Quality Assurance (NCQA)** assess and award compliance certifications to managed care organizations, including health maintenance organizations. Public agencies sometimes require accreditation by a private body as a condition of licensure, or they may accept accreditation as a substitute for their own inspection or certification programs. The next section discusses the more commonly known accreditation organizations.

The Joint Commission

The Joint Commission is a private organization created in 1951 to provide voluntary accreditation to hospitals. In 2002, the organization established its National Patient Safety Goals (NPSGs) program, to help accredited organizations address specific areas of concern in regard to patient safety. A panel of patient safety experts advises The Joint Commission on the development and updating of NPSGs. This panel, called the Patient Safety Advisory Group, is composed of nurses, physicians, pharmacists, risk managers, clinical engineers, and other professionals who have hands-on experience in addressing patient safety issues in a wide variety of healthcare settings.

National Committee for Quality Assurance

NCQA is an independent, nonprofit organization that performs quality-oriented accreditation reviews on health maintenance organizations and similar types of managed care plans. NCQA is governed by a board of directors that includes employers, consumer and labor representatives, health plan representatives, policymakers, and physicians. The purpose of NCQA is to evaluate plans and provide information that helps consumers and employers make informed decisions about purchasing health plan services. NCQA performs two distinct functions: One is the evaluation and accreditation of health plans; the other is measurement of performance.

The NCQA accreditation process involves a comprehensive review of health plan structure, policies, procedures, systems, and records. The review includes an analysis of plan documents and an on-site inspection visit by a team of expert reviewers. On the basis of the review, plans are accorded one of several possible accreditation levels: excellent, commendable, accredited, and provisional. Plans that do not meet standards are denied accreditation status.

Stop and Think

Elena Sanchez, a 42-year-old woman, lived in a large metropolitan area with several large and small hospitals. After a visit to her physician for complications of diabetes, her physician advised her that she should be admitted to one of the local hospitals for some tests and possible surgery. Elena asked her friend Teresa, a health information professional, how she should choose which hospital to go to. She preferred the one located in her neighborhood, Seacrest Memorial. Teresa told Elena that Seacrest might not be the best choice because although it was handy, it was not accredited. Why might this fact be a concern for Elena?

Accreditation Association for Ambulatory Health Care

AAAHC was formed in 1979 to assist ambulatory healthcare organizations improve the quality of care provided to patients. The accreditation decision is based on assessment of an organization's compliance with applicable standards and adherence to the policies and procedures of AAAHC. AAAHC expects substantial compliance with all applicable standards, which is assessed by at least one of the following means:

- Documented evidence
- Answers to detailed questions concerning implementation
- On-site observations and interviews by surveyors

Utilization Review Accreditation Commission

The **Utilization Review Accreditation Commission (URAC)** is an independent, nonprofit organization. Its mission is to promote continuous improvement in the quality and efficiency of healthcare delivery by achieving a common understanding of excellence among purchasers, providers, and patients through the establishment of standards, programs of education and communication, and a process of accreditation. URAC is nationally recognized as a leader in quality improvement, reviewing and auditing a broad array of healthcare service functions and systems. Their accreditation activities cover health plans, preferred provider organizations, medical management systems, health technology services, healthcare centers, specialty care, workers' compensation, medical websites, and HIPAA privacy and security compliance.

Professional Standards

Professional standards that govern U.S. hospitals typically are associated with an accrediting body such as The Joint Commission and differ from one organization to the next. The Joint Commission's Medical Staff Standard MS.6.9 requires hospitals to define (e.g., in a policy) the process for supervision of residents by licensed independent practitioners with appropriate clinical privileges. A **licensed independent practitioner** is defined as "any individual permitted by law and by the organization to provide care and services without direction or supervision, within the scope of the individual's license, and consistent with individually granted clinical privileges."

The standard also requires the medical staff to ensure that each resident is supervised in his or her patient care responsibilities by a licensed independent practitioner who has been granted clinical privileges through the medical staff process. Finally, the rules require hospitals to identify in the medical staff rules, regulations, and policies which individuals may write patient care orders, the circumstances under which they may write such orders, and what entries must be countersigned by a supervising licensed independent practitioner.

Governance

Governance, in its widest sense, refers to how any organization is run. With reference to healthcare facilities, it involves all the processes, systems, and controls that are used to safeguard the welfare of patients and the integrity of the institution. The Joint Commission's Revised Governance Standard GO.2 provides that, in addition to providing for the effective functioning of activities related to delivering quality patient care, performance improvement, risk management, medical staff credentialing, and financial management, the governing body must provide for the effective functioning of professional graduate medical education programs (e.g., by adopting policies and bylaw provisions).

Confidentiality and Privacy

Most hospital accrediting organizations, specifically The Joint Commission, include strategies for accrediting a hospital on privacy and confidentiality issues that parallel the demands of HIPAA compliance. It is important for hospital staff to understand and abide by HIPAA's Privacy Standards, including such topics as

- who qualifies as "covered entities" under the Privacy Standards
- what type of information is protected
- what HIPAA's restrictions are on the use and disclosure of PHI
- how the hospital follows the minimum necessary standard
- how the hospital implements patient rights created by the Privacy Standards
- what administrative requirements the Privacy Standards impose
- what business associates are and when the hospital needs contracts with them to disclose protected health information
- what the HIPAA preemption provisions are, and
- what penalties HHS can impose for failing to comply with the Privacy Standards.

A **covered entity** under HIPAA is a health plan, a healthcare clearinghouse, or a healthcare provider that transmits any health information in electronic form in connection with a transaction. The Privacy Rule requires a covered entity (in this case, the hospital) to make reasonable efforts to limit use of, disclosure of, and requests for PHI to the minimum necessary to accomplish the intended purpose. The minimum necessary standard is intended to make covered entities evaluate and enhance protections as needed to prevent unnecessary or inappropriate access to PHI. It is intended to reflect and be consistent with, not to override, professional judgment and standards.

The Privacy Rule is not intended to prohibit providers from talking to other providers and their patients. The following practices are considered to be permissible, if reasonable precautions are taken to minimize the chance of inadvertent disclosures to others who may be nearby (e.g., using lowered voices, talking apart):

- Healthcare staff may verbally coordinate services at hospital nursing stations.
- Nurses or other healthcare professionals may discuss a patient's condition over the phone with the patient, a provider, or a family member.
- A healthcare professional may discuss laboratory test results with a patient or other provider in a joint treatment area.
- Healthcare professionals may discuss a patient's condition during training rounds in an academic or training institution.

📁 HIPAA Tip

HIPAA regulations state that hospitals are required by law to protect the privacy of health information that may reveal a patient's identity (referred to as PHI) and to provide the patient with a written notice of privacy practice (NOPP) that describes the health information privacy practices of the hospital.

🕐 Stop and Think

Elizabeth Cotter, a 74-year-old woman, underwent a serious operation after experiencing a cardiac episode. After the surgery was completed, a nurse came to the reception area where Mrs. Cotter's family was waiting and informed them that although the procedure took longer than expected, Mrs. Cotter came through it okay and was in now in the recovery room. "You can see her as soon as she is transferred to her room, in about 30 minutes." Has there been a breach of patient confidentiality here? Why or why not?

After Mrs. Cotter returned to her room, her next-door neighbor telephoned the nurses' station to inquire as to her condition. The nurse informed the caller that although the procedure took longer than expected, and that it was "touch and go for a while," the patient was back in her room now and was expected to make a full recovery. Has there been a breach of confidentiality here? Why or why not?

Fair Treatment of Patients

In Chapter 3, we learned about **medical ethics**, which are the moral principles that govern the practice of medicine by physicians and other healthcare practitioners. When dealing with patients or healthcare users, healthcare practitioners are governed by these ethical principles and the law. Breaches of ethical rules may result in disciplinary action by employers and professional staff. Breaches of the law may result in similar disciplinary action and criminal or civil legal action against the healthcare practitioners concerned. Basic principles of medical ethics are usually regarded as

- showing respect for patient autonomy,
- not inflicting harm on patients,
- contributing to the welfare of patients, and
- providing justice and fair treatment of patients.

Ethical principles require healthcare practitioners to become advocates for their patients. The principle of justice or fairness requires medical personnel to ensure that their patients enjoy the constitutional right to equal treatment and freedom from unfair discrimination. The principle of autonomy requires medical personnel to ensure that their patients' constitutional and common law human rights to freedom and security of the individual are respected; this is safeguarded by the ethical and legal requirements of an informed consent. Respect of a patient's right to freedom of religion, beliefs, and opinions is legally required in terms of the U.S. Constitution.

A patient's right to privacy is safeguarded by the ethical and legal rules regarding confidentiality. The principle of not inflicting harm requires medical personnel to ensure that their patients' constitutional human rights to dignity, life, emergency treatment, and an environment that is not harmful to health are upheld. The principle of contributing to the welfare of patients requires medical personnel to ensure that the constitutional imperative against medical malpractice and professional negligence is not allowed.

A breach of an ethical principle or of an ethical rule or regulation formally put into effect by a professional council may be used to establish medical malpractice or professional negligence, although the breach itself may not constitute a crime or civil wrong. For a civil wrong to be proved, it would have to be shown that the health professional's conduct was also a breach of a legal obligation.

📁 HIPAA Tip

A hospital billing department is prevented from answering questions from advocates or family members who work on a patient's behalf to help pay medical bills unless the patient has signed a written authorization directing billing department employees to do so.

Imagine This!

If a physician or other healthcare practitioner negligently causes the death of a patient by breaching an ethical rule, he or she may face a criminal charge of culpable homicide or a civil action by the deceased's dependents. Marcus Sherman, a 56-year-old man, saw Dr. Edmund Pithily because of rectal bleeding. Dr Pithily performed a limited sigmoidoscopy, the results of which were negative. The patient continued to have rectal bleeding but was repeatedly reassured by the physician that he was okay. Eighteen months later, after a 25-lb weight loss, Mr. Sherman was admitted to a hospital for evaluation. He was found to have colon cancer with metastases to the liver. Despite all efforts to combat the spread of the disease, Mr. Sherman died. The physicians who reviewed his medical record judged that proper diagnostic management might have discovered the cancer when it was still curable. They attributed the advanced disease to substandard medical care. The event was considered adverse and due to negligence.

What Did You Learn?

1. What governing body licenses acute care and general hospitals?
2. List two nationally recognized organizations that play an important role in hospital accreditation.
3. What function does EMTLA serve?
4. What is the purpose of accreditation?
5. List the principles of medical ethics.

COMMON HOSPITAL PAYERS AND THEIR CLAIMS GUIDELINES

The major payers of hospital costs are much the same as those of physicians' offices and clinics. Government payers (Medicare, Medicaid, and TRICARE/CHAMPVA) typically have the largest share of claims, followed by Blue Cross and Blue Shield and managed care organizations. Other payers include private/commercial insurance companies, no-fault/liability insurance arrangements, and workers' compensation. These shares differ, however, from state to state. As stated often throughout this text, it is paramount for the health insurance professional to learn and follow the specific guidelines of each individual payer. The following subsections briefly address these major payers. For more detailed information, refer to their specific corresponding chapters.

Medicare

Medicare hospital claims are processed by nongovernment organizations or agencies that contract to serve as fiscal agents between providers (hospitals, physicians, and other healthcare providers) and the federal government. These claims processors are commonly referred to as Medicare carriers, Medicare administrative contractors (MACs), or **fiscal intermediaries** (FIs). They apply Medicare coverage rules to determine the appropriateness and medical necessity of claims.

Medicare carriers (regional companies that oversee the administration and processing of Medicare policies and claims) process Part A claims (hospital insurance) for institutional services, including inpatient hospital services as well as those provided by SNFs, home healthcare agencies, and hospice. They also process hospital outpatient claims for Medicare Part B. Examples are Blue Cross and Blue Shield, Noridian, Palmetto, and other commercial insurance companies.

Carriers are required to process claims according to government regulations. Additionally, as regional companies, they have the authority to set local policies. A Medicare carrier reviews all Medicare claims and determines whether or not each claim qualifies for reimbursement. The carrier is then responsible for developing payment policies for the states in its area. Once these local medical review policies (also known as local coverage determinations) are established, the Medicare carrier evaluates each Medicare claim to ensure that the services provided are reasonable and necessary. Additionally, Medicare carriers are responsible for

- maintaining records,
- establishing controls,
- safeguarding against fraud and abuse or excess use,
- conducting reviews and audits, and
- assisting providers and beneficiaries as needed.

HIPAA Tip

The Centers for Medicare and Medicaid Services (CMS) has instructed their Medicare carriers and intermediaries to make free or low-cost software available to providers that would enable electronic submission of HIPAA-compliant claims.

Quality Improvement Organizations

Quality improvement organizations (QIOs), formerly called peer review organizations, are groups of practicing healthcare professionals who are paid by the federal government to overview the care provided to Medicare beneficiaries and to improve the quality of services. QIOs educate and assist in the promotion of effective, efficient, and economical delivery of healthcare services to the Medicare population they serve. QIOs are discussed in more detail in Chapter 9. More information on QIOs can be found on the CMS website at http://www.cms.gov/Quality ImprovementOrgs/.

Keeping Current with Medicare

The Medicare Modernization Act of 2003 brought many new changes to the Medicare program. These new changes gave beneficiaries more choices in how they get their healthcare benefits, as follows:

- Medicare prescription drug plan (see Chapter 9), which began January 2006 (enrollment started in November 2005)
- New health plan choices, including Medicare Advantage health plans and regional preferred provider organization plans, which began in 2006
- New preventive benefits, first available January 1, 2005, including cardiovascular screening blood tests, diabetes screening tests, and "welcome to Medicare" physical examinations

The Patient Protection and Affordable Care Act of 2010 requires that most individuals have minimum health insurance. The legislation creates new public plans and expands the Medicare and Medicaid programs to include more beneficiaries while requiring that all health plans extend coverage to individuals regardless of health status.

To keep current with Medicare changes, the health insurance professional should log onto the CMS website periodically to research what is new. It is also a good idea to keep on hand a copy of the most recent edition of the beneficiary handbook, *Medicare and You,* which can be downloaded from the Internet.

Medicare Part A: Review

Part A helps provide coverage for inpatient care in hospitals, including CAHs and SNFs, but not extended care in custodial or long-term care facilities. Part A also helps cover hospice care and some home healthcare. Beneficiaries must meet certain conditions to obtain these benefits. Most individuals eligible for Medicare do not have to pay a monthly payment (premium) for Part A, because they or a spouse paid Medicare taxes while employed. If Medicare beneficiaries do not get premium-free Part A, they may be able to buy it if

- they or their spouses are not entitled to Social Security because they did not work or did not pay Medicare taxes while working and are age 65 or older or
- they are disabled but no longer get free Part A because they returned to work.

What Medicare Part A Pays

All rules about how much Medicare Part A pays depend on how many days of inpatient care the beneficiary has during what is called a **benefit period** or "spell of illness." The benefit period begins the day the individual enters the hospital or SNF as an inpatient and continues until he or she has been out of the hospital for 60 consecutive days. If the patient is in and out of the hospital or SNF several times but has not stayed out completely for 60 consecutive days, all inpatient charges for that time are figured as part of the same benefit period.

Medicare Part A pays only certain amounts of a hospital bill for any one benefit period, and the rules are slightly different depending on whether the care facility is a hospital, psychiatric hospital, or SNF, or whether care is received at home or through a hospice. Table 18-1 shows the 2011 Medicare Part A schedule outlining what Medicare pays

TABLE 18-1	2011 Medicare Part A Payment Schedule: Hospital Insurance Premiums, Deductibles, and Coinsurance
IF YOU HAVE	**IN 2011, YOU WILL PAY A MONTHLY PREMIUM OF**
0-29 quarters of Social Security credits	$450
30-39 quarters of Social Security credits	$248
40 or more quarters of Social Security credits	$0
Inpatient hospital deductible	$1,132
Inpatient hospital coinsurance	$283 per day for days 61-90 $566 per day for days 91-150 $0 Beyond 150 days
Skilled nursing facility coinsurance	$0 First 20 days $141.50 per day for days 21-100 $0 beyond 100 days

versus the deductible and coinsurance amounts for which the patient/beneficiary is responsible.

How Medicare Part A Payments Are Calculated

Medicare payments are calculated through the use of the **prospective payment system (PPS),** which is Medicare's acute care payment method for inpatient care. PPS rates are set at a level intended to cover costs for treating a typical inpatient in a given **diagnosis-related group (DRG).** DRG is a coding system that groups related diagnoses and their associated medical or surgical treatments. Payments for each hospital are adjusted for differences in area wages, teaching activity, care to the poor, and other factors. Hospitals also may receive additional payments to cover extra costs associated with **outliers** (atypical patients) in each DRG. The CMS uses the DRG system to determine the amount that Medicare would reimburse hospitals and other designated providers for the delivery of inpatient services. Each DRG corresponds to a specific patient condition, and each has a pre-established fixed amount that is paid for any patient in the DRG category. PPS and DRGs are discussed at length in Chapter 17.

Medicare Severity-Adjusted System

One of the most significant changes in DRG methodology since 1983 is the **Medicare Severity-Adjusted (MS-DRG) System.** CMS implemented this modified DRG methodology effective October 1, 2007. The new inpatient prospective payment system (IPPS) rule is intended to match hospital payments more closely with the costs of patient care and the patient's condition(s) by placing the most seriously ill patients into the highest-paying DRGs (within the DRG set) for any specific procedure. This change benefits large, urban, and teaching hospitals that have patients whose cases are more complex but provides fewer resources to smaller community and rural hospitals that treat more "routine" patients.

To keep current on recent and proposed changes to IPPS, visit the Evolve site.

IPPS 3-Day Payment Window

Diagnostic outpatient services provided to a patient by the admitting hospital within 3 calendar days prior to and including the date of the inpatient admission are considered to be inpatient services and should be included in the inpatient MS-DRG payment, unless there is no Part A coverage. The 3-day payment window is discussed in more detail later in this chapter, under the heading "72-Hour Rule."

Medicaid

Each state's Medicaid program determines the method it uses to pay for hospital inpatient services. Most states base reimbursement for hospital inpatient services on a PPS that includes DRGs and **per diems** (actual costs per day), and they provide a single payment to the hospital with no separate payment for specific services such as imaging agents and other drugs and supplies. Some states use other reimbursement methods, such as cost-based payments, state-specific fee schedules, or a percentage of charges. Many Medicaid programs also adjust payments to reflect a hospital's **case mix** (reported data including patient demographic information such as age, sex, county of residence, and race/ethnicity; diagnostic information; treatment information; disposition; total charges; and expected source of payment) or the intensity of care required by patients treated at the facility.

Medicaid reimbursement for outpatient services varies from state to state as well, and there is a significant variation in Medicaid payment amounts among states; however, Medicaid programs typically pay less than other insurers.

Chapter 8 provides more detailed information on the Medicaid program.

TRICARE

Typically, patients covered under TRICARE (a healthcare program of the United States Department of Defense Military Health System, which provides civilian health benefits for military personnel, military retirees, and their dependents, including some members of the Reserve Component) are required to use a military treatment facility if one is located near them. If a military treatment facility is unavailable or cannot provide the inpatient care needed, the patient must ask for a **nonavailability statement (NAS)**. As discussed in Chapter 10, an NAS is certification from a military hospital stating that it cannot provide the necessary care. For all inpatient admissions covered by TRICARE (except bona fide emergencies), an NAS is required. An NAS is valid for a hospital admission that occurs within 30 calendar days after it is issued and remains valid from the date of admission until 15 days after discharge for any follow-up treatment that is related directly to the admission. It is usually the patient's responsibility to provide a copy of the NAS to the hospital

and to each physician providing services to the patient. Each paper claim submitted to TRICARE must be accompanied by a copy of the NAS; hospital personnel should advise patients to keep the original of the NAS for their files and provide only copies to the hospital and physician offices as needed.

The NAS system is automated for facilities that use **electronic claims submission (ECS)**. This means that, instead of mailing paper copies of the NAS to the TRICARE carrier, the treating facility can enter the NAS electronically into the **Defense Enrollment Eligibility Reporting System (DEERS)** computer database.

An NAS is no longer required for outpatient procedures; however, to avoid claims rejection or delays, the patient or the treating facility should check with the TRICARE carrier for details on obtaining advance authorization before any procedures are done. Providers of care—whether or not they participate in TRICARE—-are required to obtain these advance authorizations.

Inpatient TRICARE payments are calculated using the same PPS as Medicare, and the DRG-based payment is the TRICARE allowable charge regardless of the billed amount. TRICARE also uses the same conversion factors as Medicare; however, the formulas are not identical to those used by the CMS. As a result, the final calculation result may differ slightly from that calculated by Medicare. Reimbursement rates and methods are subject to change per Department of Defense (DoD) guidelines.

TRICARE patients usually are required to pay a portion of the bill (**cost sharing**) directly to the hospital at the time of discharge. Copies of the *TRICARE Handbook* should be available from the hospital admitting department or the patient financial services office. For more detailed information on TRICARE, refer to Chapter 10.

CHAMPVA

CHAMPVA (a health benefits program in which the Department of Veterans Affairs (VA) shares the cost of certain healthcare services and supplies with eligible beneficiaries) uses the same DRG-based PPS as that used by TRICARE. As mentioned previously, this reimbursement system is modeled on Medicare's PPS and applies to hospital inpatient services in all 50 states, the District of Columbia, and Puerto Rico. Current DRG weights and ratios are available in the *TRICARE Reimbursement Manual*. The manual also offers a DRG calculator.

CHAMPVA typically pays the allowed amount less the beneficiary cost share, which is the lesser of
- the annual adjusted per day amount multiplied by the number of inpatient days or
- 25% of the hospital's billed charges or
- the DRG rate (in applicable inpatient facilities),

When the DRG rate does not apply, CHAMPVA pays 75% of the billed amount for covered services and supplies.

Hospitals participating in Medicare must accept the CHAMPVA-determined allowable amount for inpatient services as payment in full. Although many of the procedures in the CHAMPVA DRG-based payment system are similar or identical to those for Medicare, the actual payment amounts differ in some cases. This is because the Medicare program is designed for a beneficiary population older than 65 years, whereas many CHAMPVA beneficiaries are considerably younger than 65 and generally healthier. Services such as obstetrics and pediatrics are rare for Medicare beneficiaries but common for CHAMPVA beneficiaries.

SNFs also are paid through the use of the Medicare PPS. SNF PPS rates cover all routine, ancillary, and capital costs of covered SNF services. SNF admissions require preauthorization when TRICARE or CHAMPVA is the primary payer. SNF admissions for children younger than 10 years and CAH swing beds are exempt from SNF PPS and their costs are reimbursed on the basis of billed charges or negotiated rates. The swing bed concept allows a hospital to use its beds interchangeably for acute care or post-acute care. A **swing bed** agreement allows a change in reimbursement status. The patient "swings" from receiving acute care services and reimbursement to receiving skilled nursing services and reimbursement usually without a change of facility.

As with most third-party payers, TRICARE and CHAMPVA reimbursement rates are subject to change on an annual basis. Health insurance professionals working in inpatient hospital facilities should keep current TRICARE and CHAMPVA provider manuals on hand.

Blue Cross and Blue Shield

Inpatient hospitalization reimbursement for patients covered under Blue Cross and Blue Shield (BCBS) policies differs from region to region and depends on the benefit coverage outlined in the individual or group contract. With most BCBS policies, coverage is provided for hospital charges for a semiprivate room and most other customary, or ancillary, inpatient services up to a specific number of days, depending on the policy. Patients must usually satisfy a deductible amount, which can be $50 to $5000, and must pay a specific percentage, or copayment, of the charges—usually 10% to 20%—before reimbursement begins. Many BCBS policies have an out-of-pocket limit that the patient is responsible for, and this limit depends on the policy. Some policies also have a payment cap—a per-incident or lifetime limit on reimbursement and/or an out-of-pocket limit that limits the amount the patient has to pay.

As with most third-party payers, preauthorization is necessary for inpatient hospitalization and some outpatient procedures and diagnostic testing. Although preauthorization is ultimately the patient's responsibility, most healthcare facilities are willing to make the necessary telephone call to obtain preauthorization for the required services. The telephone number to call for preauthorization is generally listed on the back of the patient's healthcare identification (ID) card. That is the main reason for making a photocopy of both sides of the ID card. As with other third-party payers, the health insurance professional should be aware of the guidelines of the BCBS member organization before submitting claims.

Most hospitals in the United States are in the category of **Blue Cross and Blue Shield member hospitals**—that is, they have contracted as participating providers with the BCBS member organization. Member hospitals must accept the BCBS allowable fee as payment in full and, after the initial deductible and copayment are met, cannot bill the patient for any remaining charges. For nonmember hospitals—that is, hospitals that do not contract with BCBS—reimbursement is limited in that way. As with physician charges, nonparticipating hospitals can balance bill; that is, they can charge the patient for any charges above the allowable fee that BCBS does not pay.

BCBS fees for facility services are established using a variety of methods, as follows:
- Per case allowances (DRG or ambulatory payment classification [APC])
- Per diem allowances
- Percent of charges
- Resource-based relative value scale (RVRBS)

See Chapter 6 for more details on BCBS. The health insurance professional should refer to the provider payment manual or contact the particular carrier for the specific inpatient and outpatient fee calculations used for the facility in question.

Private Insurers

Most private insurers negotiate contracts with facilities regarding hospital inpatient payment methods. These contracts are typically negotiated annually. Many private payers use the DRG system to reimburse hospital inpatient services. Other common payment arrangements used by private insurers are per diems, percentage of allowable charges, and negotiated rates for specific treatments. Table 18-2 summarizes the payment mechanism by type of payer and setting of care.

❓ What Did You Learn?

1. List the major hospital payers.
2. What benefits are included in Medicare Part A?
3. Many Medicaid programs adjust payments to reflect a hospital's *case mix*. What does this term mean?
4. What reimbursement system does CHAMPVA use for inpatient charges?
5. Explain the *swing bed* concept.

NATIONAL UNIFORM BILLING COMMITTEE AND THE UB-04

The UB-04, also known as Form CMS-1450, is the paper claim form used by institutional providers (e.g., hospitals, skilled nursing facilities, home health agencies, etc.) for billing third party payers (Fig. 18-2). The Administrative Simplification Compliance Act (ASCA), however, prohibits

TABLE 18-2	Payment Mechanism by Type of Payer and Setting of Care		
TYPE OF PAYER	**FREESTANDING IMAGING CENTER/ PHYSICIAN SERVICES**	**HOSPITAL OUTPATIENT DEPARTMENTS**	**HOSPITAL INPATIENT**
Medicare	RBRVS physician fee schedule	APCs	DRGs
Private insurance	RBRVS-based fee schedule	Percentage of charges	DRGs
	Other fee schedule	Negotiated rates	Per diems
	Discounted charges	Preset per diem/per-visit rates	Percentage of charges
	Capitated rates		Negotiated rates
Medicaid	RBRVS-based fee schedule	State-specific fee schedule	DRGs
	Other fee schedule	Preset per diem/per-visit rates	Per diems
		Percentage of charges	Cost-based

APC, ambulatory payment classification; DRG, diagnosis-related group; RBRVS, resource-based relative value scale

payment of initial Medicare claims for services or supplies that were not billed electronically unless the provider meets the ASCA "exceptions" or has been granted a waiver. The ASCA X12N 837 Institutional (837I version 5010) claim format is the electronic version of the UB-04 form used by providers who submit claims electronically.

The **National Uniform Billing Committee (NUBC)** is responsible for the design and printing of the UB-04 form. The NUBC is a voluntary, multidisciplinary committee that develops data elements for claims and claim-related transactions and is composed of all major national provider and payer organizations (including Medicare).

An example of a completed UB-04 claim form along with the step-by-step completion guidelines can be found in Appendix C. To learn more about the UB-04 and to download a copy of the *Medicare Claims Processing Manual*, Internet-Only Manual Publication (IOM Pub) 100-04, visit the Evolve site.

Additional information is available to subscribers of the *Official UB-04 Data Specifications Manual*. Visit the NUBC website at http://www.nubc.org/ to subscribe.

HIPAA Tip

HIPAA standards allow the submission of paper-based claims and the use of paper-based remittances. HIPAA requires, however, that the electronic transaction and code set standards be followed whenever transactions are conducted electronically. Under the Administrative Simplification Compliance Act of 2001, physician practices with 10 or more full-time equivalent (FTE) employees, and institutional facilities with 25 or more FTE employees are required to submit Medicare claims electronically.

UB-04 Data Specifications

Data elements, identified as necessary for claims processing, in most cases are assigned designated spaces on the UB-04 form. The designated spaces are referred to as **form locators**,

and each one has a unique number. Other elements that are occasionally necessary are incorporated into general fields that use assigned codes, codes and dates, and codes and amounts. This built-in flexibility of the data set is intended to promote the greatest use of the data set and to eliminate the need for attachments to the billing form. The data specifications manual identifies the national requirements for preparing Medicare, Medicaid, military, Blue Cross and Blue Shield, and commercial insurance claims.

837I: Electronic Version of the UB-04 Form

As mentioned, the current version of the electronic institutional claim is the ASCA X12N 837I version 5010. The file format conforms to the data elements that are required on the paper UB-04. Health insurance professionals should become familiar with the upgrade to version 5010 (which accommodates the new ICD-10 codes) and should be able to recognize the difference between the electronic version and the current paper UB-04.

Data Layout of the 837I

The data layout of an 837I file may look confusing at first because of the electronic format, but the data are basically the same as in the UB-04 or the CMS-1500 form. The overall data stream of an 837I file is known as a **transaction set**, which is divided into sections with each section providing a specific kind of information.

Every section of the transaction set contains data segments. A segment name is two or three alphabetical characters that begin each line of detail. In the example shown in Fig. 18-3, the segments names are in **bold**.

Each segment contains data elements that are the same as the data provided by each individual form locator position on the UB-04 claim form. The number of elements varies depending on the purpose of the segment. Data elements are separated by asterisks (delimiters). In the example shown

Fig. 18-2 Blank UB-04 claim form.

```
ISA*00*                    *00*                    *ZZ*000001063          *ZZ*NDDHSMED
*040812*1504*U*00401*000101537*1*P*
GS*HC*000001063*NDDHSMED*20040812*1504*101537*X*004010X096A1
ST*837*0001
BHT*0019*00*101537*20040812*1504*CH
REF*87*004010X096A1
```

Fig. 18-3 Example of a transaction set section.

```
ISA*00*                    *00*                    *ZZ*000001063          *ZZ*NDDHSMED
*040812*1504*U*00401*000101537*1*P*
GS*HC*000001063*NDDHSMED*20040812*1504*101537*X*004010X096A1
ST*837*0001
BHT*0019*00*101537*20040812*1504*CH
REF*87*004010X096A1
```

Fig. 18-4 Example showing data elements in a segment.

in Fig. 18-4, the ST segment has two elements and the BHT segment has six elements.

Electronic claims are typically submitted in batches to the third party payer, who in turn, generates a 997—another type of electronic file. The 997 is an electronic response to the 837I and indicates whether the 837I transmission was accepted or rejected. If the file passed, it contains an "A" for accepted; it contains an "R" if it was rejected (Fig. 18-5).

In order to confirm whether batches were accepted or rejected by an insurer, the health insurance professional must be able to identify which batches passed and which batches failed. He or she must also be able to match the claims rejected on the 997 to the 837I file.

What Did You Learn?

1. What is the basic function and role of the NUBC?
2. Name the standard paper claim form used for inpatient hospitalization.
3. What are the designated spaces called on this universal claim form?
4. The name of the UB-04 electronic file is _____.
5. The overall data stream of the electronic UB-04 file is known as a(n) _____

STRUCTURE AND CONTENT OF THE HOSPITAL HEALTH RECORD

The information included in a hospital health record is similar to that for a physician's office or medical clinic record. It begins with demographic information—patient's name, address, age, sex, occupation, and insurance information—collected on admission.

Every time a patient receives healthcare, a record of the observations, medical or surgical interventions, and treatment outcomes is generated and maintained. This record includes information that the patient provides concerning symptoms and medical history, the results of examinations, radiology reports, laboratory test results, diagnoses, and treatment plans. Medical records and health information technicians organize and evaluate these records for completeness and accuracy.

The patient health record is the property of the hospital, and hospitals do not automatically provide a copy of a patient's health record upon discharge. If the record (or any part of it) is released, it first must be completed by all physicians involved in the patient's care prior to being copied and released to the patient. This process can take up to 30 days, after which the patient may receive a copy, normally for a fee. Patient-related information may be released to a physician or medical facility for follow-up care of the patient when needed, usually free of charge.

```
ISA*00*        *00*       *ZZ*NDDHSMED       *ZZ*000001063
*040812*1717*U*00401*000000011*0*P*>
GS*FA*NDDHSMED*000001063*20040812*1717*9*X*004010X096A1
ST*997*0001
AK1*HC*101537
AK2*837*0001
AK5*A   (Accepted File)
AK9*A*1*1*1   (Accepted File)
SE*6*0001
ST*997*0002
```

Fig. 18-5 Example of a 997 electronic file.

Standards in Hospital Electronic Medical Records

An **electronic medical record (EMR)** is a computerized version of the paper medical record. The EMR is an evolving technology that is being adopted by healthcare facilities as part of an ongoing trend to maximize efficiency and streamline functioning.

The increasing demand for quality care in the midst of rising competition has made hospitals maximize utilization of technology in the overall processes of day-to-day operations. Not only corporate but also small stand-alone and mid-size hospitals have become aware that the adoption of a well-functioning and efficient computerized hospital information system is an important and integral part of efficient hospital management. Hospitals have been gradually introducing EMRs over the past several years. Until recently, however, only large corporate hospitals were utilizing fully functional EMR applications, whereas most other hospitals use a combination of EMRs and paper-based records.

An EMR system is a complex system consisting of critical information that typically has the following key features:

- Patient's clinical information: medical history, prescriptions, allergies, diagnosis, reports, etc.
- Clinical decision support databases: databases that help in making decisions during prescription writing, drug-to-allergy database, etc.
- Orders management: order entry, retrieval, result reviewing, etc.
- Work flow management: managing processes such as appointment viewing, check-in of patients, and review.
- Security features: for maintaining security and confidentiality of critical information.
- Electronic prescription tool: a tool for writing and managing prescriptions
- Patient's financial records: service bills, receipts, etc.

When EMR is being introduced to the hospital environment, it is critical to establish a hospital information system (HIS), prepare and involve various internal and external individuals and/or groups that have a stake in a successful outcome, and define a clear implementation path for the EMR system. All components of EMR must be able to integrate with other existing information systems in the hospital. Other major factors to consider include:

- Ease of use: Most critical, as EMR will be used mostly by clinicians, some of whom can be rather hesitant in adopting new technology to be used in parallel with their care services.
- System interoperability: Capable enough to interface and interact with other information systems.
- Standardization: Standard compliance to avoid data loss/inconsistency when interacting with other systems.
- Work flow capacities: Ideally only full-solution systems should be adopted.
- The sales team of the vendor: A good fit is crucial for success, because the relationship between vendor and institution is frequently long-term.

- Vendor services: Good post-sales and maintenance support services are crucial.

EMR benefits a hospital because it

- Provides faster accessibility to records
- Requires less storage space
- Affords security of information
- Offers anytime, anywhere accessibility (e.g., remote access from handheld devices)
- Is easier to manage than paper-based records

The necessity for implementing basic information systems in hospitals is evident, so more hospitals are adopting them; however, the reluctance of the key users of these systems (e.g., the physicians) still remains a big challenge for hospitals. Investment cost and personnel training are other key factors impeding widespread adoption of EMR.

Standard Codes and Terminology

Information for inpatient health records consists of many different kinds of data, such as narrative progress notes, laboratory test results, radiology reports, history and physical examination reports, operative reports, and discharge summaries. Data come from many sites, including physician offices, hospitals, nursing facilities, public health departments, and pharmacies. Because various providers exist for each kind of data and site of care, standards for terminology are an essential requirement for a computer-based patient record that spans more than one provider's domain.

The important goal is to have an acceptable code system for each kind of data. It is unnecessary (and may be undesirable) to have all of the codes come from a single master code system, because computers can integrate multiple code systems easily.

In addition to a universal coding system, there must be a common language combining data structures and grammar so that meaningful coded messages can be sent between computer-based patient record systems. The federal government and other organizations are working on measures that would make development of such a common language possible.

💬 What Did You Learn?

1. What is an EMR?
2. List at least five items of demographic information that are typically collected when a patient is hospitalized.
3. What type of information does an inpatient health record consist of?
4. List the patient data domains used by the CPRI code system.

INPATIENT HOSPITAL/FACILITY CODING

Hospitals generate insurance claims for many third-party payers. To perform this task effectively, the health insurance professional or the health information technician must have expert knowledge of the coding and payment systems that these payers use. Hospital coding is similar to that which done in a physician's office; however, some guidelines differ significantly. The following sections provide a brief overview of both the ICD-9-CM (Volume 3) as well as the ICD-10-PCS systems for coding inpatient hospital procedures. It is a good idea that the health insurance professional have a working knowledge of both coding methods, since ICD-9 is currently in use but will likely change over ICD-10-PCS in the near future.

ICD-9-CM (Volume 3) Codes for Inpatient Hospital Procedures

ICD-9-CM Volume 3 is used to assign codes to inpatient hospital procedures. They are required for inpatient hospital Medicare Part A claims. (HCPCS codes are used for reporting procedures on Medicare Part B and other claim types.) Inpatient hospital claims require reporting the **principal procedure** if a significant procedure occurred during the hospitalization. The principal procedure is the procedure performed for definitive treatment, rather than for diagnostic or exploratory purposes, or that which was necessary to manage a complication. It is also the procedure most closely related to the principal diagnosis. The principal procedure code shown on the billing form must be the full ICD-9-CM Volume 3 procedure code including all 4-digit codes where applicable. Codes for reporting procedures other than the principal procedure are reported using the full ICD-9-CM Volume 3 procedure codes as well, including all 4 digits where applicable. Five significant procedures other than the principal procedure may be reported on the UB-04 claim form. ICD-9-CM diagnosis and procedure codes are available on the CMS website and accessible through the Evolve site.

Organization of ICD-9-CM Volume 3

Like ICD-9-CM Volume 1 and 2, Volume 3 contains an Alphabetic Index and a Tabular List, and the formats of the two sections are the same as Volumes 1 and 2. Guidelines for locating the correct procedure code involve first locating the procedure in the Alphabetic Index and then cross-referencing it to the Tabular List where the code selection is confirmed. In the Buck 2012 manual, main terms in the Volume 3 Index are in red font.

Example: Tonsillectomy 28.2 with adenoidectomy 28.3

Classification of Procedures in ICD-9 Volume 3

The following list is the general index of surgical procedures in ICD-9 Volume 3, based on numerical order:
Procedures And Interventions, Not Elsewhere
 Classified (00.0)
Operations On The Nervous System (01-05)
Operations On The Endocrine System (06-07)
Operations On The Eye (08-16)
Other Miscellaneous Diagnostic And Therapeutic
 Procedures (17)

Operations On The Ear (18-20)
Operations On The Nose, Mouth, And Pharynx (21-29)
Operations On The Respiratory System (30-34)
Operations On The Cardiovascular System (35-39)
Operations On The Hemic And Lymphatic System (40-41)
Operations On The Digestive System (42-54)
Operations On The Urinary System (55-59)
Operations On The Male Genital Organs (60-64)
Operations On The Female Genital Organs (65-71)
Obstetrical Procedures (72-75)
Operations On The Musculoskeletal System (76-84)
Operations On The Integumentary System (85-86)
Miscellaneous Diagnostic And Therapeutic Procedures
 (87-99)

Code Sets Used for Inpatient Hospital/Facility Claims in ICD-10-PCS

There are two code sets used for coding hospital/facility claims: ICD-10-PCS is used for reporting inpatient procedures only, and ICD-10-CM is used in all health treatment facilities, including both inpatient and outpatient, for coding diagnoses. The federal government mandates that all payers and providers adopt the ICD-10 coding system for services provided on or after the compliance date, which has been extended from October 1, 2013 to October 1, 2014, or they will be ineligible to receive reimbursement on claims. As mentioned in an earlier chapter, it is strongly recommended that students check the CMS website periodically at http://cms.gov/icd10/ to keep abreast of any further changes to this compliance date. ICD-9 coding will be used until ICD-10 is officially in place. The following paragraphs provide a brief explanation of the ICD-10-PCS coding system. ICD-10-CM was discussed at length in Chapter 12.

> ### 📁 HIPAA Tip
>
> All covered entities under HIPAA (health plans, payers, providers, clearinghouses) must implement the ICD-10 codes by the compliance date. The codes must be supported by medical documentation.

ICD-10-PCS

The ICD-10-PCS is a code set designed by 3M Health Information Management for CMS to replace Volume 3 of ICD-9-CM for inpatient procedure reporting. It is significantly different from ICD-9-CM Volume 3 and from Current Procedural Terminology (CPT) codes. Approximately 87,000 ICD-10-PCS procedure codes replace the nearly 4,000 ICD-9 procedure codes. It is important to keep in mind that ICD-10-PCS will not affect coding of physician services in offices and/or clinics. However, healthcare providers should be aware that documentation requirements under ICD-CM-PCS are quite different, so inpatient medical record documentation will be affected by this change.

Like ICD-10-CM codes, ICD-10-PCS codes contain seven characters, which can be numbers or letters and are based on the type of procedure performed, the approach, body part, and other characteristics. Each alphanumeric character has a specific meaning or value, depending on its place in the grouping.

Notable improvements in the ICD-10-PCS coding system include the following:

- Unique codes to differentiate approach, e.g., type of vessel, and type of repair
- Codes that define resource differences and outcomes that describe exactly what was done to the patient
- No diagnostic information is included
- Limited use of the "not-otherwise-specified"(NOS) option
- Elimination of the "not-elsewhere-classified" (NEC) option, except for new devices
- Use of standard terminology; each term is assigned a specific meaning

Structure of ICD-10-PCS Codes

The seven-digit ICD-10-PCS structure provides precision and expandability that is lacking in the former three- to four-digit ICD-9-CM procedure codes. Like ICD-10-CM, which we learned about in Chapter 12, ICD-10-PCS has a **multiaxial structure**, with each code character having the same meaning within the specific procedure section and across procedure sections to the extent possible. The first position always indicates one of the 17 procedure section values. Each of the seven characters can have up to 34 different values or definitions.

Important Note: ICD-10-PCS defines the term procedure as "the complete specification of the seven characters." Each procedure is divided into specific sections that identify the general type of procedure, with the first character (either a number or a letter) designating the section.

The new structure of ICD-10-PCS code is as follows:

- Each can be alphabetical (not case-sensitive) or numeric
  - Numbers zero through 9 are valid values
  - Letters O and I are not valid values, eliminating confusion with 0 and 1
- Each character defines a specific aspect of the procedure. The first character defines the section name related to type or location of service. Characters 2 through 7 have a standard meaning within each section but may have different meanings across sections. As shown below, the character 2-7 classification categories change depending on the value of the section in character 1

Section 0 - Medical and Surgical Categories

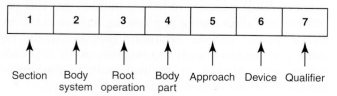

- In Section 5 Imaging Procedures categories 3, 5 and 6 represent different category types that describe detail aspects relative only to imaging type procedures.

Section 5 - Imaging Procedures

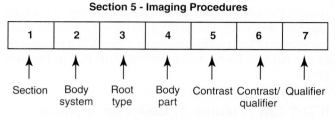

- In Section D Laboratory Procedures categories 2 through 7 contain values that describe the variants of lab procedures.

Section D - Laboratory Procedures

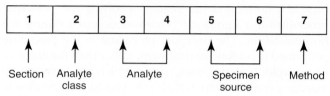

Format of the ICD-10-PCS

There are currently three separate divisions in the ICD-10-PCS system: (1) The Tabular List, (2) the Index, and (3) the List of Codes. Each section of the manual is meant to assist healthcare providers and coders in their search for the correct and complete procedure codes. It is very important that the codes used for billing, reimbursement, and reporting purposes are consistent and accurate, because they are constantly being monitored and audited by both public and private insurers. Fig. 18-6 is a partial page from the ICD-10-PCS index, and Fig. 18-7 is a sample table from the Medical and Surgical section of the ICD-10-PCS manual.

More information on ICD-10-PCS, including an informative PowerPoint presentation that describes the coding system, can be found on the Evolve site. Detailed instructions for coding inpatient hospital procedures are provided on the CMS website.

Selecting the Principal Diagnosis

The health insurance professional or coder must identify key elements or words for possible use as the **principal diagnosis**. The principal diagnosis is defined in the Uniform Hospital Discharge Data Set (UHDDS) as "that condition established after study to be chiefly responsible for occasioning the admission of the patient to the hospital for care." The UHDDS definitions are used by hospitals to report inpatient data elements in a standardized manner. Accurate principal diagnosis selection is critical to ensure that patient encounters are grouped under the proper MS-DRGs and facilities receive appropriate reimbursement.

A

Abdominal aortic plexus *see* Nerve, Abdominal Sympathetic
Abdominal esophagus *see* Esophagus, Lower
Abdominohysterectomy
  see Excision, Uterus 0UB9
  see Resection, Uterus 0UT9
Abdominoplasty
  see Alteration, Wall, Abdominal 0W0F
  see Repair, Wall, Abdominal 0WQF
  see Supplement, Wall, Abdominal 0WUF
Abductor hallucis muscle
  see Muscle, Foot, Right
  see Muscle, Foot, Left
Ablation *see* Destruction
Abortion
  Products of Conception 10A0
  Abortifacient 10A07ZX
  Laminaria 10A07ZW
  Vacuum 10A07Z6
Abrasion *see* Extraction
Accessory cephalic vein
  see Vein, Cephalic, Right
  see **Vein, Cephalic, Left**
Accessory obturator nerve *see* **Plexus, Lumbar**
Accessory phrenic nerve *see* Nerve, Phrenic
Accessory spleen *see* Spleen
Acetabulectomy
  see Excision, Lower Bones 0QB
  see Resection, Lower Bones 0QT
Acetabulofemoral joint
  see Joint, Hip, Right
  see Joint, Hip, Left
Acetabuloplasty
  see Repair, Lower Bones 0QQ
  see Replacement, Lower Bones 0QR

Acetabuloplasty *(Continued)*
  see Supplement, Lower Bones 0QU
Achilles tendon
  see Tendon, Lower Leg, Left
  see Tendon, Lower Leg, Right
Achillorrhaphy *see* Repair, Tendons 0LQ
Achillotenotomy, achillotomy
  see Division, Tendons 0L8
  see Drainage, Tendons 0L9
Acromioclavicular ligament
  see Bursa and Ligament, Shoulder, Right
  see Bursa and Ligament, Shoulder, Left
Acromion (process)
  see Scapula, Left
  see Scapula, Right
Acromionectomy
  see Excision, Upper Joints 0RB
  see Resection, Upper Joints 0RT
Acromioplasty
  see Repair, Upper Joints 0RQ
  see Replacement, Upper Joints 0RR
  see Supplement, Upper Joints 0RU
Activities of Daily Living Assessment F02
Activities of Daily Living Treatment F08
Acupuncture
  Breast
    Anesthesia 8E0H300
    No Qualifier 8E0H30Z
  Integumentary System
    Anesthesia 8E0H300
    No Qualifier 8E0H30Z
Adductor brevis muscle
  see Muscle, Upper Leg, Left
  see Muscle, Upper Leg, Right
Adductor hallucis muscle
  see Muscle, Foot, Left
  see Muscle, Foot, Right

Adductor longus muscle
  see Muscle, Upper Leg, Right
  see Muscle, Upper Leg, Left
Adductor magnus muscle
  see Muscle, Upper Leg, Right
  see Muscel, Upper Leg, Left
Adenohypophysis *see* **Gland, Pituitary**
Adenoidectomy
  see Excision, Adenoids 0CBQ
  see Resection, Adenoids 0CTQ
Adenoidotomy *see* Drainage, Adenoids 0C9Q
Adhesiolysis *see* Release
Administration
  Blood products *see* Transfusion
  Other substance *see* Introduction
Adrenalectomy
  see Excision, Endocrine System 0GB
  see Resection, Endocrine System 0GT
Adrenalorrhaphy *see* Repair, Endocrine System 0GQ
Adrenalotomy *see* Drainage, Endocrine System 0G9
Advancement
  see Reposition
  see Transfer
Airway
  Insertion of device in
    Esophagus 0DH5
    Mouth and Throat 0CHY
    Nasopharynx 09HN
  Removal of device from
    Esophagus 0DP5
    Mouth and Throat 0CPY
    Nose 09PK
  Revision of device in

Fig. 18-6 Partial page from the Index of the ICD-10-PCS (International Classification of Diseases, 10th revision, Procedure Coding System).

Section	O	Medical and Surgical
Body System	D	Gastrointestinal System
Operation	J	Inspection: Visually and/or manually exploring a body part

Body Part	Approach	Device	Qualifier
0 Upper intestinal tract **6** Stomach **D** Lower intestinal tract	**0** Open **3** Percutaneous **4** Percutaneous endoscopic **7** Via natural or artificial opening **8** Via natural or artificial opening endoscopic **X** External	**Z** No device	**Z** No qualifier
U Omentum **V** Mesentery **W** Peritoneum	**0** Open **3** Percutaneous **4** Percutaneous endoscopic **X** External	**Z** No device	**Z** No qualifier

Fig. 18-7 Sample table from Medical and Surgical section of ICD-10-PCS (International Classification of Diseases, 10th revision, Procedure Coding System).

Sometimes documentation describes symptoms, signs, and ill-defined conditions that are not linked to a specific disease. Some body system categories include codes for non-specific conditions. The code for a breast lump is found in the Tabular Listing under "Diseases of the Genitourinary System," under the subcategory "Disorders of the Breast," and would be properly coded as N63, "unspecified lump in breast." These codes, rather than codes for more specific disorders, should be used when the only facts available are the patient's signs and symptoms. Box 18-1 lists guidelines for coding inpatient hospital diagnoses.

It is very important for hospital personnel to properly code the diagnoses and procedures, because that information is what determines what DRG Medicare assigns to the

Box 18-1

Guidelines for Coding Inpatient Hospital Diagnoses

- Select the diagnoses that require coding according to current coding and reporting requirements for inpatient services.
- Select the diagnoses that require coding according to current coding and reporting requirements for hospital-based outpatient services.
- Interpret conventions, formats, instructional notations, tables, and definitions of the classification system to select diagnoses, conditions, problems, or other reasons for the encounter that require coding.
- Sequence diagnoses and other reasons for the encounter according to notations and conventions of the classification system and standard data set definitions.

- Determine whether signs, symptoms, or manifestations require separate code assignments.
- Determine whether the diagnostic statement provided by the healthcare provider does not allow for more specific code assignments.
- Recognize when the classification system does not provide a precise code for the condition documented (e.g., residual categories or nonclassified syndromes).
- Assign supplementary codes to indicate reasons for the healthcare encounter other than illness or injury.
- Assign supplementary codes to indicate factors other than illness or injury that influence the patient's health status.
- Assign supplementary codes to indicate the external cause of an injury, adverse effect, or poisoning.

patient. Reimbursement rates are determined by the DRG, so incorrectly coded diagnoses can dramatically affect reimbursement. The importance of consistent, complete documentation in the medical record cannot be overemphasized. Without such documentation, the application of all coding guidelines is a difficult, if not impossible, task. For two good websites that discuss principal diagnosis assignment and secondary diagnosis assignment, see the Websites to Explore section at the end of the chapter.

⭐ Imagine This!

Dr. Ezra Blake admits Paul Faro, who has an inoperable bowel malignancy, to the hospital for acute blood loss anemia. Mr. Faro receives a transfusion of four units of packed cells. In this case, the principal diagnosis is acute blood loss anemia, and the bowel cancer is an additional diagnosis. Later that same day, Dr. Blake admits Imogene Ferrell to the hospital for a local complication due to an ovarian malignancy. In this case, the cancer is the principal diagnosis. When more than one diagnosis meets the criteria for principal diagnosis, the coder should use the diagnosis that accounts for most of the services provided and code that as the primary diagnosis. When more than one condition is listed that pertains to similar and contrasting conditions, the coder should select the diagnosis that is the condition that resulted in the admission and for which most of the services were provided. If one of the diagnoses is ruled out during the hospitalization, it should not be used for coding. When original treatment plans are not completed during the course of the encounter or

admission, the reason for admission or encounter is still used as the principal or primary diagnosis.

For clarification, see International Classification of Diseases, 10th revision, Clinical Modification Guideline G: Complications of Surgery and Other Medical Care.

🕐 Stop and Think

Consider the case in which a physician admits a patient with obstruction of the ureter secondary to a metastasis (spread) from a previously resected colon carcinoma. Surgeons place a urinary stent to relieve the obstruction with no other therapy provided for the metastasis. In this case, what would be the principal diagnosis? Would there be a second diagnosis? If so, what would it be?

National Correct Coding Initiative

CMS implemented the **National Correct Coding Initiative** in 1996 to control improper coding that leads to inappropriate increased payment for healthcare services. The HHS program uses Medicare guidelines. The agency uses National Correct Coding Initiative edits to evaluate billing of Healthcare Common Procedure Coding System (HCPCS) codes by Medicare providers in postpayment review of providers' claims. Table 18-3 shows commonly used insurer claim forms and coding systems by setting of care. For assistance in billing, providers may access the National Correct Coding Initiative edit information online at the CMS website listed under Websites to Explore.

TABLE 18-3   Commonly Used Insurer Claim Forms and Coding Systems by Setting of Care

COMPONENTS OF CLAIMS	FREESTANDING IMAGING CENTER/ PHYSICIAN SERVICES	HOSPITAL OUTPATIENT DEPARTMENTS	HOSPITAL INPATIENT
Claim form	CMS-1500	CMS-1450 (UB-04)	CMS-1450 (UB-04)
Patient diagnoses	ICD-10-CM	ICD-10-CM	ICD-10-CM
Procedures	CPT	CPT Revenue	ICD-10-PCS Revenue
Drugs, supplies, and certain contrast agents	HCPCS (when appropriate)	HCPCS (when appropriate) Revenue	Revenue

CPT, Current Procedural Terminology; HCPCS, Healthcare Common Procedure Coding System; ICD-10-CM, International Classification of Diseases, 10th revision, Clinical Modification; ICD-10-PCS, ICD-10, Procedural Coding System.

Recent Rule Changes Affecting Hospital Billing

In 2009, HHS announced the adoption of two new rules to implement updated HIPAA standards. The first rule modifies the standard medical data code sets for coding diagnoses and inpatient hospital procedures by adopting the ICD-10-CM for diagnosis coding and ICD-10-PCS for inpatient hospital procedure coding. These new code sets replace the current ICD-9-CM, Volumes 1 and 2, and the ICD-9-CM, Volume 3, for diagnosis and procedure codes, respectively. The implementation date for ICD-10-CM and ICD-10-PCS is currently set for October 1, 2013, for all covered entities. HHS has announced its intent to delay this date; however, so periodically check the site http://www.cms.gov/icd10 for compliance date updates.

Second, HHS is adopting X12 Version 5010 and National Council for Prescription Drug Programs, Inc. (NCPDP) Version D.0 for HIPAA transactions. In this rule, the compliance date for all HIPAA-covered entities was January 1, 2012, which gave the industry time to test the standards, to ensure that systems were appropriately updated, and to test between trading partners before the compliance date. The compliance date for the Medicaid subrogation standard was also January 1, 2012, except for small health plans, which had until January 1, 2013, to come into compliance.

Version 5010 accommodates the new ICD-10 code sets and has an earlier compliance date than ICD-10 in order to ensure adequate testing time for the healthcare industry. These two important changes apply to all HIPAA-covered entities, including health plans, healthcare clearinghouses, and certain healthcare providers.

For further information on both rules, visit the Evolve site.

The 72-Hour Rule

The **72-hour rule** states that all services provided for Medicare patients within 72 hours of the hospital admission are considered to be part of the inpatient services and are to be billed on one claim. This rule is part of Medicare's PPS.

We learned in the previous chapter that under the Medicare PPS, hospitals are paid a predetermined rate for each hospital admission. Clinical information is used to classify each patient into a DRG. Such information includes the principal diagnosis, complications and comorbidities, surgical procedures, and age, gender, and discharge disposition of the patient.

The 72-hour rule has been amended in accordance with the Preservation of Access to Care Act of 2010. The CMS "final rule" states that on or after June 25, 2010, all diagnostic services (except for ambulance and maintenance renal dialysis services) provided on the date of the beneficiary's inpatient admission are considered to be related and must be bundled with the charges for the inpatient stay. Outpatient nondiagnostic services provided during the applicable payment window that are unrelated to the admission, and that are covered by Medicare Part B, should be billed separately to Medicare Part B.

Acute care hospitals require the 72-hour rule. Other facilities, such as long-term care hospitals, rehabilitation hospitals, and psychiatric hospitals, require a comparable 24-hour rule. Critical access hospitals are excluded from both 72-hour and 24-hour provisions.

For updates on the 72-hour rule, visit the Evolve site.

OUTPATIENT HOSPITAL CODING

Outpatient hospital coding includes ICD-10-CM for coding diagnoses and CPT-4 for coding procedures and services as well as HCPCS, when applicable. Section IV of the ICD-10-CM Official Guidelines for Coding Reporting contains the official diagnostic coding and reporting guidelines for outpatient services. These guidelines can be downloaded from the links found on the Evolve site.

Hospital Outpatient Prospective Payment System

In response to the rapidly rising Medicare expenditures for outpatient services and large copayments being made by Medicare beneficiaries, Congress mandated that the CMS develop a **hospital outpatient prospective payment** system (HOPPS) and reduce beneficiary copayments. This payment system was implemented August 1, 2000, and is used by CMS to reimburse for hospital outpatient services.

Ambulatory Payment Classification Coding

Ambulatory payment classification (APC) is the grouping system that the CMS developed for facility reimbursement of hospital outpatient services. This system of coding and reimbursement for services was introduced by Congress in the 1997 Balanced Budget Act and implemented by CMS in August 2000 in hospital outpatient settings. It is intended to simplify the outpatient hospital payment system, ensure the payment is adequate to compensate hospital costs, and implement deficit reduction goals of the CMS.

The APC system works as follows: All covered outpatient services are assigned to an APC group. Each group of procedure codes within an APC must be similar clinically and with regard to the use of resources. The payment rate associated with each APC is determined by multiplying the relative weight for the APC by a conversion factor, which translates the relative weights into dollar amounts. To account for geographical differences, the labor portion of the payment rate is adjusted by the hospital wage index. The HOPPS allows for additional payments for certain pass-throughs and for outlier cases involving high-cost services. **Pass-throughs** are temporary payments for specified new technologies, drugs, devices, and biologics for which costs were unavailable when APC payment rates were calculated.

The APC payment rate is the total amount the hospital receives from Medicare and the beneficiary. These rates are updated annually and take effect in January of the following year. Under the HOPPS, it is possible for more than one APC to be assigned during a single visit, in contrast with the inpatient PPS, in which only one DRG can be assigned per discharge. The importance of capturing, coding, and billing all allowable services provided should be stressed so that no possible revenue goes unbilled. HOPPS APC payments are determined totally on the basis of CPT-4/HCPCS code assignment, rather than ICD-10-PCS procedure codes, which are used for coding inpatient PPS.

In November 2000, the *Federal Register* published the HOPPS interim final rule (65 FR 67797). CMS publishes the Medicare Physician Fee Schedule and the HOPPS annually in the *Federal Register*.

To learn more about HOPPS and APCs, visit the Evolve site.

? What Did You Learn?

1. What manuals are used for coding hospital claims?
2. Define *principal diagnosis*.
3. How is the principal diagnosis determined?
4. What are APCs, and in what setting are they used?
5. Explain the term pass-through in the context it is used in this chapter.

THE HOSPITAL BILLING PROCESS: UNDERSTANDING THE BASICS

The hospital billing process begins when the patient registers for inpatient or outpatient admission. Although this procedure may differ from one institution to another, certain processes remain constant. Registration may be accomplished in person, by telephone, or via the Internet. At the time of registration, the patient typically must provide personal and insurance information. Boxes 18-2 and 18-3 list the data elements for hospital claim forms and outpatient claim forms.

As we learned in previous chapters, preauthorization or precertification is necessary for most inpatient hospital admissions. In the case of emergency admission when preauthorization is impossible, most insurers allow 48 hours for notification of hospitalization.

A certain amount of patient education goes hand in hand with hospital admission. Hospital staff members should inform patients of their rights and responsibilities. Typical patient responsibilities include an obligation for patients to

- provide a complete medical history and any information pertaining to their health;
- be responsible for their actions if they refuse any treatment or do not follow physician's orders;
- report perceived risks in their care and unexpected changes in their condition to the physician or other healthcare providers;
- report any perceived or identified safety issues related to their care or the physical environment to the physician or other healthcare providers;
- ask questions when they do not understand what they have been told about their care or what they are expected to do regarding their care;
- ensure that the financial obligations of their hospital care are fulfilled as promptly as possible;
- follow hospital rules and regulations regarding patient care and conduct; and
- be considerate of the rights of other patients and hospital personnel.

Informed Consent

Informed consent is the process by which a fully informed patient can participate in choices about his or her healthcare. It originates from the legal and ethical rights a patient has to direct what happens to his or her body and from the ethical duty of the physician to involve the patient in his or her healthcare.

The most important goal of informed consent is that the patient has an opportunity to be a knowledgeable participant in his or her healthcare decisions. Informed consent typically includes a discussion of the following elements:

- Nature of the decision or procedure
- Reasonable alternatives to the proposed intervention
- Relevant risks, benefits, and uncertainties related to each alternative

Box 18-2

Standard Data Elements: Hospital Claim Forms

Patient Characteristics
Patient identifier (unique to each hospital or care facility)
Name (last, first, middle initial)
Address (street, city, state, ZIP Code)
Date of birth
Gender
Marital status

Provider Characteristics
Hospital/facility identifier (unique)
Physician identifier (unique only for Medicare claims)
Diagnostic and treatment information
Admissions date
Admissions status
Admissions diagnosis code
Condition code
Diagnosis code
Description of service
Service date
Service units
Principal and other diagnoses (up to 6)
Principal and other procedures (up to 5)

Date of procedure
Emergency code

Insurance/Payment Information
Insurance group numbers (differ for each health plan)
Group name
Insured's name
Relationship to insured
Employer name
Employer location
Covered period
Treatment authorization codes
Payer
Total charges
Noncovered charges
Prior payments
Amount due from patient
Revenue codes
Healthcare Common Procedure Coding System (HCPCS)/rates

Courtesy U.S. Department of Health and Human Services, Centers for Medicare and Medicaid Services.

Box 18-3

Standard Data Elements: Outpatient Claim Forms

Patient Characteristics
Patient identifier (Social Security number or other identifier)
Name (last, first, middle initial)
Address (street, city, state, ZIP Code)
Date of birth
Gender
Marital status
Telephone number
Other health insurance coverage

Provider Characteristics
Physician identifier (tax identifier or other plan-specific identifier)
Physician's employer identification number

Diagnostic and Treatment Information
Date of encounter
Illness
Emergency
Admission and discharge dates
Diagnosis or nature of illness
Diagnosis code
Place of service
Procedure code

Description of services and supplies
Date patient able to return to work
Date of disability

Insurance/Payment Information
Payer's identifier (e.g., Medicare or Medicaid)
Group name
Insured's name
Insured's identification number
Insured's group number
Address and telephone number of insured
Relationship to insured
Employer name
Employer location
Covered period
Treatment authorization codes
Accept assignment
Total charges
Amount paid
Prior payments
Balance due

Courtesy U.S. Department of Health and Human Services, Centers for Medicare and Medicaid Services.

- Assessment of patient understanding
- Acceptance of the intervention by the patient

For the patient's consent to be valid, he or she must be considered competent to make the decision at hand, and this consent must be voluntary. Ideally, the physician should make it clear to the patient that he or she is participating in a decision, not merely signing a form. With this understanding, the informed consent process should be seen as an invitation to participate in healthcare decisions. The patient's understanding of what is about to occur is equally as important as the information provided; the discussion should be carried out in layperson's terms, and the patient's understanding should be assessed along the way.

If it is determined that a patient is incapacitated or incompetent to make healthcare decisions in his or her best interest, a **surrogate** (someone with legal authority to make decisions or speak on the patient's behalf) decision maker must speak for the patient. A specific hierarchy of appropriate decision makers is defined by law in most states. If no appropriate surrogate decision maker is available, the physician is expected to act in the best interest of the patient until a surrogate is found or appointed.

Stop and Think

Joseph Mason, a 68-year-old black man, was admitted to Broadmoor Medical Center with complaints of "tightness in his chest" and difficulty breathing. Dr. Ethan VanDerVoort, a cardiologist, visited Joseph in his hospital room and informed him that the results of his heart catheterization and other tests showed 80% blockage in a major artery of his heart. "We'll be putting a stent in the artery to open it up, allowing the blood to resume normal flow," Dr. VanDerVoort informed him. "Afterwards, you'll be as good as new." He patted the patient's arm and left the room.

Did Dr. VanDerVoort follow the rules of "informed consent" in this brief conversation with Mr. Mason? If not, what elements of a full informed consent scenario were ignored? How might Dr. VanDerVoort have approached this patient regarding his planned remedy for the patient's heart problem?

Present on Admission (POA)

As required by law effective October 1, 2007, all general acute-care healthcare providers must identify whether a diagnosis was present upon an inpatient admission. This concept was mandated as a result of many concerns about quality healthcare and overpaying by the government because of hospital errors. After many years of planning, the present on admission indicator (POA) was added to the UB-04 form for inpatient Medicare claims.

Hospital Charges

Hospital charges are typically divided into two types, facility charges (room and board) and ancillary charges, such as radiology, laboratory, and pharmacy. Professional charges—fees charged by the attending and/or consulting physicians—are billed separately and are not considered a part of the hospital bill.

Hospital Charge Description Master

Hospital charges can be determined in multiple ways, but the main goal is to capture costs for performing procedures and services. To facilitate the goal, every hospital has what is known as a **charge description master** (CDM) or charge master. A CDM is a listing of every type of procedure and service the hospital can provide to its patients, including procedures, pharmaceuticals, supplies, and even room charges. CDMs help make the billing process run more smoothly and accurately. Table 18-4 shows an example of a CDM.

Each item on a CDM is pre-coded with certain information, such as price, procedure code, and revenue codes. Some have modifiers, which are more specific indicators to insurance companies regarding the type of procedure that was performed. Some hospitals are now listing their prices on the Internet in a move known as **pricing transparency**.

Electronic Claims Submission (ECS)

Most hospitals now submit claims electronically rather than using the UB-04 paper claim. Specifically, claims for Medicare Part A reimbursement must be submitted electronically using the current HIPAA-compliant transaction standards.

TABLE 18-4	Example of a CDM					
CHARGE DESCRIPTION	CPT/HCPCS CODE	REVENUE CODE	CHARGE	DEPARTMENT CODE	CHARGE CODE	CHARGE STATUS
Nasal bone x-ray	70160	320	150.00	15	2214111000	12/1/2001
Thyroid sonogram	76536	320	250.00	15	2110110000	1/1/2003
Echo encephalogram	76506	320	1,500.00	15	2326222111	7/1/2005

CPT, Current Procedural Terminology; HCPCS, Healthcare Common Procedure Coding System.

The HIPAA's administrative simplification (AS) act governs the electronic process of health insurance claims. The purpose of HIPAA-AS is to standardize transactions as much as possible. Each transaction, however, has different data elements that are treated differently by various payers.

Before submitting claims electronically to any payer or clearinghouse, the facility must successfully complete enrollment, certification, and testing processes and obtain the necessary software and identifiers needed for claims submission.

For example, to transmit claims electronically with Wellmark (a Blue Cross and Blue Shield fiscal intermediary [FI]), the facility must obtain a Wellmark identifying number, that is, a submitter number, and pre-approval for electronic data interchanges (EDI). This involves completing registration and authorization forms.

The next step is for the facility to become certified, which involves sending a test transaction for a review of HIPAA-AS compliance. If the test is successful, the facility receives a certificate verifying that it was successful in completing a HIPAA-compliant electronic transaction using the new version 5010 standards.

Providers submitting electronic claims must do so in a format that either is HIPAA-compliant or can be translated into a HIPAA-compliant format. Most hospitals submit claims electronically using the 837I electronic version of the UB-04 form.

As discussed in an earlier chapter, ECS offers numerous benefits to all participants in the claims submission process. ECS is considered to be the most efficient and effective means of processing claims, ensuring swift adjudication and payment to providers, because it reduces claims processing time from start to finish. The ECS process allows providers to use applicable computer software programs to submit claims to a central location, such as a clearinghouse, via a World Wide Web interface that sends the claims to the carriers' system for processing. (Electronic claims also can be sent directly to a third-party payer.)

ECS avoids the sorting and keying process, allowing the claim data to be available immediately to the payer's system. Additionally, providers who submit claims electronically can check their claims to ensure that the data have passed basic edits and can resolve any claim data errors that may prevent the claim from being paid. ECS also provides an audit trail of claims that have failed preliminary edits. Providers can receive information about certain problems on submitted claims within a few hours instead of a few weeks. When problems or errors are detected they can be corrected, and the claim can be resubmitted immediately. When providers track submissions, make corrections, and resubmit claims online, they receive payment much more quickly than with paper filing.

Providers may use special software created by specific third-party payers or software developed to their particular needs by outside vendors to submit claims electronically. In addition to quicker payments receipt, some other advantages of ECS are:

- Claims can be submitted 7 days a week (including holidays)
- Providers receive front-end acknowledgement of claims acceptance
- Electronic remittance advice (ERA) allows automatic payment posting
- Electronic funds transfer (EFT) makes payments immediately accessible
- Electronic claims reports are provided with each submission

For more detailed information on electronic billing, visit the Evolve site.

What Did You Learn?

1. What is a chargemaster?
2. Explain *pricing transparency*.
3. Providers submitting electronic claims must do so in what type of format?
4. Identify four advantages of ECS.

Health Information Management (HIM) Systems

A hospital patient accounting system is a suite of integrated computer applications that allows healthcare facilities to manage patient records more efficiently and optimize reimbursement while ensuring regulatory compliance. This process is commonly referred to as **health information management (HIM)**. HIM systems are responsible for coding and abstracting all patient charts and releasing them for billing. Integration with other encoder products improves coding accuracy and typically features a specially designed HIM report generator. In addition to ERA management, HIM systems generally include software components that can handle functions such as:

- Patient registration
- Eligibility verification
- Claims management
- Accounts receivable
- Collections

Payment Management

The **electronic remittance advice** automates the process of receiving payments from third party payers. Electronic payments for hospital charges are automatically posted to a patient's file within the hospital financial management system. The ERA automates manual keying of explanation of benefits (EOB); provides details on how claims were paid and/or why they were denied; and helps improve business office workflow and productivity.

Revenue cycle management systems, utilized in most hospitals, manage patient information while simultaneously automating the billing process. They allow users to "work" a patient stay from beginning to end, from the initial registration process, through the charge entry, patient and insurance billing, payment entry, collecting, bad debt management, and reporting phases.

Hospital financial accounting management systems help streamline patient services, minimize rejected claims, and speed up reimbursement while, ideally, improving patient satisfaction and overall revenue cycle performance. Fig. 18-8 shows a flowchart of the hospital billing process.

> ### ❓ What Did You Learn?
>
> 1. Define a hospital patient accounting system and what it does.
> 2. Name the software components included in a typical HIM system.
> 3. What is an ERA?
> 4. List the steps of the hospital billing cycle.

HIPAA-HOSPITAL CONNECTION

As mentioned previously, HIPAA's Administrative Simplification and Compliance Act required providers, with limited exceptions, to submit all initial Medicare claims for reimbursement electronically on or after October 16, 2003. The act further stipulated that no payment may be made under Part A or Part B of the Medicare Program for any expenses incurred for items or services for which a claim is submitted in a nonelectronic form. Consequently, unless a provider fits one of the exceptions listed here, any paper claim submitted to Medicare would not be paid. In addition, if it is determined that the provider is in violation of the statute or rule, he or she may be subject to claim denials, overpayment recoveries, and applicable interest on overpayments. The exceptions to this ECS requirement include the following:

- A small provider—a provider billing a Medicare fiscal intermediary that has fewer than 25 full-time equivalent employees or a physician, practitioner, or supplier with fewer than 10 full-time equivalent employees that bills a Medicare carrier

- A dentist
- A participant in a Medicare demonstration project in which paper claim filing is required because of the inability of the Applicable Implementation Guide, adopted under HIPAA, to report data essential for the demonstration
- A provider that conducts mass immunizations such as flu injections and may be permitted to submit paper roster bills
- A provider that submits claims when more than one other payer is responsible for payment before Medicare payment
- A provider that furnishes services only outside the United States
- A provider experiencing a disruption in electricity and communication connections that are beyond its control
- A provider that can establish that an "unusual circumstance" exists and that therefore precludes electronic submission of claims electronically

> ### 📁 HIPAA Tip
>
> Hospitals can achieve HIPAA compliance successfully by meeting all of the government guidelines and requirements related to physical security, contingency plans, standard electronic transaction processes, and integrity controls as well as implementing the most advanced scenario of secure methods of data transmission and storage to ensure proper handling of patient accounts and other health-related information.

> ### ❓ What Did You Learn?
>
> 1. What is HIPAA's rule on Medicare claims submission?
> 2. List the exceptions to this rule.

BILLING COMPLIANCE

The creation of a compliance program is a major initiative of the Office of the Inspector General (OIG) in its effort to engage the private healthcare community in preventing the submission of erroneous claims and combating fraudulent conduct. In the past several years, the OIG has developed and issued compliance program guidelines directed at a variety of segments in the healthcare industry. The development of these types of compliance program guidelines is based on the belief that a healthcare provider can use internal controls to monitor adherence to applicable statutes, regulations, and program requirements more efficiently. A compliance program usually consists of the following elements:

- An internal compliance review or "legal audit" of the provider's operations (often focused in one or more targeted areas, such as billing practices)
- Identification of practices that are improper, illegal, or potentially abusive

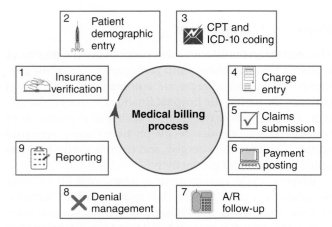

Fig. 18-8 Example of a hospital billing flowchart. A/R, Current Procedural Terminology (CPT); International Classification of Diseases (ICD) 10th revision.

- Drafting of an appropriate code of conduct for management and staff
- Appointment of a compliance officer and compliance oversight committee
- Implementation of a hotline or some other manner of reporting mechanism
- Development and implementation of a training program for relevant staff
- Design of appropriate disciplinary sanctions for violations of the plan
- Securing of continuing compliance through proper dissemination of new regulations and carrier or intermediary directives and statutes
- Periodic audits of the provider's practices and procedures to ensure continued compliance

On the basis of the success of this program, providers may wish to expand their compliance review to other areas such as U.S. Occupational Safety and Health Administration or U.S. Food and Drug Administration compliance, as appropriate.

A meaningful compliance plan addresses more than just billing procedures. Because this chapter focuses on hospital billing, we will take a closer look at **billing compliance**. Billing compliance begins with the gathering of complete and accurate information during the admission and registration interview. Most problems with claims originate in the claim development process: from the initial physician order, to the moment a patient presents in the facility, to the admission/registration process, to the clinical areas of patient care and the associated documentation, to coding, and finally to billing. A good comprehensive billing compliance program should give hands-on admissions, registration, and billing personnel as well as others within the organization involved in the claims development process an appropriate level of information relating to the "full-circle process" and instruction relating to compliance standards.

HIPAA Tip

It is recommended that hospitals periodically evaluate HIPAA rules to ensure that they are still in compliance. Experts suggest that administrative efficiencies gained from compliance in the long run would have a positive financial impact on hospitals and health systems.

What Did You Learn?

1. What is the purpose of a billing compliance program?
2. List at least seven of the nine elements of a billing compliance program.
3. Where does billing compliance begin?
4. What three areas should be included in a comprehensive billing compliance program?

CAREER OPPORTUNITIES IN HOSPITAL BILLING

Medical records and health information technicians held more than 172,000 jobs in 2008, and 37% of all jobs were in hospitals. The rest were mostly in offices of physicians, nursing care facilities, outpatient care centers, and home healthcare services. Insurance firms that deal in health matters employ a few health information technicians to tabulate and analyze health information. Public health departments also hire technicians to supervise data collection from healthcare institutions and to assist in research.

Training, Other Qualifications, and Advancement

Medical records and health information technicians entering the field typically have associate degrees from community colleges or career programs. In addition to general education, coursework includes medical terminology, anatomy and physiology, legal aspects of health information, coding and abstraction of data, statistics, database management, quality improvement methods, and computer science. Applicants can improve their chances of admission into a program by taking biology, chemistry, health, and computer science courses in high school.

Hospitals sometimes advance promising health information clerks to jobs as medical records and health information technicians, although this practice may be less common in the future. Experienced medical records and health information technicians can advance in one of several ways—by specializing, by furthering their education, or by managing. Many senior technicians specialize in coding, particularly Medicare coding, or in cancer registry. More commonly, however, advancement requires 2 to 4 years of job experience, completion of a hospital's in-house training program, or acquiring specialized education or credentialing such as certification in a health information management program.

Most employers prefer to hire **registered health information technicians (RHITs)**, who are required to pass a written examination offered by the American Health Information Management Association. To take the examination, an individual must graduate from a 2-year associate degree program accredited by the Commission on Accreditation of Allied Health Education Programs (CAAHEP) of the American Medical Association. Technicians trained in non–CAAHEP-accredited programs or on the job are not eligible to take the American Health Information Management Association examination. CAAHEP has accredited 182 programs for health information technicians. Technicians who specialize in coding may obtain voluntary certification.

In medical records and health information departments of large facilities, an experienced technician may advance to section supervisor, overseeing the work of the coding, correspondence, or discharge sections. A senior technician with RHIT credentials may become director or assistant director of a medical records and health information department in a small facility. In larger institutions, the director is usually an administrator, with a bachelor's degree in medical records and health information administration.

The American Health Information Management Association (AHIMA) and the American Academy of Professional Coders (AAPC) offer certification in various coding proficiencies. To learn more about certification, visit the Evolve site.

Job Outlook

Job prospects are good. Employment of hospital billing specialists and medical records and health information technicians is expected to grow much faster than the average for all occupations through 2012, owing to rapid growth in the number of medical tests, treatments, and procedures that will be increasingly scrutinized by third-party payers, regulators, courts, and consumers.

Although employment growth in hospitals may not keep pace with growth in other healthcare industries, many new jobs nevertheless will be created. The fastest employment growth and the greatest number of new jobs are expected to occur in offices of physicians, owing to increasing demand for detailed records, especially in large group practices. Rapid growth is also expected in nursing care facilities, home healthcare services, and outpatient care centers. Additional job openings will result from the need to replace technicians who retire or leave the occupation permanently. Table 18-5 lists common certifications and their requirements and other career opportunities in hospital billing.

The *Career Guide 2010-2011 Promising Careers that Don't Require Four Years of College* can be downloaded from the link on the Evolve site.

> ### ❓ What Did You Learn?
>
> 1. What type of coursework should a student expect to complete when entering into a medical records or health information technologic field?
> 2. What are the career opportunities for health information clerks or technicians?
> 3. What is the job outlook?

SUMMARY CHECKPOINTS

▶ Today's modern hospital is a place where sick or injured individuals receive healthcare. It also provides continuing education for practicing physicians and serves the function of an institution of higher learning for entire communities. If it is a teaching hospital, clinical education is provided to the entire spectrum of healthcare professionals. The hospital also might conduct investigational studies and perform research in medical sciences.

▶ A goal of the entire healthcare system is to reduce costs and, at the same time, to be more responsive to customers (patients).

TABLE 18-5	Certifications and Their Requirements and Other Career Opportunities in Hospital Billing
CERTIFICATION	**REQUIREMENTS**
Registered Health Information Administrator (RHIA)	Successfully completing an approved baccalaureate or post-baccalaureate program and passing a national RHIA certification examination
Registered Health Information Technician (RHIT)	Obtaining an associate degree in an approved health information technology program and passing a national certification examination
Certified Coding Specialist (CCS)	Passing a national coding examination measuring medical terminology, disease processes, pharmacology, and the application of ICD-10-CM and CPT surgery coding systems
Certified Coding Specialist— Physician-based (CCS-P)	Passing a national coding examination measuring medical terminology, disease processes, pharmacology, and the application of ICD-10-CM, CPT, and HCPCS level II coding systems
Certified Professional Coder— Hospital (CPC-H)	Passing a national coding examination measuring proficiencies in coding procedures and diagnoses on medical claims in the outpatient setting
Certified Coding Associate (CCA)	Passing a national coding examination measuring understanding of entry-level coding applications including medical terminology, disease processes, pharmacology, and ICD-10-CM and CPT medical record coding
Other Career Opportunities	
Admissions coordinator Discharge planner Medical records clerk Medical records technician	

TABLE 18-5	Certifications and Their Requirements and Other Career Opportunities in Hospital Billing—cont'd

CERTIFICATION	REQUIREMENTS
Medical secretary	
Medical transcriptionist	
Nutrition educator	
Transplant coordinator	
Tumor registrar	
Unit coordinator	

CPT, Current Procedural Terminology; HCPCS, Healthcare Common Procedure Coding System; ICD-10-CM, International Classification of Diseases, 10th revision, Clinical Modification.

▶ The major types of healthcare facilities are as follows:
- Acute care facilities
- Subacute care facilities
- ASCs
- SNFs
- Long-term care facilities
- Hospice

▶ All acute care or general hospitals must be licensed by the state in which they are located to provide care within the minimum health and safety standards established by regulation and rule. HHS enforces the standards by periodically conducting surveys of these facilities. Hospitals may seek accreditation by nationally recognized accrediting agencies such as The Joint Commission and the AOA. Surveys conducted by The Joint Commission and AOA are based on guidelines developed by each of these organizations.

▶ Common hospital payers are as follows:
- Medicare
- Medicaid
- TRICARE/CHAMPVA
- Blue Cross and Blue Shield
- Private (commercial) insurers

▶ The health insurance professional must be aware of individual payer guidelines for accurate and timely claims completion. Current guidelines can be found on the payers' websites, or provider manuals may be acquired by contacting the payer or its fiscal intermediary/carrier.

▶ The UB-04 is the standard claim form used for inpatient hospitalization. Data elements necessary for claims processing in most cases are assigned designated spaces on the form called "form locators." There are 81 form locators, and each has a unique number. Applicable information is entered into these form locators using a numeric, alphabetical, alphanumeric, or text-based format. The electronic equivalent to the UB-04 is the 837I.

▶ The information included in a hospital health record begins with demographic information—patient's name,

address, age, sex, occupation—collected on admission. Every time a patient receives healthcare, a record is maintained of the observations, medical or surgical interventions, and treatment outcomes. This record includes information that the patient provides concerning his or her symptoms and medical history, the results of examinations, radiology reports and laboratory test results, diagnoses, and treatment plans.

▶ The hospital billing process begins when the patient registers for inpatient/outpatient admission. Hospital charges are recorded for room and board, each procedure performed, medications, laboratory tests, x-rays (if applicable), and miscellaneous service charges.

▶ Although hospital coding is similar to that done in a physician's office, there are some significant differences. Two code sets are used for coding hospital/facility claims: ICD-10-PCS is used for reporting inpatient procedures only, and ICD-10-CM is used in all health treatment facilities, both inpatient and outpatient, for coding diagnoses. Additionally, hospital coders use the "principal diagnosis," which is defined as the condition determined to be chiefly responsible for the patient's admission to the facility. HCPCS codes are used for reporting procedures on Medicare Part B and other claim types. Outpatient hospital coding includes ICD-10-CM and CPT-4/HCPCS codes when applicable.

▶ The billing data that are being submitted to Medicare and other payers are examined carefully for accuracy and completeness. It is crucial that the health insurance professional responsible for hospital billing thoroughly understands the instructions relating to the correct completion of the UB-04, possesses an insight as to how the data elements interact, and comprehends what the payers do with the data when they are adjudicating a claim. Data quality, coding, and billing compliance are crucial things to consider in the submission of inpatient and outpatient claims. Staying abreast of current rules and regulations is a multidepartment responsibility, as is keeping aware of the quality of documentation, coding, and billing. Compliance cannot be viewed as a one-step process; it must be considered an ongoing effort by every member of the healthcare team.

▶ Advantages of submitting hospital claims using ECS include the following:
- Increased cash flow
- Quicker turnaround for payment than with paper claims
- Availability to submit claims 7 days a week (including holidays)
- Front End Acknowledgment Report—confirmation verifying the acceptance of claims
- Availability of ERA for faster posting of payments
- Availability of electronic funds transfer for paperless process
- Ability to generate a variety of reports

▶ A compliance program typically consists of the following elements:
- An internal compliance review or "legal audit" of the provider's operations (often focused in one or more targeted areas, such as billing practices)
- Identification of practices that are improper, illegal, or potentially abusive
- Drafting of an appropriate code of conduct for management and staff
- Appointment of a compliance officer and compliance oversight committee
- Implementation of a hotline or some other manner of reporting mechanism
- Development and implementation of a training program for relevant staff
- Design of appropriate disciplinary sanctions for violations of the plan

- Securing of continuing compliance through proper dissemination of new regulations and carrier or intermediary directives and statutes
- Periodic audits of the provider's practices and procedures to ensure continued compliance

▶ Many career opportunities may be found under the umbrella of hospital billing. Careers that require completion of a specific program and successful passing of a certification examination include the following:
- Registered Health Information Administrator (RHIA)
- Registered Health Information Technician (RHIT)
- Certified Coding Specialist (CCS)
- Certified Coding Specialist–Physician-based (CCS-P)
- Certified Coding Associate (CCA)
- Certified Professional Coder (CPC)
- Certified Professional Coder–Outpatient Hospital (CPC-H)

▶ Other career opportunities that may or may not require special education or certification (or both) include the following:
- Admissions coordinator
- Discharge planner
- Medical records clerk
- Medical records technician
- Medical secretary
- Medical transcriptionist
- Nutrition educator
- Transplant coordinator
- Tumor registrar
- Unit coordinator

⟳ CLOSING SCENARIO

After working in Broadmoor Medical Center's Billing Department for several months, Brittany has learned the various stages of hospital billing. Previously, she worked in a small medical office where she was in charge of all billing and claims submission. At Broadmoor, a much larger facility, work is more specialized, and Brittany's tasks center on Medicare claims submissions.

Broadmoor's Billing Department is part of the Health Information Management Department, which employs nearly 100 individuals. There are numerous opportunities for advancement within the Health Information Management Department, and after an employee has completed 6 months of orientation and training, he or she can apply for a position that offers better pay; however, a promotion comes with more responsibility. Brittany has decided to continue her education at Deerfield Community College and eventually acquire a bachelor's degree in health information management. She is confident that with all the job opportunities Broadmoor Medical Center offers, she will be able to achieve her long-term career goals at this medical facility.

⊖ WEBSITES TO EXPLORE

- For live links to the following websites, please visit the Evolve site at
http://evolve.elsevier.com/Beik/today/

- The website for the CMS home page is
http://www.cms.hhs.gov/
- For more information on TRICARE and CHAMPVA reimbursement, visit the following website and peruse the TRICARE Reimbursement Manual:
http://www.tricare.mil/

- For a PowerPoint Presentation on TRICARE for Life, use the following URL:
  http://www.narmc.amedd.army.mil/kacc/Tricare/TFL_BRIEFING.pdf/
- Refer to the CMS ICD-10-CM Official Guidelines for Coding and Reporting at
  http://www.cms.gov/ICD10/Downloads/7_Guidelines10cm2010.pdf/
- For extensive information on hospital compliance and payment monitoring program, log on to IPRO's website at
  http://www.ipro.org/
- To download the ICD-10-PCS Coding Guidelines, go to
  http://www.cms.gov/ICD10/Downloads/PCS_2012_guidelines.pdf/
- For more information on the ICD-10-PCS coding system, go to
  http://www.cms.gov/ICD10/Downloads/PCS2011guidelines.pdf/
- For additional information on certification, log on to the American Association of Professional Coders (AAPC) website: http://www.aapc.com/certification/
- For further information for the two new HIPAA rules, log on to the CMS website, using one of the following websites:
  http://www.cms.hhs.gov/ElectronicBillingEDITrans/18_5010D0.asp/
  http://www.cms.gov/ICD10/11a_Version_5010.asp/
- The revised portion of the *Medicare Claims Processing Manual,* Chapter 25 (Completing and Processing the CMS 1450 Data Set) and Sections 70 (Uniform Bill-Form CMS-1450 [UB-04]) and 71 (General Instructions for Completion of Form CMS-1450 [UB-04]) (Attachment A) contain detailed instructions for completing the form.
- To learn about recent developments in billing and claims related transactions, log on to the following website:
  http://www.nubc.org/
- To see the entire dialogue of the ASTM standard EMRs, use the following URL and key "E1384" in the site search:
  http://www.astm.org
- To learn more about HOPPS and APCs, explore the following website:
  http://www.cms.gov/IdentifiableDataFiles/03_HospitalOPPS.asp/
- The 835 Health Care Claim Payment/Advice Companion Guide may be downloaded from

http://hrsa.dshs.wa.gov/DSHSHIPAA/attachments/pdf/835CG103009.pdf
- The CMS 835 Companion Document is available at
  http://www.cignamedicare.com/
- A PowerPoint presentation explaining 837 Professional and Institutional Changes 4010A1 to 5010 can be downloaded from
  www.nhia.org/documents/20060800837Pand837IChngs40105010NUBC-NUCCPrsnt.ppt/
- HIPAA's transaction code sets can be located at
  http://www.cignamedicare.com/HIPAA/code_sets.html#3/
- Peruse the following websites for career opportunities in healthcare technology:
  http://www.ahima.org/careers/intro.html/
  http://www.aapc.com/medical-coding-jobs/
- Two good websites that discuss principal diagnosis assignment and secondary diagnosis assignment are as follows:
  http://www.climjocomd.com/download/codingprinciples.pdf/
  http://projects.ipro.org/index/inpatient_coding/
- An example chart of revenue codes for PA PROMISe fee-for-service providers can be found at
  http://www.dpw.state.pa.us/omap/provinf/promhb/PDF/promBGub04_IRCdskref.pdf/

Author's Note: Websites change frequently. If any of these URLs is unavailable, use applicable guide words in your Internet search to acquire additional information on the various subjects listed.

REFERENCES AND RESOURCES

Carr RF: *Hospital.* 2009, NIKA Technologies, Inc., for VA Office of Construction & Facility Management (CFM). Revised by the WBDG Health Care Subcommittee, http://www.wbdg.org/design/hospital.php#emerg/.

U.S. Department of Health and Human Services, Centers for Medicare and Medicaid Services: *Transactions and Code Sets Regulations,* 2009. http://www.cms.hhs.gov/TransactionCodeSetsStands/02_TransactionsandCodeSetsRegulations.asp#TopOfPage/.

U.S. Department of Labor, Bureau of Labor Statistics: *Occupational Outlook Handbook, 2008-09 Edition,* Medical Records and Health Information Technicians. http://www.bls.gov/oco/ocos103.htm/.

Sample Blank CMS-1500 (08/05)

Fig. A-1 Blank CMS-1500 (08/05) form.

BECAUSE THIS FORM IS USED BY VARIOUS GOVERNMENT AND PRIVATE HEALTH PROGRAMS, SEE SEPARATE INSTRUCTIONS ISSUED BY APPLICABLE PROGRAMS.

NOTICE: Any person who knowingly files a statement of claim containing any misrepresentation or any false, incomplete or misleading information may be guilty of a criminal act punishable under law and may be subject to civil penalties.

REFERS TO GOVERNMENT PROGRAMS ONLY

MEDICARE AND CHAMPUS PAYMENTS: A patient's signature requests that payment be made and authorizes release of any information necessary to process the claim and certifies that the information provided in Blocks 1 through 12 is true, accurate and complete. In the case of a Medicare claim, the patient's signature authorizes any entity to release to Medicare medical and nonmedical information, including employment status, and whether the person has employer group health insurance, liability, no-fault, worker's compensation or other insurance which is responsible to pay for the services for which the Medicare claim is made. See 42 CFR 411.24(a). If item 9 is completed, the patient's signature authorizes release of the information to the health plan or agency shown. In Medicare assigned or CHAMPUS participation cases, the physician agrees to accept the charge determination of the Medicare carrier or CHAMPUS fiscal intermediary as the full charge, and the patient is responsible only for the deductible, coinsurance and noncovered services. Coinsurance and the deductible are based upon the charge determination of the Medicare carrier or CHAMPUS fiscal intermediary if this is less than the charge submitted. CHAMPUS is not a health insurance program but makes payment for health benefits provided through certain affiliations with the Uniformed Services. Information on the patient's sponsor should be provided in those items captioned in "insured", i.e., items 1a, 4, 6, 7, 9, and 11.

BLACK LUNG AND FECA CLAIMS

The provider agrees to accept the amount paid by the Government as payment in full. See Black Lung and FECA instructions regarding required procedure and diagnosis coding systems.

SIGNATURE OF PHYSICIAN OR SUPPLIER (MEDICARE, CHAMPUS, FECA AND BLACK LUNG)

I certify that the services shown on this form were medically indicated and necessary for the health of the patient and were personally furnished by me or were furnished incident to my professional service by my employee under my immediate personal supervision, except as otherwise expressly permitted by Medicare or CHAMPUS regulations.

For services to be considered as "incident" to a physician's professional service, 1) they must be rendered under the physician's immediate personal supervision by his/her employee, 2) they must be an integral, although incidental part of a covered physician's service, 3) they must be of kinds commonly furnished in physician's offices, and 4) the services of nonphysicians must be included on the physician's bills.

For CHAMPUS claims, I further certify that I (or any employee) who rendered services am not an active duty member of the Uniformed Services or a civilian employee of the United State Government or a contract employee of the United States Government, either civilian or military (refer to 5 USC 5336). For Black-Lung claims, I further certify that the services performed were for a Black Lung-related disorder.

No Part B Medicare benefits may be paid unless this form is received as required by existing law and regulations (42 CFR 424.32).

NOTICE: Any one who misrepresents or falsifies essential information to receive payment from Federal funds requested by this form may upon conviction be subject to fine and imprisonment under applicable Federal laws.

NOTICE TO PATIENT ABOUT THE COLLECTION AND USE OF MEDICARE, CHAMPUS, FECA, AND BLACK LUNG INFORMATION
(PRIVACY ACT STATEMENT)

We are authorized by CMS, CHAMPUS and OWCP to ask you for information needed in the administration of the Medicare, CHAMPUS, FECA, and Black Lung programs. Authority to collect information is in section 205(a), 1862, 1872 and 1874 of the Social Security Act as amended, 42 CFR 411.24(a) and 424.5(a) (6), and 44 USC 3101;41 CFR 101 et seq and 10 USC 1079 and 1086; 5 USC 8101 et seq; and 30 USC 901 et seq; 38 USC 613; E.O. 9397.

The information we obtain to complete claims under these programs is used to identify you and to determine your eligibility. It is also used to decide if the services and supplies you received are covered by these programs and to insure that proper payment is made.

The information may also be given to other providers of services, carriers, intermediaries, medical review boards, health plans, and other organizations or Federal agencies, for the effective administration of Federal provisions that require other third parties payers to pay primary to Federal program, and as otherwise necessary to administer these programs. For example, it may be necessary to disclose information about the benefits you have used to a hospital or doctor. Additional disclosures are made through routine uses for information contained in systems of records.

FOR MEDICARE CLAIMS: See the notice modifying system No. 09-70-0501, titled, 'Carrier Medicare Claims Record' published in the <u>Federal Register</u>, Vol. 55 No. 177, pages 37549, Wed. Sept. 12, 1990, or as updated and republished.

FOR OWCP CLAIMS: Department of Labor, Privacy Act of 1974, "Republication of Notice of Systems of Records," <u>Federal Register</u> Vol. 55 No. 40, Wed. Feb. 28, 1990, See ESA-5, ESA-6, ESA-12, ESA-13, ESA-30, or as updated and republished.

FOR CHAMPUS CLAIMS: <u>PRINCIPLE PURPOSE(S):</u> To evaluate eligibility for medical care provided by civilian sources and to issue payment upon establishment of eligibility and determination that the services/supplies received are authorized by law.

<u>ROUTINE USE(S):</u> Information from claims and related documents may be given to the Dept. of Veterans Affairs, the Dept. of Health and Human Services and/or the Dept. of Transportation consistent with their statutory administrative responsibilities under CHAMPUS/CHAMPVA; to the Dept. of Justice for representation of the Secretary of Defense in civil actions; to the Internal Revenue Service, private collection agencies, and consumer reporting agencies in connection with recoupment claims; and to Congressional Offices in response to inquiries made at the request of the person to whom a record pertains. Appropriate disclosures may be made to other federal, state, local, foreign government agencies, private business entities, and individual providers of care, on matters relating to entitlement, claims adjudication, fraud, program abuse, utilization review, quality assurance, peer review, program integrity, third-party liability, coordination of benefits, and civil and criminal litigation related to the operation of CHAMPUS.

<u>DISCLOSURES:</u> Voluntary; however, failure to provide information will result in delay in payment or may result in denial of claim. With the one exception discussed below, there are no penalties under these programs for refusing to supply information. However, failure to furnish information regarding the medical services rendered or the amount charged would prevent payment of claims under these programs. Failure to furnish any other information, such as name or claim number, would delay payment of the claim. Failure to provide medical information under FECA could be deemed an obstruction.

It is mandatory that you tell us if you know that another party is responsible for paying for your treatment. Section 1128B of the Social Security Act and 31 USC 3801-3812 provide penalties for withholding this information.

You should be aware that P.L. 100-503, the "Computer Matching and Privacy Protection Act of 1988", permits the government to verify information by way of computer matches.

MEDICAID PAYMENTS (PROVIDER CERTIFICATION)

I hereby agree to keep such records as are necessary to disclose fully the extent of services provided to individuals under the State's Title XIX plan and to furnish information regarding any payments claimed for providing such services as the State Agency or Dept. of Health and Human Services may request.

I further agree to accept, as payment in full, the amount paid by the Medicaid program for those claims submitted for payment under that program, with the exception of authorized deductible, coinsurance, co-payment or similar cost-sharing charge.

SIGNATURE OF PHYSICIAN (OR SUPPLIER): I certify that the services listed above were medically indicated and necessary to the health of this patient and were personally furnished by me or my employee under my personal direction.

NOTICE: This is to certify that the foregoing information is true, accurate and complete. I understand that payment and satisfaction of this claim will be from Federal and State funds, and that any false claims, statements, or documents, or concealment of a material fact, may be prosecuted under applicable Federal or State laws.

According to the Paperwork Reduction Act of 1995, no persons are required to respond to a collection of information unless it displays a valid OMB control number. The valid OMB control number for this information collection is 0938-0008. The time required to complete this information collection is estimated to average 10 minutes per response, including the time to review instructions, search existing data resources, gather the data needed, and complete and review the information collection. If you have any comments concerning the accuracy of the time estimate(s) or suggestions for improving this form, please write to: CMS, N2-14-26, 7500 Security Boulevard, Baltimore, Maryland 21244-1860.

Fig. A-1—cont'd

The reader should visit the following website frequently, in order to keep up-to-date on any changes to the 1500 paper form and/or the instructions for its completion. http://www.nucc.org

CMS-1500 Claim Forms and Completion Instructions

BLUE CROSS AND BLUE SHIELD OF XY
PO BOX 1212
DUBUQUE XT 44444-1212

HEALTH INSURANCE CLAIM FORM

1. MEDICARE (Medicare #) MEDICAID (Medicaid #) TRICARE CHAMPUS (Sponsor's SSN) CHAMPVA (Member ID#) GROUP HEALTH PLAN (SSN or ID) [X] FECA BLK LUNG (SSN) OTHER (ID)	1a. INSURED'S I.D. NUMBER (For Program in Item 1) XQQ001BC1234
2. PATIENT'S NAME (Last Name, First Name, Middle Initial) BERTRAND MILDRED P	3. PATIENT'S BIRTH DATE MM 03 DD 18 YY 1956 SEX M [ ] F [X]	4. INSURED'S NAME (Last Name, First Name, Middle Initial) SAME
5. PATIENT'S ADDRESS (No., Street) 2001 WEST MAPLE STREET	6. PATIENT RELATIONSHIP TO INSURED Self [X] Spouse [ ] Child [ ] Other [ ]	7. INSURED'S ADDRESS (No., Street)

CITY MIDDLETOWN STATE XT 8. PATIENT STATUS Single [X] Married [ ] Other [ ] CITY STATE

ZIP CODE 12345 TELEPHONE (Include Area Code) (555) 234 8888 Employed [X] Full-Time Student [ ] Part-Time Student [ ] ZIP CODE TELEPHONE (INCLUDE AREA CODE) ( )

9. OTHER INSURED'S NAME (Last Name, First Name, Middle Initial) 10. IS PATIENT'S CONDITION RELATED TO: 11. INSURED'S POLICY GROUP OR FECA NUMBER

a. OTHER INSURED'S POLICY OR GROUP NUMBER a. EMPLOYMENT? (CURRENT OR PREVIOUS) YES [ ] NO [X] a. INSURED'S DATE OF BIRTH MM DD YY SEX M [ ] F [ ]

b. OTHER INSURED'S DATE OF BIRTH MM DD YY SEX M [ ] F [ ] b. AUTO ACCIDENT? PLACE (State) YES [ ] NO [X] b. EMPLOYER'S NAME OR SCHOOL NAME

c. EMPLOYER'S NAME OR SCHOOL NAME c. OTHER ACCIDENT? YES [ ] NO [X] c. INSURANCE PLAN NAME OR PROGRAM NAME

d. INSURANCE PLAN NAME OR PROGRAM NAME 10d. RESERVED FOR LOCAL USE d. IS THERE ANOTHER HEALTH BENEFIT PLAN? YES [ ] NO [X] *If yes,* return to and complete item 9 a-d.

READ BACK OF FORM BEFORE COMPLETING & SIGNING THIS FORM.
12. PATIENT'S OR AUTHORIZED PERSON'S SIGNATURE I authorize the release of any medical or other information necessary to process this claim. I also request payment of government benefits either to myself or to the party who accepts assignment below.
SIGNED SIGNATURE ON FILE DATE

13. INSURED'S OR AUTHORIZED PERSON'S SIGNATURE I authorize payment of medical benefits to the undersigned physician or supplier for services described below.
SIGNED

14. DATE OF CURRENT: MM 01 DD 21 YY XX ILLNESS (First symptom) OR INJURY (Accident) OR PREGNANCY(LMP) 15. IF PATIENT HAS HAD SAME OR SIMILAR ILLNESS. GIVE FIRST DATE MM DD YY 16. DATES PATIENT UNABLE TO WORK IN CURRENT OCCUPATION FROM MM DD YY TO MM DD YY

17. NAME OF REFERRING PHYSICIAN OR OTHER SOURCE R L JONES M D 17a. 17b. NPI 1234567890 18. HOSPITALIZATION DATES RELATED TO CURRENT SERVICES FROM MM DD YY TO MM DD YY

19. RESERVED FOR LOCAL USE 20. OUTSIDE LAB? YES [ ] NO [X] $ CHARGES

21. DIAGNOSIS OR NATURE OF ILLNESS OR INJURY. (RELATE ITEMS 1,2,3 OR 4 TO ITEM 24E BY LINE)
1. N39 0 3.
2. 4.

22. MEDICAID RESUBMISSION CODE ORIGINAL REF. NO.

23. PRIOR AUTHORIZATION NUMBER

24. A. DATE(S) OF SERVICE From MM DD YY To MM DD YY	B. PLACE OF SERVICE	C. EMG	D. PROCEDURES, SERVICES, OR SUPPLIES (Explain Unusual Circumstances) CPT/HCPCS MODIFIER	E. DIAGNOSIS POINTER	F. $ CHARGES	G. DAYS OR UNITS	H. EPSDT Family Plan	I. ID. QUAL.	J. RENDERING PROVIDER ID. #
1	01 24 XX 01 24 XX	11		99202	1	50 00	1		NPI	1234567890
2	01 24 XX 01 24 XX	11		81002	1	15 00	1		NPI	1234567890
3									NPI	
4									NPI	
5									NPI	
6									NPI	

25. FEDERAL TAX I.D. NUMBER 42 1898989 SSN [ ] EIN [X] 26. PATIENT'S ACCOUNT NO. 3201 27. ACCEPT ASSIGNMENT? (For govt. claims, see back) YES [X] NO [ ] 28. TOTAL CHARGE $ 65 00 29. AMOUNT PAID $ 30. BALANCE DUE $

31. SIGNATURE OF PHYSICIAN OR SUPPLIER INCLUDING DEGREES OR CREDENTIALS (I certify that the statements on the reverse apply to this bill and are made a part thereof.) R L Jones MD
SIGNED *R L Jones* DATE 012520XX

32. SERVICE FACILITY LOCATION INFORMATION
BROADMOOR MEDICAL CLINIC
4353 PINE RIDGE DRIVE
MILTON XY 12345-0001
a. X100XX1000 b.

33. BILLING PROVIDER INFO & PH # (555) 6567890
BROADMOOR MEDICAL CLINIC
4353 PINE RIDGE DRIVE
MILTON XY 12345-0001
a. X100XX1000 b.

Fig. B-1 (Bertrand): Blue Cross and Blue Shield; no secondary.

Sample claim forms are for example only. Diagnostic and Procedural codes are subject to annual updates. Keep up-to-date on changes made by NUCC for universal claims completion instructions.

Fig. B-2 (Marsalis): Medicaid; no secondary.

1500	MEDICARE CARRIER
HEALTH INSURANCE CLAIM FORM	STREET ADDRESS OR PO BOX NUMBER
APPROVED BY NATIONAL UNIFORM CLAIM COMMITTEE 08/05	CITY STATE ZIP

CARRIER

[ ][ ] PICA | PICA [ ][ ]

1. MEDICARE [X] (Medicare #) MEDICAID [ ] (Medicaid #) TRICARE CHAMPUS [ ] (Sponsor's SSN) CHAMPVA [ ] (Member ID#) GROUP HEALTH PLAN [ ] (SSN or ID) FECA BLK LUNG [ ] (SSN) OTHER [ ] (ID)	1a. INSURED'S I.D. NUMBER (For Program in Item 1) 181401234A
2. PATIENT'S NAME (Last Name, First Name, Middle Initial) MARTINSON FREDERICK T	3. PATIENT'S BIRTH DATE MM 10 DD 18 YY 1940 SEX M [X] F [ ]	4. INSURED'S NAME (Last Name, First Name, Middle Initial)
5. PATIENT'S ADDRESS (No., Street) 2300 PARNELL AVENUE	6. PATIENT RELATIONSHIP TO INSURED Self [ ] Spouse [ ] Child [ ] Other [ ]	7. INSURED'S ADDRESS (No., Street)
CITY MILTON	STATE XY	8. PATIENT STATUS Single [ ] Married [X] Other [ ]	CITY	STATE
ZIP CODE 12345	TELEPHONE (Include Area Code) (555) 234 0001	Employed [ ] Full-Time Student [ ] Part-Time Student [ ]	ZIP CODE	TELEPHONE (Include Area Code) ( )

PATIENT AND INSURED INFORMATION

9. OTHER INSURED'S NAME (Last Name, First Name, Middle Initial)	10. IS PATIENT'S CONDITION RELATED TO:	11. INSURED'S POLICY GROUP OR FECA NUMBER NONE
a. OTHER INSURED'S POLICY OR GROUP NUMBER	a. EMPLOYMENT? (Current or Previous) YES [ ] NO [X]	a. INSURED'S DATE OF BIRTH MM DD YY SEX M [ ] F [ ]
b. OTHER INSURED'S DATE OF BIRTH MM DD YY SEX M [ ] F [ ]	b. AUTO ACCIDENT? PLACE (State) YES [ ] NO [X]	b. EMPLOYER'S NAME OR SCHOOL NAME
c. EMPLOYER'S NAME OR SCHOOL NAME	c. OTHER ACCIDENT? YES [ ] NO [X]	c. INSURANCE PLAN NAME OR PROGRAM NAME
d. INSURANCE PLAN NAME OR PROGRAM NAME	10d. RESERVED FOR LOCAL USE	d. IS THERE ANOTHER HEALTH BENEFIT PLAN? YES [ ] NO [ ] If yes, return to and complete item 9 a-d.

READ BACK OF FORM BEFORE COMPLETING & SIGNING THIS FORM.	
12. PATIENT'S OR AUTHORIZED PERSON'S SIGNATURE I authorize the release of any medical or other information necessary to process this claim. I also request payment of government benefits either to myself or to the party who accepts assignment below. SIGNED SIGNATURE ON FILE DATE	13. INSURED'S OR AUTHORIZED PERSON'S SIGNATURE I authorize payment of medical benefits to the undersigned physician or supplier for services described below. SIGNED

14. DATE OF CURRENT: MM DD YY ILLNESS (First symptom) OR INJURY (Accident) OR PREGNANCY(LMP)	15. IF PATIENT HAS HAD SAME OR SIMILAR ILLNESS. GIVE FIRST DATE MM DD YY	16. DATES PATIENT UNABLE TO WORK IN CURRENT OCCUPATION FROM MM DD YY TO MM DD YY
17. NAME OF REFERRING PROVIDER OR OTHER SOURCE	17a. [ ] 17b. NPI	18. HOSPITALIZATION DATES RELATED TO CURRENT SERVICES FROM MM DD YY TO MM DD YY
19. RESERVED FOR LOCAL USE		20. OUTSIDE LAB? YES [ ] NO [X] $ CHARGES
21. DIAGNOSIS OR NATURE OF ILLNESS OR INJURY (Relate Items 1, 2, 3 or 4 to Item 24E by Line) 1. I10 ____ 2. ____ 3. ____ 4. ____		22. MEDICAID RESUBMISSION CODE ORIGINAL REF. NO. 23. PRIOR AUTHORIZATION NUMBER

PHYSICIAN OR SUPPLIER INFORMATION

24. A. DATE(S) OF SERVICE From MM DD YY To MM DD YY	B. PLACE OF SERVICE	C. EMG	D. PROCEDURES, SERVICES, OR SUPPLIES (Explain Unusual Circumstances) CPT/HCPCS MODIFIER	E. DIAGNOSIS POINTER	F. $ CHARGES	G. DAYS OR UNITS	H. EPSDT Family Plan	I. ID. QUAL.	J. RENDERING PROVIDER ID. #
1	01 25 XX 01 25 XX	11		99213	1	75 00	1		NPI	1234567890
2									NPI	
3									NPI	
4									NPI	
5									NPI	
6									NPI	

25. FEDERAL TAX I.D. NUMBER 42 1898989 SSN [ ] EIN [X]	26. PATIENT'S ACCOUNT NO. 2774	27. ACCEPT ASSIGNMENT? (For govt. claims, see back) YES [X] NO [ ]	28. TOTAL CHARGE $ 75 00	29. AMOUNT PAID $	30. BALANCE DUE $
31. SIGNATURE OF PHYSICIAN OR SUPPLIER INCLUDING DEGREES OR CREDENTIALS (I certify that the statements on the reverse apply to this bill and are made a part thereof.) R L JONES MD 012620XX SIGNED R L JONES MD DATE	32. SERVICE FACILITY LOCATION INFORMATION BROADMOOR MEDICAL CLINIC 4353 PINE RIDGE DRIVE MILTON XY 12345-0001 a. X100XX1000 b.	33. BILLING PROVIDER INFO & PH # (555) 6567890 BROADMOOR MEDICAL CLINIC 4353 PINE RIDGE DRIVE MILTON XY 12345-0001 a. X100XX1000 b.

NUCC Instruction Manual available at: www.nucc.org

APPROVED OMB-0938-0999 FORM CMS-1500 (08/05)

Fig. B-3 (Martinson): Medicare (simple).

1500

HEALTH INSURANCE CLAIM FORM

APPROVED BY NATIONAL UNIFORM CLAIM COMMITTEE 08/05

MEDICARE CARRIER

STREET ADDRESS OR PO BOX NUMBER

CITY STATE ZIP CODE

CARRIER

PICA   PICA

1. MEDICARE	MEDICAID	TRICARE CHAMPUS	CHAMPVA	GROUP HEALTH PLAN	FECA BLK LUNG	OTHER	1a. INSURED'S I.D. NUMBER (For Program in Item 1)
X (Medicare #)	X (Medicaid #)	(Sponsor's SSN)	(Member ID#)	(SSN or ID)	(SSN)	(ID)	233991110D

2. PATIENT'S NAME (Last Name, First Name, Middle Initial)
ATKINSON PRICILLA M

3. PATIENT'S BIRTH DATE   MM 11 DD 04 YY 1934   SEX M ☐ F ☒

4. INSURED'S NAME (Last Name, First Name, Middle Initial)

5. PATIENT'S ADDRESS (No., Street)
52 SUNSET CIRCLE

6. PATIENT RELATIONSHIP TO INSURED
Self ☐ Spouse ☐ Child ☐ Other ☐

7. INSURED'S ADDRESS (No., Street)

CITY MILTON   STATE XY

8. PATIENT STATUS
Single ☒ Married ☐ Other ☐

CITY   STATE

ZIP CODE 12345   TELEPHONE (Include Area Code) (555) 234 5454

Employed ☐ Full-Time Student ☐ Part-Time Student ☐

ZIP CODE   TELEPHONE (Include Area Code) ( )

9. OTHER INSURED'S NAME (Last Name, First Name, Middle Initial)

10. IS PATIENT'S CONDITION RELATED TO:

11. INSURED'S POLICY GROUP OR FECA NUMBER
NONE

a. OTHER INSURED'S POLICY OR GROUP NUMBER

a. EMPLOYMENT? (Current or Previous)
YES ☐ NO ☒

a. INSURED'S DATE OF BIRTH MM DD YY   SEX M ☐ F ☐

b. OTHER INSURED'S DATE OF BIRTH MM DD YY   SEX M ☐ F ☐

b. AUTO ACCIDENT?   PLACE (State)
YES ☐ NO ☒

b. EMPLOYER'S NAME OR SCHOOL NAME

c. EMPLOYER'S NAME OR SCHOOL NAME

c. OTHER ACCIDENT?
YES ☐ NO ☒

c. INSURANCE PLAN NAME OR PROGRAM NAME

d. INSURANCE PLAN NAME OR PROGRAM NAME

10d. RESERVED FOR LOCAL USE

d. IS THERE ANOTHER HEALTH BENEFIT PLAN?
YES ☐ NO ☐ If yes, return to and complete item 9 a-d.

READ BACK OF FORM BEFORE COMPLETING & SIGNING THIS FORM.

12. PATIENT'S OR AUTHORIZED PERSON'S SIGNATURE I authorize the release of any medical or other information necessary to process this claim. I also request payment of government benefits either to myself or to the party who accepts assignment below.

SIGNED SIGNATURE ON FILE   DATE

13. INSURED'S OR AUTHORIZED PERSON'S SIGNATURE I authorize payment of medical benefits to the undersigned physician or supplier for services described below.

SIGNED

14. DATE OF CURRENT: MM DD YY ILLNESS (First symptom) OR INJURY (Accident) OR PREGNANCY(LMP)

15. IF PATIENT HAS HAD SAME OR SIMILAR ILLNESS. GIVE FIRST DATE MM DD YY

16. DATES PATIENT UNABLE TO WORK IN CURRENT OCCUPATION
FROM MM DD YY   TO MM DD YY

17. NAME OF REFERRING PROVIDER OR OTHER SOURCE
R L JONES MD

17a.
17b. NPI 1234567890

18. HOSPITALIZATION DATES RELATED TO CURRENT SERVICES
FROM MM DD YY   TO MM DD YY

19. RESERVED FOR LOCAL USE

20. OUTSIDE LAB? $ CHARGES
YES ☐ NO ☒

21. DIAGNOSIS OR NATURE OF ILLNESS OR INJURY (Relate Items 1, 2, 3 or 4 to Item 24E by Line)
1. M08 80   3.
2.   4.

22. MEDICAID RESUBMISSION CODE   ORIGINAL REF. NO.

23. PRIOR AUTHORIZATION NUMBER

24. A. DATE(S) OF SERVICE From MM DD YY	To MM DD YY	B. PLACE OF SERVICE	C. EMG	D. PROCEDURES, SERVICES, OR SUPPLIES (Explain Unusual Circumstances) CPT/HCPCS	MODIFIER	E. DIAGNOSIS POINTER	F. $ CHARGES	G. DAYS OR UNITS	H. EPSDT Family Plan	I. ID. QUAL.	J. RENDERING PROVIDER ID. #
1 01 24 XX	01 24 XX	11		99214		1	115 00	1		NPI	1234567890
2 01 24 XX	01 24 XX	11		J0800		1	25 00	1		NPI	1234567890
3										NPI	
4										NPI	
5										NPI	
6										NPI	

25. FEDERAL TAX I.D. NUMBER SSN EIN
42 1898989   ☒

26. PATIENT'S ACCOUNT NO.
2340

27. ACCEPT ASSIGNMENT? (For govt. claims, see back)
☒ YES ☐ NO

28. TOTAL CHARGE $ 140 00

29. AMOUNT PAID $

30. BALANCE DUE $

31. SIGNATURE OF PHYSICIAN OR SUPPLIER INCLUDING DEGREES OR CREDENTIALS
(I certify that the statements on the reverse apply to this bill and are made a part thereof.)

R L JONES MD   012520XX

SIGNED R L JONES MD   DATE

32. SERVICE FACILITY LOCATION INFORMATION
BROADMOOR MEDICAL CLINIC
4353 PINE RIDGE DRIVE
MILTON XY 12345-0001
a. X100XX1000   b.

33. BILLING PROVIDER INFO & PH # (555) 6567890
BROADMOOR MEDICAL CLINIC
4353 PINE RIDGE DRIVE
MILTON XY 12345-0001
a. X100XX1000   b.

NUCC Instruction Manual available at: www.nucc.org

APPROVED OMB-0938-0999 FORM CMS-1500 (08/05)

Fig. B-4 (Atkinson): Medicare/Medicaid.

1500

HEALTH INSURANCE CLAIM FORM

APPROVED BY NATIONAL UNIFORM CLAIM COMMITTEE 08/05

MEDICARE CARRIER
STREET ADDRESS OR PO BOX NUMBER
CITY STATE ZIP

CARRIER →

[ ] PICA   PICA [ ]

1. MEDICARE	MEDICAID	TRICARE CHAMPUS	CHAMPVA	GROUP HEALTH PLAN	FECA BLK LUNG	OTHER	1a. INSURED'S I.D. NUMBER (For Program in Item 1)
[X] (Medicare #)	[ ] (Medicaid #)	[ ] (Sponsor's SSN)	[ ] (Member ID#)	[X] (SSN or ID)	[ ] (SSN)	[ ] (ID)	343668110A

2. PATIENT'S NAME (Last Name, First Name, Middle Initial)
FREEMAN OZWALD N

3. PATIENT'S BIRTH DATE   MM 10 | DD 16 | YY 1933   SEX M [X] F [ ]

4. INSURED'S NAME (Last Name, First Name, Middle Initial)

5. PATIENT'S ADDRESS (No., Street)
1111 DOBSON CREEK ROAD

6. PATIENT RELATIONSHIP TO INSURED
Self [X] Spouse [ ] Child [ ] Other [ ]

7. INSURED'S ADDRESS (No., Street)

CITY   MILTON   STATE XY

8. PATIENT STATUS
Single [ ] Married [X] Other [ ]

CITY   STATE

ZIP CODE   12345   TELEPHONE (Include Area Code) (555) 234 3321

Employed [ ] Full-Time Student [ ] Part-Time Student [ ]

ZIP CODE   TELEPHONE (Include Area Code) (   )

9. OTHER INSURED'S NAME (Last Name, First Name, Middle Initial)
SAME

10. IS PATIENT'S CONDITION RELATED TO:

11. INSURED'S POLICY GROUP OR FECA NUMBER
NONE

a. OTHER INSURED'S POLICY OR GROUP NUMBER
MGAP 274805022F

a. EMPLOYMENT? (Current or Previous)
[ ] YES [X] NO

a. INSURED'S DATE OF BIRTH MM | DD | YY   SEX M [ ] F [ ]

b. OTHER INSURED'S DATE OF BIRTH MM | DD | YY   SEX M [ ] F [ ]

b. AUTO ACCIDENT?   PLACE (State)
[ ] YES [X] NO

b. EMPLOYER'S NAME OR SCHOOL NAME

c. EMPLOYER'S NAME OR SCHOOL NAME

c. OTHER ACCIDENT?
[ ] YES [X] NO

c. INSURANCE PLAN NAME OR PROGRAM NAME

d. INSURANCE PLAN NAME OR PROGRAM NAME
XYSRBLUE678

10d. RESERVED FOR LOCAL USE

d. IS THERE ANOTHER HEALTH BENEFIT PLAN?
[ ] YES [ ] NO   If yes, return to and complete item 9 a-d.

READ BACK OF FORM BEFORE COMPLETING & SIGNING THIS FORM.
12. PATIENT'S OR AUTHORIZED PERSON'S SIGNATURE I authorize the release of any medical or other information necessary to process this claim. I also request payment of government benefits either to myself or to the party who accepts assignment below.

SIGNED SIGNATURE ON FILE   DATE

13. INSURED'S OR AUTHORIZED PERSON'S SIGNATURE I authorize payment of medical benefits to the undersigned physician or supplier for services described below.

SIGNED SIGNATURE ON FILE

14. DATE OF CURRENT: MM | DD | YY   ◄ ILLNESS (First symptom) OR INJURY (Accident) OR PREGNANCY(LMP)

15. IF PATIENT HAS HAD SAME OR SIMILAR ILLNESS. GIVE FIRST DATE MM | DD | YY

16. DATES PATIENT UNABLE TO WORK IN CURRENT OCCUPATION
FROM MM | DD | YY   TO MM | DD | YY

17. NAME OF REFERRING PROVIDER OR OTHER SOURCE
MARILOU LUCERO MD

17a.
17b. NPI 2907511822

18. HOSPITALIZATION DATES RELATED TO CURRENT SERVICES
FROM MM | DD | YY   TO MM | DD | YY

19. RESERVED FOR LOCAL USE

20. OUTSIDE LAB? $ CHARGES
[ ] YES [X] NO

21. DIAGNOSIS OR NATURE OF ILLNESS OR INJURY (Relate Items 1, 2, 3 or 4 to Item 24E by Line)
1. R07 9   3.
2.   4.

22. MEDICAID RESUBMISSION CODE   ORIGINAL REF. NO.

23. PRIOR AUTHORIZATION NUMBER

24. A. DATE(S) OF SERVICE From MM DD YY To MM DD YY	B. PLACE OF SERVICE	C. EMG	D. PROCEDURES, SERVICES, OR SUPPLIES (Explain Unusual Circumstances) CPT/HCPCS MODIFIER	E. DIAGNOSIS POINTER	F. $ CHARGES	G. DAYS OR UNITS	H. EPSDT Family Plan	I. ID. QUAL.	J. RENDERING PROVIDER ID. #
1	01 24 XX 01 24 XX	11		99214	1	115 00	1		NPI	2907511822
2	01 24 XX 01 24 XX	11		93350	1	175 00	1		NPI	2907511822
3	01 24 XX 01 24 XX	11		93017	1	55 00	1		NPI	2907511822
4									NPI	
5									NPI	
6									NPI	

25. FEDERAL TAX I.D. NUMBER   SSN [ ] EIN [X]
42 1898989

26. PATIENT'S ACCOUNT NO.
2544

27. ACCEPT ASSIGNMENT? (For govt. claims, see back)
[X] YES [ ] NO

28. TOTAL CHARGE $ 345 00

29. AMOUNT PAID $

30. BALANCE DUE $

31. SIGNATURE OF PHYSICIAN OR SUPPLIER INCLUDING DEGREES OR CREDENTIALS (I certify that the statements on the reverse apply to this bill and are made a part thereof.)

MARILOU LUCERO MD   012520XX

SIGNED MARILOU LUCERO MD DATE

32. SERVICE FACILITY LOCATION INFORMATION
BROADMOOR MEDICAL CLINIC
4353 PINE RIDGE DRIVE
MILTON XY 12345-0001
a. X100XX1000   b.

33. BILLING PROVIDER INFO & PH # (555) 6567890
BROADMOOR MEDICAL CLINIC
4353 PINE RIDGE DRIVE
MILTON XY 12345-0001
a. X100XX1000   b.

NUCC Instruction Manual available at: www.nucc.org

APPROVED OMB-0938-0999 FORM CMS-1500 (08/05)

Fig. B-5 (Freeman): Medicare/Medigap.

EDU BENEFITS INC
15055 144TH AV SUITE 6B
GRANITE FALLS XT 34567

HEALTH INSURANCE CLAIM FORM

1. MEDICARE MEDICAID TRICARE CHAMPUS CHAMPVA GROUP HEALTH PLAN FECA BLK LUNG OTHER	1a. INSURED'S I.D. NUMBER (For Program in Item 1)
[X] (Medicare #) [ ] (Medicaid #) [ ] (Sponsor's SSN) [ ] (Member ID#) [X] (SSN or ID) [ ] (SSN) [ ] (ID)	222553320A

2. PATIENT'S NAME (Last Name, First Name, Middle Initial)	3. PATIENT'S BIRTH DATE SEX	4. INSURED'S NAME (Last Name, First Name, Middle Initial)
FRANKLIN ALMA L	05 02 1941 M [ ] F [X]	FRANKLIN JOSEPH P

5. PATIENT'S ADDRESS (No., Street)	6. PATIENT RELATIONSHIP TO INSURED	7. INSURED'S ADDRESS (No., Street)
89 BRIDGEWAY	Self [ ] Spouse [X] Child [ ] Other [ ]	SAME
CITY STATE	8. PATIENT STATUS	CITY STATE
MILTON XT	Single [ ] Married [X] Other [ ]	
ZIP CODE TELEPHONE (Include Area Code)	Employed [X] Full-Time Student [ ] Part-Time Student [ ]	ZIP CODE TELEPHONE (INCLUDE AREA CODE)
12345 (555) 234 1009		( )

9. OTHER INSURED'S NAME (Last Name, First Name, Middle Initial)	10. IS PATIENT'S CONDITION RELATED TO:	11. INSURED'S POLICY GROUP OR FECA NUMBER
		XWT8739995
a. OTHER INSURED'S POLICY OR GROUP NUMBER	a. EMPLOYMENT? (CURRENT OR PREVIOUS) [ ] YES [X] NO	a. INSURED'S DATE OF BIRTH SEX 06 27 1938 M [X] F [ ]
b. OTHER INSURED'S DATE OF BIRTH SEX MM DD YY M [ ] F [ ]	b. AUTO ACCIDENT? PLACE (State) [ ] YES [X] NO	b. EMPLOYER'S NAME OR SCHOOL NAME FLINT RIVER SCHOOL DISTRICT
c. EMPLOYER'S NAME OR SCHOOL NAME	c. OTHER ACCIDENT? [ ] YES [X] NO	c. INSURANCE PLAN NAME OR PROGRAM NAME EDU BENEFITS INC
d. INSURANCE PLAN NAME OR PROGRAM NAME	10d. RESERVED FOR LOCAL USE	d. IS THERE ANOTHER HEALTH BENEFIT PLAN? [ ] YES [ ] NO If yes, return to and complete item 9 a-d.

READ BACK OF FORM BEFORE COMPLETING & SIGNING THIS FORM.
12. PATIENT'S OR AUTHORIZED PERSON'S SIGNATURE I authorize the release of any medical or other information necessary to process this claim. I also request payment of government benefits either to myself or to the party who accepts assignment below.

SIGNED SOF   DATE _____

13. INSURED'S OR AUTHORIZED PERSON'S SIGNATURE I authorize payment of medical benefits to the undersigned physician or supplier for services described below.

SIGNED SOF

14. DATE OF CURRENT: ILLNESS (First symptom) OR INJURY (Accident) OR PREGNANCY(LMP) 01 16 XX	15. IF PATIENT HAS HAD SAME OR SIMILAR ILLNESS. GIVE FIRST DATE MM DD YY	16. DATES PATIENT UNABLE TO WORK IN CURRENT OCCUPATION FROM 01 16 XX TO 01 24 XX
17. NAME OF REFERRING PHYSICIAN OR OTHER SOURCE RONALD K PEPPERDINE MD	17a. 17b. NPI 3256654001	18. HOSPITALIZATION DATES RELATED TO CURRENT SERVICES FROM TO
19. RESERVED FOR LOCAL USE		20. OUTSIDE LAB? $ CHARGES [ ] YES [X] NO

21. DIAGNOSIS OR NATURE OF ILLNESS OR INJURY. (RELATE ITEMS 1,2,3 OR 4 TO ITEM 24E BY LINE)	22. MEDICAID RESUBMISSION CODE ORIGINAL REF. NO.
1. R09.1 3. ___.___	
2. ___.___ 4. ___.___	23. PRIOR AUTHORIZATION NUMBER

24. A. DATE(S) OF SERVICE From / To		B. PLACE OF SERVICE	C. EMG	D. PROCEDURES, SERVICES, OR SUPPLIES (Explain Unusual Circumstances) CPT/HCPCS	MODIFIER	E. DIAGNOSIS POINTER	F. $ CHARGES	G. DAYS OR UNITS	H. EPSDT Family Plan	I. ID. QUAL.	J. RENDERING PROVIDER ID. #
1	01 20 XX 01 20 XX	11		99203		1	55 00	1		NPI	1234567890
2	01 20 XX 01 20 XX	11		71023		1	90 00	1		NPI	1234567890
3										NPI	
4										NPI	
5										NPI	
6										NPI	

25. FEDERAL TAX I.D. NUMBER SSN EIN	26. PATIENT'S ACCOUNT NO.	27. ACCEPT ASSIGNMENT? (For govt. claims, see back)	28. TOTAL CHARGE	29. AMOUNT PAID	30. BALANCE DUE
42 1898989 [X]	3322	[X] YES [ ] NO	$ 145 00	$ 00 00	$

31. SIGNATURE OF PHYSICIAN OR SUPPLIER INCLUDING DEGREES OR CREDENTIALS (I certify that the statements on the reverse apply to this bill and are made a part thereof.)	32. SERVICE FACILITY LOCATION INFORMATION	33. BILLING PROVIDER INFO & PH # (555) 6567890
R L Jones MD *R L Jones* SIGNED 012520XX DATE	BROADMOOR MEDICAL CLINIC 4353 PINE RIDGE DRIVE MILTON XY 12345-0001	BROADMOOR MEDICAL CLINIC 4353 PINE RIDGE DRIVE MILTON XY 12345-0001
	a. X100XX1000 b.	a. X100XX1000 b.

Fig. B-6 (Franklin): Group with Medicare secondary.

1500

HEALTH INSURANCE CLAIM FORM

APPROVED BY NATIONAL UNIFORM CLAIM COMMITTEE 08/05

TRICARE CARRIER NAME

STREET ADDRESS OR PPO NUMBER

CITY STATE ZIP CODE

		CARRIER

PICA | | PICA |

1. MEDICARE (Medicare #)	MEDICAID (Medicaid #)	TRICARE CHAMPUS [X] (Sponsor's SSN)	CHAMPVA (Member ID#)	GROUP HEALTH PLAN (SSN or ID)	FECA BLK LUNG (SSN)	OTHER (ID)	1a. INSURED'S I.D. NUMBER (For Program in Item 1) 321549876

2. PATIENT'S NAME (Last Name, First Name, Middle Initial) SINCLAIR EMILY J	3. PATIENT'S BIRTH DATE MM 04 DD 17 YY 2003 SEX M [X] F	4. INSURED'S NAME (Last Name, First Name, Middle Initial) SINCLAIR PARKER L

5. PATIENT'S ADDRESS (No., Street) 1344 ARGYLE COURT	6. PATIENT RELATIONSHIP TO INSURED Self [ ] Spouse [ ] Child [X] Other [ ]	7. INSURED'S ADDRESS (No., Street) APO 53555J

CITY MILTON	STATE XY	8. PATIENT STATUS Single [X] Married [ ] Other [ ]	CITY NEW YORK	STATE NY

ZIP CODE 12345	TELEPHONE (Include Area Code) (555) 234 4111	Employed [ ] Full-Time Student [ ] Part-Time Student [X]	ZIP CODE 22222	TELEPHONE (Include Area Code) ( )

9. OTHER INSURED'S NAME (Last Name, First Name, Middle Initial)	10. IS PATIENT'S CONDITION RELATED TO:	11. INSURED'S POLICY GROUP OR FECA NUMBER

a. OTHER INSURED'S POLICY OR GROUP NUMBER	a. EMPLOYMENT? (Current or Previous) YES [ ] NO [X]	a. INSURED'S DATE OF BIRTH MM 10 DD 08 YY 1984 SEX M [X] F [ ]

b. OTHER INSURED'S DATE OF BIRTH MM DD YY SEX M [ ] F [ ]	b. AUTO ACCIDENT? PLACE (State) YES [ ] NO [X]	b. EMPLOYER'S NAME OR SCHOOL NAME

c. EMPLOYER'S NAME OR SCHOOL NAME	c. OTHER ACCIDENT? YES [ ] NO [X]	c. INSURANCE PLAN NAME OR PROGRAM NAME

d. INSURANCE PLAN NAME OR PROGRAM NAME	10d. RESERVED FOR LOCAL USE	d. IS THERE ANOTHER HEALTH BENEFIT PLAN? YES [ ] NO [X] *If yes,* return to and complete item 9 a-d.

READ BACK OF FORM BEFORE COMPLETING & SIGNING THIS FORM.

12. PATIENT'S OR AUTHORIZED PERSON'S SIGNATURE I authorize the release of any medical or other information necessary to process this claim. I also request payment of government benefits either to myself or to the party who accepts assignment below.

SIGNED **SIGNATURE ON FILE**   DATE

13. INSURED'S OR AUTHORIZED PERSON'S SIGNATURE I authorize payment of medical benefits to the undersigned physician or supplier for services described below.

SIGNED

14. DATE OF CURRENT: MM 01 DD 18 YY XX ◄ ILLNESS (First symptom) OR INJURY (Accident) OR PREGNANCY(LMP)	15. IF PATIENT HAS HAD SAME OR SIMILAR ILLNESS. GIVE FIRST DATE MM DD YY	16. DATES PATIENT UNABLE TO WORK IN CURRENT OCCUPATION FROM MM DD YY TO MM DD YY

17. NAME OF REFERRING PROVIDER OR OTHER SOURCE MARILOU LUCERO MD	17a.	18. HOSPITALIZATION DATES RELATED TO CURRENT SERVICES FROM MM DD YY TO MM DD YY
	17b. NPI 2907511822	

19. RESERVED FOR LOCAL USE	20. OUTSIDE LAB? YES [ ] NO [X] $ CHARGES

21. DIAGNOSIS OR NATURE OF ILLNESS OR INJURY (Relate Items 1, 2, 3 or 4 to Item 24E by Line) 1. J12 9 3. 2. 4.	22. MEDICAID RESUBMISSION CODE ORIGINAL REF. NO.
	23. PRIOR AUTHORIZATION NUMBER 0221558766

24. A. DATE(S) OF SERVICE						B. PLACE OF SERVICE	C. EMG	D. PROCEDURES, SERVICES, OR SUPPLIES (Explain Unusual Circumstances)		E. DIAGNOSIS POINTER	F. $ CHARGES	G. DAYS OR UNITS	H. EPSDT Family Plan	I. ID. QUAL.	J. RENDERING PROVIDER ID. #
From MM	DD	YY	To MM	DD	YY			CPT/HCPCS	MODIFIER						
01	19	XX	01	19	XX	21		99221		1	250 00	1		NPI	2907511822
01	20	XX	01	21	XX	21		99231		1	150 00	2		NPI	2907511822
01	22	XX	01	22	XX	21		99238		1	110 00	1		NPI	2907511822
														NPI	
														NPI	
														NPI	

25. FEDERAL TAX I.D. NUMBER 42 1898989 SSN [ ] EIN [X]	26. PATIENT'S ACCOUNT NO. 2343	27. ACCEPT ASSIGNMENT? (For govt. claims, see back) [X] YES [ ] NO	28. TOTAL CHARGE $ 660 00	29. AMOUNT PAID $	30. BALANCE DUE $

31. SIGNATURE OF PHYSICIAN OR SUPPLIER INCLUDING DEGREES OR CREDENTIALS (I certify that the statements on the reverse apply to this bill and are made a part thereof.) MARILOU LUCERO MD 012520XX SIGNED *MARILOU LUCERO MD* DATE	32. SERVICE FACILITY LOCATION INFORMATION BROADMOOR MEDICAL CENTER 4990 PINE RIDGE CIRCLE MILTON XY 12345-0001 a. X100XX1111 b.	33. BILLING PROVIDER INFO & PH # (555) 6567890 BROADMOOR MEDICAL CLINIC 4353 PINE RIDGE DRIVE MILTON XY 12345-0001 a. X100XX1000 b.

NUCC Instruction Manual available at: www.nucc.org

APPROVED OMB-0938-0999 FORM CMS-1500 (08/05)

PATIENT AND INSURED INFORMATION

PHYSICIAN OR SUPPLIER INFORMATION

Fig. B-7 (Sinclair): TRICARE simple.

1500

HEALTH INSURANCE CLAIM FORM

APPROVED BY NATIONAL UNIFORM CLAIM COMMITTEE 08/05

VA HEALTH ADMIN CENTER

PO BOX 65024

DENVER CO 80206-9024

CARRIER

| | PICA | | | | | | | | PICA | |

1. MEDICARE (Medicare #)	MEDICAID (Medicaid #)	TRICARE CHAMPUS (Sponsor's SSN)	CHAMPVA [X] (Member ID#)	GROUP HEALTH PLAN (SSN or ID)	FECA BLK LUNG (SSN)	OTHER (ID)	1a. INSURED'S I.D. NUMBER (For Program in Item 1) 223558890	

2. PATIENT'S NAME (Last Name, First Name, Middle Initial)
SALISBURY THEODORE V

3. PATIENT'S BIRTH DATE MM 08 DD 11 YY 1957   SEX M [X] F

4. INSURED'S NAME (Last Name, First Name, Middle Initial)
SAME

5. PATIENT'S ADDRESS (No., Street)
2659 WEST LINCOLN

6. PATIENT RELATIONSHIP TO INSURED
Self [X] Spouse Child Other

7. INSURED'S ADDRESS (No., Street)

CITY MILTON   STATE XY

8. PATIENT STATUS
Single [X] Married Other

CITY   STATE

ZIP CODE 12345   TELEPHONE (Include Area Code) (555) 234 3222

Employed   Full-Time Student   Part-Time Student

ZIP CODE   TELEPHONE (Include Area Code) ( )

9. OTHER INSURED'S NAME (Last Name, First Name, Middle Initial)

10. IS PATIENT'S CONDITION RELATED TO:

11. INSURED'S POLICY GROUP OR FECA NUMBER

a. OTHER INSURED'S POLICY OR GROUP NUMBER

a. EMPLOYMENT? (Current or Previous) YES [X] NO

a. INSURED'S DATE OF BIRTH MM DD YY   SEX M   F

b. OTHER INSURED'S DATE OF BIRTH MM DD YY   SEX M   F

b. AUTO ACCIDENT?   PLACE (State) YES [X] NO

b. EMPLOYER'S NAME OR SCHOOL NAME
USN RET

c. EMPLOYER'S NAME OR SCHOOL NAME

c. OTHER ACCIDENT? YES [X] NO

c. INSURANCE PLAN NAME OR PROGRAM NAME

d. INSURANCE PLAN NAME OR PROGRAM NAME

10d. RESERVED FOR LOCAL USE

d. IS THERE ANOTHER HEALTH BENEFIT PLAN?
YES [X] NO   If yes, return to and complete item 9 a-d.

READ BACK OF FORM BEFORE COMPLETING & SIGNING THIS FORM.
12. PATIENT'S OR AUTHORIZED PERSON'S SIGNATURE I authorize the release of any medical or other information necessary to process this claim. I also request payment of government benefits either to myself or to the party who accepts assignment below.

SIGNED SOF   DATE

13. INSURED'S OR AUTHORIZED PERSON'S SIGNATURE I authorize payment of medical benefits to the undersigned physician or supplier for services described below.

SIGNED

PATIENT AND INSURED INFORMATION

14. DATE OF CURRENT: MM DD YY ◄ ILLNESS (First symptom) OR INJURY (Accident) OR PREGNANCY(LMP)

15. IF PATIENT HAS HAD SAME OR SIMILAR ILLNESS. GIVE FIRST DATE MM DD YY

16. DATES PATIENT UNABLE TO WORK IN CURRENT OCCUPATION MM DD YY   FROM   TO

17. NAME OF REFERRING PROVIDER OR OTHER SOURCE
BENNETT V ASPELMYER PA

17a.
17b. NPI 8822343451

18. HOSPITALIZATION DATES RELATED TO CURRENT SERVICES MM DD YY   FROM   TO

19. RESERVED FOR LOCAL USE

20. OUTSIDE LAB? YES [X] NO $ CHARGES

21. DIAGNOSIS OR NATURE OF ILLNESS OR INJURY (Relate Items 1, 2, 3 or 4 to Item 24E by Line)

1. N40 0   3.

2.   4.

22. MEDICAID RESUBMISSION CODE   ORIGINAL REF. NO.

23. PRIOR AUTHORIZATION NUMBER

24. A. DATE(S) OF SERVICE						B. PLACE OF SERVICE	C. EMG	D. PROCEDURES, SERVICES, OR SUPPLIES (Explain Unusual Circumstances) CPT/HCPCS	MODIFIER	E. DIAGNOSIS POINTER	F. $ CHARGES		G. DAYS OR UNITS	H. EPSDT Family Plan	I. ID. QUAL.	J. RENDERING PROVIDER ID. #
From MM	DD	YY	To MM	DD	YY											
01	23	XX	01	23	XX	21		52601		1	1200	00	1		NPI	1234567890
															NPI	
															NPI	
															NPI	
															NPI	
															NPI	

25. FEDERAL TAX I.D. NUMBER 42 1898989   SSN EIN [X]

26. PATIENT'S ACCOUNT NO. 2466

27. ACCEPT ASSIGNMENT? (For govt. claims, see back) [X] YES NO

28. TOTAL CHARGE $ 1200 00

29. AMOUNT PAID $

30. BALANCE DUE $

31. SIGNATURE OF PHYSICIAN OR SUPPLIER INCLUDING DEGREES OR CREDENTIALS
(I certify that the statements on the reverse apply to this bill and are made a part thereof.)

R L JONES MD   012520XX

SIGNED R L JONES MD   DATE

32. SERVICE FACILITY LOCATION INFORMATION
BROADMOOR MEDICAL CENTER
4990 PINE RIDGE CIRCLE
MILTON XY 12345-0001

a. X100XX1111   b.

33. BILLING PROVIDER INFO & PH # (555) 6567890
BROADMOOR MEDICAL CLINIC
4353 PINE RIDGE DRIVE
MILTON XY 12345-0001

a. X100XX1000   b.

PHYSICIAN OR SUPPLIER INFORMATION

NUCC Instruction Manual available at: www.nucc.org

APPROVED OMB-0938-0999 FORM CMS-1500 (08/05)

Fig. B-8 (Salisbury): CHAMPVA.

WORKERS COMP CARRIER

STREET ADDRESS OR PPO BOX

CITY STATE ZIP

1500

HEALTH INSURANCE CLAIM FORM

APPROVED BY NATIONAL UNIFORM CLAIM COMMITTEE 08/05

| | PICA | | | | | | | | PICA | |

1. MEDICARE (Medicare #) | MEDICAID (Medicaid #) | TRICARE CHAMPUS (Sponsor's SSN) | CHAMPVA (Member ID#) | GROUP HEALTH PLAN (SSN or ID) | FECA BLK LUNG (SSN) | OTHER [X] (ID)

1a. INSURED'S I.D. NUMBER (For Program in Item 1)
C94FPP29930

2. PATIENT'S NAME (Last Name, First Name, Middle Initial)
PORTER JAMES B

3. PATIENT'S BIRTH DATE MM 03 DD 10 YY 1968 SEX M [X] F

4. INSURED'S NAME (Last Name, First Name, Middle Initial)
COMPUTER SOLUTIONS LLC

5. PATIENT'S ADDRESS (No., Street)
23411 SOUTH 12TH AVENUE

6. PATIENT RELATIONSHIP TO INSURED
Self Spouse Child Other [X]

7. INSURED'S ADDRESS (No., Street)
4591 PRIME CIRCLE

CITY DODGEVILLE STATE XY

8. PATIENT STATUS
Single Married [X] Other

CITY LINCOLN STATE XY

ZIP CODE 12367 TELEPHONE (Include Area Code) (555) 456 9981

Employed [X] Full-Time Student Part-Time Student

ZIP CODE 12470 TELEPHONE (Include Area Code) (555) 822 0010

9. OTHER INSURED'S NAME (Last Name, First Name, Middle Initial)

10. IS PATIENT'S CONDITION RELATED TO:

11. INSURED'S POLICY GROUP OR FECA NUMBER

a. OTHER INSURED'S POLICY OR GROUP NUMBER

a. EMPLOYMENT? (Current or Previous) YES NO

a. INSURED'S DATE OF BIRTH MM DD YY SEX M F

b. OTHER INSURED'S DATE OF BIRTH MM DD YY SEX M F

b. AUTO ACCIDENT? YES NO PLACE (State)

b. EMPLOYER'S NAME OR SCHOOL NAME

c. EMPLOYER'S NAME OR SCHOOL NAME

c. OTHER ACCIDENT? YES NO

c. INSURANCE PLAN NAME OR PROGRAM NAME

d. INSURANCE PLAN NAME OR PROGRAM NAME

10d. RESERVED FOR LOCAL USE

d. IS THERE ANOTHER HEALTH BENEFIT PLAN? YES NO *If yes*, return to and complete item 9 a-d.

READ BACK OF FORM BEFORE COMPLETING & SIGNING THIS FORM.
12. PATIENT'S OR AUTHORIZED PERSON'S SIGNATURE I authorize the release of any medical or other information necessary to process this claim. I also request payment of government benefits either to myself or to the party who accepts assignment below.

SIGNED _____ DATE _____

13. INSURED'S OR AUTHORIZED PERSON'S SIGNATURE I authorize payment of medical benefits to the undersigned physician or supplier for services described below.

SIGNED _____

14. DATE OF CURRENT: MM 01 DD 25 YY XX ILLNESS (First symptom) OR INJURY (Accident) OR PREGNANCY(LMP)

15. IF PATIENT HAS HAD SAME OR SIMILAR ILLNESS. GIVE FIRST DATE MM DD YY

16. DATES PATIENT UNABLE TO WORK IN CURRENT OCCUPATION FROM MM 01 DD 25 YY XX TO MM 02 DD 24 YY XX

17. NAME OF REFERRING PROVIDER OR OTHER SOURCE
R L JONES MD

17a.
17b. NPI 1234567890

18. HOSPITALIZATION DATES RELATED TO CURRENT SERVICES FROM MM DD YY TO MM DD YY

19. RESERVED FOR LOCAL USE

20. OUTSIDE LAB? YES [X] NO $ CHARGES

21. DIAGNOSIS OR NATURE OF ILLNESS OR INJURY (Relate Items 1, 2, 3 or 4 to Item 24E by Line)

1. G56 02
2. _____ . _____
3. _____ . _____
4. _____ . _____

22. MEDICAID RESUBMISSION CODE ORIGINAL REF. NO.

23. PRIOR AUTHORIZATION NUMBER

24. A. DATE(S) OF SERVICE From MM DD YY	To MM DD YY	B. PLACE OF SERVICE	C. EMG	D. PROCEDURES, SERVICES, OR SUPPLIES (Explain Unusual Circumstances) CPT/HCPCS	MODIFIER	E. DIAGNOSIS POINTER	F. $ CHARGES	G. DAYS OR UNITS	H. EPSDT Family Plan	I. ID. QUAL.	J. RENDERING PROVIDER ID. #
1	01 25 XX	01 25 XX	11		99213		1	75 00	1		NPI	1234567890
2											NPI	
3											NPI	
4											NPI	
5											NPI	
6											NPI	

25. FEDERAL TAX I.D. NUMBER SSN EIN [X]
42 1898989

26. PATIENT'S ACCOUNT NO.
3451WC

27. ACCEPT ASSIGNMENT? (For govt. claims, see back)
[X] YES NO

28. TOTAL CHARGE $ 75 00

29. AMOUNT PAID $

30. BALANCE DUE $

31. SIGNATURE OF PHYSICIAN OR SUPPLIER INCLUDING DEGREES OR CREDENTIALS (I certify that the statements on the reverse apply to this bill and are made a part thereof.)

R L JONES MD 012520XX
SIGNED *R L JONES MD* DATE

32. SERVICE FACILITY LOCATION INFORMATION
BROADMOOR MEDICAL CLINIC
4353 PINE RIDGE DRIVE
MILTON XY 12345-0001
a. X100XX1000 b.

33. BILLING PROVIDER INFO & PH # (555) 6567890
BROADMOOR MEDICAL CLINIC
4353 PINE RIDGE DRIVE
MILTON XY 12345-0001
a. X100XX1000 b.

NUCC Instruction Manual available at: www.nucc.org

APPROVED OMB-0938-0999 FORM CMS-1500 (08/05)

Fig. B-9 (Porter): Workers' compensation.

TABLE B-1	Step-by-Step Medicaid Claims Instructions
Block 1a	Enter the Medicaid recipient's ID number.
Block 2	Enter the name of the Medicaid recipient exactly as it appears on the ID card, keying the last name first, followed by the middle name and middle initial (if one is listed). Use the correct OCR guidelines.
Block 3	Enter the patient's birth date (using the MM DD YYYY format with spaces), and enter an "X" in the appropriate gender box.
Block 4	This block is left blank.
Block 5	Enter the patient's complete mailing address as indicated on lines 1 and 2 in this block. When keying the telephone number, use spaces rather than dashes or parentheses.
Blocks 6-9d	These blocks are typically left blank on Medicaid "simple" claims.
Blocks 10a-c	Key an "X" in the appropriate boxes to indicate whether or not the claim is a result of an auto or other accident or was related to employment. In the case of an auto accident, key the 2-letter state code to indicate the state in which the accident occurred.
Block 10d	This block is usually left blank. Check with your fiscal intermediary (FI) for special situations.
Blocks 11-11d	Leave these blocks blank.
Blocks 12-13	Leave these blocks blank (signatures are normally not required on Medicaid claims).
Blocks 14-16	Leave these blocks blank.
Block 17	Enter the full name and credentials of the referring or ordering provider when applicable.
Block 17a	Leave this block blank.
Block 17b	Enter the national provider identifier (NPI) of the referring or ordering provider if one is reported in Block 17. If none, leave this blank.
Block 18	If the claim is for inpatient hospital services, enter the admission and discharge dates using either the mm cc yy or the MM DD YYYY format. If the patient is still hospitalized, leave the "To" block blank. If no hospitalization, leave this blank.
Block 19	Check the guidelines of your Medicaid FI.
Block 20	Enter an "X" in the "NO" block. Outside laboratory facilities must bill Medicaid directly.
Block 21	Enter the patient's diagnosis or diagnoses using ICD-10-CM codes, listing the primary diagnosis first. There is space for 4 codes, which should be listed in priority order.
Block 22	If this is a resubmission, enter the applicable Medicaid code.
Block 23	If preauthorization was required, enter this number (consult the specific Medicaid guidelines for your state).
Block 24a	Enter each date of service on a separate line. Enter the month, day, and year in the MMDDYY or the MMDDYYYY (no spaces) format for each service. Medicaid does not allow "date ranging for consecutive services."
Block 24b	Enter the applicable place of service (POS) code.
Block 24c	This block is conditionally required. Enter an "X" or an "E" as appropriate for services performed as a result of a medical emergency. If not an emergency service, leave this blank.
Block 24d	Enter the code number using appropriate 5-digit CPT/HCPCS procedure code and a 2-digit modifier, when applicable. If using an unlisted procedure code (ending in "-99"), a complete description of the procedure must be provided as a separate attachment.
Block 24e	Link the procedure code back to the appropriate diagnosis code in Block 21 by indicating the applicable number assigned to the diagnosis (1, 2, 3, or 4).
Block 24f	Enter the amount charged for the service. Do not use dollar signs or decimal points.
Block 24 g	Enter the number of days or units for each single visit.
Block 24 h	Consult your local Medicaid guidelines. Enter an "E" if the service was performed under the Early and Periodic Screening Diagnosis and Treatment (EPSDT) program. Enter an "F" for Family Planning services.
Block 24i	As of May 23, 2007, this is usually not reported. Consult your Medicaid FI for specific guidelines.

Continued

TABLE B-1	Step-by-Step Medicaid Claims Instructions—cont'd
Block 24j	Enter the rendering provider's NPI number in the lower (unshaded) portion of this block. In the case of a service provided "incident to" the service of a physician or nonphysician practitioner, when the person who ordered the service is not supervising, enter the PIN of the supervisor in the shaded portion. (Check with your Medicaid FI for specific guidelines in this block.)
Block 25	Enter the 9-digit federal tax employer identification number (EIN) assigned to that provider (or group) with a space instead of a hyphen after the first 2 digits, and check the appropriate box in this field. In the case of an unincorporated practice or a sole practitioner, the provider's Social Security number is typically used.
Block 26	Enter the patient's account number as assigned by the provider's computerized accounting system.
Block 27	Place an "X" in the "YES" box.
Block 28	Enter the total charges for all services listed in column 24f.
Blocks 29-30	Leave these blocks blank.
Block 31	Enter the signature of the provider, or his or her representative and initials, and the date the form was signed. The signature may be typed, stamped, or handwritten. Make sure no part of the signature falls outside of the block.
Block 32	Key the name and address of the location where services were provided, and enter the Medicaid provider number on the last line of this block. Check for updated changes with your Medicaid FI (some Medicaid FIs do not require this block to be reported if services were provided in the provider's office [which appears in Block 33] or in the patient's home).
Block 32a	Enter the NPI of the service facility in Block 32. *Note:* Only report a Service Facility Location NPI when the NPI is different from the Billing Provider NPI.
Block 32b	As of May 23, 2007, this block is usually not reported; however, you should consult the specific guidelines of the Medicaid FI in your state to be sure.
Block 33	Enter the name, address, Zip Code, and telephone number of the facility providing services. Do not include a hyphen or a space in the telephone number.
Block 33a	Effective May 23, 2007, the NPI of the billing provider or group must be reported here.
Block 33b	As of May 23, 2007, Block 33b is normally not reported; however, consult the guidelines of your state Medicaid FI to be sure.

These instructions are somewhat generic. It is important to use the specific, up-to-date CMS-1500 claims completion instructions of your local carrier.

TABLE B-2	CMS-1500 Claim Form Instructions for Medicare

Throughout these instructions, the following formats are used to report dates:

MM|DD|YY or MM|DD|CCYY—indicates that a space must be reported between month, day, and year. This space is delineated by a dotted vertical line on the CMS-1500 claim form.

MMDDYY or MMDDCCYY—indicates that no space must be reported between month, day, and year. The date must be reported as one continuous number.

Block 1	Show the type of health insurance coverage applicable to this claim by checking the appropriate box (e.g., if a Medicare claim is being filed, check the Medicare box).
Block 1a	Enter the patient's Medicare HICN whether Medicare is the primary or secondary payer (do not include spaces or hyphens).
Block 2	Enter the patient's last name, first name, and middle initial, if any, *exactly* as shown on the patient's Medicare card.
Block 3	Enter the patient's 8-digit birth date (MM|DD|CCYY) and sex.
Block 4	For Medicare simple claims, leave this block blank. If the patient has insurance primary to Medicare, through the patient's or spouse's employment or any other source, list the name of the insured here. When the insured and the patient are the same, enter the word "SAME."

TABLE B-2	CMS-1500 Claim Form Instructions for Medicare—cont'd
Block 5	On the first line, enter the patient's street address; the second line, the city and 2-letter state code; the third line, the Zip Code and phone number.
Block 6	Check the appropriate box for the patient's relationship to the insured when Block 4 is completed. If Medicare is the primary insurance, leave this block blank.
Block 7	Complete this block only when Blocks 4 and 11 are completed. Enter the insured's address and telephone number. When the address is the same as the patient's, enter the word "SAME."
Block 8	On Medicare simple claims, leave this block blank. Check the appropriate box for the patient's marital status and whether employed or a student, when applicable.
Block 9	Enter the last name, first name, and middle initial of the enrollee in a Medigap policy, if it is different from that shown in Block 2. Otherwise, enter the word "SAME." If no Medigap benefits are assigned, leave this block blank. This field may be used in the future for supplemental insurance plans.* If the patient has no insurance primary or secondary to Medicare, Blocks 9 through 9d are left blank.
Block 9a	Enter the policy or group number of the Medigap insured preceded by MEDIGAP, MG, or MGAP. Block 9d must be completed if you enter a policy or group number in Block 9a.
Block 9b	Enter the Medigap insured's 8-digit birth date (MMDDCCYY) and sex.
Block 9c	Leave this block blank if a Medigap PAYERID is entered in Block 9d. Otherwise, enter the claims processing address of the Medigap insurer. Use an abbreviated street address, 2-letter postal code, and Zip Code copied from the Medigap insured's Medigap ID card. *For example:* 1257 Anywhere Street, Baltimore, MD 21204 is shown as "1257 Anywhere St MD 21204."
Block 9d	Enter the 9-digit (alpha-numeric and up to 9-digit) PAYERID number of the Medigap insurer. If no PAYERID number exists, enter the Medigap insurance program or plan name. If you are a PAR facility and the beneficiary wants Medicare payment data forwarded to a Medigap insurer under a mandated Medigap transfer, all of the information in Blocks 9, 9a, 9b, and 9d must be complete and accurate. Otherwise, the Medicare carrier cannot forward the claim information to the Medigap insurer.
Blocks 10a-10c	Check "YES" or "NO" to indicate whether employment, auto liability, or other accident involvement applies to one or more of the services described in Block 24. For auto accidents, enter the 2-letter state code in which the accident occurred. Any block checked "YES" indicates there may be other insurance primary to Medicare. If any items in this block are checked "YES," identify primary insurance information in Block 11.
Block 10d	**Use this Block exclusively for Medicaid (MCD) information.** If the patient is entitled to Medicaid, enter the patient's Medicaid number preceded by MCD. *This Medicare carrier does not use this field.*
Block 11	This block must be completed on Medicare claims. By doing so, the provider acknowledges having made a good faith effort to determine whether Medicare is the primary or secondary payer. If there is insurance primary to Medicare for the service date on the claim, enter the insured's policy or group number and proceed to Blocks 11a-11c. Note: Enter the appropriate information in Block 11c if insurance primary to Medicare is indicated in Block 11. If there is no insurance primary to Medicare, enter the word "NONE" and proceed to Block 12.† If the insured reports a terminating event with regard to insurance that had been primary to Medicare (e.g., insured retired), enter the word "NONE" and proceed to Block 12. Circumstances under which Medicare payment may be secondary to other insurance include group health plan coverage; working aged; disability (large group health plan); end-stage renal disease; no fault and/or other liability; work-related illness/injury; workers' compensation, black lung; and veterans benefits. If Medicare is secondary, enter the insured's policy or group number within the confines of the box, or if there is no insurance primary to Medicare, enter the word "NONE."
Block 11a	Enter the insured's 8-digit birth date (MM|DD|CCYY) and sex if different from that in Block 3. *If entered as a 6-digit date, use hyphens or other punctuation, called "delimiters." If entered as an 8-digit date, do not use delimiters. This item is mandatory if a policy or group number is submitted in Block 11 and is different from the date in Block 3.*
Block 11b	Enter employer's name, if applicable. If there is a change in the insured's insurance status (e.g., retired), enter either a 6-digit (MM|DD|YY) or an 8-digit (MM|DD|CCYY) retirement date preceded by the word "RETIRED." *Please add employer's address and phone number to attached copy of EOB. This item is mandatory if a policy or group number is submitted in Block 11.*

Continued

TABLE B-2	CMS-1500 Claim Form Instructions for Medicare—cont'd
Block 11c	Enter the 9-digit PAYERID number of the primary insurer. If no PAYERID number exists, enter the complete primary payer's program or plan name. If the primary payer's EOB does not contain the claims processing address, record the primary payer's claims processing address directly on the EOB. Include the telephone number of the primary payer. **This item is mandatory if a policy or group number appears in Block 11.**
Block 11d	Leave this block blank. It is normally not required by Medicare; however, check with your local carrier for specific guidelines.
Block 12	The patient or authorized representative must sign and enter a 6-digit date (MM|DD|YY), 8-digit date (MM|DD|CCYY), or an alphanumeric date (e.g., January 1, 1998) unless a signature is on file.‡ *If entered as a 6-digit date, use delimiters. If entered as an 8-digit date, do not use delimiters.* "Signature on file" (SOF) indicators should be on the signature line, immediately following the word "signed." If the signature is not in the correct area, the information may be missed, and the claim could be denied.
Block 13	Leave this block blank for Medicare simple claims. A signature in this block authorizes payment of mandated Medigap benefits to the PAR if required Medigap information is included in Block 9 and its subdivisions. The patient or his or her authorized representative signs this item, or the signature must be on file as a separate Medigap authorization. The Medigap assignment on file in the PAR of the service/supplier's office must be insurer specific. It may state that the authorization applies to all occasions of service until it is revoked. "Signature on file" (SOF) indicators should be on the signature line, immediately following the word "signed." If the signature is not in the correct area, the information may be missed, and the claim would not be crossed over to the Medigap insurance company. Block 13 is mandatory when the provider is PAR, and Medigap information is submitted in Blocks 9-9d.
Block 14	Enter either a 6-digit (MM|DD|YY) or an 8-digit (MM|DD|CCYY) date of current illness, injury, or pregnancy.
Block 15	Leave this block blank. It is not required by Medicare.
Block 16	If the patient is employed and is unable to work in current occupation, enter 6-digit (MM|DD|YY) or 8-digit (MM|DD|CCYY) date when the patient is unable to work. An entry in this field may indicate employment-related insurance coverage. Refer to Blocks 10a and 11c. *Block 16 is mandatory if Blocks 10a and 11c are completed.*
Block 17	Enter the name of the referring or ordering physician if the service or item was ordered or referred by a physician. **Referring physician**—a physician who requests an item or service for the beneficiary for which payment may be made under the Medicare program. **Ordering physician**—a physician or, when appropriate, a nonphysician practitioner who orders nonphysician services for the patient. Examples of services that might be ordered include diagnostic laboratory tests, clinical laboratory tests, pharmaceutical services, durable medical equipment, and services incident to the service of the physician or nonphysician practitioner. If there is no referring or ordering physician or other healthcare provider, leave blank.
Blocks 17a and b	An entry in Block 17a is no longer required. If a referring/ordering provider is listed in Block 17, his or her NPI must be entered in Block 17b. If Block 17 is blank, leave Block 17b blank also. When a claim involves multiple referring or ordering physicians, a separate CMS-1500 form must be used for each referring/ordering physician. Effective May 23, 2007, the UPIN in Block 17a is *not* to be reported. Instead, the NPI must be reported in Block 17b when a service was ordered or referred by a physician.
Block 18	Enter a 6-digit (MM|DD|YY) or an 8-digit (MM|DD|CCYY) date when a medical service is furnished as a result of, or subsequent to, a related hospitalization. *Note:* The only block in which an 8-digit date is mandatory is Block 3 (patient's birth date). Either 6-digit or 8-digit dates can be used throughout the rest of the claim form; however, the date format chosen must be consistent.
Block 19	Enter either a 6-digit or an 8-digit date when the patient was last seen and the NPI of his or her attending physician when an independent physical or occupational therapist submits claims or a physician providing routine foot care submits claims. If this does not apply, leave blank.
Block 20	Complete this block when billing for diagnostic tests subject to purchase price limitations. Enter the purchase price under charges if the "YES" block is checked. A "YES" check indicates that an entity other than the one billing for the service performed the diagnostic test. A "NO" check indicates that "no purchased tests are included on the claim." When "YES" is checked, Block 32 must be completed.
Block 21	Enter the patient's diagnosis/condition. All providers must use an ICD-10-CM code number and code to the highest level of specificity. *Enter four codes in priority order (primary, secondary condition).*
Block 22	Leave this block blank; it is not required by Medicare.

TABLE B-2	CMS-1500 Claim Form Instructions for Medicare—cont'd
Block 23	Enter the quality improvement organization (QIO) prior authorization number for procedures requiring QIO prior approval or the investigational device exemption (IDE) number when an investigational device is used in a U.S. Food and Drug Administration (FDA)–approved clinical trial. Enter the 10-digit Clinical Laboratory Improvement Act (CLIA) certification number for laboratory services billed by an entity performing CLIA-covered procedures. When a physician provides services to a beneficiary residing in an SNF and the services were rendered to an SNF beneficiary outside of the SNF, the physician shall enter the Medicare facility provider number of the SNF in item 23. *Note:* Item 23 can contain only one condition. Any additional conditions should be reported on a separate CMS-1500 form. If none of this is applicable, leave Block 23 blank.
Block 24a	Enter a 6-digit or 8-digit (MMDDCCYY) date for each procedure, service, or supply. When "from" and "to" dates are shown for a series of identical services, enter the number of days or units in column G. This is a required field. The claim will be returned as unprocessable if a date of service extends more than 1 day and a valid "to" date is not present.
Block 24b	Enter the appropriate place of service code for each item used or service performed. This is a required field. *Note:* When a service is rendered to a hospital inpatient, use the "inpatient hospital" code.
Block 24c	Medicare providers are not required to complete this item.
Block 24d	Enter the procedures, services, or supplies using the appropriate 5-digit CPT or CMS HCPCS code. When applicable, show HCPCS code modifiers. When reporting an "unlisted procedure code" or a "not otherwise classified" (NOC) code, include a narrative description in item 19 if a coherent description can be given within the confines of that box. Otherwise, an attachment should be submitted with the claim. This is a required field.
Block 24e	Enter the diagnosis code reference number as shown in item 21 to relate the date of service and the procedures performed to the primary diagnosis. Enter only one reference number per line item. When multiple services are performed, enter the primary reference number for each service—1, 2, 3, or 4. This is a required field. If a situation arises where two or more diagnoses are required for a procedure code (e.g., Pap smears), the provider shall reference only one of the diagnoses in item 21.
Block 24f	Enter the charge for each listed service. Do not use decimals, dashes, or lines.
Block 24 g	Enter the number of days or units. This field is most commonly used for multiple visits, units of supplies, anesthesia minutes, or oxygen volume. If only one service is performed, enter the number 1.
Block 24 h	Leave this block blank; it is not required by Medicare.
Block 24i	Enter the ID qualifier 1 C in the shaded portion for Medicare claims.
Block 24j	Effective May 23, 2007, enter the rendering provider's NPI number in the lower portion. In the case of a service-provided "incident to" the service of a physician or nonphysician practitioner, when the person who ordered the service is not supervising, enter the PIN of the supervisor in the shaded portion.
Block 25	Enter the provider of service or supplier Federal Tax ID (EIN) or Social Security number. The participating provider of service or supplier Federal Tax ID number is required for a mandated Medigap transfer.
Block 26	Enter the patient's account number assigned by the provider's accounting system. This field is optional to assist the provider in patient identification.
Block 27	Check the appropriate block to indicate whether the provider accepts assignment of Medicare benefits. If Medigap is indicated in item 9 and Medigap payment authorization is given in item 13, the provider of service or supplier shall also be a Medicare participating provider of service or supplier and accept assignment of Medicare benefits for all covered charges for all patients.
Block 28	Enter total of all charges in item 24 f. Do not use decimals, dashes, or lines.
Block 29	Enter the total amount the patient paid on the covered services only. Leave blank if no payment has been made.
Block 30	Leave this block blank; it is not required by Medicare.
Block 31	Enter the provider's signature or his or her representative and either the 6-digit or the 8-digit date or alpha-numeric date (e.g., January 1, 2007) the form was signed. Computer-generated signatures are acceptable.
Block 32	Medicare requires name, address, and Zip Code of the facility where services were performed other than those furnished in POS 12 (Home). Medicare does not allow "SAME" to be entered in this block. Purchased tests must have the supplier name, address, Zip Code and PIN. For a certified mammography screening center, enter a 6-digit FDA-approved number.

Continued

TABLE B-2	CMS-1500 Claim Form Instructions for Medicare—cont'd
Block 32a	Only report a Service Facility Location NPI when the NPI is different from the Billing Provider NPI.
Block 32b	As of May 23, 2007, Block 32b is not to be reported. *Note:* Some Medicare carriers require providers of service (i.e., physicians) to enter the supplier's PIN when billing for purchased diagnostic tests. Check with the Medicare carrier in your area for specific instructions.
Block 33	Enter the provider's billing name, address, Zip Code, and telephone number.
Block 33a	Effective May 23, 2007, the NPI of the billing provider or group must be reported here.
Block 33b	As of May 23, 2007, Block 33b is not to be reported.

*Note: Only PARs are to complete Block 9 and its subdivisions and only when the beneficiary wishes to assign his or her benefits under a Medigap policy to the participating physician or supplier. PARs must enter information required in Block 9 and its subdivisions if requested by the patient. PARs sign an agreement with Medicare to accept assignment of benefits for all Medicare patients. A claim for which a beneficiary elects to assign his or her benefits under a Medigap policy to a participating physician/supplier is called a *mandated Medigap transfer.* Do not list other supplemental coverage in Block 9 and its subdivisions at the time a Medicare claim is filed. Other supplemental claims are forwarded automatically to the private insurer if the private insurer contracts with the carrier to send Medicare claim information electronically. If there is no such contract, the beneficiary must file his or her own supplemental claim.

†Note: For a paper claim to be considered for Medicare Secondary Payer benefits, a copy of the primary payer's EOB notice must be attached to the claim form. If a policy or group number is entered, an EOB *must* be attached.

‡Note: In lieu of signing the claim, the patient may sign a release of information statement to be retained in the provider's file. If the patient is physically or mentally unable to sign, a representative may sign on the patient's behalf. In this case, the statement's signature line must indicate the patient's name followed by "by," the representative's name, address, relationship to the patient, and the reason the patient cannot sign. The authorization is effective indefinitely unless the patient or the patient's representative revokes this arrangement. The patient's signature authorizes release of medical information necessary to process the claim. It also authorizes payment of benefits to the provider of service or supplier, when the provider of service or supplier accepts assignment on the claim. When an illiterate or physically handicapped enrollee signs by mark, a witness must enter his or her name and address next to the mark.

From the CMS: Available at: http://www.cms.hhs.gov/transmittals/downloads/R735CP.pdf.

These instructions are somewhat generic. It is important to use the specific, up-to-date CMS-1500 claims completion instructions of your local MAC.

TABLE B-3	Instructions for Filing TRICARE/CHAMPVA Paper Claims
Block 1	Required. Place an "X" in the TRICARE CHAMPUS box for TRICARE claims; place an "X" in the CHAMPVA for CHAMPVA claims.
Block 1a	Required. Enter the sponsor's Social Security number (not the beneficiary's unless they are the same). If the beneficiary is a NATO beneficiary, enter "NATO" here.
Block 2	Required. Enter the patient's last name, first name, and middle initial (if any) *exactly* as shown on the TRICARE or CHAMPVA ID card.
Block 3	Required. Enter the patient's 8-digit birth date (MM DD YYYY) as shown on the ID card, and place an "X" in the appropriate box indicating sex.
Block 4	Required. Enter the sponsor's last name, first name, and middle initial, or if the sponsor and the patient are the same, enter the word "SAME."
Block 5	Required. Enter the complete address of the patient's place of residence at the time of service and the telephone number. Do not use post office box numbers. For rural addresses, indicate the box number and rural route or 911E number.
Block 6	Required. If the beneficiary is the sponsor, indicate "SELF" or provide the relationship to the sponsor. If "other" is checked, indicate how the beneficiary is related to the sponsor (e.g., former spouse). *Note:* Parents, parents-in-law, stepparents, and any grandchildren who are not adopted are not eligible for TRICARE despite the fact that they may have a military ID card. Be sure to check the back of the dependent beneficiary's ID card to ensure it indicates authorization for civilian/TRICARE benefits.
Block 7	Required. Enter the address of the active duty sponsor's duty station or the retiree's mailing address. If the address is the same as the beneficiary's, enter "SAME." If "SAME" is entered in Block 4, leave this block blank. If the sponsor resides overseas, enter the APO/FPO address.
Block 8	Required. Check the appropriate box for the patient's marital status and whether employed or a student.

TABLE B-3	Instructions for Filing TRICARE/CHAMPVA Paper Claims—cont'd
Block 9	Enter the name of the insured if different from that shown in Block 2. If the beneficiary is covered by a spouse's insurance, Blocks 11a-d should be used to show other health insurance held by the beneficiary. If there is no other health insurance (OHI), leave Blocks 9a-d blank. *Note:* Block 11d should be completed before determining the need for completing Blocks 9a-d. If Block 11d is checked "YES," Blocks 9a-d must be completed before claims processing as follows:
Block 9a	Provide the policy number/group number of the other insured's policy.
Block 9b	Enter the other insured's date of birth, and check the appropriate box for sex.
Block 9c	Enter the name of the employer or name of the school.
Block 9d	Enter the name of the insurance plan or the program name where the individual has OHI coverage. If the other coverage is truly supplemental to TRICARE (Medicaid or a plan specifically stating it is supplemental to TRICARE), enter the name and the word "SUPPLEMENTAL" in this block.
Blocks 10a-c	Required. Check "YES" or "NO" to indicate whether employment, auto liability, or other accident involvement applies to one or more of the services described in Block 24. Provide information concerning potential third-party liability. The claims processor will send a DD form 2527, "Statement of Personal Injury— Possible Third Party Liability," to the beneficiary if the diagnosis code or codes indicate such.
Block 10d	Conditionally required. Use this block to indicate that other health insurance is attached, if this is the case.
Block 11	Conditionally required. If the beneficiary has OHI, enter the policy/group number here. Indicate if the beneficiary is covered by Medicare; otherwise, leave blank. Blocks 9a-d should be used to report other coverage held by family members that includes coverage of the beneficiary.
Block 11a	Conditionally required. If the beneficiary has OHI, enter the date of birth and sex if different from Block 3.
Block 11b	Conditionally required. Enter the employer or school name, if applicable. For CHAMPVA claims, if the patient is retired, indicate the branch of service followed by "RET."
Block 11c	Conditionally required. Enter the OHI plan or program name. If the beneficiary is covered by a supplemental policy (Medicaid or a policy specifically stating it is supplemental to TRICARE), indicate "SUPPLEMENTAL."
Block 11d	Required. Indicate if there is or is not another health benefit plan that is primary to TRICARE. The beneficiary may be covered under a plan held by a spouse, a parent, or some other person. If this block is checked "YES," Blocks 9a-d must be completed.
Block 12	Required. "SIGNATURE ON FILE" or "SOF" can be used here if the beneficiary's signature is on file in the provider's office (and on a document that includes a release of information statement). If not on file, the beneficiary must sign and date Block 12. If the patient is younger than 18 years old, either parent should sign the claim unless the services are confidential. If the patient is older than 18 years old but cannot sign the claim, the person who signs must be the legal guardian or, in the absence of a legal guardian, a spouse or parent of the patient. The signer should write the beneficiary's name in Block 12, followed by the word "by" and his or her own signature. A statement must be attached giving the signer's full name, address, relationship to the beneficiary, and the reason the signer is unable to sign. Also, documentation must be attached showing the signer's appointment as legal guardian or power of attorney.
Block 13	Leave blank for TRICARE and CHAMPVA claims. Claims checks are forwarded to PAR and nonPAR accepting assignment. On nonPAR claims, benefit checks are mailed to the patient.
Block 14	Conditionally required. Enter the date of current illness, injury, or pregnancy, if it is documented in the health record. Remember to be consistent with date format.
Block 15	Conditionally required. If it is documented in the health record that the patient has had the same or similar condition previously, enter that date here.
Block 16	Conditionally required. If the patient is employed and unable to work in his or her current occupation, enter the date when patient was unable to work. *Note:* An entry in this field may indicate employment-related insurance coverage.
Block 17	Conditionally required. Enter the name and address of the entity that referred the patient to the provider of services identified on the claim. This is required for all charges for a consultation or the claims processor will have to pay the claim at the rate for the lowest category of office visit. If the beneficiary was referred from an MTF, enter the name of the MTF, and attach a copy of the military referral form (DD 2161 or SF 513). If none of these conditions are applicable, leave blank.

Continued

TABLE B-3	Instructions for Filing TRICARE/CHAMPVA Paper Claims—cont'd
Block 17a-17b	Effective May 23, 2007, Block 17a is no longer reported, and the NPI of the provider entered in Block 17 must be reported in Block 17b. If there was no referring/ordering provider or if the other guidelines are as described for Block 17, leave blank.
Block 18	Conditionally required. If the patient was hospitalized as an inpatient, enter the "from" and "to" dates here.
Block 19	Not required. Leave blank.
Block 20	Conditionally required. Indicate whether laboratory work was done outside of the provider's office, and if so, enter the total amount charged by the laboratory for work being reported on the claim. Check "NO" if no laboratory work was done.
Block 21	Required. Enter the patient's diagnosis/condition using an ICD-10-CM code number or numbers if more than one diagnosis exists.
Block 22	Not required. Leave blank.
Block 23	Conditionally required. Enter the prior authorization number if the services require preauthorization/preadmission review.
Block 24a	Required. Enter the month, day, and year for each procedure/service or supply. If "from" and "to" dates are shown here for a series of identical services, enter the total number of units in Block 24g.
Block 24b	Required. Enter the appropriate 2-digit numeric place of service (POS) code. For the list of applicable codes, log on to http://www.findacode.com/cms1500-claim-form/cms1500-place-of-service-codes.html.
Block 24c	This block is conditionally required. Enter an "X" or an "E" as appropriate for services performed as a result of a medical emergency.
Block 24d	Required. Enter the appropriate CPT/HCPCS code for each service. If using one of the "not elsewhere classified" codes, you must supply a narrative description of the service/supply.
Block 24e	Required. Enter the appropriate diagnosis reference code (1, 2, 3, 4) as shown in Block 21 to relate to each service/procedure. If multiple services/procedures were performed, enter the diagnosis code reference number for each service/procedure.
Block 24f	Required. Enter the charge for each listed service. Include the cents with dollar amounts. *For example, $24.00 should be entered as 24 00 rather than $24. Dashes, decimal points, or lines should not be used in this item.*
Block 24 g	Required. Provide the days or units for each line item. This block should be used for multiple visits for identical services, number of miles, units of supplies, or oxygen volume. If anesthesia, provide the beginning and end time of administration, time in minutes, or 15-minute units.
Block 24 h	Not required. Leave blank.
Block 24i	Conditionally required. Enter the appropriate ID qualifier if local TRICARE/CHAMPVA guidelines require an entry here.
Block 24j	Effective May 23, 2007, enter the provider's NPI number in the lower, unshaded portion. In the case of a service provided incident to the service of a physician or nonphysician practitioner, when the person who ordered the service is not supervising, enter the PIN of the supervisor in the shaded portion.
Block 25	Required. Enter the 9-digit federal tax ID (EIN) assigned to that provider (or group), and check the appropriate box. In the case of an unincorporated practice or a sole practitioner, the provider's Social Security number is typically used.
Block 26	Conditionally required. Enter the patient's account number assigned by the provider of service's or supplier's accounting system.
Block 27	Required. PARs and nonPARs accepting assignment should check this box "YES." Failure to complete this box or if the "X" is outside the box means assignment was not accepted. To accept assignment under TRICARE guidelines means that the provider will accept the TRICARE-determined allowed amount as payment in full for services. If a provider does not accept assignment, payment and the EOB go to the beneficiary *only*. The provider would not be given any information on the claim other than receipt. On claims where assignment is not accepted, the provider may collect only up to 115% of the TRICARE-determined allowed amount for the services.
Block 28	Required. Enter total charges for the services (i.e., total of all charges in Block 24f). Use the same formatting as that explained in Block 24 f.

TABLE B-3	Instructions for Filing TRICARE/CHAMPVA Paper Claims—cont'd
Block 29	Required. Enter the amount received by the provider or supplier from OHI. If no payment was made by the primary payer, an EOB should be attached to the claim indicating why the primary payer made no payment. If the primary payer is Medicare or an HMO, an EOB should be attached whether payment was made or not. Any payment received from the beneficiary should not be included in this box. If no payment was received, this block is left blank.
Block 30	Not required. Leave blank.
Block 31	Required. This block must contain the signature of the provider or that of his or her authorized representative and date. If someone other than the provider of services signs on the provider's behalf, there should be a notarized statement on file with the claims processor indicating the provider's permission to accept someone else's signature. This "representative" should sign his or her name and title so as not to be confused with the actual provider.
Block 32	Only report a Service Facility Location NPI when the NPI is different from the Billing Provider NPI.
Block 32a	Enter the NPI of the service facility.
Block 32b	As of May 23, 2007, Block 32b is no longer reported. Follow the specific guidelines of the TRICARE fiscal intermediary.
Block 33	Enter the name, complete address, and telephone number (including area code) of the provider's physical office.
Block 33a	Effective May 23, 2007, the NPI of the billing provider must be reported here.
Block 33b	Effective May 23, 2007, Block 33b is no longer reported.

These instructions are somewhat generic. It is important to use the specific, up-to-date CMS-1500 claims completion instructions of your regional contractor or CHAMPVA claims VA center in Denver, Colorado.

TABLE B-4	Step-by-Step Guidelines for Workers' Compensation Claims
Block 1	"Other" should be checked for workers' compensation claims, unless the claim is for patients who are receiving Black Lung benefits.
Block 1a	Enter the claim number if one has been assigned (check your state's requirements for this block if no claim number has been assigned, or use the patient's Social Security number).
Block 2	Use the same guidelines as with all other carriers.
Block 3	Indicate the patient's 8-digit birth date and sex.
Block 4	The *employer's name* is entered here as the "insured."
Block 5	Use the same guidelines as with all other carriers.
Block 6	Check "OTHER."
Block 7	Enter the address of the insurance company/corporation.
Block 8	Check "EMPLOYED." Consult your local state guidelines regarding whether or not it is necessary to indicate marital status because requirements vary from state to state.
Block 9	For most claims, leave Blocks 9 through 9d blank. If there is a question as to whether or not the injury/illness falls under workers' compensation, enter the applicable information for the patient's other insurance if your state guidelines require this information.
Blocks 9a-d	Leave blank or follow state guidelines.
Block 10a	Check "YES" to indicate that the injury occurred while the patient was on the job.
Blocks 10b-c	Check "NO."
Block 10d	Leave blank.
Blocks 11-11c	Leave blank.
Block 11d	Normally, this is left blank; however, if the workers' compensation case is pending, check with your local state agency's guidelines as to whether or not this box would be checked "YES."

Continued

TABLE B-4	Step-by-Step Guidelines for Workers' Compensation Claims—cont'd
Blocks 12-13	No signature is required.
Block 14	Enter the 6-digit or 8-digit date that the injury occurred or the date on which the illness first was noticed by the patient (this date must coincide with the employer's First Report of Injury and the provider's First Report of Treatment). *Note:* Remember to be consistent with the date format.
Block 15	If a date is documented in the patient's record, indicate it in this block; otherwise, leave blank.
Block 16	Enter the first full day the patient was unable to perform his or her job duties to the first day the patient is back to work (this should be documented in the provider's First Report of Treatment).
Block 17	Enter the name (first name, middle initial, last name) and credentials of the professional who referred, ordered, or supervised the services or supplies on the claim. Do not use periods or commas within the name. A hyphen can be used for hyphenated names. For laboratory and x-ray claims, enter the name of the physician who ordered the diagnostic services.
Blocks 17a-b	If the name of a healthcare professional was reported in 17, enter his or her NPI in 17b. Block 17a is not to be reported after May 23, 2007, unless the payer's or state agency's guidelines say differently.
Block 18	Use the same guidelines as with all other carriers.
Block 19	Leave blank.
Block 20	Use the same guidelines as with all other carriers.
Block 21	Use the same guidelines as with all other carriers.
Blocks 22-23	Leave blank.
Blocks 24a-j	Use the same guidelines as with all other carriers, or consult the appropriate state agency's guidelines.
Block 25	Use the same guidelines as with all other carriers.
Block 26	Use the same guidelines as with all other carriers.
Block 27	Leave blank; this is not applicable because all workers' compensation payments go to the provider.
Block 28	Use the same guidelines as with all other carriers.
Block 29-30	Leave blank.
Block 31	Use the same guidelines as with all other carriers.
Block 32	Key the name and address of the location where services were provided.
Block 32a	Only report a Service Facility Location NPI when the NPI is different from the Billing Provider NPI.
Block 32b	Block 32b is no longer reported after May 23, 2007. Follow the specific guidelines of the applicable workers' compensation carrier.
Block 33	Enter the name, address, Zip Code, and telephone number of the billing provider.
Block 33a	Effective May 23, 2007, the NPI of the billing provider or group must be reported here.
Block 33b	Effective May 23, 2007, Block 33b is no longer reported. Follow the specific guidelines of the applicable workers' compensation carrier.

These instructions are somewhat generic. It is important to use the specific, up-to-date CMS-1500 claims completion instructions of the appropriate workers' compensation address.

UB-04 Claim Form and Completion Instructions

Access the following website to download instructions and keep up-to-date on Medicare's guidelines for completing the UB-04 http://www.ub04.net/downloads/Medicare_Pub_Ch_25.pdf

1 Iowa Mercy	2		3a PAT. CNTL # KELSEY		4 TYPE OF BILL
4461 Kers Mill			b. MED. REC. # KELSEY		
Springfield KY 12345			5 FED. TAX NO. 3664021CC	6 STATEMENT COVERS PERIOD FROM THROUGH	7

8 PATIENT NAME a Jones, Ron	9 PATIENT ADDRESS a 6161 Briarwood				
b	b Springfield			c KY d 12345	e

10 BIRTHDATE	11 SEX	12 DATE	ADMISSION 13 HR 14 TYPE 15 SRC	16 DHR	17 STAT	18 19 20 21	CONDITION CODES 22 23 24 25 26 27 28	29 ACDT STATE	30
03251975	M								

31 OCCURRENCE CODE DATE	32 OCCURRENCE CODE DATE	33 OCCURRENCE CODE DATE	34 OCCURRENCE CODE DATE	35 OCCURRENCE SPAN CODE FROM THROUGH	36 OCCURRENCE SPAN CODE FROM THROUGH	37

38 Ronald Jones
      6161 Briarwood
      Springfield, KY 12345

39 CODE VALUE CODES AMOUNT	40 CODE VALUE CODES AMOUNT	41 CODE VALUE CODES AMOUNT
a		
b		
c		
d		

42 REV. CD	43 DESCRIPTION	44 HCPCS/RATE/HIPPS CODE	45 SERV. DATE	46 SERV. UNITS	47 TOTAL CHARGES	48 NON-COVERED CHARGES	49	
1	EMERGENCY DEPT VISIT, 3 KEY CO		0709XX	1.00	66 23			1
2								2
3								3
4								4
5								5
6								6
7								7
8								8
9								9
10								10
11								11
12								12
13								13
14								14
15								15
16								16
17								17
18								18
19								19
20								20
21								21
22								22
23	PAGE 1 OF 1	CREATION DATE 0709XX TOTALS ➡			66 23			23

50 PAYER NAME	51 HEALTH PLAN ID	52 REL. INFO	53 ASG. BEN.	54 PRIOR PAYMENTS	55 EST. AMOUNT DUE	56 NPI	
A XYZ Insurance		Y	Y				A
B						57 OTHER	B
C						PRV ID	C

58 INSURED'S NAME	59 P. REL	60 INURED'S UNIQUE ID	61 GROUP NAME	62 INSURANCE GROUP NO.	
A Ronald Jones	01	999-00-5432		8503Y	A
B					B
C					C

63 TREATMENT AUTHORIZATION CODES	64 DOCUMENT CONTROL NUMBER	65 EMPLOYER NAME	
A			A
B			B
C			C

66 DX 723.1	A	B	C	D	E	F	G	H	68
	I	J	K	L	M	N	O	P	Q

69 ADMIT DX	70 PATIENT REASON DX a b c	71 PPS CODE	72 ECI	73

74 PRINCIPAL PROCEDURE CODE DATE	a OTHER PROCEDURE CODE DATE	b OTHER PROCEDURE CODE DATE	76 ATTENDING NPI 67805027	QUAL
c OTHER PROCEDURE CODE DATE	d OTHER PROCEDURE CODE DATE	e OTHER PROCEDURE CODE DATE	LAST Cardi, MD	FIRST Perry
			77 OPERATING NPI	QUAL

80 REMARKS	81CC a		76 ...

77 OPERATING	NPI		QUAL
	LAST		FIRST
78 OTHER	NPI		QUAL
	LAST		FIRST
79 OTHER	NPI		QUAL
	LAST		FIRST

UB-04 CMS-1450   APPROVED OMB NO.   THE CERTIFICATIONS ON THE REVERSE APPLY TO THIS BILL AND ARE MADE A PART HEREOF.

Fig. C-1 Completed UB-04 claim form for a Medicare Part A patient.

Completion guidelines for the UB-04 may differ slightly from state to state or carrier to carrier. An example of a 2012 claims completion guidelines for the UB-04 form can be accessed using the following website: http://www.idmedicaid.com

| TABLE C-1 | UB-04 Claim Form Completion Guidelines |

UB-04 FIELD	INSTRUCTIONS
1	*(Untitled) Provider Name, Address, and Telephone Number*—Required. Enter the provider name, city, state, and Zip Code. The post office box number or street name and number may be included. Phone or fax number or both are desired.
2	*(Untitled) Pay-To Name, Address, and Secondary Identification Fields*—Required when the pay-to name and address information is different than the billing provider information in FL 1. If used, the minimum entry is the provider name, address, city, state, and Zip Code.
3a	*Patient Control Number*—Enter the patient's alphanumeric control number if assigned and required for reference purposes.
3b	*Medical/Health Record Number*—Enter the number assigned to the patient's medical/health record by the provider.
4	*Type of Bill*—Required. Follow Medicare guidelines to complete this field.
5	*Federal Tax Number*—Required. Enter the provider of service Federal Tax ID (EIN).
6	*Statement Covers Period (From-Through)*—Required. Enter the beginning and ending dates of service.
7	*Untitled*—Not used.
8a	*Patient's Name (Last Name, First Name, Middle Initial)*—Required. Enter the patient's last name, first name, and middle initial, if any, as it appears on the Sterling card.
8b	*(Untitled) Patient ID*—Enter the patient ID if different than the subscriber/insured's ID.
9	*Patient's Address*—Required. Enter the patient's full mailing address including street number and name, post office box number or RFD, city, state, and Zip Code.
10	*Patient Birth Date*—Required. Enter the patient's birth date.
11	*Patient Sex*—Required. Enter "M" for male or "F" for female.
12	*Admission/Start of Care Date*—Required for inpatient, SNF, and home health. Enter the date the patient was admitted for care or start of care.
13	*Admission Hour*—Not required.
14	*Type of Admission/Visit*—Required for inpatient and SNF. Enter the code indicating priority of admission according to Medicare guidelines.
15	*Source of Admission*—Required for inpatient and outpatient. Enter the code indicating the source of admission according to Medicare guidelines.
16	*Discharge Hour*—Not required.
17	*Patient Status*—Required for all inpatient, SNF, home health, and outpatient hospital services. Follow Medicare guidelines to complete this field.
18	*Condition Codes*—Conditional. Follow Medicare guidelines to complete this field.
19	*Condition Codes*—Conditional. Follow Medicare guidelines to complete this field.
20	*Condition Codes*—Conditional. Follow Medicare guidelines to complete this field.
21	*Condition Codes*—Conditional. Follow Medicare guidelines to complete this field.
22	*Condition Codes*—Conditional. Follow Medicare guidelines to complete this field.
23	*Condition Codes*—Conditional. Follow Medicare guidelines to complete this field.
24	*Condition Codes*—Conditional. Follow Medicare guidelines to complete this field.
25	*Condition Codes*—Conditional. Follow Medicare guidelines to complete this field.
26	*Condition Codes*—Conditional. Follow Medicare guidelines to complete this field.
27	*Condition Codes*—Conditional. Follow Medicare guidelines to complete this field.
28	*Condition Codes*—Conditional. Follow Medicare guidelines to complete this field.
29	*Accident State*—Not used.

Continued

TABLE C-1	UB-04 Claim Form Completion Guidelines—cont'd
UB-04 FIELD	**INSTRUCTIONS**
30	*Untitled*—Not used.
31	*Occurrence Codes and Dates*—Conditional. Follow Medicare guidelines to complete these fields.
32	*Occurrence Codes and Dates*—Conditional. Follow Medicare guidelines to complete these fields.
33	*Occurrence Codes and Dates*—Conditional. Follow Medicare guidelines to complete these fields.
34	*Occurrence Codes and Dates*—Conditional. Follow Medicare guidelines to complete these fields.
35	*Occurrence Span Code and Dates*—Conditional. Follow Medicare guidelines to complete these fields.
36	*Occurrence Span Code and Dates*—Conditional. Follow Medicare guidelines to complete these fields.
37	*Untitled*—Not used.
38	*Responsible Party Name/Address*—Not required.
39	*Value Codes and Amounts*—Conditional. Follow Medicare guidelines to complete these fields.
40	*Value Codes and Amounts*—Conditional. Follow Medicare guidelines to complete these fields.
41	*Value Codes and Amounts*—Conditional. Follow Medicare guidelines to complete these fields.
42	*Revenue Codes*—Required. Enter the appropriate revenue codes to identify specific accommodation or ancillary charges or both.
43	*Revenue Description*—Enter a narrative description or abbreviation for each corresponding revenue code.
44	*HCPCS/Rates/HIPPS/Rate Codes*—Conditional. Report HCPCS where required for Medicare billing. On inpatient hospital bills, the accommodation rate is shown here. HIPPS rate code is reported here.
45	*Service Date*—Conditional. Report service dates where required for Medicare billing.
46	*Units of Service*—Required. Enter the number of days, visits, procedures, or tests as applicable for the corresponding service in accordance with Medicare guidelines.
47	*Total Charges*—Enter the charge for each listed service.
48	*Noncovered Charges*—Enter the total noncovered charges pertaining to the corresponding revenue code.
49	*Untitled*—Not used.
50	*Payer Identification*—Required. Enter "Sterling Life Insurance" on line A if Sterling Option I, Sterling Option II, or Sterling—Partners—Montana has been identified as the primary payer.
51	*Health Plan ID*—Enter the national health plan identifier when one is established.
52	*Release of Information Certification Indicator*—Required. A "Y" should be entered to indicate a signed statement permitting release of data to other organizations has been received from the patient to adjudicate the claim.
53	*Assignment of Benefits Certification Indicator*—Not used.
54	*Prior Payments*—Enter the total amount the patient paid on covered services only.
55	*Estimated Amount Due from Patient*—Not used.
56	*National Provider ID (NPI)*— Required, effective May 23, 2007.
57	*Other Provider ID*—Use this field to report other provider identifiers as assigned by a health plan (legacy number) before May 23, 2007.
58	*Insured's Name*—Required. Enter the patient's name as it appears on the Sterling card in accordance with Medicare guidelines.
59	*Patient's Relationship to Insured*—Enter "18" (Self) for all Sterling patients.
60	*Insured's Unique ID*—Required. Enter the patient's ID number as it appears on the Sterling card. Starts with an "N …."
61	*Insurance Group Name*—Enter the plan that is on the Sterling Card: Sterling Option I, Sterling Option II, or Sterling—Partners—Montana.
62	*Insurance Group Number*—Not required.

TABLE C-1	UB-04 Claim Form Completion Guidelines—cont'd
UB-04 FIELD	**INSTRUCTIONS**
63	*Treatment Authorization Code*—Follow Medicare guidelines to complete this field.
64	*Document Control Number (DCN)*— Follow Medicare guidelines to complete this field.
65	*Employer Name*—Follow Medicare guidelines to complete this field.
66	*Diagnosis and Procedure Code Qualifier (ICD Version Indicator)*—Follow Medicare guidelines to complete this field.
67	*Principal Diagnosis Code*—Required for inpatient and outpatient hospital services. Enter the patient's diagnosis/condition according to Medicare guidelines. Report diagnosis to the highest level of specificity.
67a-67q	*Other Diagnosis Codes*—Conditional. Enter up to 8 other diagnoses that coexisted in addition to the principal diagnosis as an additional or secondary diagnosis. Report diagnoses to the highest level of specificity. Sterling will ignore data submitted in 67i-67q.
68	*Untitled*—Not used.
69	*Admitting Diagnosis*—Required for inpatient and selective outpatient hospital services. Enter the patient's diagnosis/condition according to Medicare guidelines. Report diagnosis to the highest level of specificity.
70a-70c	*Patient's Reason for Visit*—Not used.
71	*Prospective Payment System (PPS) Code*—Not used.
72	*External Cause of Injury (ECI) Code*—Not used.
73	*Untitled*—Not used.
74	*Principal Procedure Code and Date*—Required for inpatient. Enter the principal procedure code and corresponding date according to Medicare guidelines. Report the full ICD-10-PCS procedure code, including all required digits where applicable.
74a-74e	*Other Procedure Codes and Dates*—Required for inpatient. Enter up to 5 significant procedures other than the principal procedure and corresponding dates according to Medicare guidelines. Report the full ICD-10-PCSprocedure code, including all required digits where applicable.
75	*Untitled*—Not used.
76	*Attending Provider Name and Identifiers (Including NPI)*—Required. Enter the NPI and name of the attending physician on inpatient bills or the physician who requested the outpatient services.
77	*Operating Provider Name and Identifiers (Including NPI)*—Not used.
78 and 79	*Other Provider Name and Identifiers (Including NPI)*—Not used.
80	*Remarks*—Enter any remarks needed to provide information that is necessary for payment but not provided elsewhere on the claim.
81	*Code-Code Field*—Required. Providers submitting claims for their primary facility and its subparts report their taxonomy code on all their claims submitted. The taxonomy code assists in crosswalking from the NPI of the provider to each of its subparts when a provider has chosen not to apply for a unique national provider number for those subparts individually.

Glossary

7th character – Certain ICD-10-CM categories require an extension to provide further specificity about the condition being coded. The applicable 7th character is required for all codes within the category or as the notes indicate in the Tabular instructions. This extension may be a number or letter and must always be the 7th character. If a code that requires a 7th character is not 6 characters long, a placeholder "X" must be used to fill in the empty characters.

72-hour rule – Rule, part of Medicare's prospective payment system, that states that all services provided for Medicare patients within 72 hours of hospital admission are considered part of the inpatient services and are to be billed on one claim.

A

abandoning – Ceasing to provide care.

abuse – Improper or harmful procedures or methods of doing business that are contradictory to accepted business practices.

acceptance – When the insurance company agrees to accept the individual for benefits coverage, or when the policy is issued.

accepting assignment – Process wherein healthcare providers agree to accept the amount paid by the carrier as payment in full (after the patient satisfies his or her cost-sharing responsibilities as outlined in the insurance policy).

accountability – Responsibility the healthcare profession has to patients so that a feeling of confidence exists between patient and provider.

Accountable Care Organization (ACO) – Network of physicians and hospitals that works together and accepts collective responsibility for the cost and quality of care delivered to a specific number of Medicare beneficiaries for a minimum of at least 3 years; similar to a health maintenance organization (HMO).

accounts receivable – Total amount of money owed from all patient ledgers.

accounts receivable aging report – Report showing how long invoices, or patient accounts, have been outstanding, typically illustrated using variable periods (e.g., 30 days, 60 days).

accreditation – Voluntary process through which an organization is able to measure the quality of its services and performance against nationally recognized standards. Accreditation is the process by which a private or public agency evaluates and recognizes (certifies) an institution as fulfilling applicable standards.

Accreditation Association for Ambulatory Health Care (AAAHC) – Formed in 1979 to help ambulatory healthcare organizations improve the quality of care provided to patients. An accreditation decision is based on a careful and reasonable assessment of an organization's compliance with applicable standards and adherence to the policies and procedures of the AAAHC.

activities of daily living (ADLs) – Behaviors related to personal care that typically include bathing, dressing, eating, toileting, getting in or out of a bed or a chair, and walking.

actuarial value – Percentage of total average costs for covered benefits that a plan covers.

acute care – Involves assessing and treating sudden or unexpected injuries and illnesses.

acute care facility – Facility that is equipped and staffed to respond immediately to a critical situation.

acute condition – When a patient's medical state becomes unstable.

adjudicated – How a decision was made regarding the payment of an insurance claim.

adjudication – Process of a carrier reviewing a claim and deciding on its payment.

administrative services organization (ASO) – Organization that provides a wide variety of health insurance administrative services for groups that have chosen to self-fund their health benefits.

Administrative Simplification and Compliance Act (ASCA) – Act under the Health Insurance Portability and Accountability Act (HIPAA) that requires health plans and healthcare clearinghouses to use certain standard transaction formats and code sets for the electronic transmission of health information.

advance beneficiary notice (ABN) – Form that Medicare requires all healthcare providers to use when Medicare does not pay for a service. Patients must sign the form to acknowledge that they understand they have a choice about their healthcare in the event that Medicare does not pay.

allowable charges – Fees Medicare allows for a particular service or supply.

alternate billing cycle – Billing system that incorporates the mailing of a partial group of statements at spaced intervals during the month.

ambulatory payment classification (APC) – Service classification system that the Centers for Medicare and Medicaid Services (CMS) developed for facility reimbursement of hospital outpatient services. It is intended to simplify the outpatient hospital payment system, ensure the payment is adequate to compensate hospital costs, and implement deficit-reduction goals of the CMS.

ambulatory surgery centers (ASCs) – Facilities where surgeries are performed that do not require hospital admission. ASCs provide a cost-effective and convenient environment that may be less stressful than what many hospitals offer.

Americans with Disabilities Act (ADA) – Act that protects the civil rights of individuals with disabilities. Equal opportunity provisions pertain to employment, public accommodation, transportation, state and local government services, and telecommunications.

ancillary – Staff members of the medical team including nurses, medical assistants, health insurance professionals, and technicians.

appeal(s) – To request or petition that a decision be re-examined. Medicare regulations allow providers and beneficiaries who are dissatisfied with a Medicare determination (of a fee-for-service claim) to request that the determination be reconsidered through the appeals process.

application (skills) – Ability to use computer hardware and software including Windows and Microsoft Word (or similar word-processing software) and the ability to use the Internet.

ASCII (American Standard Code for Information Interchange) – Most common format used for text files in computers and on the Internet.

assign benefits – When a patient affixes his or her signature to a document that states that the patient agrees to have the insurance carrier pay benefits directly to the healthcare provider. This also can be done by signing Block 13 of the CMS-1500 claim form.

assignment of benefits – Arrangement by which a patient requests that his or her health insurance benefit payments be made directly to a designated person or facility such as a physician or a hospital.

autonomy – Working without direct supervision; having the flexibility of choices. In health insurance, the freedom to choose what medical expenses would be covered.

average length of stay (ALOS) – Predetermined number of days of approved hospital stay assigned to an individual diagnosis-related group.

B

balance billing – Practice of billing patients for any balance left after deductibles, coinsurance, and insurance payments have been made.

basic health insurance – Insurance that includes hospital room and board and inpatient hospital care, some hospital services and supplies such as x-ray studies and medicine, surgery, and some physician visits.

beneficiary – Individual who has health insurance through the Medicare, Medicaid, or TRICARE programs.

Beneficiary Complaint Response Program – Program that handles complaints by Medicare beneficiaries (or their representatives) made either in writing or by telephone. A case manager is assigned to work with the beneficiary from start to finish, keeping the beneficiary informed throughout the review process about the status of the complaint.

Beneficiary Notices Initiative – Medicare beneficiaries and providers have certain rights and protections related to financial liability under the fee-for-service (FFS) Medicare and Medicare Advantage (MA) programs. These financial liability and appeal rights and protections are communicated to beneficiaries through notices given by providers.

benefit cap – Maximum benefit amount paid for any one incident or any one year.

benefit period – Duration of time during which a Medicare beneficiary is eligible for Part A benefits for services incurred in a hospital or a skilled nursing facility (SNF) or both. A benefit period begins the day an individual is admitted to a hospital or SNF and ends when the beneficiary has not received care in a hospital or SNF for 60 consecutive days.

billing compliance – Following a specific set of rules and regulations in the gathering of complete and accurate information leading to patient billing and the claims development process.

billing cycle – The period when medical offices send statements to patients, usually every 30 days.

billing services – Companies that offer services to healthcare facilities including billing processes and claims filing. Many billing services take on the responsibility of keeping up with rapidly changing Medicare and other healthcare-related laws.

binds – When the insurance company agrees to accept the individual for benefits.

biological – Drugs or medicinal preparations obtained from animal tissue or other organic sources.

birthday rule – Informal procedure used in the health insurance industry to help determine which health plan is considered "primary," when individuals (usually children) are listed as dependents on more than one health plan. The health plan of the parent whose birthday comes first in the calendar year would be considered the primary plan.

Black Lung Benefits Act – Act that provides compensation for miners with black lung (pneumoconiosis). This act requires liable mine operators to award disability payments and establishes a fund administered by the Secretary of Labor that provides disability payments to miners when the mine operator is unknown or unable to pay.

BlueCard Program – Program that links independent Blue Plans so that members and their families can obtain healthcare services while traveling or working anywhere in the United States, receiving the same benefits they would receive if they were at home.

BlueCard Worldwide – Provides Blue Plan members inpatient and outpatient coverage at no additional cost in more than 200 foreign countries. Hospitals participating in BlueCard Worldwide are located in major travel destinations and business centers around the world.

Blue Cross and Blue Shield Federal Employee Program (FEP) – Program that provides coverage for several million federal government employees, retirees, and their dependents.

Blue Cross and Blue Shield member hospitals – Hospitals that have contracted as participating providers with the Blue Cross and Blue Shield Association member organization. Member hospitals must accept the Blue Cross and Blue Shield allowable fee as payment in full and cannot bill the patient for any remaining charges after the initial deductible and copayment are met.

breach of confidentiality – When confidential information is disclosed to a third party without patient consent or court order.

budget period – Almost any medical bills that the applicant or the applicant's family still owes or that were paid in the months for which Medicaid is sought.

business associate – Defined by the Health Insurance Portability and Accountability Act (HIPAA) as an individual or corporate "person" who performs on behalf of the covered entity any function or activity involving the use or disclosure of protected health information and is not a member of the workforce of the covered entity.

C

cafeteria plan – Type of plan that deducts the cost of the plan (premium) from the employee's wages before withholding taxes are deducted, allowing employees the option of pretax payroll deduction for some insurance premiums, unreimbursed medical expenses, and child or dependent care expenses.

capitation – Common method of reimbursement used primarily by health maintenance organizations in which the provider or medical facility is paid a fixed, per capita amount for each individual enrolled in the plan, regardless of how many or few services the patient uses.

carriers – Claims processors that apply Medicare coverage rules to determine the appropriateness and medical necessity of claims. Also called fiscal intermediaries.

carve out – Eliminating a certain specialty of health services from coverage under the healthcare policy.

case mix adjustment – Reported data that include patient demographic information such as age, sex, county of residence, and race/ethnicity; diagnostic information; treatment information; disposition; total charges; and expected source of payment.

casual employee – Employee who is not entitled to paid holiday or sick leave, has no expectation of ongoing employment, and for whom each engagement with the employer constitutes a separate contract of employment. Casual employees often receive a higher rate of pay to compensate for a lack of job security and benefits.

catastrophic cap (cat cap) – Maximum cost limit placed on covered medical bills under TRICARE. The cat cap is the monetary limit that a family of an active duty member would have to pay in any given year.

categorically needy – Typically used to describe low-income families with children; individuals receiving Supplemental Security Income; pregnant women, infants, and children with incomes less than a specified percent of the federal poverty level; and Qualified Medicare Beneficiaries.

category – Codes in the tabular section of Current Procedural Terminology (CPT) are formatted using four classifications: section, subsection, subheading, and category. "Category" is the most definitive classification and aids in selecting the applicable code.

Category III codes – Established by the American Medical Association as a set of temporary CPT codes for emerging technologies, services, and procedures where data collection is necessary to substantiate widespread use or for the U.S. Food and Drug Administration approval process.

Centers for Medicare and Medicaid Services (CMS) – An agency within the US Department of Health & Human Services responsible for administration of Medicare (the federal health insurance program for seniors) and Medicaid (the federal needs-based program). CMS also oversees the Children's Health Insurance Program (CHIP), the Health Insurance Portability and Accountability Act (HIPAA) and the Clinical Laboratory Improvement Amendments (CLIA), among other services.

certification – Culmination of a process of formal recognition of the competence possessed by an individual.

CHAMPUS Maximum Allowable Charge – TRICARE allowable charge. The amount on which TRICARE figures a beneficiary's cost-share (coinsurance) for covered charges.

CHAMPVA for Life (CFL) – Benefits for covered medical services designed for spouses or dependents of veterans who are age 65 or older and enrolled in Medicare Parts A and B. The benefit is payable after Medicare pays its share.

charge description master (CDM) – Listing of every type of procedure and service the hospital can provide to patients including procedures, pharmaceuticals, supplies, and room charges. CDMs help make the billing process run more smoothly and accurately.

chief complaint (CC) – The reason why the patient is seeing the physician. Also called presenting problem.

Children's Health Insurance Program (CHIP) – Enacted as part of the Balanced Budget Act of 1997, CHIP provides federal matching funds for states to implement health insurance programs for children in families that earn too much to qualify for Medicaid but too little to afford private health coverage reasonably.

Civilian Health and Medical Program of the Department of Veterans Affairs (CHAMPVA) – Healthcare benefits program for qualifying dependents and survivors of veterans, whereby the Department of Veterans Affairs (VA) shares the cost of covered healthcare services and supplies with eligible beneficiaries. There is no cost to beneficiaries when they receive healthcare treatment at a VA facility.

Civilian Health and Medical Program of the Uniformed Services (CHAMPUS) – Military healthcare program that existed for more than 30 years until it was replaced with TRICARE in 1998.

claims adjustment reason codes – Codes that detail the reason why an adjustment was made to a healthcare claim payment by the payer. These codes are used in the electronic remittance advice and the standard paper remittance advice.

claims clearinghouse – Company that receives claims from different healthcare providers and specializes in consolidating the claims so that they can send one transmission containing batches of claims to each third-party payer. A clearinghouse is typically an independent, centralized service available to healthcare providers for the purpose of simplifying medical insurance claims submission for multiple carriers.

claims processor – Facility that handles TRICARE claims for healthcare received within a particular state or region.

clean claims – Claims that can be processed for payment quickly without being returned, when all of the information necessary for processing the claim has been entered on the claim form, and the information is correct.

clearinghouse – Business entity that specializes in consolidating claims received from providers and transmitting them in batches to each respective third-party payer.

Clinical Laboratory Improvement Act (CLIA) – Program that Congress established in 1988 to regulate quality standards for all laboratory testing done on humans to ensure the safety, accuracy, reliability, and timeliness of patient test results regardless of where the test was performed.

closed panel HMO – Multispecialty group practice in which other healthcare providers in the community generally cannot participate.

CMS-1500 claim form – Standard insurance form used by all government and most commercial insurance payers.

code – In healthcare, a group of numbers or a combination of alphanumeric characters or both used to provide uniform identification of a disease, disorder, symptom, morbidity, and mortality and a medical procedure.

code sets – Data elements used to document uniformly the reasons why patients are seen and the procedures or services or both provided to them during their healthcare encounters.

coinsurance – Type of cost sharing between the insurance provider and the policyholder. After the deductible has been met, the insurance provider pays a certain percentage of the bill and the policyholder pays the remaining percentage.

collection agency – Organization that obtains or arranges for payment of money owed to a third party.

collection ratio – Total amount collected divided by the total amount charged.

combination code – A single code that is used when more than one otherwise individually classified disease is combined with another disease and one code is assigned for both, or when a single code is used to describe conditions that frequently occur together used to classify two diagnoses, a diagnosis with an associated secondary process (manifestation), or a diagnosis with an associated complication.

coming and going rule – Rule that coverage for injuries sustained while an employee is commuting to and from work is generally excluded by most state workers' compensation laws.

commercial health insurance – Any kind of health insurance paid for by somebody other than the government. Also called private health insurance.

communication – Sending and receiving of information through mutually understood speech, writing, or signs.

comorbidity – Presence of more than one disease or disorder that occurs in an individual at the same time.

competency – In the eyes of the law, parties must be mentally capable and of proper age when entering into a contractual agreement.

comprehension – Understanding the meaning (of what you have read).

comprehensive insurance – See comprehensive plan.

comprehensive plan – Type of policy that combines basic and major medical coverage into one plan.

concurrent care – When a patient receives similar services (e.g., hospital visits) by more than one healthcare provider on the same day.

confidentiality – Foundation for trust in the patient-provider relationship that concerns the communication of private and personal information from one individual to another.

consideration – Binding force in any contract that gives it legal status; the object of value that each party gives to the other.

Consolidated Omnibus Budget Reconciliation Act (COBRA) – Law passed by Congress in 1986 that gives workers who lose their health insurance benefits and their dependents the right to continue group coverage temporarily under the same group health plan sponsored by their employer in certain instances where coverage under the plan would otherwise end.

consultation – When the primary care provider sends a patient to another provider, usually a specialist, for the purpose of the consulting physician rendering his or her expert opinion regarding the patient's condition. The primary care provider does not relinquish the care of the patient to the consulting provider.

contractual write-off – When the provider agrees, through a contractual agreement, not to be paid the remaining amount of a fee after the patient has paid his or her deductible and coinsurance and all third-party payers have paid their share.

contraindication – Issue that makes a certain medical treatment or procedure inadvisable.

convention(s) – In healthcare coding, general rules and instructional notes for use of the classification independent of the guidelines

coordination of benefits (COB) – When a patient and spouse (or parent) are covered under two separate employer group policies, the total benefits an insured can receive from both group plans are limited to no more than 100% of the allowable expenses, preventing the policyholder(s) from making a profit on health insurance claims. The primary plan pays benefits up to its limit, and the secondary plan pays the difference, up to its limit.

coordination of benefits contractor – Individual who ensures that the information on the Medicare eligibility database regarding other health insurance primary to Medicare is up-to-date and accurate.

copayment – Amount of money the patient has to pay out of his or her own pocket.

correct code initiative – Part of the National Correct Coding Initiative to develop correct coding methods for the Centers for Medicare and Medicaid Services (CMS). It is intended to reduce overpayments that result from improper coding.

cost avoid(ance) – Healthcare provider bills and collects from liable third parties before sending the claim to Medicaid.

cost outliers – Atypical patients whose hospital stays are considerably shorter or longer than average.

cost sharing (share of cost) – Situation where insured individuals pay a portion of the healthcare costs, such as deductibles, coinsurance, or copayment amounts.

counseling – Service provided to the patient and his or her family that involves impressions and recommended diagnostic studies, discussion of diagnostic results, prognosis, risks and benefits of treatment, and instructions.

countable income – Amount of income left over after eliminating all items that are not considered income and applying all appropriate exclusions to the items that are considered income.

covered charges – Allowed services, supplies, and procedures for which Medicare and TRICARE (and most other insurers) would pay. Covered charges include medical and psychological services and supplies that are considered appropriate care and are generally accepted by qualified professionals to be reasonable and adequate for the diagnosis and treatment of illness, injury, pregnancy, or mental disorders or for well-child care.

covered entity – Health plan, healthcare clearinghouse, or healthcare provider who transmits any health information in electronic form in connection with a transaction.

covered expenses – Charges incurred that qualify for reimbursement under the terms of the policy contract.

CPT-5 – Ongoing project by the American Medical Association to make improvements in the structure and processes of Current Procedural Terminology (CPT) codes to reflect the coding demands of the current healthcare system and to address challenges presented by the Health Insurance Portability and Accountability Act (HIPAA).

credible coverage – Basic benefits offered by the Medicare Part D Prescription Drug Plan. A Medicare beneficiary who does not choose to enroll in a Part D Plan must acquire a "certificate of credible coverage" to avoid a penalty if he or she decides to sign up after the open-enrollment period.

critical care – Constant attention (either at bedside or immediately available) by a physician in a medical crisis.

custodial care – Nonmedical care that helps individuals with activities of daily living (bathing dressing, toileting, preparation of special diets, and self-administration of medication) that does not require constant attention of specially trained medical personnel.

D

daily journal – Chronologic record of all patient transactions including previous balances, charges, payments, and current balances for that day. Also called a day sheet.

deductible – Certain amount of money that the patient must pay each year toward his or her medical expenses before health insurance benefits begin.

default code – Code listed next to a main term in the ICD-10-CM Index representing the condition most commonly associated with the main term or the unspecified code for the condition.

defendant – Party being sued in a lawsuit.

Defense Enrollment Eligibility Reporting System (DEERS) – Computerized data bank that lists all active and retired military service members. The data bank is checked before processing claims to ensure that patients are eligible for TRICARE benefits.

de-identified – When identifiable elements are removed from information that could be linked to a particular individual.

demand bills – Under Medicare rules, a beneficiary, on receiving notification of noncoverage, has the right to request that a fiscal intermediary review that determination.

demographic information – Information such as name, address, Social Security number, and employment.

denial notice – Explanation that a local coverage decision does not cover a certain item or service.

diagnosis – Determination of the nature of a cause of disease; the art of distinguishing one disease from another.

diagnosis-related group (DRG) – System of classifying hospital inpatient cases into categories with similar use of the facility's resources. Under this system, a hospital is paid a predetermined lump sum amount, regardless of the costs involved, for each Medicare patient treated and discharged.

dial-up(s) – Form of Internet access to establish a dialed connection to an Internet service provider (ISP) via telephone lines.

diligence – Persistence; the ability to stick with a task until it is finished.

direct claim submission – Submitting claims directly to an insurance carrier. Also called direct data entry (DDE) claims.

direct contract model – Health maintenance organization (HMO) similar to an individual practice association except that the HMO contracts directly with the individual physicians. The HMO recruits a variety of community healthcare providers—primary care and specialists.

direct data entry (DDE) claims – Claims that are submitted directly to an insurance carrier.

disability income insurance – Form of health insurance that replaces a portion of earned income when an individual is unable to perform the requirements of his or her job because of injury or illness that is not work related.

disability insurance – Type of insurance that provides a stated weekly or monthly payment for lost income resulting from accidents or sickness or both that are not work related.

disbursements journal – Listing of all expenses paid out to vendors such as building rent, office supplies, and salaries.

discounted fee-for-service – When a healthcare provider offers services at rates that are lower than the usual, customary, and reasonable fees.

disproportionate share – Payment adjustment to compensate hospitals for the higher operating costs they incur in treating a large share of low-income patients.

disproportionate share hospitals – Facilities that receive additional payments to ensure that communities have access to certain high-cost services such as trauma and emergency care and burn services.

donut hole – Officially referred to as the Medicare Part D coverage gap, the donut hole is the difference between the initial coverage limit and the catastrophic coverage threshold. After a Medicare beneficiary exceeds the prescription drug coverage limit, he or she is financially responsible for the entire cost of prescription drugs until the expense reaches the catastrophic coverage threshold.

downcoding – When claims are submitted with outdated, deleted, or nonexistent Current Procedural Terminology (CPT) codes, and the payer assigns a substitute code it thinks best fits the services performed, resulting in a decreased payment. Also, downcoding can result when Evaluation and Management service levels do not match up with diagnostic codes.

DRG grouper – A computer software program that takes the coded information and identifies the patient's diagnosis-related group (DRG) category.

dual coverage (Medi-Medi) – When aged or disabled (or both) individuals who are very poor are covered under the Medicaid and Medicare programs, these individuals may receive Medicare services for which they are entitled and other services available under that state's Medicaid program.

dual eligibles – Patients who are eligible for Medicaid and Medicare coverage. See dual coverage (Medi-Medi).

durable power of attorney – Relative (or other person) who has been named as an agent to handle the patient's affairs if the patient becomes incapacitated.

E

E codes – ICD-9-CM codes that begin with the letter "E" and describe the circumstance causing an injury, not the nature of the injury, and therefore should not be used as a principal diagnosis. Supplementary Classification of External Causes of Injury and Poisoning - E800 to E999.

Early and Periodic Screening, Diagnosis, and Treatment (EPSDT) program – Child health component of Medicaid developed to fit the standards of pediatric care and to meet the special physical, emotional, and developmental needs of low-income children.

earned income – Income from employment.

egregious – Conspicuously negligent.

electronic claims clearinghouse – Business entity that receives claims from several medical facilities and consolidates these claims so that one transmission containing multiple claims can be sent to each insurance carrier. A clearinghouse serves as an intermediary between medical practices and insurance companies, facilitating the electronic exchange of information between the facilities.

electronic claims submission (ECS) – Process that allows providers to use computers and applicable software programs to submit claims to a central location such as a clearinghouse via a Web interface. The Web interface sends the claims to the carrier system for processing.

electronic data interchange (EDI) – Electronic transfer of information in a standard format between two entities. EDI allows business entities to exchange information and transact business in a rapid and cost-effective way.

electronic funds transfer (EFT) – System wherein money is moved electronically between accounts or organizations. In the case of insurance claims, when claims are submitted electronically, many carriers transfer the payments directly into the provider's bank account rather than mailing a check, making the funds instantly usable.

electronic media claim (EMC) – Instead of filing a claim on a paper claim form, claim information is entered into a computer and electronically transferred to a computer system (e.g., using a modem and a telephone line).

electronic medical record (EMR) – Electronic file wherein patients' health information is stored in a computer system. Synonymous terms for an EMR include electronic patient record, electronic health record, and computerized patient record.

electronic protected health information (e-PHI) – Identifiable health information that is protected under the HIPAA Privacy Rule in electronic form.

electronic remittance advice (ERA) – One of several different types of electronic formats rather than a paper document. Payments can be posted automatically to patient accounts, allowing the health insurance professional to update accounts receivable much more quickly and accurately than if he or she had to post the payments manually.

electronic remittance notice (ERN) – Electronic data file commonly referred to as the "835" that can be downloaded into a biller's computer via a modem. The 835 shows claims that have been paid with the dollar amounts and shows claims denied with the reason for denial.

emancipated minor – Individual older than 16 years and younger than 18 years who is living separate and apart from his or her parents and not receiving any financial support from them (except by court order or benefits to which the youth is entitled [i.e., Social Security]); living beyond the parent's custody and control; and not in foster care.

emergency care – Care given in a hospital emergency department.

Emergency Medical Treatment and Labor Act (EMTLA) – Act that requires any hospital to respond to a person's emergent medical condition by determining the nature of the condition. If an emergent condition exists, it must be treated to the best of the facility's ability regardless of ability to pay. Patients may be transferred as appropriate after stabilization of the condition.

emergent medical condition – Onset of a health condition that requires immediate medical attention.

Employee Retirement Income Security Act of 1974 (ERISA) – Federal law that sets minimum standards for pension plans in private industry, which is how most self-insured employers fund their programs.

employer identification number (EIN) – Nine-digit number assigned to employers by the Internal Revenue Service. Business entities that pay wages to one or more employees are required to have an EIN as their taxpayer identifying number.

employment network – Public agency or private organization that has agreed to provide services under the Ticket to Work program guidelines.

encounter form – Multipurpose billing form used by most providers that can be customized to medical specialties and preprinted with more common diagnoses and procedures. Also called a superbill, routing form, or patient service slip.

end-stage renal disease (ESRD) – Permanent kidney disorders requiring dialysis or transplant.

enrollees – Individuals who are covered under a managed care plan.

enrollment process – Process through which medical offices usually must go before they can submit claims. The process typically involves completing and returning electronic data interchange setup requirement forms so that the business entity that is to receive the claims can create a compatible information file about the practice in its computer system so that claims can be processed.

entity/entities – Individual, business organization, or some kind of an economic unit that controls resources, incurs obligations, and engages in business activities.

eponyms – Diseases, procedures, or syndromes named for individuals who discovered or first used them.

Equal Credit Opportunity Act – Act stating that a business entity may not discriminate against a credit applicant on the basis of race, color, religion, national origin, age, sex, or marital status.

ERISA plans – Certain type of plan typically established by self-insured employers that provides benefits to employees in the form of life, disability, health insurance, severance pay, and pension plans. Benefits are funded through the purchase of insurance policies or through the establishment of trusts, paid for by the employer or the employer and employee together. The money is invested, and the employer takes a tax deduction for its contribution to the trust. If an employer maintains an ERISA pension plan, the federal ERISA law sets strict minimum standards on how the assets are managed and paid out.

errata – List of errors and their corrections made to a document shortly after the original text is published.

essential modifiers – Indented terms listed under a main term, used to describe different anatomical sites, etiology, or clinical types. Essential modifiers must be a part of the documented diagnosis.

established patient – Person who has been treated previously by the healthcare provider, regardless of location of service, within the past 3 years.

ethics – Code of conduct of a particular group of people or culture.

etiology – Cause or origin of a disease or condition.

etiquette – Following the rules and conventions governing correct or polite behavior in society in general or in a particular social or professional group or situation.

Evaluation and Management (E & M) codes – Codes found at the beginning of the CPT manual that represent the services provided directly to the patient during an encounter that do not involve an actual procedure.

exacerbation – Worsening or an increase in the severity of a disease or its signs and symptoms.

exclusions – Illnesses or injuries not covered by the health insurance policy.

exemption(s) – When a business organization (or individual) is not required to purchase workers' compensation insurance for employees because of a specific classification of business type or the fact that it has a minimal number of employees. (Exemption criteria vary from state to state.)

explanation of benefits (EOB) – Document prepared by the carrier that gives details of how the claim was adjudicated. It typically includes a comprehensive listing of patient information, dates of service, payments, or reasons for nonpayment. See remittance advice (RA).

eZ TRICARE – Electronic claims filing process wherein providers can upload batches of claims directly from their practice management systems using a variety of claims processing formats.

F

face-to-face time – Time that the healthcare provider spends in direct contact with a patient during an office visit, which includes taking a history, performing an examination, and discussing results.

Fair Credit Billing Act – Set of procedures or steps that business entities (medical practices) must follow if a customer claims that they made a mistake in their billing.

Fair Credit Reporting Act – Law that gives consumers the right to a copy of their credit reports. The law is intended to protect consumers from having their eligibility for credit damaged by incomplete or misleading credit report information.

Fair Debt Collection Practices Act – Act that prohibits certain abusive methods used by third-party collectors or bill collectors hired to collect overdue bills.

Federal Employees Health Benefits (FEHB) Program – Health insurance coverage the government pays for its own civilian employees.

Federal Employment Compensation Act (FECA) – Act that provides workers' compensation for nonmilitary federal employees. FECA covers medical expenses resulting from a disability and provides compensation for survivors of employees who are killed while on the job or who die from a job-related illness or condition.

Federal Employment Liability Act (FELA) – Under this act, states in which railroads are engaged in interstate commerce are liable for injuries to their employees if they have been negligent.

Federal Insurance Contributions Act (FICA) – Act that provides for a federal system of old-age, survivors, disability, and hospital insurance.

federal poverty level (FPL) – Income standards that are updated annually and that serve as one of the eligibility factors for various state and federal assistance programs (e.g., Supplemental Security Income).

fee-for-service (FFS) – Traditional type of healthcare policy whereby the provider charges a specific fee (typically the usual, customary, and reasonable fee) for each service rendered and is paid that fee by the patient or by the patient's insurance carrier. See indemnity (fee-for-service) and indemnity insurance.

financial means test – Detailed and comprehensive questionnaire that establishes financial need to receive Supplemental Security Income.

first-listed diagnosis – Main condition treated or investigated during the outpatient (ambulatory) encounter. In cases where there is no definitive diagnosis, the main symptom or sign, abnormal findings, or problem is reported as the first-listed diagnosis; this replaces the outdated term "primary diagnosis."

first party (party of the first part) – In legal language, the patient in the implied contract between the physician and patient.

fiscal intermediary (FI) (fiscal agent) – Commercial insurer or agent that contracts with the U.S. Department of Health and Human Services for the purpose of processing and administering Part A Medicare claims for the reimbursement of healthcare coverage. A fiscal intermediary also may provide consultative services or serve as a center for communication with providers and make audits of providers' needs.

flexible spending account (FSA) – IRS Section 125 cafeteria plan. The cost of the plan (premium) is deducted from the employee's wages before withholding taxes are deducted, allowing employees the option of pretax payroll deduction for some insurance premiums, unreimbursed medical expenses, and child or dependent care expenses.

form locators – Assigned designated spaces on UB-92 form for data elements necessary for claims processing. Each one has a unique number.

for-profit hospitals – When a hospital's monetary income is greater than its expenses.

fraud – Defined by the National Health Care Anti-Fraud Association as an intentional deception or misrepresentation that the individual or entity makes, knowing that the misrepresentation could result in some unauthorized benefit to the individual or the entity or to another party.

G

General Equivalence Mappings (GEMs) – Tool developed by various organizations that can be used like a two-way translation dictionary to assist with the conversion of ICD-9-CM codes to ICD-10 or the conversion of ICD-10 codes back to ICD-9-CM.

general hospital – Hospital that is set up to handle the care of many kinds of disease and injury. A general hospital is usually the major healthcare facility in a region and typically has an emergency department to deal with immediate threats to health and the capacity to dispatch emergency medical services.

general journal – Chronologic listing of transactions, with a specific format for recording each transaction. Each transaction is recorded separately and consists of a date, all accounts that receive a debit entry, all accounts that receive a credit entry, and a clear description of each transaction.

general ledger – Permanent history of all financial transactions from day one of the life of a practice. A general ledger can be used to prepare a range of periodic financial statements such as income statements, balance sheets, or both.

geographic practice cost index (GPCI) – Used by Medicare to adjust for variance in operating costs of medical practices located in different parts of the United States.

governance – Refers to how any organization is run. With reference to healthcare facilities, it includes all the processes, systems, and controls used to safeguard the welfare of patients and the integrity of the institution.

grandfathered group insurance – Group health insurance coverage plan in which employees were enrolled before the enactment of the Patient Protection and Affordable Care Act (PPACA). Grandfathered group insurance health plans are exempt from most of the reforms under the PPACA.

grievance – Written complaint submitted by an individual covered by the plan concerning claims payment, reimbursement, policies, or quality of health services.

group contract – Contract of insurance made with a company, a corporation, or other groups of common interest wherein all employees or individuals (and their eligible dependents) are insured under a single policy. Everyone receives the same benefits.

group insurance – Contract between an insurance company and an employer (or other entity) that covers eligible employees or members. Group insurance is generally the least expensive kind of insurance, and in many cases, the employer pays part or all of the cost.

group model – Health maintenance organization (HMO) that contracts with independent, multispecialty physician groups who provide all healthcare services to its members. Physician groups usually share the same facility, support staff, medical records, and equipment.

group plan – One insurance policy that covers a group of people.

guarantor – Person who is responsible for, or agrees to pay, someone else's debt if the individual defaults on a financial obligation. In health insurance, if the patient is a minor, the guarantor would typically be a parent or an adult legally responsible for the patient.

H

HCFA Common Procedure Coding System (HCPCS) – Developed by the Health Care Financing Administration to provide a uniform language that accurately describes medical, surgical, and diagnostic services, serving as an effective means for reliable nationwide communication among physicians, insurance carriers, and patients.

HCPCS codes – Descriptive terms with letters or numbers or both used to report medical services and procedures for reimbursement. HCPCS codes provide a uniform language to describe medical, surgical, and diagnostic services. These codes are used to report procedures and services to government and private health insurance programs, and reimbursement is based on the codes reported.

Health Care Financing Administration (HCFA) – See Centers for Medicare and Medicaid Services.

Health Care Quality Improvement Program – Program created to improve health outcomes of all Medicare beneficiaries regardless of personal characteristics, physical location, or setting.

healthcare service plans – Plans normally underwritten by Blue Cross and Blue Shield, which were initially involved in paying claims for indemnity carriers; however, more recently, many healthcare service plans have developed managed care products to compete with companies offering managed care plans.

health insurance – See medical insurance.

health insurance claim number (HICN) – Number assigned to a Medicare beneficiary that allows the health insurance professional to look at the patient's identification card and immediately determine the level of coverage. The number is in the format of 9 digits, usually the beneficiary's Social Security number, followed by one alpha character.

Health Insurance Exchange – Model intended to create a more organized and competitive market for health insurance by offering a choice of plans with common rules governing how the plan is offered and its cost and providing information to help consumers understand better the choices available to them.

health insurance policy premium – Monthly (or quarterly) fee paid by the policyholder.

Health Insurance Portability and Accountability Act (HIPAA) – Legislation passed in 1996 that includes a privacy rule creating national standards to protect personal health information and that requires most employer-sponsored group health insurance plans to accept transfers from other group plans without imposing a preexisting condition clause.

health maintenance organization (HMO) – Organization that provides its members with basic healthcare services for a fixed price and for a given time period.

Health Maintenance Organization (HMO) Act – Act passed by Congress in 1973 that provided grants to employers who set up HMOs.

health record – Clinical, scientific, administrative, and legal document of facts containing statements relating to a patient. It incorporates scientific data and scientific events in chronologic order regarding the case history, clinical examination, investigative procedures, diagnosis, treatment of the patient, and his or her response to the treatment. Also called medical record.

health savings account (HSA) – Special tax shelter that works in conjunction with a low-cost, high-deductible health insurance policy to provide comprehensive healthcare coverage at the lowest possible net cost for individuals who qualify. HSAs are set up for the purpose of paying medical bills, allowing individuals to make tax-deferred contributions to personal retirement funds. See also medical savings account (MSA).

HIPAA-covered entities – Consist of healthcare providers, health plans (including employer-sponsored plans), and healthcare clearinghouses (including billing agents). Covered entities must comply with Health Insurance Portability and Accountability Act (HIPAA) rules for any health or medical information of identifiable individuals.

HMO with point-of-service (POS) option – Health maintenance organization (HMO) member is allowed to see providers who are not in the HMO network and receive services from specialists without first going through a primary care physician; however, the plan pays a smaller portion of the bill than if the member had followed regular HMO procedures. The member also pays a higher premium and a higher copayment each time the option is used.

home health prospective payment system (HH PPS) – Fixed payment for home health services.

hospice – Facility or service that provides care for terminally ill patients and support to their families, either directly or on a consulting basis with the patient's physician. The emphasis is on symptom control and support before and after death.

hospital outpatient prospective payment system (HOPPS) – Payment system developed by the Centers for Medicare and Medicaid Services (CMS), sometimes referred to as OPPS, that was implemented August 1, 2000, and is used to reimburse for hospital outpatient services and reduce Medicare beneficiary copayments.

I

iatrogenic effects – Symptom or illness in a patient brought on unintentionally by a physician's activity, manner, or therapy.

identifiers – Numbers used in the administration of health care to distinguish individual healthcare providers, health plans, employers, and patients. Identifiers are intended to simplify administrative processes such as referrals and billing, improve the accuracy of data, and reduce costs.

implied contract – Unwritten contract between a healthcare provider and a patient that has all the components of a legal contract and is just as binding.

implied promises – Promises that are neither spoken nor written but are implicated by the individuals' actions and performance.

incidental disclosure – Type of privacy exposure that is specifically allowed under Health Insurance Portability and Accountability Act (HIPAA) (e.g., if two patients in the reception room happen to know each other).

indemnify – To reimburse or make payment for a loss.

indemnity (fee-for-service) – Traditional healthcare insurance where patients can choose any provider or hospital they want (including specialists) and change physicians at any time. The insured (or policyholder) pays a periodic fee called a premium, which is based on the policy type and coverage. The patient also pays a certain amount of money up front each year toward his or her medical expenses, known as the deductible, before the insurance company begins paying benefits.

indemnity insurance – The "standard" type of health insurance individuals can purchase. It provides comprehensive major medical benefits and allows insured individuals to choose any physician or hospital when seeking medical care. See indemnity (fee-for-service).

indented code – Codes that refer to the common portion of the procedure listed in the preceding entry.

indigent – People who are poor and deprived, typically without sufficient resources to take care of their daily needs. "Medically indigent" refers to an individual who does not have health insurance and who is not eligible for other healthcare coverage such as Medicaid, Medicare, or private health insurance.

individual practice association (IPA) – Individual healthcare providers who provide all the needed healthcare services for a health maintenance organization (HMO).

informed consent – The process by which a fully informed patient can participate in choices about his or her healthcare. This concept originates from the legal and ethical rights patients have to direct what happens to their bodies and from the ethical duty of physicians to involve patients in their healthcare.

initial claims – Claims submitted for reimbursement under Medicare, including claims with paper attachments; demand bills; claims where Medicare is the secondary payer and there is only one primary payer; claims submitted to a Medicare fee-for-service carrier or fiscal intermediary for the first time including resubmitted, previously rejected claims; and nonpayment claims.

initiative – Readiness and ability to take action.

"in-kind" income – As opposed to cash, food, clothing, shelter, or something you can use to get food (e.g., food stamps).

inpatient – Patient who has been formally admitted to a hospital for diagnostic tests, medical care and treatment, or a surgical procedure, typically staying overnight.

inpatient rehabilitation facility prospective payment system (IRF PPS) – Reimbursement system activated by the Centers for Medicare and Medicaid Services (CMS) in 2001. Reimbursement is based on the hospital stay, beginning with an admission to the rehabilitation hospital or unit and ending with discharge from that facility.

instrumental activities of daily living – Activities that generally include using the telephone, shopping, preparing meals, keeping house, doing laundry, doing yard work, managing personal finances, and managing medications.

insurance – Written agreement (policy) between two entities, whereby one entity (the insurance company) promises to pay a specific sum of money to a second entity (often an individual or another company) if certain specified undesirable events happen.

insurance billing cycle – Interaction between a healthcare provider and a third-party payer. The cycle begins when a patient visits a healthcare provider where a medical record is created or an existing one is updated and can take several days to several months to complete, depending on the number of exchanges in communication required.

insurance cap – Limit to the amount of money a policyholder has to pay out of pocket for any one incident or in any one year. The cap is reached when out-of-pocket expenses for deductibles and coinsurance total a certain amount.

insurance claims register (log) – Columnar sheet used to record claims information. This is used as an alternative to a suspension file.

insured – Individual who is covered by an insurer.

insurer – Insuring party.

integrity – Having honest, ethical, and moral principles.

intermediaries – See fiscal intermediary (FI) (fiscal agent).

International Classification of Diseases, 9th Revision, Clinical Modification (ICD-9-CM) – Three-volume coding system that provided a method of classifying morbidity data for the indexing of medical records, medical case reviews, ambulatory and other medical care programs, and basic health statistics before the introduction of ICD-10 system.

International Classification of Diseases, 10th Revision (ICD-10) – Updated version of the ICD manual, released in three volumes from 1992-1994. ICD-10 provides increased clinical detail and addresses information regarding previously classified diseases and new diseases discovered since the ninth revision.

interstate commerce – Trade that involves more than one state.

J

job deconditioning – When an individual psychologically or physically loses his or her ability to perform normal job duties at the previous level of expertise as a result of being absent from work.

Joint Commission, The – Private organization created in 1951 to provide voluntary accreditation to hospitals. The purpose of The Joint Commission is to encourage the attainment of uniformly high standards of institutional medical care by establishing guidelines for the operation of hospitals and other health facilities and conducting survey and accreditation programs.

K

key components – Main elements that establish the level in Evaluation and Management coding (history, examination, and complexity in medical decision making).

L

labor component – Represents labor cost variations among different areas of the United States.

late effects (sequelae) – Residual conditions produced after the acute phase of an illness or injury has ended.

laterality – Side of the body on which surgery was performed or which side of the body is affected.

Level I (codes) – American Medical Association (AMA) Physicians' CPT codes. Five-digit codes, accompanied by descriptive terms, are used for reporting services performed by healthcare professionals. Level I codes are developed and updated annually by the AMA.

Level II (codes) – National codes used to report medical services, supplies, drugs, and durable medical equipment not contained in the Level I codes. Codes begin with a single letter, followed by 4 digits. Level II codes supersede Level I codes for similar encounters, Evaluation and Management services, or other procedures and represent the portion of procedures involving supplies and materials. Level II codes are developed and updated annually by the Centers for Medicare and Medicaid Services (CMS) and their contractors.

Level III (codes) – Descriptors developed by local Medicare contractors for use by physicians, practitioners, providers, and suppliers in completion of claims for payment. Level III codes are used on a limited basis.

licensed independent practitioner – Defined by The Joint Commission as "any individual permitted by law and by the organization to provide care and services, without direction or supervision, within the scope of the individual's license and consistent with individually granted clinical privileges."

lifetime maximum cap – Amount after which the insurance company does not pay any more of the charges incurred.

lifetime (one-time) release of information form – Form that the beneficiary may sign, authorizing a lifetime release of information, instead of signing an information release form annually.

litigious – Quick to take legal action (bring lawsuits).

local coverage determinations (LCDs) – medical-necessity documents that focus exclusively on whether a service is reasonable and necessary according to the ICD-9-CM code for that particular Current Procedural Terminology (CPT) procedure code.

Longshore and Harbor Workers' Compensation Act – Act that provides workers' compensation to specified employees of private maritime employers.

long-term care facilities – Facilities that provide care for adults who are chronically ill or disabled and are no longer able to manage in independent living situations.

long-term care hospital prospective payment system (LTCH PPS) – Discharge-based prospective payment system for long-term care hospitals that replaces the former fee-for-service or cost-based system.

long-term disability – Helps replace income for up to 5 years or until the disabled individual turns 65.

M

maintenance of benefits (MOB) – Allows patients to receive benefits from all health insurance plans under which they are covered, while maintaining their cost-sharing responsibilities (coinsurance/copay amounts) on these coverages and ensuring that the total combined payment from all sources is never more than the total charge for the services.

main term(s) – In diagnostic coding, the identifying word (or words) of a diagnosis that when located in the Index to Diseases (Volume 2) aids in locating the correct diagnosis code. Main terms are conditions, nouns, adjectives, and eponyms and are always printed in boldface type for ease of reference.

major medical insurance – Insurance that includes treatment for long-term, high-cost illnesses or injuries and inpatient and outpatient expenses.

managed care organizations – Healthcare delivery system that attempts to keep costs down by "managing" the care to eliminate unnecessary treatment and reduce expensive hospital care. The most familiar models are health maintenance organizations (HMOs) and preferred provider organizations (PPOs).

managed care plan – Plan composed of a group of providers who share the financial risk of the plan or who have an incentive to deliver cost-effective, quality service.

managed healthcare – Any system of health payment or delivery arrangements in which the health plan attempts to control or coordinate the use of health services by its enrolled members to contain health expenditures, improve quality, or both. Under managed healthcare plans, patients see designated providers, and benefits are paid according to the structure of the managed care plan.

mandated Medigap transfer – Claim for which a beneficiary elects to assign his or her benefits under a Medigap policy to a participating physician or supplier.

mandated services – Certain basic services that must be offered to the categorically needy population in any state Medicaid program.

manifestations – Signs or symptoms of a disease.

Maternal and Child Health Services – Federal-state partnership under the Title V Block Grant enacted to achieve the goal to improve the health of all mothers and children consistent with the health status goals and national health objectives established by the Secretary of the U.S. Department of Health and Human Services.

Medicaid – Combination federal and state medical assistance program designed to provide comprehensive and quality medical care for low-income families with special emphasis on children, pregnant women, elderly adults, disabled individuals, and parents with dependent children who have no other way to pay for healthcare. Coverage varies from state to state.

Medicaid contractor – Commercial insurer contracted by the U.S. Department of Health and Human Services for the purpose of processing and administering Medicaid claims.

Medicaid integrity contractors – Private companies that conduct audit-related activities under contract to the Medicaid Integrity Group (MIG), the component within the Centers for Medicare and Medicaid Services (CMS) that is charged by the U.S. Department of Health and Human Services with carrying out the Medicaid Integrity Program (MIP).

Medicaid secondary claim – Type of claim that occurs when the beneficiary has two healthcare coverages—medical insurance coverage (e.g., commercial or group policies) or dual coverage with traditional (original) Medicare enrollment. In such cases, Medicaid is the payer of last resort.

Medicaid "simple" claim – When the patient has Medicaid coverage only and no secondary insurance.

medical ethics – Code of conduct for the healthcare profession. Basic principles usually include showing respect for patient autonomy, not inflicting harm on patients, contributing to the welfare of patients, and providing justice and fair treatment of patients.

medical etiquette – Following the rules and conventions governing correct or polite behavior in the healthcare profession.

medical record – See health record.

medical insurance – Insurance that covers part (or all) of the financial expenses incurred as a result of medical procedures, services, and certain supplies performed or provided by healthcare professionals if and when an individual becomes sick or injured. Also known as health insurance.

medically necessary – Medical services, procedures, or supplies that are reasonable and necessary for the diagnosis or treatment of a patient's medical condition, in accordance with the standards of good medical practice, performed at the proper level, and provided in the most appropriate setting.

medically needy – Individuals who do not qualify in the categorically needy program (because of excess income or resources) but need help to pay for excessive medical expenses.

medical necessity (medically necessary) – For a procedure or service to qualify for payment under the medically necessary principle, it must be consistent with the diagnosis and in accordance with the standards of good medical practice, performed at the proper level, and provided in the most appropriate setting.

medical savings account (MSA) – Special tax shelter set up for the purpose of paying medical bills. Known as the Archer MSA, it is similar to an IRA and works in conjunction with a special low-cost, high-deductible health insurance policy to provide comprehensive healthcare coverage at the lowest possible net cost for individuals who qualify. MSAs are currently limited to self-employed people and employees of small businesses with less than 50 employees. Also called health savings account (HSA).

Medicare – Comprehensive federal insurance program established by Congress in 1966 that provides financial assistance with medical expenses to individuals 65 years old or older and individuals younger than 65 years with certain disabilities.

Medicare Administrative Contractor (MAC) – Private insurance companies that serve as agents of the federal government in the administration of the Medicare program, including the payment of claims.

Medicare crossover program – Process whereby beneficiary claims data are automatically transmitted (usually electronically) from a Medicare administrative contractor to a supplemental insurance policy for additional payment after Medicare has determined its obligatory payment. The process is activated when a PAR Medicare provider (1) includes a specific identifier—a COBA ID number—on the claim and (2) assigns payment benefits to that provider. Also called Medigap crossover.

Medicare gaps – Uninsured areas under Medicare with which elderly and disabled Americans need additional help.

Medicare HMOs – Network of physicians and other healthcare providers for Medicare recipients. Members or enrollees must receive care only from the providers in the network except in emergencies. This is the least expensive and most restrictive Medicare managed care plan.

Medicare hospital insurance (Medicare HI) – Medicare Part A.

Medicare limiting charge – In the original Medicare plan, the highest amount of money a Medicare beneficiary can be charged for a covered service by physicians and other healthcare suppliers who do not accept assignment. The limiting charge is 15% over Medicare's "approved amount." The limiting charge applies only to certain services and does not apply to supplies or equipment.

Medicare managed care plan – Health maintenance organization (HMO) or preferred provider organization (PPO) that uses Medicare to pay for part of its services for eligible beneficiaries. It provides all basic Medicare benefits, plus some additional coverages (depending on the plan) to fill the gaps Medicare does not pay.

Medicare-Medicaid crossover claims – In cases in which patients qualify for Medicare and Medicaid coverage, the claim is first submitted to Medicare, which pays its share, and then the claim is "crossed over" to Medicaid.

Medicare nonparticipating provider (nonPAR) – Provider or supplier who has not signed a contract with Medicare and may choose whether to accept Medicare's approved amount as payment on a case-by-case basis. If they do not accept the approved amount, the beneficiary pays the full billed amount.

Medicare Part A – Hospital insurance. Medicare Part A helps pay for medically necessary services, including inpatient hospital care, inpatient care in a skilled nursing facility (SNF), home healthcare, and hospice care.

Medicare Part A fiscal intermediary (FI) – Private organization that contracts with Medicare to pay Part A and some Part B bills. The FI determines payment to Part A facilities for covered items and services provided by the facility.

Medicare Part B – Medical (physicians' care) insurance financed by a combination of federal government funds and beneficiary premiums.

Medicare Part C (Medicare Advantage plans) – Prepaid healthcare plans that offer regular Part A and Part B Medicare coverage in addition to coverage for other services. Formerly called Medicare+Choice.

Medicare Part D (Prescription Drug Plan) – Pays a portion of prescription drug expenses and cost sharing for qualifying individuals.

Medicare participating provider (PAR) – Provider or supplier who has signed a contract with Medicare and agrees to accept the allowed amount by Medicare as payment in full.

Medicare Secondary Payer (MSP) – Term used when Medicare is not responsible for paying first because the beneficiary is covered under another insurance policy.

Medicare Secondary Payer claims – When a patient has other health insurance coverage, such as a group health policy, that payer becomes primary, and Medicare becomes the secondary payer. When the primary payer has processed the claim, a Medicare Secondary Payer claim is submitted to Medicare along with the explanation of benefits from the primary payer.

Medicare Severity Adjusted (MS-DRG) System – Centers for Medicare and Medicaid Services (CMS) new, restructured diagnosis-related group (DRG) system, which began October 1, 2007, in which DRG weights are adjusted based on the severity of a patient's condition. This new system is expected to account for the severity of a patient's condition more accurately. Previously, the Medicare system used 538 DRGs; the new system uses 745 MS-DRGs.

Medicare Summary Notice (MSN) – Monthly statement that the beneficiary receives from Medicare after a claim is filed. The statement lists Part A and Part B claims information, including the patient's deductible status.

Medicare supplement plans – Private insurance plans specifically designed to provide coverage for some of the services that Medicare does not pay, such as Medicare's deductible and coinsurance amounts and for certain services not allowed by Medicare. Also called Medigap insurance.

Medicare supplement policy – Health insurance plan sold by private insurance companies to help pay for healthcare expenses not covered by Medicare and its deductibles and coinsurance.

Medigap crossover program – See Medicare crossover program.

Medigap insurance – Policies sold by private insurance companies to fill "gaps" in the original (fee-for-service) Medicare plan coverage. Policies are specifically designed to supplement Medicare benefits. See Medicare supplement plans.

Merchant Marine Act (Jones Act) – Act that provides seamen (individuals involved in transporting goods by water between U.S. ports) with the same protection from employer negligence that the Federal Employment Liability Act provides railroad workers.

Military Health System – Total healthcare system of the U.S. uniformed services. The system includes military treatment facilities and various programs in the civilian healthcare market, such as TRICARE.

military treatment facility (MTF) – Clinic or hospital operated by the U.S. Department of Defense located on a military base that provides care to military personnel, their dependents, and military retirees and their dependents.

modified own-occupation policy – Covers workers for their own occupation as long as they are not gainfully employed elsewhere. This policy is a variation of own-occupation policies.

modifier(s) – Words that are added to main terms to supply more specific information about a patient's clinical picture. Modifiers provide the means by which the reporting healthcare provider can indicate that a service or procedure performed has been altered by some specific circumstance but has not changed its definition or code.

modifying terms – Descriptive words indented under the main term that provide further description of a procedure or service. A main term can have up to three modifying terms. In Current Procedural Terminology (CPT) coding, modifying terms often have an effect on the selection of the appropriate procedural code. See also modifier(s).

mono-spaced fonts – Fonts in which each character takes up exactly the same amount of space.

morbidity – Presence of illness or disease.

morphology – In medicine, morphology refers to the size, shape, and structure rather than the function of a given organ. For example, as a diagnostic imaging technique, ultrasound assists in the recognition of abnormal morphologies as symptoms of underlying conditions.

mortality – Deaths that occur from a disease.

multiaxial structure – Code configuration wherein each character has the same meaning within the specific procedure section and across procedure sections to the extent possible, meaning each 7-character alphanumeric code has a section corresponding to descriptive subsections, such as anatomy or surgical approach. Only the designation of the first character is fixed to a defined section. The roles of the other six characters are assigned depending on the preceding character. For a code in section 0 (medical and surgical), the codes that follow are body system, root operation, body part, approach, device, and qualifier with an actual set of codes for each succeeding character fixed by the preceding one.

N

National Committee for Quality Assurance (NCQA) – Independent, nonprofit organization that performs quality-oriented accreditation reviews on health maintenance organizations (HMOs) and similar types of managed care plans. The purpose of NCQA is to evaluate plans and to provide information that helps consumers and employers make informed decisions about purchasing health plan services.

National Correct Coding Initiative (NCCI) – Implemented by the Centers for Medicare and Medicaid Services (CMS) in 1996 to control improper coding that leads to inappropriate increased payment for healthcare services.

national provider identifier (NPI) – Standard unique identifier required by the Health Insurance Portability and Accountability Act (HIPAA) and assigned to all healthcare providers, health plans, and employers that identifies them on standard transactions. The NPI is a 10-digit "intelligence-free" number, meaning the number does not carry any information about the provider, such as the state in which he or she practices or type of specialization.

National Uniform Billing Committee (NUBC) – Created by the American Hospital Association in 1975 and includes the participation of all the major provider and payer organizations in the United States. NUBC was formed to develop a single billing form and standard data set that could be used nationwide by institutional providers and payers for handling healthcare claims.

NEC ("not elsewhere classifiable") – Abbreviation in the ICD-10-CM Index that represents "other specified." When a specific code is not available for a condition in the Index, the coder is directed to the "other specified" code in the Tabular where an NEC entry under a code identifies it as the "other specified" code.

negligence – Failure to exercise a reasonable degree of care.

neonates – Newborns 30 days old or younger.

Neoplasm – new growth, often resulting in a tumor.

network – Interrelated system of people and facilities that communicate with one another and work together as a unit. An approved list of physicians, hospitals, and other providers is created.

network model – Health maintenance organization (HMO) that has multiple provider arrangements including staff, group, or individual practice association structures.

new patient – Person who is new to the practice, regardless of location of service, or one who has not received any medical treatment by the healthcare provider or any other provider in that same office within the past 3 years.

no-fault insurance – In workers' compensation insurance, benefits are paid to the injured (or ill) worker regardless of who is to blame for the accident or injury.

nonavailability statement (NAS) – Document of certification from the military treatment facility (MTF) that says it cannot provide the specific health care that the beneficiary needs at that facility. The statements must be entered electronically in the Defense Department's DEERS computer files by the MTF.

noncovered services – Situations in which an item or service is not covered under Medicare.

nonessential modifiers – Terms in parentheses immediately following the main terms. Typically, these terms are alternative terminology for the main term and are provided to assist the coder in locating the applicable main term. Nonessential modifiers are usually not a part of the diagnostic statement.

nonlabor component – Represents a geographic calculation based on whether the hospital is located in a large urban or other area.

nonparticipating provider (nonPAR) – Provider who has no contractual agreement with the insurance carrier; the provider does not have to accept the insurance company's reimbursement as payment in full.

NOS ("not otherwise specified") – Abbreviation that is the equivalent of "unspecified," meaning that a more specific diagnosis is unavailable. Before assigning an NOS code, the coder should examine the medical record more closely or question the physician/provider for more complete documentation.

noun – One of the types of main terms used in diagnostic coding. The Index to Diseases (Volume 2 in the ICD-9-CM manual) is organized by main terms, which are always printed in boldface type for ease of reference. Main terms can be nouns (e.g., a disease, disturbance, or syndrome), adjectives, diseases, or conditions.

O

objectivity – Not influenced by personal feelings, biases, or prejudice.

observation – In Current Procedural Terminology (CPT) coding, classification for a patient who is not sick enough to qualify for acute inpatient status but requires hospitalization for a brief time.

occupational therapy – Skilled treatment for ill or injured individuals that facilitates their return to ordinary tasks around home or at work (or both) by maximizing physical potential through lifestyle adaptations, sometimes through the use of assistive devices.

OCR scannable – Documents formatted and printed in such a way that they can be "read" using a specific process referred to as "optical character recognition" (OCR). The CMS-1500 is printed using a special red ink, and when the form is scanned, everything in red "drops out," and the computer reads the information printed within the blocks.

offer – In contract law, proposition to create a contract.

ombudsman – Individual who is responsible for investigating and resolving workers' complaints against the employer or insurance company that is denying the benefits.

"one-write" system – Paper accounting system that captures all accounting information at the time a transaction occurs. It is especially useful for small practices. Also called the pegboard system.

open enrollment period – Six-month period when an individual may sign up for Medicare or Medigap policies, or both.

open panel plan – Plan in which the providers maintain their own offices and identities and see patients who belong to a health maintenance organization (HMO) and patients who do not. Healthcare providers in the community may participate if they meet certain HMO or individual practice association standards.

optical character recognition (OCR) – Recognition of printed or written text characters by a computer. See OCR scannable.

optional services – Services for which federal funding is available. States can provide as many or as few as they choose to their categorically needy population. Some of these services include dental services, clinic services, optometrist services and eyeglasses, and prescribed drugs.

other health insurance (OHI) – TRICARE-eligible beneficiary has other healthcare coverage besides TRICARE Standard, Extra, or Prime through an employer, an association, or a private insurer, or if a student in the family has a healthcare plan obtained through his or her school. Also called double coverage or coordination of benefits.

outliers – Atypical patients.

out-of-pocket maximum – After a patient has paid a certain amount of medical expenses, the usual, customary, and reasonable (allowed) fee for covered benefits is paid in full by the insurer.

outpatient – Patient who has not been officially admitted to a hospital but receives diagnostic tests or treatment in that facility or a clinic connected with it.

own-occupation policy – Covers workers who are unable to perform in the occupation or job that they were doing before the disability occurred.

P

palliative care – Care given to improve the quality of life of patients who have a serious or life-threatening disease. The goal of palliative care is to prevent or treat the symptoms of the disease and side effects caused by treatment of the disease as early and effectively as possible. Also called comfort care, supportive care, and symptom management.

paraphrase – Rephrasing or summarizing important facts in your own words.

participating provider (PAR) – Provider who contracts with the third-party payer and agrees to abide by certain rules and regulations of that carrier.

pass-throughs – Temporary payments for specified new technologies, drugs, devices, and biologicals for which costs were unavailable when calculating ambulatory payment classification payment rates.

patient information form – Form that medical offices usually require new patients to fill out. The form asks for information such as name, address, employer, and health insurance information.

patient ledger – Chronologic accounting of activities of a particular patient (or family) including all charges and payments.

patient ledger card – Accounting form on which professional service descriptions, charges, payments, adjustments, and current balance are posted chronologically.

pay and chase claims – When the state Medicaid agency pays the medical bills and then attempts to recover these paid funds from liable third parties.

payer of last resort – After all other available third-party resources meet their legal obligation to pay claims, the Medicaid program pays for the care of an individual eligible for Medicaid.

payroll journal – Listing of wages and salaries.

peer review organizations (PROs) – Groups of practicing healthcare professionals who are paid by the federal government to evaluate the care provided to Medicare beneficiaries in each state and to improve the quality of services. PROs act to educate and assist in the promotion of effective, efficient, and economical delivery of health services to the Medicare population they serve.

per diem rates – Actual costs per day.

permanent and stationary – When a condition reaches a state of maximal medical improvement.

permanent disability – Level of disability where the ill or injured employee's condition is such that it is impossible to return to work. There are two classifications of permanent disability—permanent partial disability and permanent total disability.

permanent partial disability – When a disability prevents an individual from performing one or more occupational functions but does not impair his or her capability for performing less demanding employment.

permanent total disability – When an individual's ability to work at any occupation is totally and permanently lost.

Physician Quality Reporting System (PQRS) – A reporting system, previously called the Physician Quality Reporting Initiative, established by the Tax Relief and Health Care Act (TRHCA) of 2006, which included an incentive payment for eligible professionals who satisfactorily reported data on quality measures for covered services furnished to Medicare beneficiaries. The Medicare, Medicaid, and SCHIP Extension Act of 2007 authorized a financial incentive for participation in this program.

Physicians' Current Procedural Terminology, Fifth Edition (CPT-5) – An updated version of the CPT-4 manual, developed in part by the American Medical Association, to improve existing CPT features and correct deficiencies in the current CPT-4 coding system, to respond to deficiencies encountered by emerging user needs, and to address challenges presented by Health Insurance Portability and Accountability Act (HIPAA). (Not yet universally used in the US.)

Physicians' Current Procedural Terminology, Fourth Edition (CPT-4) – Manual containing a list of descriptive terms and identifying codes used in reporting medical services and procedures performed and supplies used by physicians and other professional healthcare providers in the care and treatment of patients.

placeholder character ("X") – ICD-10-CM uses the letter "X" as a placeholder character. It has two uses: (1) As the 5th character for certain 6 character codes; "X" provides for future expansion without disturbing the 6-character structure. (2) When a code has fewer than 6 characters, and a 7th character extension is required; "X" is assigned for all characters fewer than 6 to meet the requirement of coding to the highest level of specificity.

plaintiff – Party bringing a lawsuit.

point-of-service (POS) plan – "Hybrid" type of managed care that allows patients either to use the health maintenance organization (HMO) provider or to go outside the plan and use any provider they choose. Also called open-ended HMO.

policy – Written agreement between two parties, whereby one entity (the insurance company) promises to pay a specific sum of money to a second entity (often an individual or another company) if certain specified undesirable events occur.

policyholder – Individual in whose name the policy is written; the insured.

portability – According to the Health Insurance Portability and Accountability Act (HIPAA), people with preexisting medical conditions cannot be denied health insurance coverage when moving from one employer-sponsored group healthcare plan to another.

practice management software – Type of software that deals with the day-to-day operations of a medical practice. It allows users to enter patient demographic information, schedule appointments, maintain lists of insurance payers, perform billing tasks, and generate reports.

preauthorization – Cost-containment procedure required by most managed healthcare and indemnity plans before a provider carries out specific procedures or treatments for a patient. The insured must contact the insurer before hospitalization or surgery and receive prior approval for the service. Preauthorization does not guarantee payment.

precertification – Process whereby the provider (or a member of his or her staff) contacts the patient's managed care plan before inpatient admissions and performance of certain procedures and services to verify the patient's eligibility and coverage for the planned service.

predetermination – Method used by some insurance companies to find out whether or not a specific medical service or procedure would be covered. Most insurance companies request a written statement from the healthcare provider with the specific Current Procedural Terminology (CPT) codes for the proposed procedures before providing a predetermination of benefits.

preexisting conditions – Physical or mental conditions of an insured individual that existed before the issuance of a health insurance policy or that existed before issuance and for which treatment was received. Preexisting conditions are excluded from coverage under some policies, or a specified length of time must elapse before the condition is covered.

preferred provider organization (PPO) – Group of hospitals and physicians that agree to render particular services to a group of people, generally under contract with a private insurer. These services may be furnished at discounted rates if the members receive their health care from member providers, rather than selecting a provider outside of the network.

premium – Specific sum of money paid by the insured to the insurance company in exchange for financial protection against loss.

preventive medicine – Practice that focuses on overall health and the prevention of illness. Some insurance policies pay medical expenses even if the individual is not sick or injured because it is often less costly to keep a person well or detect an emerging illness in its early stages when it is more treatable than possibly having to pay more exorbitant expenses later on should that individual become seriously ill.

pricing transparency – Sharing information so that people know upfront what their healthcare will cost. For example, some hospitals now put their prices on the Internet.

primary care manager (PCM) – Healthcare provider or a team of healthcare providers that the enrollee (under the TRICARE Prime plan) must see first for all routine medical care, similar to a primary care provider or gatekeeper in civilian managed care plans.

primary care physician (PCP) – In a preferred provider organization (PPO) plan, specific provider who oversees the member's total healthcare treatment.

principal diagnosis – Reason for admission to the acute care facility.

prioritize – To organize by importance.

privacy – Right to be left alone and to maintain individual autonomy, solitude, intimacy, and control over information about oneself.

privacy standards – Intended to define what are appropriate and inappropriate disclosures of individually identifiable health information, and how patient rights are to be protected.

privacy statement – Statement patients are asked to sign when they visit their healthcare providers. The statement includes information about who the physician or pharmacy shares health information with and why and outlines what rights patients have to access their own health information.

professional ethics – Moral principles associated with a specific vocation.

Program of All-Inclusive Care for the Elderly (PACE) – Program that provides comprehensive alternative care for noninstitutionalized elderly individuals, 55 years and older, who would otherwise be in a nursing home. A multidisciplinary team composed of a physician, nurse, therapists, dietitian, social worker, home care coordinator, and transportation supervisor completes an initial and semiannual assessment of each participant with a documented plan of treatment.

progress or supplemental report – Report that a physician must file to keep the employer and insurance carrier apprised of a patient's treatment plan, progress, and status in workers' compensation cases.

prospective payment system (PPS) – Medicare reimbursement system for inpatient hospital costs based on predetermined factors and not on individual services. Rates are set at a level intended to cover operating costs for treating a typical inpatient in a given diagnosis-related group. Payments for each hospital are adjusted for various factors such as differences in area wages, teaching activity, and care to the poor.

protected health information (PHI) – Identifiable health information that is protected under the HIPAA Privacy Rule.

provider-sponsored organization (PSO) – group of medical providers—physicians, clinics, and hospitals—that skips the insurance company middleman and contracts directly with patients. Members pay a premium and a copayment each time a service is rendered.

Q

Qualified Disabled and Working Individuals – Individuals who lose their Medicare benefits because they returned to work.

Qualified Medicare Beneficiaries – Medicare beneficiaries who qualify for certain additional benefits only if they have incomes below the federal poverty level and resources at or below twice the standard allowed under the Supplemental Security Income program.

quality improvement organization (QIO) – Program that works with consumers, physicians, hospitals, and other caregivers to refine care delivery systems to ensure patients get the right care at the right time, particularly among underserved populations. The program also safeguards the integrity of the Medicare trust fund by ensuring that payment is made only for medically necessary services, and it investigates beneficiary complaints about quality of care.

quality review study – Assessment of patient care designed to achieve measurable improvement in processes and outcomes of care. Improvements are achieved through interventions that target healthcare providers, practitioners, plans, or beneficiaries.

R

real-time claims adjudication (RTCA) – Means of electronic communication that allows instant resolution of an insurance claim including the third-party insurer's payment, adjustment, and patient responsibility.

reasonable and customary fee – Commonly charged or prevailing fee for a specific health procedure or service within a geographic area.

reciprocity – When one state allows Medicaid beneficiaries from other states (usually states that are adjacent) to be treated in its medical facilities.

Recovery Audit Contractor (RAC) – The job of an RAC is to detect and correct past improper payments so that Centers for Medicare and Medicaid Services (CMS) and carriers, fiscal intermediaries, and Medicare Administrative Contractors can implement actions that prevent future improper payments. Providers who bill Medicare on a fee-for-service basis are subject to review by RACs.

referral – Request by a healthcare provider for a patient under his or her care to be evaluated or treated or both by another provider, usually a specialist.

registered health information technicians (RHITs) – Technicians who pass a written examination offered by the American Health Information Management Association.

reimbursement – Payment to an insured individual for a covered expense or loss experienced by or on behalf of the insured.

relative value scale (RVS) – Method of determining reimbursement for medical services on the basis of establishing a standard unit value for medical and surgical procedures. RVS compares and rates each individual service according to the relative value of each unit and converts this unit value to a dollar value.

release of information – Form signed by the patient, authorizing a release of medical information necessary to complete the insurance claim form. Typically, a release of information is valid for only 1 year.

remittance advice (RA) – paper or electronic form sent by Medicare to the service provider that explains how payment was determined for a claim (or claims). Formerly called explanation of benefits (EOB).

remittance remark codes – Codes that represent nonfinancial information on a Medicare remittance advice.

remote assignment – When uniformed service members and their families are located 50 miles or more from a military treatment facility.

reserve components (RCs) – Military service members in the Army and National Guard Reserves.

residential healthcare facility – Facility for the care of individuals who do not require hospitalization and who cannot be cared for at home; nursing home.

resource-based relative value scale (RBRVS) – Method on which Medicare bases its payments for physicians' services. The federal government established RBRVS as a standardized physician payment schedule determined by the resource costs necessary to provide the service or procedure rather than on the actual fees typically charged by the physician.

resource-based relative value system – Reimbursement system designed to address the increasing cost of healthcare in the United States and try to resolve the inequities between geographic areas, time in practice, and the current payment schedule. Replaces the Medicare fee system. See resource-based relative value scale (RBRVS).

resource utilization groups (RUGs) – Used to calculate reimbursement in a skilled nursing facility (SNF) according to severity and level of care. Under the Medicare prospective payment system, patients are classified into an RUG that determines how much Medicare would pay the SNF per day for that patient.

respite care – Provides individuals such as family members with temporary relief from tasks associated with providing care in the home for frail or disabled individuals.

respondeat superior – Key principle in business law, which says that an employer is responsible for the actions of his or her employees in the course of employment.

review of systems (ROS) – In a physical examination, information gathering that involves a series of questions the provider asks the patient to identify what body parts or body systems are involved.

S

secondary claim – Claim that the secondary insurer (the insurance company who pays after the primary carrier) receives after the primary insurer pays its monetary obligations.

second party (party of the second part) – In legal language, healthcare provider in the implied contract between the physician and patient.

section – One of four classifications in the Tabular section (Volume 1) of the Current Procedural Terminology (CPT) manual. This section (e.g., Surgery or Radiology) is one of the six major areas into which all CPT codes and descriptions are categorized.

security standards – Standards that need to be developed and adopted for all health plans, clearinghouses, and providers to follow and to be required at all stages of transmission and storage of healthcare information to ensure integrity and confidentiality of the records at all phases of the process, before, during, and after electronic transmission.

see – Used as a cross-reference term in the Current Procedural Terminology (CPT) Alphabetic Index and directs the coder to an alternate main term.

self-insured/self-insurance – When the employer—not an insurance company—is responsible for the cost of medical services for its employees.

self-pay patient – Patient who may have inadequate health insurance coverage or no insurance at all.

self-referring – When a member of a managed healthcare group is allowed to receive services from specialists without first going through a primary care physician.

sequela (pl. sequelae) – Residual conditions produced after the acute phase of an illness or injury has ended. Also called late effects.

share of cost – Allows people who do not meet the income or assets requirements (medically needy) of Medicaid to qualify for assistance by using their medical expenses to spend down their income before Medicaid considers their eligibility. Qualifying patients are allowed to pay Medicaid the amount of money that is still over the Medicaid income allowance. Once this amount is paid, the patient becomes eligible for Medicaid services. Also called Payment Error Rate Measurement (PERM).

short-stay outlier – Adjustment to the federal payment rate for long-term care hospital (LTCH) stays that are considerably shorter than the average length of stay for an LTCH diagnosis-related group.

short-term disability – Coverage that pays a percentage of an individual's wages or salary if and when he or she becomes temporarily disabled.

single or specialty service plans – Health plans that provide services only in certain health specialties, such as mental health, vision, or dentistry.

skilled nursing facility (SNF) – Institution or a distinct part of an institution that is licensed or approved under state or local law and is primarily engaged in providing skilled nursing or skilled rehabilitation services to patients who need skilled medical care that cannot be provided in a custodial-level nursing home or in the patient's home.

small claims litigation – Process administered by the services at local county or district courts that makes it easy for individuals or businesses to recover legitimate debts without using expensive legal advisors. Small claims suits can be for any amount of money up to a limiting threshold that varies by state, usually $3000 to $5000.

small (entity) provider – Provider of services with fewer than 25 full-time equivalent employees or a physician, practitioner, facility, or supplier (other than a provider of services) with fewer than 10 full-time equivalent employees.

small provider of services – Hospital, critical access hospital, skilled nursing facility (SNF), comprehensive outpatient rehabilitation facility, home health agency, or hospice program with fewer than 25 full-time equivalent employees.

small supplier – Physician, practitioner, facility, or supplier with fewer than 10 full-time equivalent employees.

Social Security Disability Insurance (SSDI) – (1) Primary federal insurance program that protects workers from loss of income resulting from disability and provides monthly cash benefits to disabled workers younger than age 65 and to certain dependents. (2) Insurance program for individuals who become unable to work. It is administered by the Social Security Administration and funded by Federal Insurance Contributions Act tax withheld from workers' pay and by matching employer contributions. SSDI pays qualifying disabled workers cash and healthcare benefits.

specialist – Physician who is trained in a certain area of medicine.

special needs plan (SNP) – Type of Medicare Advantage plan designed to attract and enroll Medicare beneficiaries who fall into a certain special needs classification. There are two types of SNPs. The exclusive SNP enrolls only beneficiaries who fall into the special needs demographic. The other type is the disproportionate share SNP.

special report – Report that accompanies the claim to help determine the appropriateness and medical necessity of the service or procedure. It is required by many third-party payers when a rarely used, unusual, variable, or new service or procedure is performed.

Specified Low-Income Medicare Beneficiaries – Beneficiaries with resources similar to Qualified Medicare Beneficiaries but with slightly higher incomes.

spend down – Depleting private or family finances to the point where the individual or family becomes eligible for Medicaid assistance.

sponsor – Under the TRICARE plan, a service member, whether in active duty, retired, or deceased.

staff model – Closed panel type of health maintenance organization (HMO) in which a multispecialty group of physicians are contracted to provide healthcare to members of an HMO and are compensated by the contractor via salary and incentive programs.

stand-alone code – Current Procedural Terminology (CPT) code that contains the full description of the procedure without additional explanation.

standardized amount – Figure representing the average cost per case for all Medicare cases during the year.

standard paper remittance advice (SPRA) – Product of the standardization of the provider payment notification of the Centers for Medicare and Medicaid Services (CMS). The form was created to provide a document that is uniform in content and format and to ease the transition to the electronic remittance format.

State Children's Health Insurance Program (SCHIP) – Program that allows states to expand their Medicaid eligibility guidelines to cover more categories of children.

stop loss insurance – Protection from exorbitant medical claims. This is often used by self-insured groups.

subacute care unit – Comprehensive, highly specialized inpatient program designed for an individual who has had an acute event as a result of an illness, injury, or worsening of a disease process. It specifies a level of maintenance care where there is no urgent or life-threatening condition requiring medical treatment.

subcategory – In the Current Procedural Terminology (CPT) Evaluation and Management section, codes are divided into categories and subcategories. A category would be Office or Other Outpatient Services; a subcategory under it could be either New Patient or Established Patient. In the ICD-9-CM coding system, there are 3-digit category codes, usually followed by a 4th or 5th digit set of subcategory codes.

subheading – One of four classifications in the Tabular section (Volume 1) of the Current Procedural Terminology (CPT) manual. See subsection.

subjective information – Biased or personal information. For example, a patient's history is based on what the patient tells the healthcare provider in his or her own words.

subpoena duces tecum – Legal document that requires an individual to appear in court with a piece of evidence that can be used or inspected by the court.

subsection – One of four classifications in the Tabular section (Volume 1) of the Current Procedural Terminology (CPT) manual that divides sections further into smaller units, usually by body system.

supplemental coverage – Benefit add-ons to health plans such as vision, dental, or prescription drug coverage.

supplemental medical insurance (SMI) – See Medicare supplement plans and Medigap insurance.

Supplemental Security Income (SSI) – Program established in 1972 and controlled by the Social Security Administration that provides federally funded cash assistance to qualifying elderly and disabled poor individuals.

surrogate – Substitute.

suspension file – Series of files set up chronologically and labeled according to the number of days since the claim was submitted. This type of claims tracking system is used by offices that file paper claims.

swing beds – Changes in reimbursement status when patients "swing" from receiving acute care services and reimbursement to receiving skilled nursing services and reimbursement.

T

Tax Equity and Fiscal Responsibility Act (TEFRA) – Law enacted by Congress in 1982 to place limits on Medicare reimbursement that applies to stays in long-term acute care hospitals. After TEFRA was passed, the fee-for-service-based payment system was replaced with a prospective payment system.

telecommunication – Transmission of claim information over phone lines using a computer and a modem. This is the most common form of electronic claim transmission.

temporarily disabled – When an individual is unable to work for a short time as a result of sickness or injury (excluding job-related illnesses or injuries).

Temporary Assistance for Needy Families (TANF) – Federal-state cash assistance program for poor families, typically headed by a single parent. Formerly called Aid to Families with Dependent Children.

temporary disability – Level of disability where the worker's ability to perform his or her job responsibilities is lost for a specific period. There are two subcategories of temporary disability—temporary total disability and temporary partial disability.

temporary partial disability – When an injury or illness impairs an employee's ability to work for a limited time. The impairment is such that the individual is able to perform limited employment duties and is expected to recover fully.

temporary total disability – When a worker's ability to perform his or her job responsibilities is totally lost but on a temporary basis.

third party (party of the third part) – In legal language, the insurance company in the implied contract between the physician and the patient.

third-party administrator (TPA) – Person or organization who processes claims and performs other contractual administrative services. Often hired by self-insured groups to provide claims-paying functions.

third-party liability – Legal obligation of third parties to pay all or part of the expenditures for medical assistance furnished under a state plan.

third-party payer – Any organization (e.g., Blue Cross and Blue Shield, Medicare, Medicaid, commercial insurance company) that provides payment for specified coverages provided under the health plan.

Ticket to Work Program – Voluntary program that gives certain individuals with disabilities greater choice in selecting the service providers and rehabilitation services they need to help them keep working or get back to work. This program was created with passage of the federal Ticket to Work and Work Incentives Improvement Act of 1999.

trading partner agreement – Formal contract between Medicare Part B and a supplemental insurer.

transaction set – Collection of data that contains all the information required by the receiving system to perform a normal business transaction. An example is the overall data stream of an 837 file, which is divided into sections with each section providing a specific kind of information.

treating source – Provides the long-term medical information (called medical evidence of record), which is normally required in every claim for disability benefits.

treatment, payment, or (healthcare) operations (TPO) – To avoid interfering with an individual's access to quality health care or the efficient payment for such healthcare, the Health Insurance Portability and Accountability Act (HIPAA) Privacy Rule permits a covered entity to use and disclose protected health information, with certain limits and protections, for treatment, payment, and health care operations activities without the patient's written consent, provided that such use or disclosure is consistent with other applicable requirement of the HIPAA privacy rules.

TRICARE – Regionally based managed healthcare program for active duty personnel and eligible family members, retirees and family members younger than age 65, and survivors of all uniformed services.

TRICARE allowable charge – See CHAMPUS Maximum Allowable Charge.

TRICARE Extra – Preferred provider option through which, rather than an annual fee, a yearly deductible is charged. Healthcare is delivered through a network of civilian healthcare providers who accept payments from TRICARE and provide services at negotiated, discounted rates.

TRICARE for Life (TFL) – Comprehensive health benefits program with no monthly premium. TFL is available to uniformed services retirees, their spouses, and their survivors who are 65 or older, are Medicare-eligible, are enrolled in Medicare Part A, and have purchased Medicare Part B coverage. TFL was established by the National Defense Authorization Act.

TRICARE Management Activity – Established by the Department of Defense to oversee the TRICARE managed healthcare program and to enhance the performance of TRICARE worldwide.

TRICARE Prime – Health maintenance organization (HMO) type of plan in which enrollees receive healthcare through a military treatment facility primary care manager or a supporting network of civilian providers.

TRICARE Prime Remote – Provides healthcare coverage through civilian networks or TRICARE-authorized providers for uniformed service members and their families who are on remote assignment.

TRICARE Standard – Standard fee-for-service (indemnity) option. This program provides greater personal choice in the selection of healthcare providers, although it requires higher individual out-of-pocket costs than a managed care plan. Formerly called CHAMPUS.

TRICARE Standard Supplemental Insurance – Health benefit plans that are specifically designed to supplement TRICARE Standard benefits. Plans are frequently available from military associations or other private organizations and firms and generally pay most or all of whatever is left after TRICARE Standard has paid its share of the cost of covered healthcare services and supplies.

Truth in Lending Act – Requires the person or business entity to disclose the exact credit terms when extending credit to applicants and regulates how they advertise consumer credit.

U

UB-04 – Basic hardcopy (paper) claim form, also known as Form CMS-1450, required by the Centers for Medicare and Medicaid Services (CMS) and accepted only from institutional providers (e.g., hospitals, skilled nursing facilities [SNFs], home health agencies) that are excluded from the mandatory electronic claims submission requirement set forth in the Administrative Simplification Compliance Act.

unit/floor time – Time the physician spends on bedside care of the patient and reviewing the health record and writing orders.

unusual circumstances – Situations beyond the control of the submitting provider, such as a service interruption in the mode of submitting electronic claims or other extraordinary circumstances, which prevents claims from being submitted electronically.

usual, customary, and reasonable (UCR) – Use of fee screens to determine the lowest value of physician reimbursement based on (1) the physician's usual charge for a given procedure, (2) the amount customarily charged for the service by other physicians in the area (often defined as a specific percentile of all charges in the community), and (3) the reasonable cost of services for a given patient after medical review of the case. UCR rates are typically what an insurance carrier would allow as covered expenses.

utilization review – Method of tracking, reviewing, and giving opinions regarding care provided to patients. Utilization review evaluates the necessity, appropriateness, and efficiency of the use of healthcare services, procedures, and facilities to control costs and manage care.

Utilization Review Accreditation Commission (URAC) – Independent, nonprofit organization. Its mission is to promote continuous improvement in the quality and efficiency of healthcare delivery by achieving a common understanding of excellence among purchasers, providers, and patients through the establishment of standards, programs of education and communication, and a process of accreditation.

V

V codes – A classification of codes in ICD-9-CM provided to deal with occasions when circumstances other than a disease or injury classifiable to categories 001-999 (the main part of ICD-9) are recorded as "diagnoses" or "problems." Supplementary Classification of Factors Influencing Health Status and Contact with Health Services (V01-V91.)

vertically integrated hospitals – Hospitals that provide all levels of healthcare.

vocational rehabilitation – Retraining or physical therapy that may be necessary if an injury or illness results in a worker being unable to perform the usual duties of his or her occupation.

W

waiver – Formal (sometimes written) release from a particular rule or regulation. For example, the Secretary of the U.S. Department of Health and Human Services may grant a waiver for submitting Medicare claims electronically if the provider of services is experiencing "unusual circumstances."

workers' compensation – Type of insurance regulated by state laws that pays medical expenses and partial loss of wages for workers who are injured on the job or become ill as a result of job-related circumstances. Commonly referred to as workers' comp or WC.

X

XPressClaim – Secure, streamlined Web-based system that allows providers to submit TRICARE claims electronically and, in most cases, to receive instant results.

Index

A

AAAHC (Accreditation Association for Ambulatory Health Care), 54, 378, 379
AALL (American Association for Labor Legislation), 4t
Abandoning, of patient, 28
Abbreviations, in ICD-10 tabular list, 245
ABN (advanced beneficiary notice), 161–162, 163f
Abnormal findings, ICD-10-CM coding for, 260
Abuse
  defined, 139
  healthcare, 41–42
    by consumers, 42
    costs of, 41–42
    defining, 41–42
    examples of, 41
    prevention of, 42
    schemes for committing, 42
    who commits, 42
  in Medicaid system, 139–140
Acceptance, of contract, 28–29
Access
  to health insurance, 7–9
  to information
    through de-identification, 301–303
    through patient authorization, 301, 302f
Accountability, 36
Accountable Care Organizations (ACOs), 11, 52
Accounting methods, 304–306
  daily journal (day sheet) as, 304, 305f
  disbursements journal as, 304, 306f
  electronic software as, 305–306
  general journal as, 304
  general ledger as, 304
  "one-write" or pegboard system as, 304, 307f
  patient ledger as, 304, 307f
  payroll journal as, 304, 306f
Accounting systems, computerized, 305–306, 361–365
  generating reports in, 364–365
    accounts receivable aging report as, 364, 365f
    insurance claims aging report as, 364, 366f, 367f

Accounting systems, computerized (Continued)
    practice analysis report as, 364–365, 368f
  HIPAA and, 365–369
  managing transactions with, 362–364
    insurance carrier adjustments (contractual write-offs) in, 363–364
    posting and tracking patient charges in, 362, 363f
    processing payments in, 363, 363f
  selection of, 361–362
Accounts receivable, 304
Accreditation, 378–379
  by Accreditation Association for Ambulatory Health Care, 378, 379
  defined, 378
  by Joint Commission, 378
  by National Committee for Quality Assurance, 378–379
  by Utilization Review Accreditation Commission, 379
Accreditation Association for Ambulatory Health Care (AAAHC), 54, 378, 379
ACN (attachment control number), 80
ACOs (Accountable Care Organizations), 11, 52
Active Duty Dental Program (ADDP), 190–192
Active duty family members (ADFMs), 194
Activities of daily living (ADLs), 231, 377
  for resource utilization groups, 358–359
Actuarial value, 89
Actuaries, 10
Acute care, defined, 375
Acute care facilities, 375
Acute conditions
  defined, 375
  ICD-10-CM coding for, 250–253
Acute inpatient hospital prospective payment system, 355, 359
ADA (Americans with Disabilities Act), 231
Additional insurance, on patient information form, 67–68, 67f, 68f
Additional Low-Income Medicare Beneficiary (ALMB) Program, 132
ADDP (Active Duty Dental Program), 190–192

ADFMs (active duty family members), 194
Adjudication, 325
  Current Procedural Terminology and, 273
  defined, 323
  form for, 325, 326f
  by Medicaid, 136
  by Medicare, 172
  real-time, 334
Adjustments, insurance carrier, 363–364
ADLs (activities of daily living), 231, 377
  for resource utilization groups, 358–359
Administrative functionality, in electronic medical record, 347
Administrative services organizations (ASOs), 89–90
Administrative Simplification Compliance Act (ASCA)
  on claim submission, 63–64, 79
  on electronic transmissions, 338–339
  on Medicare claims, 165–168, 166f
  on UB-04 form, 384–385
Admission services, E & M codes for, 287
Advanced beneficiary notice (ABN), 161–162, 163f
Advancement, in hospital billing career, 399–400
Affordable Care Act, 49
  and Medicaid, 125, 125f
Aged individuals, Medicaid for, 123f
Agency for Healthcare Policy and Research (AHCPR), 115
Aging population, 299
Aging report
  accounts receivable, 364, 365f
  electronic insurance
    generation of, 364, 366f, 367f
    tracking of, 80–82, 81f
AHCPR (Agency for Healthcare Policy and Research), 115
Aid to Needy Families with Children/Reach Up (ANFC/RU), 121
Allowable charges
  under Medicare, 150
  under TRICARE, 196
Allowed services, under TRICARE, 190
ALMB (Additional Low-Income Medicare Beneficiary) Program, 132
ALOS (average length of stay), 357

Page numbers followed by *f* indicate figures; *t* tables; *b* boxes.

Alphabetic index, to ICD-10-CM, 241, 244*f*
  coding steps for, 243
  cross-references in, 243–246
  essential and nonessential modifiers in,
    242–243, 245*f*
  main terms in, 242–246, 244*f*
  parentheses in, 243–246, 247*f*
Alternate billing cycle, 78, 308
Alternative medicine, Medicare Part A
    noncoverage of, 147*t*
AMA. *See* American Medical Association
    (AMA).
Ambulatory patient groups (APGs), 358
Ambulatory payment classifications (APCs),
    238, 356*t*, 358, 394
Ambulatory surgery
  CHAMPVA coverage for, 204*t*, 205*t*
  ICD-10-CM coding for, 259–263
Ambulatory surgery centers (ASCs), 376
American Accreditation HealthCare
    Commission, 54
American Association for Labor Legislation
    (AALL), 4*t*
American Collectors Association, 314
American Medical Association (AMA)
  Code of Medical Ethics of, 39
  in origins of health insurance, 4–5, 4*t*
  Physicians' CPT codes of, 274
American National Standards Institute
    (ANSI)
  on claim attachments, 80
  on electronic data interchange, 339
  on practice management software, 366
American Recovery and Reinvestment Act
    (ARRA)
  on electronic medical records, 348
  history of, 8
  and Medicaid, 120–121
American Standard Code for Information
    Interchange (ASCII), 77
Americans with Disabilities Act (ADA), 231
Ancillary members, of medical team, 27
"and," in ICD-10-CM coding, 252
ANFC/RU (Aid to Needy Families with
    Children/Reach Up), 121
ANSI. *See* American National Standards
    Institute (ANSI).
Anthracosis, 215
APCs (ambulatory payment classifications),
    238, 356*t*, 358, 394
APGs (ambulatory patient groups), 358
Appeals, 334–335
  under CHAMPVA, 209
  due to denied claims, 334
  due to incorrect payments, 334
  under Medicare, 335
    for fee-for-service claims, 176–179,
      179*f*
    for managed care claims, 179–180,
      180*f*
  time limit for filing, 332
  under workers' compensation, 216–217

Appendices
  of Current Procedural Terminology
    manual, 276
  of HCPCS Level II coding manual, 291
Application skills, computer, 14
Appointment times, patient expectations of,
    297
ARRA. *See* American Recovery and
    Reinvestment Act (ARRA).
ASC(s) (ambulatory surgery centers), 376
ASC X12 Version 5010, for Medicare claims,
    167
ASCA. *See* Administrative Simplification
    Compliance Act (ASCA).
ASCA X12N 8371 Version 5010,
    385–387
  data elements in segment of, 385–387,
    387*f*
  data layout of, 385–387
  response to transmission of, 387, 387*f*
  transaction set section of, 385, 387*f*
ASCII (American Standard Code for
    Information Interchange), 77
ASOs (administrative services organizations),
    89–90
Assignment
  acceptance of
    with Medicaid, 138
    with TRICARE, 196
  of benefits, 67*f*, 68, 303
  of diagnosis-related groups, 357
Associate degree, 14
Associated Credit Bureaus, 314
Attachment(s), to claims, 79–80
Attachment control number (ACN), 80
Attending physician's statement, for
    disability claim, 228*f*, 230
Audits, Medicare, 175
Authorization to release information
  accessing information through, 301,
    302*f*
  for disability claim, 229*f*
  exceptions for insurance claims
    submission to, 40
  HIPAA on, 300
  legal aspects of, 33, 34*f*, 40
  "lifetime," 68
  on patient information form, 67*f*, 68
Authorized providers, TRICARE,
    194–196
Automated voice response (AVR) system, to
    verify Medicaid eligibility, 131
Autonomy, 17–18, 86
Average length of stay (ALOS), 357

B

Bachelor of Science degree, 14
Bad debt write-offs, 364
Balance billing, 55
  with Medicaid, 138
  resource-based relative value scale and,
    356–357

Balanced Budget Act (BBA)
  and home health prospective payment
    system, 360
  and Medicaid managed care, 133–134, 151
Basic coverage, 47, 86
BCBS. *See* Blue Cross and Blue Shield (BCBS).
BCBSA (Blue Cross and Blue Shield
    Association), 90
Beneficiary(ies)
  of Medicare, 69, 146
  of TRICARE, 188–189
Beneficiary Complaint Response Program,
    181
Beneficiary Notices Initiative, 181
Benefit(s)
  assignment of, 67*f*, 68
  coordination of, 55, 333
    with TRICARE, 193
  explanation of. *See* Explanation of benefits
    (EOB).
  maintenance of, 55
  standardized, 49
  summary of, 49
Benefit cap, for short-term disability policies,
    225
Benefit period, for Medicare, 150–151, 382
Bill(s), overdue, 308
Billing, 303–308
  accounting methods for, 304–306
    daily journal (day sheet) as, 304, 305*f*
    disbursements journal as, 304, 306*f*
    electronic software as, 305–306
    general journal as, 304
    general ledger as, 304
    "one-write" or pegboard system as, 304,
      307*f*
    patient ledger as, 304, 307*f*
    payroll journal as, 304, 306*f*
  assignment of benefits in, 303
  balance, 55
    with Medicaid, 138
    resource-based relative value scale and,
      356–357
  billing services for, 314, 340
  and collection, 308–311
  cost of software system for, 362
  electronic medical records and, 306–308
  hospital. *See* Hospital billing.
  keeping patient informed in, 304
  patient accounting system for, 361–362
Billing compliance, 398–399
Billing Coordinator, 17*t*
Billing cycle, 78, 308
Billing date, errors in, 136*f*
Billing errors, in Medicaid, 135–136, 136*f*
Billing services, 314, 340
Binding contract, 28
Biologicals, Medicare Part A noncoverage
    of, 147*t*
Birthday rule, 54–55, 333
Black Lung Benefits Act, 215
Blood, Medicare coverage for, 146*t*

Blue Cross, history of, 3, 4t, 90
Blue Cross and Blue Shield (BCBS), 90–94
  claims submission for, 95–96
    electronic, 95–96
    timely, 95
  deductibles for, 384
  as hospital payer, 384
  participating vs. nonparticipating providers in, 95
  preauthorization by, 384
  programs of, 91–94
    BlueCard Program and BlueCard Worldwide as, 91, 91f, 92f
    Federal Employee Program as, 91
    Federal Employees Health Benefits as, 91
    healthcare service plans as, 94
      high-deductible, 94
      indemnity (fee-for-service), 94
      managed care (HMOs and PPOs), 90, 94
      point-of-service, 94
    Medicare as, 91–94
    Medicare supplement plans as, 94
  Websites to Explore on, 100
Blue Cross and Blue Shield Association (BCBSA), 90
Blue Cross and Blue Shield (BCBS) member hospitals, 384
"Blue Plans," 90
Blue Shield, history of, 3, 90–91
BlueCard Program, 91, 91f
BlueCard Worldwide, 91, 92f
"Blues, the," 90
Bold
  in ASCA X12N 8371 version 5010, 385
  in CPT manual index, 277
Brackets, in ICD-10 tabular list, 245–246
Breach
  of confidentiality, 41
  of contract, 28
  of ethical principle, 380–381
Budget period, for Medicaid, 124–125
Bullet, in CPT manual, 278t
Business associate, 368–369

C

CAAHEP (Commission on Accreditation of Allied Health Education Programs), 399
CAC (common access card), for TRICARE eligibility, 194
Cafeteria plan, 50
CAHs (critical access hospitals), 375–376
CAP (Claims Assistant Professional), 17t
Capitation
  history of, 4t
  in HMO, 105
  in Medicaid managed care, 133
  reimbursement with, 353t, 354
Career opportunities
  for health insurance professional, 18–20
  in hospital billing, 399–400

Carrier(s)
  Medicare, 91–94, 146–147, 148f, 381
  Railroad Retirement Board, 146–147
Carrier adjustments, 363–364
Carrier direct, 80, 340, 341
  vs. claims clearinghouses, 76–77, 341–342
Carrier information, on back of insurance card, 321–322, 322f
"Carrying fee," 311
Carve-out, 90
Case-level adjustment, 359–360
Case-mix adjustment, 355
Cash disbursements journal, 304, 306f
Casual employee, 216
Catastrophic (cat) cap
  for CHAMPVA, 203
  for TRICARE, 196
Categorically needy, Medicaid for, 123f, 124
Category(ies)
  in CPT coding, 279, 280f
  in E & M coding, 281
  in HCPCS Level II coding, 290, 290f
  in ICD-10 tabular list, 242, 247f
Category II codes, 275–276
Category III codes, 276, 276f
CCA (certified coding associate), 400t
CCS (certified coding specialist), 400t
CCS-P (certified coding specialist–physician-based), 400t
CDM (charge description master), 396, 396t
Center for Medicare and Medicaid Innovation (CMI), 182
Centers for Disease Control and Prevention (CDC), Disability and Health Team of, 232–233
Centers for Medicare and Medicaid Services (CMS)
  Affordable Care Act of, 49
  claims form of. See CMS-1500 (08/05) form.
  hierarchical condition category of, 355–356
Certificate of coverage, 49
Certificate of creditable coverage, for TRICARE, 189
Certificates of Medical Necessity (CMNs), as claim attachments, 79–80
Certification
  as health insurance professional, 14, 19, 20–21
  in hospital billing, 400, 400t
  of managed care programs, 107–108
Certified coding associate (CCA), 400t
Certified coding specialist (CCS), 400t
Certified coding specialist–physician-based (CCS-P), 400t
Certified professional coder–hospital (CPC-H), 400t
CFC (Community First Choice) Option, 125
CHAMPUS (Civilian Health and Medical Programs of the Uniformed Services), 187

CHAMPUS Maximum Allowable Charge (CMAC), 190
CHAMPVA. See Civilian Health and Medical Program of the Department of Veterans Affairs (CHAMPVA).
CHAMPVA cat cap, 203
CHAMPVA for Life (CFL) program, 207, 207t
  eligibility for, 207
CHAMPVA In-house Treatment Initiative (CITI), 203, 206
CHAMPVA Meds by Mail program, 205
Charge(s)
  errors in, 136f
  hospital, 396
Charge description master (CDM), 396, 396t
Chart notes, 69–70, 70f
Chief complaint, E & M codes for, 284
Children, Medicaid for, 123f
Children's Health Insurance Program (CHIP), 9, 125–126
Chronic conditions, ICD-10-CM coding for, 250–253, 257–258
CITI (CHAMPVA In-house Treatment Initiative), 203, 206
Civilian Health and Medical Program of the Department of Veterans Affairs (CHAMPVA), 48–50, 199–207
  benefits under, 203
  cat cap for, 203
  CHAMPVA for Life program in, 207, 207t
    eligibility for, 207
  claims for, 207–208
    appeals and reconsiderations of, 209
    electronic, 207
    explanation of benefits for, 209, 210f
    filing deadlines for, 208, 208b
    paper, 208–209
  cost sharing for, 201–202, 203–205
    with no other health insurance, 203, 204t
    with other health insurance, 203, 204t
  eligibility for, 199–201
    extended, 202
    identification of, 202–203, 202f
    loss of, 201
  and HMO coverage, 206
  as hospital payer, 383–384
  in-house treatment initiative of, 203, 206
  and Medicare, 206
  Meds by Mail program of, 205
  payment summary for, 203, 205t
  preauthorization for, 203–205, 207–208
  prescription drug benefit under, 205–206
  providers under, 206–207
  and TRICARE, 206
  types of health insurance plans primary to, 206
Civilian Health and Medical Programs of the Uniformed Services (CHAMPUS), 187
  maximum allowable charge for, 190

Claim(s), 61–83, 318–336
  adjudication of, 325
    Current Procedural Terminology and, 273
    defined, 323
    form for, 325, 326f
    by Medicaid, 136
    by Medicare, 172
    real-time, 334
  appeals of, 334–335
    under CHAMPVA, 209
    due to denied claims, 334
    due to incorrect payments, 334
    under Medicare, 335
      for fee-for-service claims, 176–179,
        179f
      for managed care claims, 179–180,
        180f
    time limit for filing, 332
    under workers' compensation, 216–217
  attachments to, 79–80
  BCBS and commercial, 95–96
    electronic filing of, 95–96
    timely filing of, 95
  for CHAMPVA, 207–208
    appeals and reconsiderations of, 209
    electronic, 207
    explanation of benefits for, 209, 210f
    filing deadlines for, 208, 208b
    paper, 208–209
  clean, 79, 322–323
  CMS-1500 (08/05) form for, 21–23, 47,
    77–82
    for CHAMPVA, 208
    common errors/omissions on, 78, 78f
    completion of
      general guidelines for, 319, 320b
      instructions for, 63, 77, 406–424
    example of, 22f, 404–405
    format of, 77
    history of, 62–63, 77
    for Medicaid, 134
    for Medicare, 168–172
    optical character recognition from, 77–78
      format rules for, 77–78, 78f
    proofreading of, 79
    proposed revisions to, 63
    users of, 78–79
  common errors made on, 78, 78f, 322,
    322b
  correction of, 325, 326f
  denied, 323
    appeals of, 334
  for disability income insurance, 225–230
    attending physician's statement in,
      228f, 230
    authorization to disclose health
      information in, 229f
    employee's responsibilities in, 225–230,
      226f
    employer's responsibilities in, 227f, 230
    health insurance professional's role in,
      230

Claim(s) (Continued)
  electronic, 63
    advantages of, 75
    BCBS and commercial, 95–96
    CHAMPVA, 207
    electronic transactions and code set
      requirements for, 64
    essential information on, 66–73
      additional insurance as, 67–68, 67f, 68f
      from encounter form, 70–72, 71f, 72f,
        73f
      insurance authorization and
        assignment as, 67f, 68
      insurance information as, 66, 67f, 68f
      new patient information as, 66, 67f,
        68f
      from patient health record, 69–70, 70f
      from patient information form,
        66–68, 67f
      from patient insurance identification
        card, 66, 69, 69f
      from patient ledger card, 72–73, 74f
    HIPAA on, 21, 63–65
      electronic transactions and code set
        requirements of, 64
      exceptions in, 65, 65b, 165–167
      national identifier requirements of,
        64–65
      new 5010 standards for, 65–66, 65b
      privacy requirements of, 64
      security requirements of, 64
    hospital, 396–397
    Medicare, 165, 342–343
      exceptions to mandatory, 65, 65b,
        165–167
    national identifier requirements for,
      64–65
    privacy requirements for, 64
    process for submitting, 66–77, 340–342
      advantages of, 342
      clearinghouse for, 75–76, 340, 341f
      clearinghouse vs. direct data entry for,
        76–77, 341–342
      direct data entry for, 76, 340, 341
      enrollment in, 340
      filing methods in, 340
      for Medicare, 342–343
    security requirements for, 64
    for TRICARE, 199, 383
    UB-04, 385–387
      data elements in segment of, 385–387,
        387f
      data layout of, 385–387
      response to transmission of, 387, 387f
      transaction set section of, 385, 387f
    verifying insurance with new
      technology on, 73–75
  electronic media, 342–343
  employer identification number on, 323
  explanation of benefits for, 96, 97f
    CHAMPVA, 209, 210f
    defined, 328–329

Claim(s) (Continued)
    downcoding in, 330
    electronic, 96–98, 344
      authorization for, 344, 346f
    interpretation of, 328–330, 331f
    Medicaid, 136, 137f
    Medicare, 172–175
      electronic, 175
      standard paper, 172–175, 174f
    TRICARE, 199, 200f
    troubleshooting in, 329–330
  HIPAA on, 323
  inpatient hospital
    data elements for, 394, 395b
    electronic, 396–397
  international form for, 91, 92f
  keys to successful, 319–322, 320f
    collection and verification of patient
      information as, 320–321
    documentation as, 322
    following payer guidelines as, 322
    obtaining necessary preauthorization
      and precertification as, 321–322,
      322f
    proofreading to avoid errors as, 322, 322b
    submission of clean claim as, 322–323
  Medicaid, 134–135
    CMS-1500 form for, 134
    reciprocity of, 134–135
    resubmission of, 134
    secondary, 134, 135t
    "simple," 134
    time limit for filing, 136
  Medicare, 165–168
    Administrative Simplification
      Compliance Act on, 165–167, 166f
    appeals on, 335
      with fee-for-service, 176–179, 179f
      with managed care, 179–180, 180f
    audits of, 175
    deadline for filing, 168
    demand bills for, 165, 166f
    electronic, 165, 342–343
      exceptions to mandatory, 65, 65b,
        165–167
    electronic funds transfer for, 175, 177f
    for hospital costs, 381–384, 382t
    initial, 165
    Medicare Summary Notice for, 172–175,
      173f
    information on, 172
    for Medigap, 169, 169f, 170t
    paper
      ASCA enforcement of, 167–168
      CMS-1500 form for, 168–172
      exception criteria for, 65, 65b, 165–167
      guidelines for completion of, 168–169
    Recovery Audit Contractor Program for,
      176
    remittance advice for, 172–175
      electronic, 175, 176f
      standard paper, 172–175, 174f

Claim(s) *(Continued)*
  for secondary policy, 169–171, 333
    completion of, 170–171, 171*t*
    conditional payment for, 171
    criteria for, 169–170
    status request for, 168
    timely filing rules for, 168
    transition to ASC X12 Version 5010 for, 167
  Medicare/Medicaid crossover, 135, 171–172
  optical character recognition scanning of, 325, 325*b*
  outpatient, 394, 395*b*
  overview of, 62–63
  paper
    for CHAMPVA, 208–209
    for Medicare
      ASCA enforcement of, 167–168
      CMS-1500 form for, 168–172
      exception criteria for, 65, 65*b*, 165–167
      guidelines for completion of, 168–169
    for TRICARE, 198–199, 198*f*
    UB-04, 384–385, 386*f*
  payments on
    incorrect, 334
    posting of, 19, 330, 332*f*
    processing of, 363, 363*f*
    receiving of, 328, 330*t*
  processing of, 323–333
    appeals in, 334–335
      under CHAMPVA, 209
      due to denied claims, 334
      due to incorrect payments, 334
      under Medicare, 335
      time limit for filing, 332
      under workers' compensation, 216–217
    claims adjudication in, 325
      Current Procedural Terminology and, 273
      defined, 323
      form for, 325, 326*f*
      by Medicaid, 136
      by Medicare, 172
      real-time, 334
    flow chart for, 324*f*
    interpretation of explanation of benefits in, 328–330, 331*f*
      downcoding in, 330
      troubleshooting in, 329–330
    optical character recognition scanning in, 325, 325*b*
    posting payments in, 19, 330, 332*f*
    receiving payment in, 328, 330*t*
    for secondary claims, 333–334, 333*f*
    steps in, 324*f*
    time limits for, 330–333
    tracking in, 325–328, 327*f*
      insurance claims register system for, 328, 329*f*
      suspension file system for, 328
  rejected, 79, 323

Claim(s) *(Continued)*
  returned, 79, 323
  secondary, 333–334, 333*f*
    Medicaid, 134, 135*t*
  submission methods for, 62–63
  for Supplemental Security Income and Social Security Disability Insurance, 233–234
    health insurance professional's role in, 234
    healthcare provider's role in, 233–234
    patient's role in, 233
  tracking of, 80–82, 325–328
    electronic insurance aging report for, 80–82, 81*f*
    form for, 325–328, 327*f*
    insurance claims register system for, 328, 329*f*
    insurance log for, 80–82, 81*f*
    suspension file system for, 328
    using practice management software, 80–82, 80*f*
  for TRICARE, 197–199
    deadline for submitting, 199
    electronic, 199, 383
    explanation of benefits for, 199, 200*f*
    paper, 198–199, 198*f*
    who submits, 197–198
  uniform bill (UB-04), 384–387
    claim form and completion instructions for, 425–429
    data specifications for, 385
    electronic, 385–387
      data elements in segment of, 385–387, 387*f*
      data layout of, 385–387
      response to transmission of, 387, 387*f*
      transaction set section of, 385, 387*f*
    paper, 384–385, 386*f*
  websites on, 83, 336
  workers' compensation, 217–222
    first report of injury in, 217, 218*f*
    forms for, 222
    physician's role in, 217–220, 221*f*
    time limits for, 217
Claim adjustment reason code, 165–167
Claim attachments, 79–80
Claims Assistant Professional (CAP), 17*t*
Claims clearinghouses, 75–76, 340
  vs. direct claims, 76–77, 340
  flow chart of claim sent to, 340–341, 341*f*
  for TRICARE, 199
Claims processor, for TRICARE, 197
Claims register, 80–82, 81*f*, 328, 329*f*
Claims tracking form, 325–328, 327*f*
Class preparation, 15
Clean claims, 79, 322–323
Clearinghouses, 75–76, 340
  vs. direct claims, 76–77, 340
  flow chart of claim sent to, 340–341, 341*f*
  for TRICARE claims, 199
Clinic, 375

Clinical chart note, 69–70, 70*f*
Clinical Laboratory Improvement Amendments (CLIA) program, 182
Clinical notes, 69–70, 70*f*
Closed-panel plan, 105
CMAC (CHAMPUS Maximum Allowable Charge), 190
CMI (Center for Medicare and Medicaid Innovation), 182
CMNs (Certificates of Medical Necessity), as claim attachments, 79–80
CMS (Centers for Medicare and Medicaid Services)
  Affordable Care Act of, 49
  hierarchical condition category of, 355–356
CMS Quarterly Provider Update, 161
CMS-1450 form. *See* Uniform bill (UB-04) claim form.
CMS-1500 (08/05) form, 21–23, 47, 77–82
  for CHAMPVA, 208
  common errors/omissions on, 78, 78*f*
  completion of
    general guidelines for, 319, 320*b*
    instructions for, 63, 77, 406–424
  example of, 22*f*, 404–405
  format of, 77
  history of, 62–63, 77
  for Medicaid, 134
  for Medicare, 168–172
  optical character recognition from, 77–78
    format rules for, 77–78, 78*f*
  proofreading of, 79
  proposed revisions to, 63, 301
  users of, 78–79
COB (coordination of benefits), 55, 333
  with TRICARE, 193
COBA (Coordination of Benefits Agreement) Program, 171
COBC (Coordination of Benefits Contractor), 171
COBRA (Consolidated Omnibus Budget Reconciliation Act), 8, 29–30, 53–54
Code(s)
  in ICD-10 tabular list, 242, 247*f*
  in inpatient health records, 388
  uses of, 240–241
"Code also" note, in ICD-10 tabular list, 248–249
"Code first" note, in ICD-10-CM coding, 248
Code fragmentation, 42
Code layout, in CPT manual index, 277
Code libraries, 362
Code of Medical Ethics, 39
Code sets
  for Current Procedural Terminology, 274
  for electronic claims, 64
  HIPAA requirements for, 64, 339
  for posting and tracking of patient charges, 362
Coder, certified professional, 400*t*

Coding
  crosswalk in, 292
  Evaluation and Management (E & M).
      See Evaluation and Management
      (E & M) codes.
  HCPCS, 289–291, 290f
    HIPAA and, 292
    history of, 274
    Level II manual for, 290–291
      appendices in, 291
      index of main terms in, 290–291,
          291f
      modifiers in, 291
      table of drugs in, 291
    National Medicare Codes of, 274
    overview of, 289–291
    uses of, 274–275
    websites on, 294
  ICD-10 system for. See International
      Classification of Diseases (ICD)-10
      coding system.
  inpatient, 388–393
    E & M codes for, 281, 287
    ICD-10-PCS for, 389–390
      code structure of, 390
      format of, 390, 391f
      selecting principal diagnosis in,
          390–392, 392b
    National Correct Coding Initiative for,
        392, 393t
    National Correct Coding Initiative for,
        291–292, 392, 393t
  outpatient, 393–394
    ambulatory payment classification
        coding for, 394
    prospective payment system and,
        393–394
  for TRICARE, 196–197
Coding associate, certified, 400t
Coding specialist, 17t
  certified, 400t
  physician-based, 400t
  reporting of denied charges to, 19
Coexisting conditions, ICD-10-CM coding
    for, 258–264
Coinsurance, 47, 86
Collection
  arranging credit or payment plans for,
      308–310
    establishing credit in, 310, 310f
    with self-pay patients, 309–310
  billing cycle for, 78, 308
  collection agencies for, 314
  laws affecting, 311–312
    Equal Credit Opportunity Act as, 311
    Fair Credit Billing Act as, 311
    Fair Credit Reporting Act as, 311
    Fair Debt Collection Practices Act as,
        311–312
    Truth in Lending Act as, 311
  methods of, 312–313
    by letter, 313, 313f

Collection (Continued)
    by telephone, 312, 312f
  of patient information, 320–321
  and payment policy, 308, 309f
  problems with, 310–311
  small claims litigation for, 308, 314–315
Collection agencies, 314
Collection ratio, 304
Colons, in ICD-10 tabular list, 246
Combination codes, ICD-10-CM, 250–251
Combination records, 347
Coming and going rule, 216
Commercial health insurance, 88
  by Blue Cross and Blue Shield. See Blue
      Cross and Blue Shield (BCBS).
  claims submission for, 95–96
    electronic, 95–96
    involving secondary coverage, 96–98, 97f
    timely, 95
  coverage mandate for, 89
  defined, 88
  health insurance exchanges and, 89
  high-risk pool in, 88–89
  origins of, 7
  remittance advice for, 96, 97f
    electronic, 96–98
  self-insurance and, 89–90
  who pays for, 88
Commission on Accreditation of Allied Health
    Education Programs (CAAHEP), 399
Common access card (CAC), for TRICARE
    eligibility, 194
Communication, oral and written, 14
Community First Choice (CFC) Option, 125
Community Health Accreditation Program,
    54
Community sign-in sheet, 37–38, 73b
Comorbidity, in diagnosis-related groups,
    357
Competency, 28
Competent parties, in contract, 28–29
Complaint management, for managed care,
    108, 108f
Compliance, billing, 398–399
Comprehension, reading, 14
Comprehensive plan, 47, 86
Computer(s), 337–350
  for electronic claims, 340–342
    advantages of, 342
    clearinghouse for, 75–76, 340
      vs. direct data entry, 76–77, 341–342
      flow chart of claim sent to, 340–341,
          341f
    direct data entry for, 76, 340, 341
      vs. claims clearinghouse, 76–77,
          341–342
    enrollment in, 340
    filing methods for, 340
    for Medicare, 342–343
  for electronic claims status reports, 344,
      347f
  for electronic data interchange, 339–340

Computer(s) (Continued)
    benefits of, 339–340
    HIPAA on, 339
    history of, 339
  for electronic funds transfer, 343–344,
      345f
  for electronic medical record, 344–349
    with combination records, 347
    with digital imaging hybrid, 347
    federal funding for trials and
        "meaningful use" of, 348–349
    future of, 348
    potential issues in, 347–348
    privacy concerns with, 348
  for electronic remittance advice, 344, 346f
  HIPAA and electronic transmissions via,
      338–339
  impact on health insurance of, 338
  in transitioning to ICD-10 diagnostic
      coding system, 344
  websites on, 350
Computer software program, to verify
    Medicaid eligibility, 132
Computerized patient accounting systems,
    305–306, 361–365
  generating reports in, 364–365
    accounts receivable aging report as, 364,
        365f
    insurance claims aging report as, 364,
        366f, 367f
    practice analysis report as, 364–365,
        368f
  HIPAA and, 365–369
  managing transactions with, 362–364
    insurance carrier adjustments
        (contractual write-offs) in, 363–364
    posting and tracking patient charges in,
        362, 363f
    processing payments in, 363, 363f
  selection of, 361–362
Concurrent care, E & M coding for, 281
Condition, ICD-10-CM coding for, 256
Conditional payment, for Medicare Second
    Payer, 171
Confidentiality, 39–41
  breach of, 41
  defined, 39
  exceptions to, 40
  HIPAA regulations on, 38
  in hospitals, 379–380
  patient expectations of, 298
Consent, informed, 394–396
Consideration, in contract, 28–29
Consolidated Omnibus Budget
    Reconciliation Act (COBRA), 8, 29–30,
    53–54
Consultations
  E & M coding for, 281, 287–288
  vs. referrals, 112
Consumer(s), patients as, 299
Consumer Coalition for Quality Health
    Care, 54

Consumer Data Industry Association, 314
Contract
    binding, 28
    breach of, 28
    competent parties in, 28–29
    consideration in, 28–29
    elements of, 27–28
    implied, 28–29
    legal form of, 28–29
    legal object of, 28–29
    offer and acceptance of, 28–29
    termination of, 28
Contract law, 27–28
Contractors
    Durable Medical Equipment, 146–147
    Medicaid, 125, 126
    Medicaid integrity, 126–127
    Medicare Administrative, 91–94, 146–147,
        148f
Contractual write-offs, 363–364
Contraindication, 252
Contributing factors, E & M codes for,
    284–285, 285f
Conventions
    in CPT coding, 279
    in ICD-10-CM
        for alphabetical index, 242–243
        defined, 243
        etiology/manifestation, 248
        for tabular list, 245
Coordination of benefits (COB), 55, 333
    with TRICARE, 193
Coordination of Benefits Agreement (COBA)
    Program, 171
Coordination of Benefits Contractor
    (COBC), 171
Coordination of care, E & M codes for, 284
Copayments, 58
    for CHAMPVA, 203
    for managed care, 105
    for Medicaid, 136–138
Core courses, in insurance billing
    professional program, 14, 15b
Correct code initiative edit, 330
Correction
    of claims, 325, 326f
    of medical record, 35, 35f
Cosmetic surgery, Medicare Part A
    noncoverage of, 147t
Cost avoidance, 135
Cost outliers, 355
Cost sharing, 10
    under CHAMPVA, 201–202, 203–205
        with no other health insurance, 203,
            204t
        with other health insurance, 203, 204t
    under Medicaid, 128–129
    under Medicare, 150–151, 150t
    under TRICARE, 196–197, 196t,
        197t, 383
Counseling, E & M coding for, 281, 284
Countable income, 122

Courses, in insurance billing professional
    program, 14, 15b
Court order, exception for signed release of
    information due to, 40
Coverage
    basic, 47
    certificate of, 49
    creditable, 88
    major medical, 47
    in managed care program, 106
    standardized, 49
    summary of benefits and, 49
Coverage mandate, 89
Covered charges, under TRICARE, 190
Covered entities
    and electronic claims, 21
    HIPAA and, 300
        claim submission by, 63
        requirements for, 300–301
    in hospital billing, 379–380
    practice management software and, 368
Covered expenses, 58, 86
Covered services, under Medicare Part A,
    146, 146t
CPC-H (certified professional
    coder–hospital), 400t
CPT. See Current Procedural Terminology
    (CPT).
Credit
    arrangements for, 308–310, 310f
    laws affecting, 311–312
        Equal Credit Opportunity Act as, 311
        Fair Credit Billing Act as, 311
        Fair Credit Reporting Act as, 311
        Fair Debt Collection Practices Act as,
            311–312
        Truth in Lending Act as, 311
Creditable coverage, 88
    for Medicare Prescription Drug Plan, 152
    for TRICARE, 189
Critical access hospitals (CAHs), 375–376
Critical care services, E & M coding for, 281, 288
Cross-references
    in CPT manual, 279, 280f
    in ICD-10-CM manual alphabetic index,
        243–246
Crosswalk, 292
Current Procedural Terminology, 4th edition
    (CPT-4), 273
Current Procedural Terminology, 5th edition
    (CPT-5), 292
Current Procedural Terminology (CPT)
    coding, 273–274
    basic steps of, 279–280, 280f
    conventions, punctuation, and symbols
        used in, 279
        cross-referencing as, 279, 280f
        indented codes as, 279, 279f, 280–281
        section, subsection, subheading, and
            category as, 279, 280f
        semicolon as, 279, 279f
        stand-alone code as, 279, 279f

Current Procedural Terminology (CPT)
    coding (Continued)
    development of, 274
    Evaluation and Management (E & M)
        codes in, 281–286, 282f
        for contributing factors, 284–285, 285f
        documentation with
            importance of, 289, 289f, 290b
            requirements for, 283, 283f
        for key components, 284
            examination as, 284
            history as, 284
            medical decision making as, 284
        modifiers of, 288–289
        for prolonged services, 286, 286f
        subheadings in, 286–288
            for consultations, 287–288
            for critical care services, 288
            for emergency department services, 288
            for hospital inpatient services, 287
            for hospital observation services,
                286–287
            for nursing facility services, 288
            for office or other outpatient services,
                286, 287t
        three factors to consider with, 283–284
        vocabulary used in, 281–282
        websites on, 294
    levels of, 274–275
    manual for, 275–278
        Appendices A–N in, 276
        Category II codes in, 275–276
        Category III codes in, 276, 276f
        index to, 277
            code layout in, 277
            main terms in, 277, 277f
            modifying terms in, 277, 277f
        introduction and main sections of,
            275–278, 275f, 275t
        modifiers in, 275, 275f, 278
        special reports in, 278
        symbols used in, 277, 278t
        unlisted procedure or service in, 278
    overview of, 273–274
    purpose of, 274
    websites on, 294
Custodial care, 52–53
    under CHAMPVA, 207
Custodial services, Medicare Part A
    noncoverage of, 147t
Customary fee. See Usual, customary, and
    reasonable (UCR) rates.

D
Daily journal, 304, 305f
Dashes, in ICD-10 tabular list, 246
Data, E & M codes for, 287t
Data elements, in segment of ASCA X12N
    8371 Version 5010, 385–387, 387f
Data entry, direct, 76, 340, 341
    claims attachment with, 80
    vs. claims clearinghouse, 76–77, 341–342

Date of service, errors in, 136f
Date received, errors in, 136f
Day, errors in, 136f
Day sheet, 304, 305f
DDE (Direct Data Entry), 76, 340, 341
  claims attachment with, 80
  vs. claims clearinghouses, 76–77, 341–342
Deductibles
  for BCBS inpatient services, 384
  for CHAMPVA, 203
  for fee-for-service plans, 46–47, 86
  for HMOs, 6
"Deep pocket," 27
Default codes, in ICD-10-CM, 249
Defendant, 315
Defense Enrollment Eligibility Reporting
    System (DEERS), 188–189, 383
Deficit Reduction Act (DRA), and Medicaid
    cost sharing, 128
De-identification, accessing information
    through, 301–303
Delinquent accounts
  collection agencies for, 314
  collection by letter for, 313, 313f
  collection by telephone for, 312, 312f
  small claims litigation for, 308, 314–315
Demand bills, for Medicare, 165, 166f
Demographic information, on medical
    record, 62
Denial of benefits, under workers'
    compensation, 216–217
Denied charges, reporting of, 19
Denied claims, 323
  appeals of, 334
Dental care, 53
Dental treatment facility (DTF), TRICARE,
    190–192
Diagnosis
  principal
    in diagnosis-related groups, 357
    ICD-10-CM coding for, 251–252
  sources of, 238, 239t, 243f
  uncertain, 256–257
Diagnosis codes
  E & M, 287t
  errors in, 136f
  ICD-10-CM, 256
    uncertain, 256–257
Diagnosis-related groups (DRGs), 357–358
  assignment of, 357
  calculation of payments with, 357–358
  CHAMPVA coverage for, 204t, 205t
  functioning of, 357
  history of, 4t
  and ICD-10 diagnostic coding, 238
  long-term care, 359–360
  for Medicare, 382
  in prospective payment system, 353, 356t
Diagnosis-related groups (DRGs) grouper,
    357
Diagnostic services only, ICD-10-CM coding
    for, 258–259

Dial-ups, in claim submission, 76–77
Digital imaging hybrid, 347
Diligence, 15
Direct claim submission, 76, 340, 341
  claims attachment with, 80
  vs. claims clearinghouses, 340, 76–77
Direct contract model, of HMO, 106
Direct Data Entry (DDE), 76, 340, 341
  claims attachment with, 80
  vs. claims clearinghouses, 76–77, 341–342
Disability
  defined, 225, 230–231
  determination for workers' compensation
    of, 220
  long-term, 225
  permanent, 220
    partial, 220
    total, 220
  short-term, 225
  temporary, 220, 225
    partial, 220
    total, 220
Disability and Health Team, of Centers for
    Disease Control and Prevention,
    232–233
Disability Determination Agency, 233
Disability income insurance
  claims for, 225–230
    attending physician's statement in,
      228f, 230
    authorization to disclose health
      information in, 229f
    employee's responsibilities in, 225–230,
      226f
    employer's responsibilities in, 227f, 230
    health insurance professional's role in,
      230
  defining disability for, 225
  for long-term disability, 225
  private and employer-sponsored, 224–230
  for short-term disability, 225
  websites on, 236
Disability insurance, 49–50
  private, 49
  Social Security, 49, 231–232
    administration and funding for, 231
    eligibility for, 231
    filing claims for, 233–234
      health insurance professional's role
        in, 234
      healthcare provider's role in,
        233–234
      patient's role in, 233
    history of, 231
  workers' compensation, 49–50
Disability programs
  federal, 230–234
    Americans with Disabilities Act and, 231
    Centers for Disease Control and
      Prevention Disability and Health
      Team as, 232–233
    filing claims for, 233–234

Disability programs (Continued)
    Social Security Disability Insurance as,
      231–232
    Supplemental Security Income as, 232
    Ticket to Work Program as, 233
    state, 232
Disabled individuals, Medicaid for, 123f
Disbursements journal, 304, 306f
Discharge services, E & M codes for, 287
Discharge summaries, as claim attachments,
    79–80
Discounted fee-for-service, 353, 353t
Disease process, ICD-10-CM coding for
    conditions integral to, 250
    conditions not integral to, 250
Disproportionate share, in diagnosis-related
    group payments, 358
Disproportionate share hospitals, 129
DME (durable medical equipment)
    CHAMPVA coverage for, 204t, 205t
    Medicare Part B coverage of, 147
DME (durable medical equipment)
    contractors, 146–147
Documentation
    for claim filing, 322
    of E & M codes, 289, 289f, 290b
    importance of, 289, 289f, 290b
    requirements for, 283, 283f
    of medical record, 33–36, 35f
"Donut hole," in Medicare Part D
    (Prescription Drug Plans), 152
Double coverage, with TRICARE, 193
Downcoding
    by insurance company, 330
    by Medicare, 175
DRA (Deficit Reduction Act), and Medicaid
    cost sharing, 128
DRGs. See Diagnosis-related groups (DRGs).
DTF (dental treatment facility), TRICARE,
    190–192
Dual coverage. See Dual eligibility.
Dual eligibility, 129–130, 132, 153
    claims for, 135, 171–172
    prescription drug coverage with, 152
Durable medical equipment (DME)
    CHAMPVA coverage for, 204t, 205t
    Medicare Part B coverage of, 147
Durable Medical Equipment (DME)
    contractors, 146–147
Durable power of attorney, 41
Duties, of health insurance professional,
    17–18, 17t, 19

E
E & M codes. See Evaluation and
    Management (E & M) codes.
Early Periodic Screening, Diagnosis, and
    Treatment (EPSDT) program, 127
Earned income, 224–225
ECS (electronic claims submission), 375,
    396–397
EDI. See Electronic Data Interchange (EDI).

Education, of health insurance professional, 14, 15*b*, 19
EFMP (Exceptional Family Member Program), 193
EFT (electronic funds transfer), 343–344, 345*f*
    for Medicare, 175, 177*f*
Egregious cause, of injury or illness, 216
EIN (employer identification number), 65, 323
Electronic claims, 63
    advantages of, 75
    BCBS and commercial, 95–96
    CHAMPVA, 207
    electronic transactions and code set requirements for, 64
    essential information for, 66–73
        from encounter form, 70–72, 71*f*, 72*f*, 73*f*
        from patient health record, 69–70, 70*f*
        from patient information form, 66–68, 67*f*
            additional insurance as, 67–68, 67*f*, 68*f*
            insurance authorization and assignment as, 67*f*, 68
            insurance information as, 66, 67*f*, 68*f*
            new patient information as, 66, 67*f*, 68*f*
        from patient insurance identification card, 66, 69, 69*f*
        from patient ledger card, 72–73, 74*f*
    HIPAA on, 21, 63–65
        electronic transactions and code set requirements of, 64
        exceptions in, 65, 65*b*, 165–167
        national identifier requirements of, 64–65
        new 5010 standards for, 65–66, 65*b*
        privacy requirements of, 64
        security requirements of, 64
    hospital, 396–397
    Medicare, 165, 342–343
        exceptions to mandatory, 65, 65*b*, 165–167
    national identifier requirements for, 64–65
    privacy requirements for, 64
    process for submitting, 66–77, 340–342
        advantages of, 342
        clearinghouse for, 75–76, 340
            vs. direct data entry, 76–77, 341–342
            flow chart of claim sent to, 340–341, 341*f*
        direct data entry for, 76, 340, 341
            vs. claims clearinghouses, 76–77, 341–342
        enrollment in, 340
        filing methods for, 340
        for Medicare, 342–343
    security requirements for, 64
    for TRICARE, 199, 383
    UB-04, 385–387

Electronic claims *(Continued)*
        data elements in segment of, 385–387, 387*f*
        data layout of, 385–387
        response to transmission of, 387, 387*f*
        transaction set section of, 385, 387*f*
    verifying insurance with new technology on, 73–75
Electronic claims clearinghouses, 75–76, 340
    vs. direct claims, 340, 76–77
    flow chart of claim sent to, 340–341, 341*f*
    for TRICARE, 199
Electronic Claims Processor, 17*t*
Electronic claims receipt, 96
Electronic claims submission (ECS), 375, 396–397
Electronic Data Interchange (EDI), 339–340
    benefits of, 339–340
    defined, 21, 339
    HIPAA requirements for, 64, 339
    history of, 339
    to verify Medicaid eligibility, 132
Electronic Data Interchange (EDI) Gateway, for TRICARE, 199
Electronic encounter form, 70, 72*f*
Electronic funds transfer (EFT), 343–344, 345*f*
    for Medicare, 175, 177*f*
Electronic Health Transactions Standards, 37
Electronic insurance aging report
    generation of, 364, 366*f*, 367*f*
    tracking of, 80–82, 81*f*
Electronic media claims (EMCs), 342–343
Electronic medical records (EMRs), 306–308, 344–349
    in claims submission, 69
    combination records with, 347
    components of, 344–347
    defined, 344, 388
    digital imaging hybrid in, 347
    federal funding and "meaningful use" of, 307–308, 348–349
    future of, 348
    hospital, 388
    key features of, 388
    potential issues with, 347–348
    privacy concerns of, 348
    security of, 347
Electronic patient accounting software, 305–306
Electronic protected health information (e-PHI), 64
Electronic remittance advice (ERA), 96–98, 344
    authorization for, 344, 346*f*
    hospital, 397
    Medicare, 175
        enrolling for, 175, 176*f*
Electronic transactions, HIPAA requirements for, 64
Electronic transmissions, role of HIPAA in, 338–339
Emancipated minors, 28
EMCs (electronic media claims), 342–343

Emergency care, E & M coding for, 281
Emergency department, nonemergency use of, 129
Emergency department services, E & M coding for, 288
Emergency medical condition, 378
Emergency Medical Treatment & Labor Act (EMTALA), 129, 378
Emergency room charges, CHAMPVA coverage for, 204*t*
Emergent medical condition, 378
Employee, casual, 216
Employee liability, 27
Employee Retirement Income Security Act (ERISA), 89
Employee Retirement Income Security Act (ERISA) plans, 89
Employee's statement form, for disability claim, 225–230, 226*f*
Employer identification number (EIN), 65, 323
Employer liability, 27
Employer's statement form, for disability claim, 227*f*, 230
Employer-sponsored health insurance plans, 7
Employment network, 233
EMRs. *See* Electronic medical records (EMRs).
EMTALA (Emergency Medical Treatment & Labor Act), 129, 378
Encounter form, 70–72, 71*f*, 72*f*
Encounters for circumstances other than disease or injury, ICD-10-CM coding for, 254–256
End-stage renal disease (ESRD)
    Medicare for, 144–145
    Omnibus Budget Reconciliation Act on, 30
Enrollees, 47, 102
Enrollment
    in Medicare, 150
    for submitting claims, 340
Entitlement program, 133
Entity(ies), 1–2
    covered
        and electronic claims, 21
        HIPAA and, 300
            claim submission by, 63
            requirements for, 300–301
        in hospital billing, 379–380
        practice management software and, 368
EOB. *See* Explanation of benefits (EOB).
e-PHI (electronic protected health information), 64
EPSDT (Early Periodic Screening, Diagnosis, and Treatment) program, 127
Equal Credit Opportunity Act, 311
ERA. *See* Electronic remittance advice (ERA).
ERISA (Employee Retirement Income Security Act), 89
ERISA (Employee Retirement Income Security Act) plans, 89
Errata, 96–99

Error(s)
  in billing, 135–136, 136f
  on claims, 78, 78f, 322, 322b
  in payment, 328, 330t
ESRD (end-stage renal disease)
  Medicare for, 144–145
  Omnibus Budget Reconciliation Act on, 30
Essential modifiers, in ICD-10-CM manual alphabetic index, 242–243, 245f
Established patient, E & M coding for, 281
Ethical aspects, 25–44
  of confidentiality and privacy, 39–41
  of healthcare fraud and abuse, 41–42
  medical ethics as
    applicable to health insurance, 28–29
    and medical etiquette, 30–32, 31f
  websites on, 44
Ethical principles, in hospital, 380
  breach of, 380–381
Ethics
  defined, 30–31
  medical, 30–31, 31f
    applicable to health insurance, 28–29
    defined, 31
    in hospitals, 380–381
    and medical etiquette, 30–32, 31f
  professional, 16
Etiology, 238
Etiology/manifestation convention, in ICD-10 tabular list, 248
Etiquette, medical, 31–32
Evaluation and Management (E & M) codes, 281–286, 282f
  categories list for, 281
  for contributing factors, 284–285, 285f
  defined, 281
  documentation with
    importance of, 289, 289f, 290b
    requirements for, 283, 283f
  for key components, 284
    examination as, 284
    history as, 284
    medical decision making as, 284
  modifiers of, 288–289
  for patient status, 283
  for place of service, 283
  for prolonged services, 286, 286f
  subcategories list for, 281
  subheadings in, 286–288
    for consultations, 287–288
    for critical care services, 288
    for emergency department services, 288
    for hospital inpatient services, 287
    for hospital observation services, 286–287
    for nursing facility services, 288
    for office or other outpatient services, 286, 287t
  three factors to consider with, 283–284
  for type of service, 283
  vocabulary used in, 281–282
  websites on, 294

Exacerbation, 376
Examination, E & M codes for, 284, 287t
Exceptional Family Member Program (EFMP), 193
Exceptions to Electronic Claim Submission Requirements, 65, 65b, 165–167
Exchanges, health insurance, 11, 52, 89
"Excludes notes," in ICD-10-CM coding, 249f, 253
Exclusions, 47
Expenses, covered, 58
Explanation of benefits (EOB), 96, 97f
  CHAMPVA, 209, 210f
  defined, 328–329
  downcoding on, 330
  electronic, 96–98, 344
    authorization for, 344, 346f
  interpretation of, 328–330, 331f
  Medicaid, 136, 137f
  Medicare, 172–175
    electronic, 175
    enrolling for, 175, 176f
    standard paper, 172–175, 174f
  TRICARE, 199, 200f
  troubleshooting of, 329–330
Eye care, Medicare Part A noncoverage of, 147t
eZ TRICARE, 199

F

FA (Family Assistance) Program, 121
Face-to-face time, E & M codes for, 285
Fair Credit Billing Act (FCBA), 311
Fair Credit Reporting Act, 311
Fair Debt Collection Practices Act, 311–312
Fair treatment, of patients, 380–381
Family(ies), Medicaid for, 123f
Family Assistance (FA) Program, 121
Family plan, 69
FastAttach, 80
FCBA (Fair Credit Billing Act), 311
FECA (Federal Employment Compensation Act), 50, 215
Federal Benefit Rate (FBR), 122
Federal contributions, to Medicaid, 120–121
Federal disability programs, 230–234
  Americans with Disabilities Act and, 231
  CDC Disability and Health Team as, 232–233
  filing claims for, 233–234
  Social Security Disability Insurance as, 231–232
  Supplemental Security Income as, 232
  Ticket to Work Program as, 233
Federal Employee Program (FEP), 91
Federal Employees Health Benefits (FEHB) Program, 88, 91
Federal Employment Compensation Act (FECA), 50, 215
Federal Employment Liability Act (FELA), 50, 215
Federal False Claim Amendments Act, 30

Federal funds, for electronic medical record trials, 348–349
Federal government, role in Medicaid of, 123, 123f
Federal Insurance Contributions Act (FICA), 49, 145, 231
Federal legislation, and workers' compensation, 215
Federal poverty level (FPL), 8, 9, 121–122, 122t
Federal Privacy Act, 29
Fee(s), discussion with patient of, 304
Fee schedules, for Medicare, 354
Fee-for-service (FFS) plans, 84–100
  with basic coverage, 47, 86
  BCBS, 94
  claim form for, 47
  coinsurance in, 47, 86
  comprehensive, 47, 86
  covered expenses in, 86
  deductible in, 46–47, 86
  discounted, 353, 353t
  exclusions in, 47
  functioning of, 86–87
  insurance cap ("stop loss") in, 47, 86–87
  lifetime maximum cap in, 87
  with major medical coverage, 47, 86
  vs. managed care, 46, 85, 103f
  for Medicare, 151, 158
    appeals process for, 176–179, 179f
  origins of, 6, 10
  out-of-pocket maximum in, 47, 86–87
  overview of, 46–47, 85–86
  participating provider in, 87
  preexisting conditions in, 47, 87–88
  premiums in, 46–47, 86
  private, 104t
    for Medicare, 151, 158
    appeals process for, 176–179, 179f
  reimbursement in, 353, 353t
  traditional, 85–86
  usual, customary, and reasonable rates in, 47, 87
  websites on, 100
FEHB (Federal Employees Health Benefits) Program, 88, 91
FELA (Federal Employment Liability Act), 50, 215
FEP (Federal Employee Program), 91
FFS plans. See Fee-for-service (FFS) plans.
FI(s). See Fiscal intermediaries (FIs).
FICA (Federal Insurance Contributions Act), 49, 145, 231
Final Rule, 64–65
  in Version 5010, 65
Financial arrangement plan, 308–310, 310f
Financial issues, patient expectations of, 298
Financial means test, for Supplemental Security Income, 232
First party, 29
First report of injury, 217, 218f

First-listed condition, ICD-10-CM coding for, 253
Fiscal intermediaries (FIs)
for fee-for-service plans, 91–94
for Medicaid, 126
for Medicare, 91–94
on Medicare claims, 167
for Part A, 146–147, 148f, 381
for Part B, 150
Flexible spending account (FSA), 50–51, 51t
Floor time, E & M codes for, 285
Form locators, for UB-04 form, 385
For-profit hospitals, 375
FPL (federal poverty level), 8, 9, 121–122, 122t
Fraud
defined, 139
healthcare, 41–42
by consumers, 42
costs of, 41–42
defining, 41–42
examples of, 41
prevention of, 42
schemes for committing, 42
who commits, 42
in Medicaid system, 139–140
Medicare billing, 182
workers' compensation, 224
Fraud and Abuse Act, 30
FSA (flexible spending account), 50–51, 51t
Full-time equivalent (FTE) employees, for Medicare claims, 167

G
General Equivalence Mappings (GEMs), 344
General hospital, 375
General journal, 304
General ledger, 304
General medical examination, with abnormal findings, 260
Geographic practice cost index (GPCI), 359
Governance, 379
Grandfathering, 89
Grievance, 108
Group contract, 48, 85
advantages of, 48
disadvantages of, 48
history of, 7
Group model, of HMO, 105
Guaranteed renewable long-term disability insurance, 225
Guarantor, 62

H
HCBS (Home and Community-Based Service) waivers, 127–128
HCC (hierarchical condition category), 355–356
HCFA (Health Care Financing Administration), 62–63, 77, 274
HCFA-1500 claims form, 62–63, 77

HCPCS. See Health Care Financing Administration (HCFA) Procedure Coding System (HCPCS).
HDHP (high-deductible health plan), 94
Header words, in CPT manual, 279, 280f
Health and Human Services (HHS)
federal poverty level guidelines of, 121–122, 122t
Privacy Rule of, 64
standardized benefits and coverage rule of, 49
Health Care and Educational Reconciliation Act, 6, 30
Health Care Financing Administration (HCFA), 62–63, 77, 274
Health Care Financing Administration (HCFA) Procedure Coding System (HCPCS), 289–291, 290f
HIPAA and, 292
history of, 274
Level II manual for, 290–291
appendices in, 291
index of main terms in, 290–291, 291f
modifiers in, 291
table of drugs in, 291
National Medicare Codes of, 274
overview of, 289–291
uses of, 274–275
websites on, 294
Health dollar, sources and uses of, 5, 5f, 6f
Health information administrator, registered, 400t
Health information management (HIM) systems, 397
Health information systems, 63
Health information technicians, registered, 399, 400t
Health information technology (HIT), for Medicaid, 140
Health Information Technology for Economic and Clinical Health (HITECH) Act, 348
Health insurance
access to, 7–9
defined, 2
history of, 3–4
key issues in, 7–10
metamorphosis of, 4–7, 4t, 5f, 6f
obtaining, 7
origins of, 1–12
puzzle pieces of, 2–3, 3f
sources of, 47–48
Consolidated Omnibus Budget Reconciliation Act and, 53–54
group contract as, 48
individual policies as, 48
Medicaid as, 48
Medicare as, 48
TRICARE/CHAMPVA as, 48–50
"watchdogs" for, 54
websites on, 60

Health insurance (Continued)
standardized benefits and coverage rule for, 49
sufficient, 10
terms common to third-party carriers of, 54–58
birthday rule as, 54–55, 333
coordination of benefits as, 55
copayment as, 58
covered expenses as, 58
medical necessity as, 55, 56f
non-cancellable policy as, 58
participating vs. nonparticipating providers as, 58
primary care physician as, 58
provider as, 58
third-party payer as, 58
usual, reasonable, and customary as, 55–57
timeline for, 4t
types of, 46–47
Accountable Care Organizations as, 52
dental care as, 53
disability insurance as, 49–50
private, 49
Social Security, 49
workers' compensation, 49–50
flexible spending account as, 50–51, 51t
health insurance exchanges as, 52
health reimbursement arrangements as, 51–52, 51t
indemnity (fee-for-service), 46–47
long-term care insurance as, 52–53
managed care as, 47
medical savings account as, 50, 51t
vision care as, 53
websites on, 60
Health insurance claim form
CMS-1500 (08/05) paper, 21–23, 22f
electronic, 21
Health insurance claim number (HICN), Medicare, 162, 164t
Health insurance exchanges, 11, 52, 89
Health insurance plans, 10–11
Health insurance policy premium. See Premiums.
Health Insurance Portability and Accountability Act (HIPAA), 36–39
and career prospects of health insurance professional, 18–19, 18b
on claims, 63–65
electronic transactions and code set requirements of, 64
exceptions in, 65, 65b, 165–167
filing of, 323
national identifier requirements of, 64–65
new 5010 standards for, 65–66, 65b
privacy requirements of, 64
security requirements of, 64
compliance with, 36, 36f
developing plan for, 38–39

Health Insurance Portability and
    Accountability Act (HIPAA) (Continued)
  on creditable coverage, 88
  on electronic transmissions, 338–339
  enforcement of confidentiality regulations
      of, 38
  and HCPCS coding, 292
  and hospitals, 398
  impact of, 37–38
    on accessing information
        through de-identification, 301–303
        through patient authorization, 301,
            302f
    on authorization to release information,
        300
    on covered entities, 300
        requirements for, 300–301
    on health insurance professionals, 37,
        37f
    on patients, 37–38, 299–303
    on patient's right of access and
        correction, 301
    on private businesses, 38
    on providers, 38
  on managed care, 107, 112–115
  and military insurers, 209
  objectives of, 36
  in origins of health insurance, 4b, 8, 8b
  and practice management software,
      365–369
  on preexisting conditions, 88
  Transaction Standards of, 366
  and workers' compensation, 224
Health insurance professional(s)
  career as, 13–24
    focus of, 21
    as good choice for you, 20
    home-based, 19–20
    prospects for, 18–20
  certification as, 14, 20–21
  claim submission by. See Claims.
  defined, 14
  education of, 14, 15b
  impact of HIPAA on, 37, 37f
  job duties and responsibilities of, 17–18,
      17t
  occupational trends and future outlook
      for, 18
  preparation of, 14–17, 16t
  required skills and interests of, 14–17
  rewards of, 20
  websites on, 24
  what to expect as, 19–20
  your future as, 13–17
Health insurance "puzzle," 2–3, 3f
Health insurance "watchdogs," 54
Health maintenance organization(s)
    (HMOs), 104t, 105–106
  BCBS, 94
  CHAMPVA and, 206
  closed-panel, 105
  comparison of, 103f
  defined, 6, 105

Health maintenance organization(s) (HMOs)
    (Continued)
  direct contract model of, 106
  group model of, 105
  history of, 4t, 5–6
  individual practice association in, 106
  Medicare, 155–158
    advantages and disadvantages of,
        158–159
    with point-of-service option, 158
  mixed model of, 105
  network model of, 105
  open-ended, 106
  open-panel, 106
  staff model of, 105
Health Maintenance Organization (HMO)
    Act, 6
Health Plan Employer Data and Information
    Set (HEDIS), 107
Health record. See Medical record(s).
Health reimbursement accounts, 51–52, 51t
Health reimbursement arrangements
    (HRAs), 51–52, 51t
Health Savings Account (HSA), 50, 51t, 94
Health systems, modern, 375–377
Healthcare abuse, 41–42
  by consumers, 42
  costs of, 41–42
  defining, 41–42
  examples of, 41
  prevention of, 42
  schemes for committing, 42
  who commits, 42
Healthcare costs
  cost sharing of. See Cost sharing.
  factors affecting, 9–10, 9f
Healthcare demand, and healthcare costs, 10
Healthcare facility(ies), 375–377
  acute care, 375
  ambulatory surgery centers as, 376
  critical access hospitals as,
      375–376
  home health agencies as, 377
  hospice as, 377
  intermediate care, 377
  long-term care, 377
  other types of, 376–377, 376f
  skilled nursing, 376–377
  subacute care, 376
Healthcare fraud, 41–42
  by consumers, 42
  costs of, 41–42
  defining, 41–42
  examples of, 41
  prevention of, 42
  schemes for committing, 42
  who commits, 42
Healthcare identifiers, 64–65
Healthcare provider. See Provider(s).
Healthcare provider report, for workers'
    compensation, 217–220, 221f
Healthcare reform
  in history of health insurance, 6

Healthcare reform (Continued)
  legal and ethical side of, 30
  and managed care organizations, 116
  and Medicaid, 123
  and Medicare Advantage plans, 151
  and preexisting conditions, 87–88
Healthcare service plans, 94
Hearing aids, Medicare Part A noncoverage
    of, 147t
HEDIS (Health Plan Employer Data and
    Information Set), 107
HH PPS (home health prospective payment
    system), 356t, 360
  Medicare, 355
HHS. See Health and Human Services (HHS).
HICN (health insurance claim number),
    Medicare, 162, 164t
Hierarchical condition category (HCC),
    355–356
High severity problem, E & M codes for, 285
High-deductible health plan (HDHP), 94
High-risk pool, 7–8, 88–89
HIM (health information management)
    systems, 397
HIPAA. See Health Insurance Portability and
    Accountability Act (HIPAA).
HIPAA 5010 Transaction Standards, 300–301
HIPAA-covered entities, 300
  claim submission by, 63
  requirements for, 300–301
HIS (hospital information system), 388
History
  E & M codes for, 284, 287t
  in electronic medical record, 344
History of present illness (HPI) elements, 289
HIT (health information technology), for
    Medicaid, 140
HITECH (Health Information Technology
    for Economic and Clinical Health) Act,
    348
HMOs. See Health maintenance organization
    (s) (HMOs).
Home and Community-Based Service
    (HCBS) waivers, 127–128
Home health agencies, 377
Home health care, Medicare coverage for,
    146t
Home health prospective payment system
    (HH PPS), 356t, 360
  Medicare, 355
Home-based careers, 18, 19–20
Horizontal triangles, in CPT manual, 278t
Hospice care, 377
  Medicare coverage for, 146t
Hospital(s)
  accreditation of, 378–379
    by Accreditation Association for
        Ambulatory Health Care, 378, 379
    by Joint Commission, 378
    by National Committee for Quality
        Assurance, 378–379
    by Utilization Review Accreditation
        Commission, 379

Hospital(s) (Continued)
BCBS member, 384
confidentiality and privacy in, 379–380
critical access, 375–376
disproportionate share, 129
emerging issues with, 374–375
fair treatment of patients in, 380–381
for-profit, 375
general, 375
governance of, 379
legal and regulatory environment of, 377–381
modern, 375–377
professional standards in, 379
specialized, 375
vertically integrated, 374
Hospital billing, 372–403
career opportunities in, 399–400
job outlook for, 400, 400t
training, other qualifications, and advancement in, 399–400
compliance program for, 398–399
electronic claims submission for, 396–397
flowchart for, 398, 398f
health information management systems for, 397
HIPAA and, 398
hospital charges in, 396
charge description master for, 396, 396t
informed consent and, 394–396
payment management for, 397–398, 398f
physician office vs., 374
present on admission and, 396
process of, 394–398
recent rules affecting, 393
72-hour rule as, 393
standard data elements in, 394, 395b
UB-04 claim form for, 384–387
claim form and completion instructions for, 425–429
data specifications for, 385
electronic, 385–387
data elements in segment of, 385–387, 387f
data layout of, 385–387
response to transmission of, 387, 387f
transaction set section of, 385, 387f
paper, 384–385, 386f
websites on, 402–403
Hospital charges, 396
charge description master for, 396, 396t
Hospital coding
inpatient, 388–393
E & M codes for, 281, 287
ICD-10-PCS for, 389–390
code structure of, 390
format of, 390, 391f
selecting principal diagnosis in, 390–392, 392b
National Correct Coding Initiative for, 392, 393t

Hospital coding (Continued)
outpatient, 393–394
ambulatory payment classification coding for, 394
prospective payment system and, 393–394
physician office vs., 374
Hospital information system (HIS), 388
Hospital inpatient services
coding for, 388–393
E & M codes for, 281, 287
ICD-10-PCS for, 389–390
code structure of, 390
format of, 390, 391f
selecting principal diagnosis in, 390–392, 392b
National Correct Coding Initiative for, 392, 393t
Hospital insurance, Medicare, 146–147
covered services in, 146, 146t
eligibility for, 146
Medicare Administrative Contractors for, 146–147, 148f, 372
noncovered services in, 146, 147t
Hospital insurance (HI), Medicare, 132
Hospital observation services, E & M codes for, 286–287
Hospital outpatient prospective payment system (HOPPS), 393–394
Hospital outpatient services, 393–394
ambulatory payment classification coding for, 394
prospective payment system and, 393–394
Hospital payers, 377
Blue Cross and Blue Shield as, 384
CHAMPVA as, 383–384
Medicaid as, 383, 385t
Medicare as, 381–383
benefit period for, 382
calculation of payments under, 382
keeping current with, 381–382
Medicare Severity-Adjusted System of, 382–383
payment mechanism by setting of care for, 385t
payment schedule for, 382, 382t
and quality improvement organizations, 381
review of, 382
three-day payment window for, 383, 393
private insurers as, 384, 385t
TRICARE as, 383
Hospital registration, 394
Hospital-Issued Notice of Noncoverage (HINN), for Medicare, 181
Housekeeping services, Medicare Part A noncoverage of, 147t
HPI (history of present illness) elements, 289
HRAs (health reimbursement arrangements), 51–52, 51t
HSA (Health Savings Account), 50, 51t, 94
Human Genome Project, 4t

I
IADLs (instrumental activities of daily living), 231
Iatrogenic effects, 115
ICD-10. See International Classification of Diseases, 10th Revision (ICD-10).
Identification (ID) cards
carrier information on back of, 321–322, 322f
CHAMPVA, 202–203, 202f
Medicaid, 131, 131f
Medicare, 162, 164f
replacement of, 162–164
patient insurance, 66, 69, 69f
uniformed services, 194, 195b, 195f
Identification number, employer, 65, 323
Identifiers, HIPAA on, 339
Impending condition, ICD-10-CM coding for, 252
Implied contract, 28
Implied promises, 28–29
"In diseases classified elsewhere" notes, in ICD-10-CM coding, 248
Incidental disclosure, 37–38
"Includes notes," in ICD-10-CM coding, 252
Inclusion terms, in ICD-10-CM coding, 252
Income
countable, 122
defined, 122
"in-kind," 122
spend-down of, 124–125
Incorrect payments, 334
Indemnification, 1
Indemnity insurance plans. See Fee-for-service (FFS) plans.
Indented code, in CPT coding, 279, 279f, 280–281
Independent review organization (IRO), 108
Index
to CPT manual, 277
code layout in, 277
main terms in, 277, 277f
modifying terms in, 277, 277f
to HCPCS coding manual, 290–291, 291f
to ICD-10-CM manual, 241, 244f
coding steps for, 243
cross-references in, 243–246
essential and nonessential modifiers in, 242–243, 245f
main terms in, 242–246, 244f
parentheses in, 243–246, 247f
Indigent, 4–5
Individual policies, 7, 48
advantages of, 48
disadvantages of, 48
Individual practice association (IPA), 106
Information
access to
through de-identification, 301–303
through patient authorization, 301, 302f

Information (*Continued*)
  authorization for release of
    accessing information through, 301, 302f
    for disability claim, 229f
    exceptions for insurance claims submission to, 40
    HIPAA on, 300
    legal aspects of, 33, 34f, 40
    "lifetime," 68
    on patient information form, 67f, 68
Informed consent, 394–396
INFs (intermediate nursing facilities), E & M coding for, 288
Initial claims, for Medicare, 165
Initial hospital care, E & M codes for, 287
Initiative, 15
Injury, first report of, 217, 218f
"In-kind" income, 122
Inpatient coding, 388–393
  E & M, 281, 287
  ICD-10-PCS for, 389–390
    code structure of, 390
    format of, 390, 391f
    selecting principal diagnosis in, 390–392, 392b
  National Correct Coding Initiative for, 392, 393t
Inpatient hospital claim form, 394, 395b
Inpatient hospital prospective payment system, 355, 359
  three-day payment window for, 383, 393
Inpatient mental health services, CHAMPVA coverage for, 204t, 205t
Inpatient prospective payment system (IPPS), 355, 359
  three-day payment window for, 383, 393
Inpatient psychiatric facility prospective payment system, 355
Inpatient rehabilitation facility prospective payment system (IRF PPS), 356t, 360
  Medicare, 355
Inpatient services
  CHAMPVA coverage for, 204t, 205t
  coding for, 388–393
    E & M codes for, 281, 287
    ICD-10-PCS for, 389–390
      code structure of, 390
      format of, 390, 391f
      selecting principal diagnosis in, 390–392, 392b
    National Correct Coding Initiative for, 392, 393t
Inpatient-only treatment, exception for signed release of information for, 40
Instructional notes, in ICD-10 tabular list, 248, 248f, 249f
Instrumental activities of daily living (IADLs), 231

Insurance, defined, 1–3
Insurance authorization and assignment, on patient information form, 67f, 68
Insurance billing cycle, 78, 308
Insurance cap, 47, 86–87
Insurance carrier adjustments, 363–364
Insurance claims aging report
  generation of, 364, 366f, 367f
  tracking of, 80–82, 81f
Insurance claims register system, 80–82, 81f, 328, 329f
Insurance identification card, 66, 69, 69f
Insurance information, on patient information form, 66, 67f, 68f
Insurance law, 27–28
Insurance log, 80–82, 81f, 328, 329f
Insurance verification, with new technology, 73–75
Insured, 1, 46–47
Insurer, 1
Intangible services, 297
Integrity, 15
Intelligence free number, 64–65
Interactive Voice Response (IVR) systems, 73
Interest charges, 311
Intermediate care facilities, 377
Intermediate nursing facilities (INFs), E & M coding for, 288
International claim form, 91, 92f
International Classification of Diseases, 10th Revision, Clinical Modification (ICD-10-CM) coding system, 238
  code structure of, 241, 254t
  general and chapter-specific guidelines for, 249
    for acute and chronic conditions, 250–253
    for codes A00.0–T88.9 and Z00–Z99.89, 249–250
    for combination codes, 250–251
    for conditions integral to disease process, 250
    for conditions not integral to disease process, 250
    for impending or threatened condition, 252
    for late effects (sequelae), 251–252
    for laterality, 252
    for signs and symptoms, 250
  manual for, 241
    alphabetic index to, 241, 244f
      coding steps for, 243
      cross-references in, 243–246
      essential and nonessential modifiers in, 242–243, 245f
      main terms in, 242–246, 244f
      parentheses in, 243–246, 247f
    default codes in, 249
    morphology codes in, 248
    tabular list in, 244, 244f
      abbreviations in, 245
      "code also" note in, 248–249

International Classification of Diseases, 10th Revision, Clinical Modification (ICD-10-CM) coding system (*Continued*)
    conventions for, 245, 248f
    etiology/manifestation convention in, 248
    format and structure of codes in, 244–245, 247f
    instructional notes in, 248, 248f, 249f
    manifestation codes in, 248
    placeholder character in, 245
    punctuation in, 245
    7th character in, 245, 247f
  for outpatient services, 252–253
    for circumstances other than disease or injury, 254–256
    diagnosis, condition, problem, or other reason for encounter/visit in, 256
    for ambulatory surgery, 259–263
    for chronic diseases, 257–258
    for coexisting conditions, 258–264
    for diagnostic services only, 258–259
    for general medical examination with abnormal findings, 260
    for preoperative evaluations only, 259
    for routine health screenings, 260
    for routine prenatal visits, 260
    for therapeutic services only, 259
    with uncertain diagnosis, 256–257
    first-listed condition in, 253
    level of detail in, 254–255
      codes with 3, 4, or 5 digits in, 255–256
      use of full number of digits in, 256–257
    with observation stay, 253
    surgical, 253–257
    symptoms and signs in, 253–257
International Classification of Diseases, 10th Revision (ICD-10) coding system, 237–271
  diagnosis in, 238, 239t, 243f
  history of, 239–240, 240t
  and other coding structures, 238
  overview of, 240–241
  transition to, 238
  role of computers in, 344
  uses of, 240–241
  websites on, 260
International Classification of Diseases, 10th Revision, Procedure Classification System (ICD-10-PCS) coding system, 238, 389–390
  code structure of, 390
  format of, 390, 391f
  selecting principal diagnosis of, 390–392, 392b
Internet, as healthcare tool, 299
Internet-based eligibility check systems, 75
Interstate commerce, 215
IVR (Interactive Voice Response) systems, 73

J

Job deconditioning, 220
Job duties, of health insurance professional, 17–18, 17*t*, 19
Job outlook, for hospital billing, 400
Johnson, Lyndon B., 4–5
Joint Commission, 54
  accreditation by, 378
  on managed care, 107
Jones Act, 215
Journal
  daily, 304, 305*f*
  disbursements, 304, 306*f*
  general, 304
  payroll, 304, 306*f*

K

Kentucky Transitional Assistance Program (K-TAP), 121
Key components, E & M codes for, 284
Kimball, Justin Ford, 3, 90

L

Labor component, in diagnosis-related group payments, 358
Late effects, ICD-10-CM coding for, 251–252
Laterality, ICD-10-CM coding for, 252
LCD (local coverage determination), 162
Lead terms, in ICD-10-CM manual alphabetic index, 242–246, 244*f*
Ledger
  general, 304
  patient, 304, 307*f*
Legal aspects, 25–44
  of compliance with HIPAA, 36–39, 36*f*
  of confidentiality and privacy, 39–41
  of healthcare fraud and abuse, 41–42
  important legislation affecting health insurance as, 29–30
  insurance and contract law as, 27–28
    elements of legal contract in, 27–28
    termination of contracts in, 28
  medical law and liability as, 26–27
    applicable to health insurance, 28–29
    employee liability in, 27
    employer liability in, 27
  of medical record, 32–33, 34*f*
  websites on, 44
Legal contract
  binding, 28
  breach of, 28
  competent parties in, 28–29
  consideration in, 28–29
  elements of, 27–28
  implied, 28–29
  legal form of, 28–29
  legal object of, 28–29
  offer and acceptance of, 28–29
  termination of, 28
Legal environment, of hospitals, 377–381
Legal form, of contract, 28–29

Legal object, of contract, 28–29
Legislation
  affecting health insurance, 29–30
  and workers' compensation, 215
Length of stay, average, 357
Letter, collection by, 313, 313*f*
Level I codes, 274, 289–290
Level II codes, 274, 289–290
Level II manual, for HCPCS, 290–291
  appendices in, 291
  index of main terms in, 290–291, 291*f*
  modifiers in, 291
  table of drugs in, 291
Level III codes, 275, 289–290
Liability
  employee, 27
  employer, 27
  medical, 26–27
  third-party, Medicaid and, 135, 135*t*
Licensed independent practitioner, 379
Life expectancy, and healthcare costs, 9–10
Lifelong learning, 15–16
Lifetime maximum cap, 87
Lifetime release of information, 68, 160, 161*f*
Limiting charge, Medicare, 165
Litigation, small claims, 308, 314–315
Litigiousness, 27
"Local" codes, 275
Local coverage determination (LCD), 162
Log
  generating and maintaining of, 19
  insurance claims, 80–82, 81*f*, 328, 329*f*
Longshore and Harbor Workers' Compensation Act, 215
Long-term care diagnosis-related groups (LTC-DRGs), 359–360
Long-term care facilities (LTCFs), 377
  E & M coding for, 288
Long-term care hospital (LTCH) prospective payment system, 355, 359–360
Long-term care insurance, 52–53
Low severity problem, E & M codes for, 285
LTC-DRGs (long-term care diagnosis-related groups), 359–360
LTCFs (long-term care facilities), 377
  E & M coding for, 288
LTCH (long-term care hospital) prospective payment system, 355, 359–360

M

MACs. *See* Medicare Administrative Contractors (MACs).
Main terms
  in CPT manual index, 277, 277*f*, 279
  in HCPCS coding manual index, 290–291, 291*f*
  in ICD-10-CM manual alphabetic index, 242–246, 244*f*
Maintenance of benefits (MOB), 55
Major medical coverage, 47, 86

Managed care, 47, 101–118
  advantages of, 106
  in BCBS, 94
  certification and regulation of, 107–108
    by complaint management, 108, 108*f*
    by HIPAA, 107
    by Joint Commission, 107
    by NCQA, 107
    by URAC, 107
    by utilization review, 108
  defined, 10, 47, 102–103
  disadvantages of, 106–107
  vs. fee-for-service, 46, 85, 103*f*
  future of, 116
  HIPAA and, 112–115
  history of, 4*t*, 5–6
  impact of, 115–116
    on healthcare providers, 115–116
    on physician-patient relationship, 115
  Medicaid, 133–134
  Medicare, 151, 155–160
    appeals process for, 179–180, 180*f*
    HMOs for, 155–158
      advantages and disadvantages of, 158–159
      with point-of-service option, 158
    preferred provider organization for, 158
    provider-sponsored organization for, 158
    Special Needs Plan for, 155, 158
    types of, 155
  preauthorization in, 106, 109, 110*f*
  precertification in, 109, 111*f*
  predetermination in, 109
  principles of, 102–103, 103*f*
  referrals in, 109–112
    vs. consultations, 112
    how to obtain, 112, 113*f*
  websites on, 118
  workers' compensation and, 224
Managed care organizations (MCOs)
  functions of, 102
  healthcare reform's impact on, 116
  Medicaid, 133–134
  reimbursement with, 353
  types of, 103–106, 103*f*, 104*t*
Management, E & M codes for, 287*t*
Mandated Medigap transfer, 169
Mandated services, for Medicaid, 123–124, 124*t*
Mandatory services, for Medicaid, 123–124, 124*t*
Manifestation, 248
Manifestation codes, in ICD-10 tabular list, 248
MassHealth, 120–121
Maternal and Child Health Services, 127
MCOs. *See* Managed care organizations (MCOs).
MDS (minimum data set), for resource utilization groups, 358

Meaningful use incentives, 307–308, 348–349
"Means Test," for CHAMPVA, 203
Media intervention, and healthcare costs, 10
Medicaid, 48, 119–142
　accepting assignment with, 138
　accepting patients with, 130
　claims for, 134–135
　　CMS-1500 form for, 134
　　reciprocity of, 134–135
　　resubmission of, 134
　　secondary, 134, 135t
　　"simple," 134
　　time limit for filing, 136
　common billing errors with, 135–136, 136f
　copayments for, 136–138
　defined, 120
　eligibility for, 123, 123f
　　for categorically needy, 123f, 124
　　for medically needy, 123f, 124–125, 125f
　　verification of, 130–132
　　　automated voice response system for, 131
　　　benefits of systems for, 132
　　　computer software program for, 132
　　　electronic data interchanges for, 132
　　　Medicaid identification card for, 131, 131f
　　　point-of-sale device for, 132
　enrollment vs. spending in, 125, 125f
　evolution of, 4–5, 4t, 121–123
　　healthcare reform in, 123
　　Supplemental Security Income in, 121–123
　　　eligibility expansion for, 122–123
　　　eligibility for, 121–122, 122b, 122t
　　Temporary Assistance for Needy Families in, 121
　exception for signed release of information to, 40
　federal and state contributions to, 120–121
　fraud and abuse in, 139–140
　as hospital payer, 383, 385t
　managed care in, 133–134
　and Medicare, 132–133
　　difference between, 133, 133t
　　dual eligibles for, 129–130, 132, 153
　　special programs for, 132–133
　other programs in, 127–128
　　Early Periodic Screening, Diagnosis, and Treatment program as, 127
　　Home and Community-Based Services as, 127–128
　　　state plan option expansion of, 128
　　Maternal and Child Health Services as, 127
　　Program of All-Inclusive Care for the Elderly as, 127
　participating providers for, 130
　payment for services in, 129–130

Medicaid (Continued)
　dual eligibles in, 129–130
　medically necessary, 129
　prescription drug coverage in, 129
　preauthorization for, 138
　premiums and cost sharing for, 128–129
　　Emergency Medical Treatment & Labor Act on, 129
　　enforcement of, 129
　　for nonemergency use of emergency department, 129
　quality practices for, 140
　remittance advice for, 136, 137f
　retention, storage, and disposal of records for, 138
　services requiring prior approval in, 138
　state programs for, 120–121
　structure of, 123–127
　　Community First Choice Option in, 125
　　federal government's role in, 123, 123f
　　fiscal intermediaries in, 126
　　mandated services in, 123–124, 124t
　　Medicaid contractors in, 125, 126
　　Medicaid integrity contractors in, 126–127
　　State Children's Health Insurance Program in, 125–126
　　states' options in, 124–125, 124t
　and third-party liability, 135, 135t
　websites on, 142
Medicaid contractors, 125, 126
Medicaid Fraud Control Unit, 139
Medicaid HIPAA Compliant Concept Model (MHCCM), 123b
Medicaid identification card, 131, 131f
Medicaid integrity contractors (MICs), 126–127
Medicaid Integrity Group (MIG), 126–127
Medicaid Integrity Program (MIP), 126–127
Medi-Cal, 120–121
Medical billing and coding specialist. See Health insurance professional(s).
Medical billing services, 314
Medical billing software system, cost of, 362
Medical center, 375
Medical Claims Analyst, 17t
Medical Claims Processor, 17t
Medical Claims Reviewer, 17t
Medical Coder, 17t
Medical Collector, 17t
Medical decision making
　E & M codes for, 284, 287t
　surrogate for, 396
Medical ethics, 30–31, 31f
　applicable to health insurance, 28–29
　defined, 31
　in hospitals, 380
　and medical etiquette, 30–32, 31f
Medical etiquette, 31–32
Medical examination, with abnormal findings, 260

Medical information, authorization for release of
　accessing information through, 301, 302f
　for disability claim, 229f
　exceptions for insurance claims submission to, 40
　HIPAA on, 300
　legal aspects of, 33, 34f, 40
　"lifetime," 68
　on patient information form, 67f, 68
Medical insurance. See Health insurance.
Medical law
　applicable to health insurance, 28–29
　and liability, 26–27
Medical liability, 26–27
Medical necessity, 62
　for Medicare, 160–161
　for third-party payers, 55, 56f
Medical progress reports, for workers' compensation, 222, 223f
Medical record(s), 32–33
　access to, 33, 301
　for claim processing, 69–70, 70f
　combination, 347
　complete, 32, 69
　correction of, 35, 35f, 301
　defined, 32, 33–35
　demographic information on, 62
　documentation of, 33–36, 35f
　electronic, 306–308, 344–349
　　in claims submission, 69
　　combination records with, 347
　　components of, 344–347
　　defined, 344, 388
　　digital imaging hybrid in, 347
　　federal funding and "meaningful use" of, 307–308, 348–349
　　future of, 348
　　hospital, 388
　　key features of, 388
　　potential issues with, 347–348
　　privacy concerns of, 348
　　security of, 347
　hospital
　　electronic, 388
　　standard codes and terminology in, 388
　　structure and content of, 387–388
　ownership of, 32
　purposes of, 32
　releasing information from, 33, 34f
　retention of, 32–33
　　for Medicaid, 138
Medical record review, for Medicare, 181, 182
Medical savings account (MSA), 104t
　for Medicare, 151
　for third-party payers, 50, 51t
Medical technology, and healthcare costs, 10
Medically necessary services
　Medicaid payment for, 129
　Medicare Part A coverage for, 146

Medically needy, Medicaid for, 123f, 124–125, 125f
Medicare, 48, 143–185
  administration of, 144–145
  advanced beneficiary notice for, 161–162, 163f
  allowable charges under, 150
  BCBS and, 91–94
  benefit period for, 150–151, 382
  billing for, 164–165
    determination of fee in, 165
    participating and nonparticipating providers in, 165
    Physician Fee Schedule in, 164–165, 164t
  CHAMPVA and, 206
  changing health or prescription coverage under, 152
  claims for, 165–168
    Administrative Simplification Compliance Act on, 165–167, 166f
    appeals on, 335
      with fee-for-service, 176–179, 179f
      with managed care, 179–180, 180f
    audits of, 175
    deadline for filing, 168
    demand bills for, 165, 166f
    electronic, 165, 342–343
      exceptions to mandatory, 65, 65b, 165–167
    electronic funds transfer for, 175, 177f
    for hospital costs, 381–384, 382t
    initial, 165
    Medicare Summary Notice for, 172–175, 173f
      information on, 172
    Medicare/Medicaid Crossover, 135, 171–172
    for Medigap, 169, 169f, 170t
    paper
      ASCA enforcement of, 167–168
      CMS-1500 form for, 168–172
      exception criteria for, 65, 65b, 165–167
      guidelines for completion of, 168–169
    Recovery Audit Contractor Program for, 176
    remittance advice for, 172–175
      electronic, 175, 176f
      standard paper, 172–175, 174f
    for secondary policy, 169–171, 333
      completion of, 170–171, 171t
      conditional payment for, 171
      criteria for, 169–170
    status request for, 168
    timely filing rules for, 168
    transition to ASC X12 Version 5010 for, 167
  combination coverage with, 153–155
    Medicare Secondary Payer as, 155, 156f
    Medicare supplement (Medigap) policies as, 153–155

Medicare *(Continued)*
    crossover program for, 171
    defined, 153
    eligibility for, 153–155
    and gaps by care type, 153, 154b
    vs. Medicare Advantage, 159t
    premium for, 153
    types of, 153, 154t
    Medicare/Medicaid dual eligibility as, 129–130, 132, 153
  cost-sharing requirements of, 150–151, 150t
  determination of medical necessity for, 160–161
  diagnosis-related groups for, 382
  dual eligibility for, 119, 129–130, 153
  enrollment in, 150
    open period for, 152
  health insurance claim number for, 162, 164t
  history of, 4–5, 4t, 144–153, 145f
  as hospital payer, 381–383
    benefit period for, 382
    calculation of payments under, 382
    keeping current with, 381–382
    Medicare Severity-Adjusted System of, 382–383
    payment mechanism by setting of care for, 385t
    payment schedule for, 382, 382t
    and quality improvement organizations, 381
    review of, 382
    three-day payment window for, 383, 393
  identification card for, 162, 164f
    replacement of, 162–164
  importance of understanding, 160
  keeping current with, 381–382
  lifetime release of information form for, 160, 161f
  local coverage determination for, 162
  managed care plans under, 151, 155–160
    appeals process for, 179–180, 180f
    HMOs as, 155–158
      advantages and disadvantages of, 158–159
      with point-of-service option, 158
    preferred provider organization as, 158
    provider-sponsored organization as, 158
    Special Needs Plan as, 155, 158
    types of, 155
  and Medicaid, 132–133
    difference between, 133, 133t
    dual eligibility for, 119, 129–130, 153
    special programs for, 132–133
  medical savings account for, 151
  other plans for, 151–152
  Part A, 146–147
    benefit period for, 382
    calculation of payments for, 382
    covered services in, 146, 146t, 382
    eligibility for, 146

Medicare *(Continued)*
  Medicare Administrative Contractors for, 146–147, 148f, 372
    noncovered services in, 146, 147t
    payment schedule for, 382, 382t
    review of, 382
  Part B, 147–150, 148t
  Part C (Medicare Advantage Plans), 151
    appeals process for, 179–180, 180f
    healthcare reform impact on, 151
    hierarchical condition category for reimbursement under, 355–356
    traditional Medicare with Medigap policy *vs.*, 159t
  Part D (Medicare Prescription Drug Benefit Plan), 152, 152t
  premiums for, 147–151, 150t
  private fee-for-service plan for, 151, 158
    appeals process for, 176–179, 179f
  Program of All-Inclusive Care for the Elderly in, 152–153
  quality assurance for
    Beneficiary Complaint Response Program for, 181
    beneficiary notices initiative for, 181
    billing fraud and, 182
    Center for Medicare and Medicaid Innovation in, 182
    Clinical Laboratory Improvement Amendments Program in, 182
    Hospital-Issued Notice of Noncoverage for, 181
    Notice of Discharge and Medicare Appeal Rights for, 181
    Physician Quality Reporting System in, 182
    physician review of medical records in, 181, 182
    Quality Improvement Organizations for, 180, 181, 381
    quality review studies for, 180–182
  reimbursement system for, 354–356
    fee schedules as, 354
    prospective payment system as, 354–355
      acute inpatient hospital, 355, 359
      defined, 354
      home health, 355
      for hospital care, 382
      inpatient psychiatric facility, 355
      inpatient rehabilitation facility, 355
      long-term care hospital, 355, 359–360
      Medicare Advantage Program (CMS hierarchical condition category) as, 354, 355–356
      outpatient, 355
      skilled nursing facility, 355
    resource-based relative value scale for formula for, 357b
    transition to, 359–360
    setting payment policy for, 359
  structure of, 145–150
  website on, 184–185

Medicare Administrative Contractors
(MACs), 91–94
    on Medicare claims, 167
    for Medicare Part A, 146–147, 148f, 381
    for Medicare Part B, 150
Medicare Advantage plans, 106, 151
    appeals process for, 179–180, 180f
    healthcare reform impact on, 151
    reimbursement under, 354, 355–356
    traditional Medicare with Medigap policy
        vs., 159t
Medicare carriers, 91–94, 146–147, 148f, 381
Medicare Codes, National, 274
Medicare gaps, 153, 154b
Medicare hospital insurance (Medicare HI), 132
Medicare identification card, 162, 164f
    replacement of, 162–164
Medicare legacy IDs, 64–65
Medicare Physician Fee Schedule, 164–165,
    164t
Medicare Prescription Drug Benefit Plan,
    152, 152t
Medicare Secondary Payer (MSP), 155, 156f
    claims for, 169–171, 333–334
        completion of, 170–171, 171t
        conditional payment for, 171
        criteria for, 169–170
Medicare Severity-Adjusted Diagnosis-
    Related Group (MS-DRG) System,
    382–383
Medicare Summary Notice (MSN), 172–175,
    173f
Medicare supplement plans, 48, 94, 153–155
    claims for, 169, 169f, 170t
    crossover program for, 171
    defined, 153
    eligibility for, 153–155
    and gaps by care type, 153, 154b
    vs. Medicare Advantage, 159t
    premium for, 153
    types of, 153, 154t
Medicare-certified providers, for TRICARE, 194
Medicare/Medicaid crossover claims, 135,
    171–172
Medigap plans, 48, 94, 153–155
    claims for, 169, 169f, 170t
    crossover program for, 171
    defined, 153
    eligibility for, 153–155
    and gaps by care type, 153, 154b
    vs. Medicare Advantage, 159t
    premium for, 153
    types of, 153, 154t
Medigap transfer, mandated, 169
Medi-Medi, 129–130, 132, 153
    claims for, 135, 171–172
    prescription drug coverage with, 152
Mental health services, CHAMPVA coverage
    for, 204t, 205t
Merchant Marine Act, 215
MHCCM (Medicaid HIPAA Compliant
    Concept Model), 123b

MHS (Military Health System), 188
MICs (Medicaid integrity contractors),
    126–127
MIG (Medicaid Integrity Group), 126–127
Military carriers, 48–50, 186–212
    CHAMPVA as, 199–207
        benefits under, 203
        CHAMPVA for Life program in, 207, 207t
            eligibility for, 207
        claims for, 207–208
            appeals and reconsiderations of, 209
            explanation of benefits for, 209, 210f
            filing deadlines for, 208, 208b
            paper, 208–209
        cost sharing for, 201–202, 203–205
            with no other health insurance, 203,
                204t
            with other health insurance, 203, 204t
        eligibility for, 199–201
            extended, 202
            identification of, 202–203, 202f
            loss of, 201
        and HMO coverage, 206
        in-house treatment initiative of, 203,
            206
        and Medicare, 206
        payment summary for, 203, 205t
        preauthorization for, 203–205, 207–208
        prescription drug benefit under,
            205–206
        providers under, 206–207
        and TRICARE, 206
        types of health insurance plans primary
            to, 206
    HIPAA and, 209
    overview of, 187
    TRICARE as, 187–190
        additional programs under, 190–194,
            192f
        allowed services under, 190
        authorized providers under, 194–196
        and CHAMPVA, 206
        claims for, 197–199
            deadline for submitting, 199
            electronic, 199, 383
            explanation of benefits for, 199, 200f
            paper, 198–199, 198f
            who submits, 197–198
        coding and payment system for,
            196–197
        cost sharing for, 196–197, 196t, 197t,
            383
        dental programs under, 190–192
        eligibility for, 188–189
            losing of, 189
            verifying, 194, 195b, 195f
        ineligibility for, 189
        management activity of, 188
        Military Health System and, 188
        nonavailability statement for, 192, 383
        and other health insurance, 193
        Overseas Program of, 189

Military carriers (Continued)
        PARs and nonPARs for, 196
        program options for, 189, 190t, 191t
        regional contractors for, 188
        regional service map for, 187–188, 188f
        supplemental insurance policies under,
            193
        supplemental programs under, 193
            Exceptional Family Member Program
                as, 193
            TRICARE Plus as, 193
            TRICARE for Life program in, 193–194
                eligibility for, 193–194
        Young Adult program for, 189–190
    websites on, 212
Military Health System (MHS), 188
Military ID cards, 194, 195b, 195f
Military treatment facilities (MTFs), 188
Miners, black lung in, 215
Minimal problem, E & M codes for, 284
Minimum data set (MDS), for resource
    utilization groups, 358
Minimum essential coverage, 89
Minors, emancipated, 28
MIP (Medicaid Integrity Program), 126–127
Mixed model, of HMO, 105
MOB (maintenance of benefits), 55
Moderate severity problem, E & M codes for,
    285
Modified own-occupation policy, 225
Modifiers
    in CPT coding, 275, 275f, 278
    in E & M coding, 288–289
    essential and nonessential, in ICD-10-CM
        manual alphabetic index, 242–243,
        245f
    in HCPCS Level II coding, 291
Modifying terms, in CPT manual index, 277,
    277f
Mono-spaced fonts, 77–78
Morals, 30–31
Morphology, 249
Morphology codes, in ICD-10-CM, 248
Mortality statistics, 238
MSA. See Medical savings account (MSA).
MS-DRG (Medicare Severity-Adjusted
    Diagnosis-Related Group) System,
    382–383
MSN (Medicare Summary Notice), 172–175,
    173f
MSP. See Medicare Secondary Payer (MSP).
MTFs (military treatment facilities), 188
Multiaxial structure, 390
Multiple coding, ICD-10-CM, 250

N
NAS (nonavailability statement), TRICARE
    Standard, 192, 383
National Committee for Quality Assurance
    (NCQA), 54
    accreditation by, 378–379
    on managed care, 107

National Correct Coding Initiative (NCCI), 291–292, 392, 393t
National Council for Prescription Drug Programs, Inc. (NCPDP) Version D.0, 393
National Electronic Attachment (NEA), 80
National Healthcare Anti-Fraud Association (NHCAA), 41
National identifier, HIPAA requirements for, 64–65
National Medicare Codes, 274
National Organization of Social Security Claimants' Representatives, 233
National Patient Safety Goals (NPSGs), 378
National provider identifier (NPI), 64–65
National Provider System, 138
National Supplier Clearinghouse (NSC) identifiers, 64–65
National Uniform Billing Committee (NUBC), 77, 384–387
National Uniform Claim Committee (NUCC), 63, 77
  on Medicare claim form, 168
Nature of presenting problem, E & M codes for, 284
NCCI (National Correct Coding Initiative), 291–292, 392, 393t
NCPDP (National Council for Prescription Drug Programs, Inc.) Version D.0, 393
NCQA. See National Committee for Quality Assurance (NCQA).
NEA (National Electronic Attachment), 80
NEC ("not elsewhere classifiable"), in ICD-10 tabular list, 245
Neglect, in Medicaid system, 139–140
Negligence, 27
Network
  employment, 233
  in managed care, 102
  in Medicare, 155
Network model, of HMO, 105
Network providers, for TRICARE, 194
New patient, E & M coding for, 281
New patient information, on patient information form, 66, 67f, 68f
NHCAA (National Healthcare Anti-Fraud Association), 41
997 electronic file, 387, 387f
No cancelable long-term disability insurance, 225
NODMAR (Notice of Discharge and Medicare Appeal Rights Review), 181
No-fault insurance, 216
Nonavailability statement (NAS), TRICARE Standard, 192, 383
Non-cancellable policy, 58
Noncovered services, under Medicare Part A, 146, 147t
Non–DRG-based services, CHAMPVA coverage for, 204t, 205t
Nonessential modifiers, in ICD-10-CM manual alphabetic index, 242–243, 245f

Non-institutional TRICARE-authorized providers, 194
Nonlabor component, in diagnosis-related group payments, 358
Nonmedical services, Medicare Part A noncoverage of, 147t
Non-network providers, for TRICARE, 194–196
Nonparticipating providers (nonPARs), 58
  in fee-for-service plans, 95
  for Medicare, 165
  for TRICARE, 196
NOS ("not otherwise specified"), in ICD-10 tabular list, 245
"Not elsewhere classifiable" (NEC), in ICD-10 tabular list, 245
"Not otherwise specified" (NOS), in ICD-10 tabular list, 245
Notice of Discharge and Medicare Appeal Rights Review (NODMAR), 181
NPI (national provider identifier), 64–65
NPSGs (National Patient Safety Goals), 378
NSC (National Supplier Clearinghouse) identifiers, 64–65
NUBC (National Uniform Billing Committee), 77, 384–387
NUCC (National Uniform Claim Committee), 63, 77
  on Medicare claim form, 168
Nursing facility services, E & M coding for, 288
Nursing home. See also Skilled nursing facility(ies) (SNFs)
  as resource utilization groups, 358

O
OASDI (Old-Age, Survivors, and Disability Insurance), 231
Oath of Hippocrates, 30–32
Objectivity, 15
OBRA (Omnibus Budget Reconciliation Act), 29, 30
Observation services, E & M codes for, 286–287
Observation stay, ICD-10-CM coding for, 253
Occupational therapy, 222
Occupational trends, of health insurance professional, 18
OCESAA (Omnibus Consolidated and Emergency Supplemental Appropriations Act), 360
OCR. See Optical character recognition (OCR).
Offer, of contract, 28–29
Office for Civil Rights (OCR), 64
Office of the Inspector General (OIG), on billing compliance, 398–399
Office services, E & M codes for, 286, 287t
Office setting, patient expectations of, 297
OHI. See Other health insurance (OHI).

Old-Age, Survivors, and Disability Insurance (OASDI), 231
Ombudsman, 216
Omnibus Budget Reconciliation Act (OBRA), 29, 30
Omnibus Consolidated and Emergency Supplemental Appropriations Act (OCESAA), 360
One-time release of information, 68, 160, 161f
"One-write" system, 304, 307f
Online Workers' Compensation Service Center, 224
Open enrollment period
  for Medicare, 152
  for Medigap policies, 153–155
Open-ended HMO, 106
Open-panel plan, 106
Operative reports, as claim attachments, 79–80
OPPS (outpatient prospective payment system)
  hospital, 393–394
  Medicare, 355
Optical character recognition (OCR), 77–78
  in claim processing, 325, 325b
  format rules for, 77–78, 78f
Optical character recognition (OCR) scannable, 77
Optional services, for Medicaid, 124–125, 124t
Oregon Health Plan, 120–121
"Other," in ICD-10-CM coding, 252
Other health insurance (OHI)
  CHAMPVA with, 203, 204t
  CHAMPVA without, 203, 204t
  TRICARE and, 193
"Other specified code," in ICD-10-CM coding, 248f, 252
Outliers
  cost, 355
  for Medicare, 382
  short-stay, 359–360
Out-of-pocket maximum, 47, 86–87
Outpatient claim form, 394, 395b
Outpatient hospital coding, 393–394
  ambulatory payment classification coding for, 394
  E & M, 281
  prospective payment system and, 393–394
Outpatient prospective payment system (OPPS)
  hospital, 393–394
  Medicare, 355
Outpatient services
  CHAMPVA coverage for, 204t, 205t
  E & M codes for, 286, 287t
  ICD-10-CM coding for, 252–253
    for circumstances other than disease or injury, 254–256
    diagnosis, condition, problem, or other reason for encounter/visit in, 256
    for ambulatory surgery, 259–263

Outpatient services (*Continued*)
for chronic diseases, 257–258
for coexisting conditions, 258–264
for diagnostic services only, 258–259
for general medical examination with abnormal findings, 260
for preoperative evaluations only, 259
for routine health screenings, 260
for routine prenatal visits, 260
for therapeutic services only, 259
for uncertain diagnosis, 256–257
first-listed condition in, 253
level of detail in, 254–255
codes with 3, 4, or 5 digits in, 255–256
use of full number of digits in, 256–257
for observation stay, 253
surgical, 253–257
symptoms and signs in, 253–257
Outpatient surgery, ICD-10-CM coding for, 253–257
Overdue bills, 308
Overpayment, in Medicare, 160
Own-occupation policies, 225

P
PACE (Program of All-Inclusive Care for the Elderly), 127, 152–153
Palliative care, 374
Palmetto Government Business Administrators (PGBA), 198
Paper claims
for CHAMPVA, 208–209
CMS-1500 form for. *See* CMS-1500 (08/05) form.
for Medicare
ASCA enforcement of, 167–168
CMS-1500 form for, 168–172
exception criteria for, 65, 65*b*, 165–167
guidelines for completion of, 168–169
for TRICARE, 198–199, 198*f*
UB-04, 384–385, 386*f*
Paper encounter form, 70, 71*f*
Paperwork
in managed care program, 106
patient expectations of, 297
PAR(s). *See* Participating providers (PARs).
Paraphrasing, 15
Parentheses
in ICD-10 tabular list, 246
in ICD-10-CM manual alphabetic index, 243–246, 247*f*
Partial disability
permanent, 220
temporary, 220
Partial payment, 308
Participating providers (PARs), 58
in fee-for-service plans, 87, 95
for Medicaid, 130
for Medicare, 165
for TRICARE, 196
Party of the first part, 29
Party of the second part, 29

Party of the third part, 29
Pass-throughs, 394
Patient(s), 295–317
billing of. *See* Billing.
collection from. *See* Collection.
as consumers, 299
expectations of, 296–298
financial issues as, 298
getting comfortable with healthcare provider as, 298
honoring appointment times as, 297
patient load as, 298
privacy and confidentiality as, 298
professional office setting as, 297
relevant paperwork and questions as, 297
fair treatment of, 380–381
future trends concerning, 299
aging population as, 299
Internet as healthcare tool as, 299
patients as consumers as, 299
HIPAA impact on, 37–38, 299–303
accessing information as
through de-identification, 301–303
through patient authorization, 301, 302*f*
authorization to release information as, 300
covered entities as, 300
requirements for, 300–301
patient's right of access and correction as, 301
websites on, 317
Patient abuse, in Medicaid system, 139–140
Patient account, 362, 363*f*
Patient Account Representative, 17*t*
Patient accounting systems, computerized, 305–306, 361–365
generating reports in, 364–365
accounts receivable aging report as, 364, 365*f*
insurance claims aging report as, 364, 366*f*, 367*f*
practice analysis report as, 364–365, 368*f*
HIPAA and, 365–369
managing transactions with, 362–364
insurance carrier adjustments (contractual write-offs) in, 363–364
posting and tracking patient charges in, 362, 363*f*
processing payments in, 363, 363*f*
selection of, 361–362
Patient charges, posting and tracking of, 362, 363*f*
Patient entry screen, 68*f*
Patient examination, E & M codes for, 284, 287*t*
Patient health record. *See* Medical record(s).
Patient history
E & M codes for, 284, 287*t*
in electronic medical record, 344

Patient identification, errors in, 136*f*
Patient identification card. *See* Identification (ID) card.
Patient information
authorization to release. *See* Authorization to release information.
collection and verification of, 320–321
Patient information form, 303
for claim processing, 66–68, 67*f*
Patient insurance identification card, 66, 69, 69*f*
Patient ledger, 304, 307*f*
Patient ledger card, 72–73, 74*f*, 330, 332*f*
Patient load, patient expectations of, 298
Patient neglect, in Medicaid system, 139–140
Patient Protection and Affordable Care Act (PPACA), 30
on CHAMPVA eligibility, 201
and fee-for-service plans, 86
history of, 6
and Medicaid, 120–121
and Medicare, 382
Patient registration form, 66–68, 67*f*
Patient Safety Advisory Group, 378
Patient service slip, 70–72, 71*f*, 72*f*
Pay and chase claims, 135
Payer guidelines, for claim filing, 322
Payer of last resort, 133
Payment(s)
incorrect, 334
posting of, 19, 330, 332*f*
processing of, 363, 363*f*
receiving, 328, 330*t*
Payment Error Rate Measurement (PERM), 128
Payment management, hospital, 397–398, 398*f*
Payment plan, 308–310, 310*f*
Payment policy, 308, 309*f*
discussion with patient of, 304
Payment system, for TRICARE, 196–197
Payroll journal, 304, 306*f*
PCP. *See* Primary care physician (PCP).
PDPs (Prescription Drug Plans), Medicare, 152, 152*t*
Peer review organizations (PROs)
defined, 361
for Medicare, 180, 181
and prospective payment systems, 361
Pegboard system, 304, 307*f*
Per diem rates, 355
for Medicaid, 383
PERM (Payment Error Rate Measurement), 128
Permanent condition, in workers' compensation, 220
Permanent disability, 220
partial, 220
total, 220
Personal care, Medicare Part A noncoverage of, 147*t*
Personal care accounts, 51–52, 51*t*

Personal Responsibility and Work Opportunity Reconciliation Act, 121
Personality traits, positive, 15
PFFS plans. *See* Private fee-for-service (PFFS) plans.
PGBA (Palmetto Government Business Administrators), 198
Pharmacy services, CHAMPVA coverage for, 204*t*
PHI. *See* Protected health information (PHI).
Physical examination, E & M codes for, 284, 287*t*
Physician Fee Schedule, Medicare, 164–165, 164*t*
Physician Quality Reporting System (PQRS), 182
Physician review, of medical records, for Medicare, 181, 182
Physician-patient relationship, 28–29
impact of managed care on, 115
Physicians' CPT codes, 274
PINs (provider identification numbers), 64–65
Place of service code, errors in, 136*f*
Placeholder character, in ICD-10 tabular list, 245
Plaintiff, 315
Plus sign, in CPT manual, 278*t*
Pneumoconiosis, 215
POA (present on admission), 396
Point dash, in ICD-10 tabular list, 246–249
Point-of-sale device, to verify Medicaid eligibility, 132
Point-of-service (POS) plan, 104*t*, 106
BCBS, 94
Medicare, 158
Policy, 1–2
non-cancellable, 58
Policyholder, 46–47, 86
Portability, 36
POS plan. *See* Point-of-service (POS) plan.
Posting
of patient charges, 362, 363*f*
of payments, 19, 330, 332*f*
Postpayment audits, Medicare, 175
PPACA. *See* Patient Protection and Affordable Care Act (PPACA).
PPOs. *See* Preferred provider organizations (PPOs).
PPS. *See* Prospective payment system (PPS).
PQRS (Physician Quality Reporting System), 182
Practice analysis report, 364–365, 368*f*
Practice management software, 63
HIPAA and, 365–369
insurance information using, 68*f*
patient entry screen using, 68*f*
Preauthorization
for BCBS, 384
for CHAMPVA, 203–205, 207–208
in managed care, 106, 109, 110*f*
with Medicaid, 138
obtaining necessary, 321–322

Precertification
in managed care, 109, 111*f*
obtaining necessary, 321–322
Predetermination, in managed care, 109
Preexisting conditions, 47
in fee-for-service plans, 87–88
history of, 7, 8
in managed care, 112–114
Preferred provider organizations (PPOs), 104–105, 104*t*
BCBS, 90, 94
CHAMPVA and, 206
comparison of, 103*f*
Medicare, 158
Pregnant women, Medicaid for, 123*f*
Premiums
defined, 1
for fee-for-service plans, 46–47, 86
in managed care program, 106
for Medicaid, 128–129
for Medicare
for Medicare supplement (Medigap) policies, 153
Part B, 147–151, 150*t*
Part D (Prescription Drug Plans), 152
Prenatal visits, ICD-10-CM coding for, 260
Preoperative evaluations only, ICD-10-CM coding for, 259
Prepayment audits, Medicare, 175
Prescription drug coverage
under CHAMPVA, 205–206
in managed care program, 106
under Medicaid, 129
Prescription Drug Plans (PDPs), Medicare, 152, 152*t*
Present on admission (POA), 396
Presenting problem, E & M codes for, 284
Preventive care
in managed care program, 106
Medicare Part A noncoverage of, 147*t*
Medicare Part B coverage of, 147
Preventive medicine, 2
Pricing transparency, 396
Primary care physician (PCP), 58
in BCBS, 94
in health maintenance organization, 105
impact of managed care on, 116
in point-of-service model, 106
in preferred provider organization, 104
Principal diagnosis
in diagnosis-related groups, 357
in ICD-10 diagnosis coding, 251–252
in ICD-10-PCS coding, 390–392, 392*b*
Prior approval, with Medicaid, 138
Prioritizing, 15
Privacy, 39–41
defined, 39
of electronic medical records, 348
HIPAA requirements for, 64, 339
in hospitals, 379–380
in managed care, 106
patient expectations of, 298

Privacy Rule, 64, 379–380
practice management software and, 366–368
Privacy Standards
computers and, 339
with hospital billing, 379
legal and ethical aspects of, 37
practice management software and, 368
Privacy statement, 37
Private businesses, impact of HIPAA on, 38
Private disability insurance, 49
Private fee-for-service (PFFS) plans, 104*t*
for Medicare, 151, 158
appeals process for, 176–179, 179*f*
Private health insurance. *See* Commercial health insurance.
Private insurers, as hospital payers, 384, 385*t*
PRO(s). *See* Peer review organizations (PROs).
Problem, ICD-10-CM coding for, 256
Problem patients, 310–311
Procedural coding. *See* Current Procedural Terminology (CPT) coding.
Procedure code, errors in, 136*f*
Professional ethics, 16
Professional office setting, patient expectations of, 297
Professional services, CHAMPVA coverage for, 204*t*, 205*t*
Professional standards, for hospitals, 379
Professional standards review organization
defined, 361
for Medicare, 180, 181
and prospective payment systems, 361
Program of All-Inclusive Care for the Elderly (PACE), 127, 152–153
Progress reports, for workers' compensation, 222, 223*f*
Prolonged services, E & M codes for, 286, 286*f*
Promises, implied, 28–29
Proofreading
to avoid errors in claims, 322, 322*b*
of CMS-1500 form, 79
Prospective payment system (PPS), 353, 353*t*
acute inpatient hospital, 355, 359
three-day payment window for, 383, 393
defined, 353
home health, 356*t*, 360
Medicare, 355
inpatient psychiatric facility, 355
inpatient rehabilitation facility, 356*t*, 360
Medicare, 355
for Medicare, 354–355
acute inpatient hospital, 355, 359
defined, 354
home health, 355
for hospital care, 382
inpatient psychiatric facility, 355
inpatient rehabilitation facility, 355
long-term care hospital, 355, 359–360

Prospective payment system (PPS) (Continued)
  Medicare Advantage Program (CMS hierarchical condition category) as, 354, 355–356
  outpatient, 355
  skilled nursing facility, 355
  outpatient
    hospital, 393–394
    for Medicare, 355
  peer review organizations and, 361
Protected health information (PHI), 64
  electronic, 64
  HIPAA on, 300
  under workers' compensation, 224
Provider(s), 58
  CHAMPVA, 206–207
  impact of HIPAA on, 38
  impact of managed care on, 115–116
  in managed care program, 106
  nonparticipating, 58
    in fee-for-service plans, 95
    for Medicare, 165
    for TRICARE, 196
  participating, 58, 87, 95
    in fee-for-service plans, 87, 95
    for Medicaid, 130
    for Medicare, 165
    for TRICARE, 196
  patient expectations of getting comfortable with, 298
  TRICARE-authorized, 194–196
Provider identification numbers (PINs), 64–65
Provider-sponsored organization (PSO), 104t, 106
  Medicare, 158
Punctuation, in ICD-10 tabular list, 245

Q

QDWIs (Qualified Disabled and Working Individuals), 132
QIOs. See Quality improvement organizations (QIOs).
QI(s) (Qualified Individuals) program, 132
QMBs (Qualified Medicare Beneficiaries), 132
Qualifications, for hospital billing, 399–400
Qualified Disabled and Working Individuals (QDWIs), 132
Qualified Individuals (QIs) program, 132
Qualified Medicare Beneficiaries (QMBs), 132
Quality assurance, for Medicare
  Beneficiary Complaint Response Program for, 181
  beneficiary notices initiative for, 181
  billing fraud and, 182
  Center for Medicare and Medicaid Innovation in, 182
  Clinical Laboratory Improvement Amendments Program in, 182

Quality assurance, for Medicare (Continued)
  Hospital-Issued Notice of Noncoverage for, 181
  Notice of Discharge and Medicare Appeal Rights for, 181
  Physician Quality Reporting System in, 182
  physician review of medical records in, 181, 182
  Quality Improvement Organizations for, 180, 181, 381
  quality review studies for, 180–182
Quality improvement organizations (QIOs)
  defined, 361
  for Medicare, 180, 181, 381
  and prospective payment systems, 361
Quality practices, in Medicaid, 140
Quality review studies, for Medicare, 180–182
Questions, patient expectations of, 297

R

RA. See Remittance advice (RA).
RAC (Recovery Audit Contractor) Program, 176
Railroad Retirement Board Carriers (RRBC), 146–147
RBRVS. See Resource-based relative value scale (RBRVS).
Real-time claims adjudication (RTCA), 334
"Reason codes," 136
Reason for encounter/visit, ICD-10-CM coding for, 256
Reasonable and customary fee. See Usual, customary, and reasonable (UCR) rates.
Rebilling, 308
Reciprocity, with Medicaid, 134–135
Recovery Audit Contractor (RAC) Program, 176
Referral(s)
  defined, 109–112
  E & M coding for, 281–283
  form for, 112, 113f
  in health maintenance organization, 105
  in managed care, 109–112
    vs. consultations, 112
    how to obtain, 112, 113f
  in point-of-service model, 106
  in preferred provider organization, 104
Regional contractors, for TRICARE, 188
Register, claims, 80–82, 81f, 328, 329f
Registered health information administrator (RHIA), 400t
Registered health information technicians (RHITs), 399, 400t
Registration, hospital, 394
Regulation, of managed care programs, 107–108
Regulatory environment, of hospitals, 377–381
Rehabilitation, vocational, 220

Reimbursement
  computerized accounting systems for, 361–365
    generating reports in, 364–365
      accounts receivable aging report as, 364, 365f
      insurance claims aging report as, 364, 366f, 367f
      practice analysis report as, 364–365, 368f
    HIPAA and, 365–369
    managing transactions with, 362–364
      insurance carrier adjustments (contractual write-offs) in, 363–364
      posting and tracking patient charges in, 362, 363f
      processing payments in, 363, 363f
    selection of, 361–362
  defined, 352
  methods of, 353–354, 353t
  websites on, 371
Reimbursement Specialist, 17t
Reimbursement systems, 351–371
  ambulatory payment classification as, 356t, 358
  capitation as, 353t, 354
  diagnosis-related groups for, 356t, 357–358
    assignment of, 357
    calculation of payments with, 357–358
    functioning of, 357
    in prospective payment system, 353
  fee-for-service as, 353, 353t
    discounted, 353, 353t
  with managed care organizations, 353
  for Medicare, 354–356
    fee schedules as, 354
    prospective payment system as, 354–355
      acute inpatient hospital, 355, 359
      defined, 354
      home health, 355
      inpatient psychiatric facility, 355
      inpatient rehabilitation facility, 355
      long-term care hospital, 355, 359–360
      Medicare Advantage Program (CMS hierarchical condition category) as, 354, 355–356
      outpatient, 355
      skilled nursing facility, 355
    resource-based relative value scale as formula for, 357b
    transition to, 359–360
    setting payment policy for, 359
  other, 356–359, 356t
  prospective payment system as, 353, 353t
    acute inpatient hospital, 355, 359
      three-day payment window for, 383, 393
    home health, 356t, 360
    Medicare, 355

Reimbursement systems *(Continued)*
  inpatient psychiatric facility, 355
  inpatient rehabilitation facility, 356*t*, 360
    Medicare, 355
  long-term care hospital, 355, 359–360
  for Medicare, 354–355
    acute inpatient hospital, 355, 359
    defined, 354
    home health, 355
    inpatient psychiatric facility, 355
    inpatient rehabilitation facility, 355
    long-term care hospital, 355, 359–360
    Medicare Advantage Program (CMS
      hierarchical condition category)
      as, 354, 355–356
    outpatient, 355
    skilled nursing facility, 355
  peer review organizations and, 361
  relative value scale for, 356
  resource-based, 356–357
    for Medicare, 357*b*, 359–360
  relative value units for, 353, 353*t*
  resource utilization groups for, 356*t*,
    358–359
  significance to health insurance
    professional of, 360–361
  understanding of, 352–354
Rejected claims, 79, 323
Relative value scale (RVS), 356
  resource-based, 356–357
    for Medicare, 357*b*, 359–360
Relative value units (RVUs), 164, 353, 353*t*,
  356
Release of medical information,
    authorization for
  accessing information through, 301, 302*f*
  for disability claim, 229*f*
  exceptions for insurance claims
    submission to, 40
  HIPAA on, 300
  legal aspects of, 33, 34*f*, 40
  "lifetime," 68
  on patient information form, 67*f*, 68
Remark codes
  for Medicaid claims, 136
  for Medicare claims, 165–167
Remittance advice (RA), 96, 97*f*
  CHAMPVA, 209, 210*f*
  defined, 328–329
  downcoding on, 330
  electronic, 96–98, 344
    authorization for, 344, 346*f*
    hospital, 397
    Medicare, 175
      enrolling for, 175, 176*f*
  interpretation of, 328–330, 331*f*
  Medicaid, 136, 137*f*
  Medicare, 172–175
    electronic, 175
      enrolling for, 175, 176*f*
    standard paper, 172–175, 174*f*
  TRICARE, 199, 200*f*

Remittance advice (RA) *(Continued)*
  troubleshooting of, 329–330
Remittance notice. *See* Remittance advice
  (RA).
Report(s), 364–365
  aging
    accounts receivable, 364, 365*f*
    insurance claims
      generation of, 364, 366*f*, 367*f*
      tracking of, 80–82, 81*f*
  generation of, 364–365
  operative, as claim attachments, 79–80
  practice analysis, 364–365, 368*f*
  special, CPT coding for, 278
  for workers' compensation
    healthcare provider, 217–220, 221*f*
    medical progress, 222, 223*f*
    progress, 222, 223*f*
    supplemental, 222, 223*f*
Residential healthcare facilities, as resource
  utilization groups, 358
Resource utilization groups (RUGs), 356*t*,
  358–359
Resource-based relative value scale (RBRVS),
  356–357
  change from fee-for-service to, 164
  formula for calculating, 357*b*
  transition to, 359–360
Respite care, 377
Respondeat superior, 27
Responsibilities, of health insurance
  professional, 17–18, 17*t*, 19
Resubmission, of Medicaid claims, 134
Returned claims, 79
Revenue cycle management systems, 398, 398*f*
RHIA (registered health information
  administrator), 400*t*
RHITs (registered health information
  technicians), 399, 400*t*
Risk, E & M codes for, 287*t*
Roles, of health insurance professional,
  17–18, 17*t*
Roosevelt, Theodore, 4–5
Routine health screenings, ICD-10-CM
  coding for, 260
Routing form, 70–72, 71*f*, 72*f*
RRBC (Railroad Retirement Board Carriers),
  146–147
RTCA (real-time claims adjudication), 334
RUGs (resource utilization groups), 356*t*,
  358–359
RVS. *See* Relative value scale (RVS).
RVUs (relative value units), 164, 353, 353*t*,
  356

S
Safety-net providers, 120
Schedule, time management, 16*t*
SCHIP (State Children's Health Insurance
  Program), 125–126
Screenings, routine health, ICD-10-CM
  coding for, 260

Second party, 29
Secondary claims
  Medicaid, 134, 135*t*
  processing of, 333–334, 333*f*
Secondary coverage, commercial claims
  involving, 96–98, 97*f*
Secondary Payer, Medicare. *See* Medicare
  Secondary Payer (MSP).
Sections
  in CPT coding, 279, 280*f*
  of HCPCS Level II codes, 290, 290*f*
Security, 39–40
  HIPAA requirements for, 64, 339
Security Rule, 64
Security standards, 339
*Security Standards for the Protection of Electronic
  Protected Health Information*, 64
See, cross-referencing with, in CPT manual,
  279, 280*f*
Self-insurance, 89–90
  Employee Retirement Income Security Act
    and, 89
  single or specialty service plans for, 90
  third-party administrators/administrative
    service organizations for, 89–90
Self-limiting problem, E & M codes for, 285
Self-pay patients, 309–310
Self-referring method, 158
Semicolon, in CPT coding, 279, 279*f*
Sequelae, ICD-10-CM coding for, 251–252
7th character, in ICD-10 tabular list, 245, 247*f*
72-hour rule, 383, 393
Severity-Adjusted Diagnosis-Related Group
  System, for Medicare, 382–383
Short-stay outlier, 359–360
Sign(s), ICD-10-CM coding for, 250, 253–257
Signature, errors in, 136*f*
"Signature on file" statement, 169, 169*f*
Sign-in sheet, 37–38, 73*b*
"Simple" claim, Medicaid, 134
Single service plans, 90
Skilled nursing facility(ies) (SNFs), 376–377
  billing for, 384
  E & M coding for, 288
  as resource utilization groups, 358
Skilled nursing facility (SNF) care
  under CHAMPVA, 207, 207*t*
  Medicare coverage for, 146*t*
Skilled nursing facility prospective payment
  system (SNF PPS), 355
SLMBs (Specified Low-Income Medicare
  Beneficiaries), 132
Small claims litigation, 308, 314–315
Small provider, 65–66, 79, 343
  for Medicare claims, 167
Small supplier, 65–66, 79, 343
SMI (supplemental medical insurance), 132
SNFs. *See* Skilled nursing facility(ies) (SNFs).
SNP (Special Needs Plan), Medicare, 155, 158
Social Security Act, 4*t*
Social Security benefits, Supplemental
  Security Income and, 122, 122*b*

Social Security Disability Insurance (SSDI), 49, 231–232
  administration and funding for, 231
  eligibility for, 231
  filing claims for, 233–234
    health insurance professional's role in, 234
    healthcare provider's role in, 233–234
    patient's role in, 233
  history of, 231
Social Security Number, on patient information form, 66
Software
  billing, cost of, 362
  electronic patient accounting, 305–306
  practice management, 63
    HIPAA and, 365–369
    insurance information using, 68f
    patient entry screen using, 68f
    to verify Medicaid eligibility, 132
Special Needs Plan (SNP), Medicare, 155, 158
Special reports, CPT coding for, 278
Specialist, 105
Specialized hospitals, 375
Specialty service plans, 90
Specified Low-Income Medicare Beneficiaries (SLMBs), 132
Spend-down, of income, 124–125
Sponsor
  in CHAMPVA, 201–202
  in TRICARE, 188–189
SPR (standard paper remittance) advice, 137f
  Medicare, 172–175, 174f
SPRA (standard paper remittance advice), 137f
  Medicare, 172–175, 174f
SSDI. See Social Security Disability Insurance (SSDI).
SSI. See Supplemental Security Income (SSI).
Staff model, of HMO, 105
Stand-alone code, in CPT coding, 279, 279f
Standard paper remittance (SPR) advice (SPRA), 137f
  Medicare, 172–175, 174f
Standard X12 transactions, 65
Standardized amount, in diagnosis-related group payments, 357–358
Standardized benefits and coverage rule, 49
Standards and Guidelines for the Accreditation of Managed Care Organizations, 107
Standards for Privacy of Individually Identifiable Health Information, 64
State Children's Health Insurance Program (SCHIP), 125–126
State contributions, to Medicaid, 120–121
State programs
  for disabilities, 232
  for Medicaid, 120–121
  for uninsured, 9
Statement, 70–72, 73f, 74f
Stationary condition, in workers' compensation, 220

"Stop loss" insurance, 47, 86–87, 90
Study, learning how to, 15
Subacute care facilities, 376
Subcategories
  in E & M coding, 281
  in ICD-10 tabular list, 242, 247f
Subheadings
  in CPT coding, 279, 280f
  of E & M code section, 286–288
Subjective information, patient history as, 284
Subpoena duces tecum, 40
Subsection, in CPT coding, 279, 280f
Subsequent hospital care, E & M codes for, 287
Summary Notice, Medicare, 172–175, 173f
Summary of benefits and coverage, 49
Superbill, 70–72, 71f, 72f
Supplemental coverage, 90
Supplemental Insurance, TRICARE Standard, 193
Supplemental medical insurance (SMI), 132
Supplemental reports, for workers' compensation, 222, 223f
Supplemental Security Income (SSI), 121–123, 232
  administration and funding for, 232
  disability program of, 49
  eligibility for, 121–122, 122b, 122t, 232
    expansion of, 122–123
  filing claims for, 233–234
    health insurance professional's role in, 234
    healthcare provider's role in, 233–234
    patient's role in, 233
Surrogates
  for intangible services, 297
  for medical decision making, 396
Suspension file system, for claims tracking, 328
Swing bed agreement, 384
Swipe terminals, 75
Symbols, in CPT manual, 277, 278t
Symptoms, ICD-10-CM coding for, 250, 253–257

T
Table of drugs, in HCPCS Level II coding manual, 291
Tabular list
  in CPT manual, 279, 280f
  in ICD-10-CM manual, 244, 244f
    abbreviations in, 245
    "code also" note in, 248–249
    conventions for, 245, 248f
    etiology/manifestation convention in, 248
    format and structure of codes in, 244–245, 247f
    instructional notes in, 248, 248f, 249f
    manifestation codes in, 248
    placeholder character in, 245
    punctuation in, 245
    7th character in, 245, 247f

TAC (TRICARE allowable charge), 196
TANF (Temporary Assistance for Needy Families), 121
Tangible items, 297
Tax Equity and Fiscal Responsibility Act (TEFRA), 29, 354
TDCC (Transportation Data Coordinating Committee), 339
Telecommunications, 340
Telephone, collection by, 312, 312f
Temporary Assistance for Needy Families (TANF), 121
Temporary disability, 220, 225
  partial, 220
  total, 220
TennCare, 120–121
Termination, of contract, 28
Text characters, optical character recognition of, 77
Text files, optical character recognition of, 77
TFL (TRICARE for Life), 191t, 193–194
  eligibility for, 193–194
Therapeutic services only, ICD-10-CM coding for, 259
Third party, 29
Third party only (TPO) billing, 33
Third-party administrators (TPAs), 89–90
Third-party carriers, terms common to, 54–58
Third-party liability, Medicaid and, 135, 135t
Third-party payer, 58, 62, 85
Threatened condition, ICD-10-CM coding for, 252
Three-day rule, 383, 393
Ticket to Work Program, 233
  functioning of, 233
  purpose of, 233
Time, E & M codes for, 285, 285f
  prolonged, 286, 286f
Time limits, for claims processing, 330–333
Time management schedule, 16t
Timely filing
  of BCBS and commercial claims, 95
  of CHAMPVA claims, 208, 208b
  of Medicaid claims, 136
  of Medicare claims, 168
  of workers' compensation claims, 217
TLAC (TRICARE Latin America/Canada), 189
TMA (TRICARE Management Activity), 187–188
TOP (TRICARE Overseas Program), 189
Total charge, errors in, 136f
Total disability
  permanent, 220
  temporary, 220
TPAs (third-party administrators), 89–90
TPO (treatment, payment, or healthcare operations), information disclosed for, 300
TPO (third party only) billing, 33
TPRADFM (TRICARE Prime Remote for Active Duty Family Members), 191t

Tracking
  of claims, 80–82, 325–328
    electronic insurance aging report for,
      80–82, 81f
    form for, 325–328, 327f
    insurance claims register system for,
      328, 329f
    insurance log for, 80–82, 81f
    suspension file system for, 328
    using practice management software,
      80–82, 80f
  of patient charges, 362, 363f
Trading partners, 21
Training, in hospital billing, 399–400
Training program, for health insurance
  professional, 14, 15b, 19
Transaction capability, in electronic medical
  record, 347
Transaction management, 362–364
  insurance carrier adjustments (contractual
    write-offs) in, 363–364
  posting and tracking patient charges in,
    362, 363f
  processing payments in, 363, 363f
Transaction set, in ASCA X12N 8371 version
  5010, 385
Transaction Standards, HIPAA, 366
Transportation, non-emergency, Medicare
  Part A noncoverage of, 147t
Transportation Data Coordinating
  Committee (TDCC), 339
TRD (TRICARE Retiree Dental Program), 192
Treating source, 233–234
Treatment, payment, or healthcare
  operations (TPO), information disclosed
  for, 300
Triangle, in CPT manual, 278t
TRICARE, 48–50, 187–190
  allowed services under, 190
  authorized providers under, 194–196
  and CHAMPVA, 206
  claims for, 197–199
    deadline for submitting, 199
    electronic, 199, 383
    explanation of benefits for, 199, 200f
    paper, 198–199, 198f
    who submits, 197–198
  coding and payment system for, 196–197
  cost sharing for, 196–197, 196t, 197t, 383
  eligibility for, 188–189
    losing of, 189
    verification of, 194, 195b, 195f
  as hospital payer, 383
  ineligibility for, 189
  management of, 187–188
  Military Health System and, 188
  and other health insurance, 193
  PARs and nonPARs for, 196
  programs under
    additional, 190–194, 192f
    dental, 190–192
    options for, 189, 190t, 191t

TRICARE (Continued)
  supplemental, 193
    Exceptional Family Member Program
      as, 193
    TRICARE Plus as, 193
  TRICARE Extra as, 190, 191t, 192f
  TRICARE for Life as, 191t, 193–194
    eligibility for, 193–194
  TRICARE Overseas Program as, 189
  TRICARE Prime as, 190, 191t, 192f
  TRICARE Prime Remote as, 191t
  TRICARE Reserve Select as, 191t
  TRICARE Retired Reserve as, 191t
  TRICARE Standard as, 190, 191t
    comparison of, 192f
    nonavailability statement for, 192,
      383
    supplemental insurance with, 193
  TRICARE Young Adult Program as,
    189–190
  US Family Health Plan as, 191t
  regional contractors for, 188
  regional service map for, 187–188, 188f
  supplemental insurance policies under, 193
TRICARE allowable charge (TAC), 196
TRICARE Eurasia-Africa, 189
TRICARE Extra program, 190, 191t, 192f
TRICARE for Life (TFL), 191t, 193–194
  eligibility for, 193–194
TRICARE Latin America/Canada (TLAC), 189
TRICARE Management Activity (TMA),
  187–188
TRICARE Overseas Program (TOP), 189
TRICARE Pacific, 189
TRICARE Plus, 193
TRICARE Prime program, 190, 191t, 192f
TRICARE Prime Remote for Active Duty
  Family Members (TPRADFM), 191t
TRICARE Prime Remote program, 191t
TRICARE Reserve Select (TRS), 191t
TRICARE Retired Reserve (TRR), 191t
TRICARE Retiree Dental Program (TRD), 192
TRICARE Standard program, 190, 191t
  comparison of, 192f
  nonavailability statement for, 192, 383
  supplemental insurance with, 193
TRICARE Young Adult (TYA) Program,
  189–190
TRICARE-authorized providers, 194–196
TRR (TRICARE Retired Reserve), 191t
TRS (TRICARE Reserve Select), 191t
Truth in Lending Act, 311
TYA (TRICARE Young Adult) Program,
  189–190

U
UB-04 claim form. See Uniform bill (UB-04)
  claim form.
UCR (usual, customary, and reasonable)
  rates, 47, 55–57, 87, 353
UHDDS (Uniform Hospital Discharge Data
  Set), 390

Unbundling, of charges, 42
Uncertain diagnosis, ICD-10-CM coding for,
  256–257
"Under 10" rule, 65–66, 66b, 79, 79b
Undertreatment, in managed care, 106
Undesirable events, 1–2
Uniform bill (UB-04) claim form, 384–387
  claim form and completion instructions
    for, 425–429
  data specifications for, 385
  electronic, 385–387
    data elements in segment of, 385–387,
      387f
    data layout of, 385–387
    response to transmission of, 387, 387f
    transaction set section of, 385, 387f
  paper, 384–385, 386f
  websites on, 402–403
Uniform Hospital Discharge Data Set
  (UHDDS), 390
Uniformed services ID card, 194, 195b, 195f
Uninsured
  identification of, 8–9
  state programs for, 9
Unique provider identification numbers
  (UPINs), 64–65
Unit(s), errors in, 136f
Unit time, E & M codes for, 285
Universal claim form. See CMS-1500 (08/05)
  form.
Unlisted procedure or service, CPT coding
  for, 278
Unnecessary procedures, in managed care
  program, 106
"Unspecified codes," in ICD-10-CM coding,
  248f, 252
Unusual circumstances, 343
UPINs (unique provider identification
  numbers), 64–65
URAC (Utilization Review Accreditation
  Commission), 54, 379
  on managed care, 107
US Family Health Plan (USFHP), 191t
"Use additional code" note, in ICD-10-CM
  coding, 248
"Use it or lose it" rule, 50–51
Usual, customary, and reasonable (UCR)
  rates, 47, 55–57, 87, 353
Utilization management, for managed care,
  108
Utilization review, of managed care, 108
Utilization Review Accreditation
  Commission (URAC), 54, 379
  on managed care, 107

V
Verification
  of insurance, with new technology, 73–75
  of Medicare eligibility, 130–132
    automated voice response system for,
      131
    benefits of systems for, 132

Verification *(Continued)*
    computer software program for, 132
    electronic data interchanges for, 132
    Medicaid ID card for, 131, 131*f*
    point-of-sale device for, 132
  of patient information, 320–321
  of TRICARE eligibility, 194, 195*b*, 195*f*
Vertically integrated hospitals, 374
Vision care, 53
  Medicare Part A noncoverage of, 147*t*
Vocational rehabilitation, 220

W

Waiting periods, for workers' compensation,
    220–222
Waivers, 79
  Medicaid Home and Community-Based
    Service, 127–128
"Watchdogs," health insurance, 54

"Wellness" exams, Medicare Part B coverage
    of, 147
"with," in ICD-10-CM coding, 252
Workers' compensation, 49–50, 214–224
  appeals under, 216–217
  benefits under, 216
    denial of, 216–217
    waiting periods for, 220–222
  claims for, 217–222
    first report of injury in, 217, 218*f*
    forms for, 222
    physician's role in, 217–220, 221*f*
    time limits for, 217
  defined, 214
  determination of disability in, 220
  eligibility for, 215–217
  exception for signed release of
    information in cases of, 40
  exemptions from, 216
  federal legislation and, 215

Workers' compensation *(Continued)*
  fraud involving, 224
  HIPAA and, 224
  history of, 214–215
  and managed care, 224
  Online Workers' Compensation Service
    Center for, 224
  progress reports in, 222, 223*f*
  sources of, 215
  special billing notes on, 222–224
  for vocational rehabilitation, 220
  websites on, 236
Write-offs
  bad debt, 364
  contractual, 363–364

X

"X," in ICD-10 tabular list, 242
XPressClaim, for TRICARE, 199